Magnetic Resonance Imaging

METHODS IN MOLECULAR MEDICINE™

John M. Walker, SERIES EDITOR

Magnetic Resonance Imaging

Methods and Biologic Applications

Edited by

Pottumarthi V. Prasad

Department of Radiology
Evanston Northwestern Healthcare, Evanston
and Feinberg School of Medicine at Northwestern University
Chicago, IL

HUMANA PRESS ✳ TOTOWA, NEW JERSEY

Photocopy Authorization Policy:

Printed in the United States of America. 10 9 8 7 6 5 4 3 2 1

eISBN 1-59745-010-3
ISSN 1543-1894

Library of Congress Cataloging-in-Publication Data

Magnetic resonance imaging : methods and biologic applications / edited by Pottumarthi V. Prasad.
    p. ; cm. -- (Methods in molecular medicine, ISSN 1543-1894 ; 124)
  Includes bibliographical references and index.
  ISBN 1-58829-397-1 (alk. paper)
  1. Magnetic resonance imaging. [DNLM: 1. Magnetic Resonance Imaging--methods. 2. Biomedical Research--methods. 3. Magnetic Resonance Spectroscopy--methods. WN185 M19595 2006] I. Prasad, Pottumarthi V. II. Series.
  RC78.7.N83M3435 2006
  616.07'548--dc22

                               2005022802

To Raji, Supritha, and Omkar

Preface

The concept of spatially localized nuclear magnetic resonance (now called magnetic resonance imaging or MRI) evolved in the early 1970s. Like many developments in science, these early suggestions were considered esoteric and it took almost a decade before industry recognized their diagnostic potential. Over the last two decades, MRI has matured into a versatile diagnostic imaging modality within radiology, and is accepted as the gold-standard in several areas by virtue of its exquisite anatomical depiction of soft tissue. The recent Nobel Prize in Physiology or Medicine was awarded to two scientists responsible for the development of nuclear magnetic resonance into an imaging technique. Not surprisingly, neither is a medical professional: Professor Paul Lauterbur is a chemist, and Professor (Sir) Peter Mansfield, a physicist. The applications of their work also extend well beyond the field of clinical diagnosis and into the realm of basic science, in particular biology.

A major strength of MRI is its sensitivity to a plethora of physiological factors. This makes MRI extraordinarily versatile, and provides a fertile ground for innovative academic research into novel applications. Coupled with technological advancements in basic hardware, it has led to an expanding role for MRI as an experimental tool. A unique attribute of MRI is its capacity for translation all the way from cellular suspensions to in vivo human studies. MRI is no longer considered only as a clinical diagnostic imaging modality, but also as a key tool in biological research. This is evidenced by the fact that all major academic universities currently have active basic science MRI facilities in addition to clinical research MRI centers. The major pharmaceutical companies have also invested in imaging divisions that include MRI.

The primary objective of *Magnetic Resonance Imaging: Methods and Biologic Applications* is to introduce MRI to biological scientists. Chapter 1 provides an overall introduction of MRI to a relative novice. Dr. Storey has taken a tremendous interest and spared no effort in putting this chapter together. The technical and mathematical details were kept to a minimum without compromising the description of the various concepts involved. The specific technical challenges that MRI faces when applied to microscopic resolutions are discussed in Chapter 2. Each of the succeeding chapters highlights unique attributes of MRI and introduces current works-in-progress in newly evolving areas of molecular and cellular imaging. Methodological details are provided where possible. We have focused on three major features of MRI and organized the chapters along these lines:

1. Exquisite anatomical detail.

    Chapters 3 and 4 discuss the applications of MRI to developmental biology and mouse phenotyping. Chapter 5 illustrates the use of diffusion tensor imaging, a technique that is unique to MRI, for understanding fiber architecture and its relationship to brain function.

2. The ability to provide information regarding the "functional status" of tissue by using endogenous contrast mechanisms.

    At least two endogenous contrast mechanisms have evolved for routine use in evaluating brain function based on regional blood flow. These are discussed in Chapters 6 and 7. The same mechanisms have also been applied to the kidney, as discussed in Chapter 8. Magnetic resonance spectroscopy also provides unique biochemical signatures that can be used to evaluate functional or physiological status of tissue, as discussed in Chapter 9. A major advantage of MRI is that it is noninvasive, allowing anatomical and physiological investigations of healthy subjects. Another important aspect of any diagnostic imaging modality is its ability to characterize pathophysiology. Chapters 10 and 11 discuss the application of MRI to neuropathology and tumor biology. Since drug development is intricately related to pathophysiology, there is major interest in the pharmaceutical industry in using imaging methods both for preclinical and clinical testing purposes. Chapter 12 illustrates the role of MRI within the pharmaceutical industry.

3. The ability to use exogenous contrast material to extract information regarding the spatial distribution, tissue function, metabolic activity, or monitoring of gene expression.

    Exogenous contrast agents have become a key feature of diagnostic MRI, and it can be argued that the next revolution in MRI lies in the development of novel contrast materials. A notable milestone was the demonstration of hyperpolarized noble gas imaging, which has applications in functional assessment of the lung (Chapter 13). Recently, contrast materials have been developed for noninvasive evaluation of tissue pH (Chapter 14). Manganese-enhanced MRI (MEMRI) has also been shown to provide a unique probe of physiology and pathophysiology and is discussed in Chapter 15. This is one of the few chapters in this book that follow the customary Methods for Molecular Medicine protocols format.

    In the last five years, terms such as molecular and cellular imaging have entered the vocabulary. This refers not to imaging of individual molecules (which is beyond the resolution of NMR), but to imaging of such processes as metabolic activity or gene expression that occur on a molecular level. Chapters 16 and 17 discuss the concepts of targeted contrast agents and "molecular switches." Finally Chapter 18 provides a hands-on approach to cellular labeling using super-paramagnetic iron oxide contrast agents.

Though the initial intent was that *Magnetic Resonance Imaging: Methods and Biologic Applications* be directed towards biological scientists who may wish to use MRI as a tool in their own research, it became apparent as the contents evolved that even MRI specialists may find the book useful for its methods-oriented chapters. As evidenced by the author list, MRI research involves scientists of very different educational and professional backgrounds. The field is now sufficiently mature that no single MRI scientist or expert can be familiar with all aspects of imaging applications, and it is hoped that each reader may find some aspects of this book useful.

I would like to take this opportunity to thank the entire group of outstanding authors for their valued contributions, as well as my family for their patience and understanding during the course of this project.

Pottumarthi V. Prasad

Contents

Contributors

ERIC T. AHRENS • *Department of Biological Sciences and the Pittsburgh NMR Center for Biomedical Research, Carnegie Mellon University, Pittsburgh, PA*

JEFF W. M. BULTE • *MR Research Division, Russell H. Morgan Department of Radiology and Radiological Science; Institute for Cell Engineering, Johns Hopkins University School of Medicine, Baltimore, MD*

SAVERIO CAPUANO • *Pittsburgh Development Center, Magee–Women's Research Institute, Pittsburgh, PA*

SHELTON D. CARUTHERS • *Cardiovascular MR Labs, Division of Cardiology, Washington University in St. Louis, Missouri; MRI Clinical Science, Philips Medical Systems, Cleveland, OH*

SUDEEP CHANDRA • *Department of Imaging Sciences, Millennium Pharmaceuticals Inc., Cambridge, MA*

X. JOSETTE CHEN • *Department of Medical Biophysics, University of Toronto; Mouse Imaging Centre, Integrative Biology, Hospital for Sick Children, Toronto, Ontario, Canada*

RICK M. DIJKHUIZEN • *Department of Medical Imaging, Image Sciences Institute, University Medical Center Utrecht, Utrecht, The Netherlands*

BARJOR GIMI • *Russell H. Morgan Department of Radiology and Radiological Sciences, Johns Hopkins University School of Medicine, Baltimore, MD*

MICHAEL HORN • *Center for Bio-Imaging, Sahlgrenska Academy, Gothenburg University, Göteborg, Sweden*

FAHMEED HYDER • *Magnetic Resonance Research Center, Departments of Diagnostic Radiology and Biomedical Engineering, Section of Bioimaging Sciences, Yale University, New Haven, CT*

IKUHIRO KIDA • *Department of Biophysics, Research Institute for Electronic Science, Hokkaido University, Sapporo, Japan*

GREGORY M. LANZA • *Cardiovascular MR Labs, Division of Cardiology, Washington University in St. Louis, MO*

ANGELIQUE LOUIE • *Department of Biomedical Engineering, University of California, Davis, CA*

SUSUMU MORI • *MR Research Division, Russell H. Morgan Department of Radiology and Radiological Science; F.M. Kirby Research Center for Functional Brain Imaging, Kennedy Krieger Institute, Baltimore, MD*

Vu M. Mai • *Department of Radiology, Evanston Northwestern Healthcare, Evanston, and Feinberg School of Medicine at Northwestern University, Chicago, IL*

Arvind P. Pathak • *Russell H. Morgan Department of Radiology and Radiological Science, Johns Hopkins University School of Medicine, Baltimore, MD*

Robia G. Pautler • *Department of Molecular Physiology and Biophysics, Baylor College of Medicine, Houston, TX*

Pottumarthi V. Prasad • *Department of Radiology, Evanston Northwestern Healthcare, Evanston, and Feinberg School of Medicine at Northwestern University, Chicago, IL*

Natarajan Raghunand • *Arizona Cancer Center, University of Arizona, Tucson, AZ*

Gerald P. Schatten • *Pittsburgh Development Center, Magee-Women's Research Institute, Pittsburgh, PA*

Matthew D. Silva • *Department of Imaging Sciences, Millennium Pharmaceuticals Inc., Cambridge, MA*

Hyagriv N. Simhan • *Pittsburgh Development Center, Magee-Women's Research Institute, Pittsburgh, PA*

Mangala Srinivas • *Department of Biological Sciences and the Pittsburgh NMR Center for Biomedical Research, Carnegie Mellon University, Pittsburgh, PA*

Pippa Storey • *Department of Radiology, Evanston Northwestern Healthcare, Evanston, and Feinberg School of Medicine at Northwestern University, Chicago, IL*

Samuel A. Wickline • *Cardiovascular MR Labs, Division of Cardiology, Washington University in St. Louis, MO*

Donald S. Williams • *Imaging, Merck & Co. Inc., West Point, PA*

Patrick M. Winter • *Cardiovascular MR Labs, Division of Cardiology, Washington University in St. Louis, MO*

Jiangyang Zhang • *MR Research Division, Russell H. Morgan Department of Radiology and Radiological Science; Department of Biomedical Engineering, Johns Hopkins University School of Medicine, Baltimore, MD*

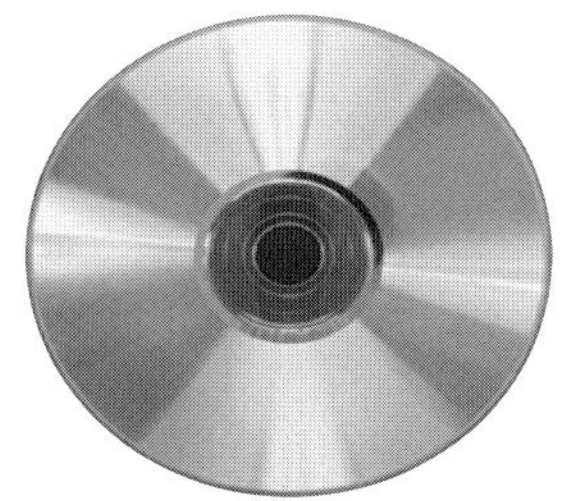

COMPANION CD

All illustrations may be found on the Companion CD attached to the inside back cover. The image files are organized into folders by chapter number and are viewable in most web browsers. The CD is compatible with both Apple Macintosh and Windows® operating systems.

I

INTRODUCTION

1

Introduction to Magnetic Resonance Imaging and Spectroscopy

Pippa Storey

Summary

This chapter provides a brief introduction to the principles and practice of magnetic resonance imaging and spectroscopy. Its goal is to equip researchers in the life sciences with a basic understanding of the capabilities and limitations of magnetic resonance techniques, and a command of the terminology used in more technical publications, including the methods sections of this book. Magnetic resonance is extremely versatile, and this introductory chapter attempts to provide an indication of its current range of applications, as well as emerging possibilities. Many of the applications mentioned here are described in greater detail in the later chapters. It is hoped that this introduction may provide some guidance to the reader in navigating the rest of the book, and in identifying ways to exploit magnetic resonance imaging and spectroscopy in his or her own research.

Key Words: Magnetic resonance; imaging; spectroscopy; spin; gyromagnetic ratio; precession; Larmor frequency; chemical shift; pulse sequence; free induction decay; spin echo; gradient echo; frequency-encoding; phase-encoding; contrast agent; metabolite; proton; carbon-13; phosphorus; fluorine.

Introduction

Magnetic resonance imaging (MRI) and spectroscopy (MRS) provide noninvasive tools to investigate the internal anatomy and physiology of living subjects and ex vivo preparations. They exploit the phenomenon of nuclear magnetic resonance (MR), whereby atomic nuclei exposed to a strong magnetic field absorb and reemit electromagnetic waves at a characteristic or 'resonant' frequency, which falls in the radio frequency (RF) range. Because there are no known adverse effects from either the strong magnetic fields or the radio waves, MRI and MRS are considered safe for human studies and longitudinal animal experiments. They are also extremely versatile, because of the wealth of information contained in the signal, regarding both the gross struc-

From: *Methods in Molecular Medicine, Vol. 124*
Magnetic Resonance Imaging: Methods and Biologic Applications
Edited by: P. V. Prasad © Humana Press Inc., Totowa, NJ

tural properties of the tissue and its biochemistry. The techniques used to elicit and analyze the signal can be readily tailored to amplify the factors of interest, providing high-resolution images of specific structures, such as arteries, lesions, and white matter tracts, and detailed assays of tissue metabolites. Although MRI has traditionally been regarded as a tool for anatomical depiction, and MRS as a physiological probe, the disciplines are gradually converging as investigators develop new means to image functional properties on the one hand, and to obtain spatially localized spectra on the other. This chapter provides a brief introduction to the principles of MRI and MRS, and an explanation of the terminology and techniques that will be encountered in later chapters. More comprehensive treatments can be found in other texts *(1–7)*.

1. Principles of Magnetic Resonance

The term magnetic resonance (MR), in the context of imaging and spectroscopy, is shorthand for nuclear magnetic resonance (NMR). The word nuclear is frequently dropped, particularly in medical applications, because of its inappropriate connotations of high-energy processes such as fission (splitting of nuclei) and radioactivity (decay of unstable nuclei). NMR is unrelated to either of these processes, and is actually a very low-energy phenomenon, involving the absorption and emission of radio frequency (RF) waves. At the intensities used in MR scanners, the radio waves are not believed to pose any risk to humans or animals.

Because the resonant frequency of the nuclei is an extremely precise measure of the local magnetic field, it provides a very sensitive probe of their molecular environment. In this capacity, MR has long been used in chemistry for the analysis of molecular structure and interactions, and for the identification of chemical compounds. Only recently (since the early 1970s) has it been applied to in vivo spectroscopy and imaging.

The purpose of the present section is to describe the origin and detection of the MR signal, the fundamental limits on its amplitude, and the means by which it conveys information about tissue structure and biochemistry.

1.1. Behavior of Nuclei in a Magnetic Field

The phenomenon of NMR derives from the fact that certain nuclei possess tiny magnetic moments, similar to that of a common bar magnet (**Fig. 1**). In the presence of an applied magnetic field, the magnetic moments undergo a rotational motion known as precession, which is analogous to the slow wobble exhibited by a spinning top or gyroscope. The explanation of nuclear precession lies in the relationship between the magnetic moment of the nucleus and its intrinsic spin.

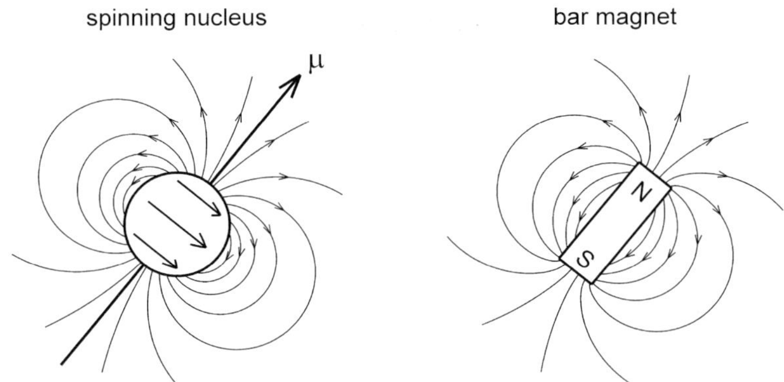

Fig. 1. Nuclei with nonzero spin possess a magnetic moment, **μ**, and produce a tiny magnetic field analogous to that of a bar magnet. The arrows on the nucleus itself indicate its direction of spin, whereas the curved lines surrounding the nucleus and the bar magnet depict their magnetic fields.

1.1.1. Nuclear Spin and Magnetic Moment

Spin is a fundamental property of certain nuclei, notably hydrogen, that contain unpaired protons or neutrons. Although spin is an essentially quantum mechanical property, it can be visualized as the rotation of the nucleus about its own axis, similar to that of a gyroscope. Because the nucleus is positively charged, its spin entails a circulation of charge, analogous to a tiny current loop. From electromagnetism, it is known that a current loop behaves much like a bar magnet, producing its own magnetic field, and experiencing a turning force or 'torque' in the presence of another magnet. The circulation of charge associated with the nuclear spin similarly endows the nucleus with a magnetic moment. The nucleus therefore produces its own tiny magnetic field, and is subject to a torque in the presence of an external field. The torque attempts to turn the magnetic moment of the nucleus into alignment with the external field, where its energy is a minimum.

1.1.2. Larmor Precession

Because the magnetic moment of the nucleus is derived from its spin, the orientation of the magnetic moment is locked to the spin axis. This is expressed through the equation:

$$\mu = \gamma \mathbf{I}, \qquad [1]$$

where **μ** is the magnetic moment of the nucleus and **I** is its spin. Note that each is a vector quantity (as indicated by the bold script), and thus has both magni-

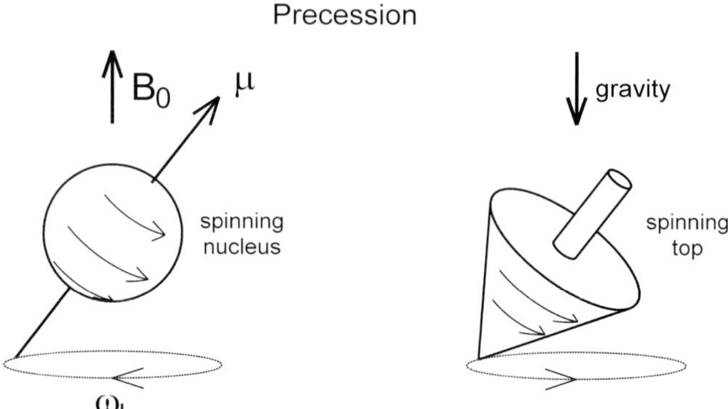

Fig. 2. In the presence of an external magnetic field, $\mathbf{B_0}$, nuclei with nonzero spin precess about the field, just as a spinning top precesses about gravity. (Note that the direction of precession is different in the two cases, because the fields are opposite.)

tude and direction. The direction of $\mathbf{I}$ is given by the spin axis. $\boldsymbol{\mu}$ is parallel to $\mathbf{I}$ and determines the orientation of the nucleus' intrinsic magnetic field (**Fig. 1**). The factor γ is known as the gyromagnetic ratio, and is a property of the nucleus.

Because the magnetic moment of the nucleus is parallel to its spin, any change in the direction of the magnetic moment requires a corresponding re-orientation of the spin axis. A similar situation exists with a gyroscope; any reorientation of the gyroscope is necessarily accompanied by a change in the direction of its spin axis. The result is that when a gyroscope is subjected to a gravitational field it does not immediately fall over but instead remains upright, albeit with a slow wobble about the vertical known as precession. Similarly, when a nucleus is subjected to a magnetic field, its magnetic moment does not simply swing into alignment with the field but instead precesses about the direction of the field, as depicted in **Fig. 2**.

1.1.3. Larmor Frequency

The frequency at which the nucleus precesses about the magnetic field is known as the Larmor frequency, ω_L. It can be shown from classical mechanics that the value of the Larmor frequency is proportional to the strength of the magnetic field, B_0, and the gyromagnetic ratio of the nucleus:

$$\omega_L = \gamma B_0. \tag{2}$$

The values of γ for some of the nuclei commonly used in biological studies are shown in **Table 1**. The most important of these nuclei for magnetic reso-

Table 1
Some of the Nuclear Isotopes Used in Biological Applications of Magnetic Resonance Imaging and Spectroscopy[a]

Nuclear isotope	Natural abundance (%)	Spin	$\gamma/2\pi$ (MHz/T)
^{1}H	99.98	$\frac{1}{2}$	42.58
^{2}H	0.015	1	6.53
^{3}He	0.00014[b]	$\frac{1}{2}$	−32.44
^{7}Li	92.6	$\frac{3}{2}$	16.5
^{13}C	1.11	$\frac{1}{2}$	10.71
^{14}N	99.6	1	3.1
^{15}N	0.36	$\frac{1}{2}$	−4.3
^{19}F	100	$\frac{1}{2}$	40.05
^{23}Na	100	$\frac{3}{2}$	11.26
^{31}P	100	$\frac{1}{2}$	17.23
^{39}K	93.1	$\frac{3}{2}$	2.0
^{129}Xe	26.44	$\frac{1}{2}$	−11.84

[a]Isotopes are listed with their natural abundance, nuclear spin, and gyromagnetic ratio, γ.
[b]The helium-3 used in magnetic resonance studies is derived from the decay of tritium (^{3}H).

nance imaging (MRI) is hydrogen, because it is present throughout the body in water and fat. Many of the other nuclei that are prevalent in the body, such as carbon-12 and oxygen-16, do not exhibit MR because they have no net spin.

As **Table 1** indicates, the values of the gyromagnetic ratio for nuclei of interest lie in the range of megahertz (MHz) per tesla (T), where tesla is a unit of magnetic field strength. Because the field strengths typically used in MR scanners are on the order of a few tesla, the Larmor frequencies fall in the megahertz, or RF, regime.

1.1.4. Chemical Shift

The net magnetic field experienced by the nucleus is a sum of the external field applied to the tissue and the much smaller fields generated by the electrons surrounding the nucleus. These additional fields alter the precession frequency of the nucleus by a tiny fraction known as the chemical shift. The value of the chemical shift is characteristic of the molecular group in which the nucleus resides, and thus provides a distinctive signature for each metabolite. By analyzing the frequencies present in the MR signal, the investigator can identify the metabolites in the tissue and estimate their concentration. This procedure forms the basis of magnetic resonance spectroscopy (MRS), discussed in **Subheading 4.**

1.1.5. Summary

- Nuclei with unpaired protons or neutrons possess magnetic moments, which precess about the direction of an applied magnetic field.
- The frequency of precession is known as the Larmor frequency ω_L, and depends on the nucleus and the strength of the local magnetic field.
- The local magnetic field is modified by the molecular environment of the nucleus, producing a fractional change in its Larmor frequency known as the chemical shift.

1.2. Excitation and Signal Detection

Each nucleus with nonzero spin generates its own tiny magnetic field, whose strength and orientation are characterized by the nuclear magnetic moment (**Fig. 1**). As the nucleus precesses about $\mathbf{B}_0$, its magnetic moment rotates at the Larmor frequency ω_L, producing an oscillating magnetic field. The net magnetic field oscillations generated by all the nuclei in the sample can be detected with an RF receiver coil, and constitute the MR signal. The signal will be zero, however, unless a macroscopic number of the nuclei are precessing in synchrony. In the present section, we will show how this can be achieved by means of an RF excitation.

1.2.1. Nuclear Magnetization

The magnetic field of a nucleus is a complicated function of space (**Fig. 1**) but is uniquely specified by its magnetic moment, $\boldsymbol{\mu}$. The net magnetic field of all the nuclei in a given volume of tissue can similarly be specified by the vector sum of their magnetic moments. The sum is known as the nuclear magnetization, and denoted $\mathbf{M}$. The component of $\mathbf{M}$ that lies in the transverse plane (perpendicular to the static field $\mathbf{B}_0$) rotates at the Larmor frequency, ω_L, as the nuclei precess. This produces an oscillating magnetic field that can be detected with an RF receiver coil. The receiver coil consists essentially of one or more loops of wire, through which lines of magnetic flux may pass. As the transverse magnetization rotates, the magnetic flux through the loop oscillates, inducing a small alternating voltage in the coil. The MR signal is thus proportional to the transverse component of $\mathbf{M}$.

At equilibrium, the nuclei precess with random phases, as shown in **Fig. 3**. The transverse components of their magnetic moments, therefore, cancel out, and produce no detectable signal. There is, however, a small net magnetization, $\mathbf{M}_0$, in the longitudinal direction (parallel to $\mathbf{B}_0$). It cannot be detected directly, because it does not oscillate. It is necessary for producing the signal, however, as we will soon show.

The equilibrium magnetization arises because the nuclei exhibit a slight preference for being aligned along the direction of the external magnetic field. This

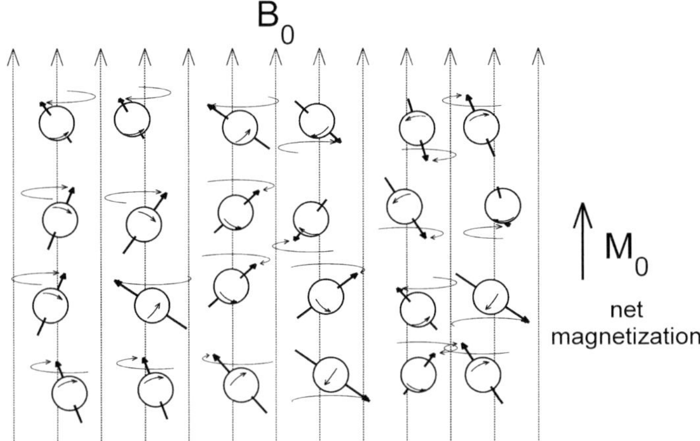

Fig. 3. At equilibrium, the nuclei precess about $\mathbf{B}_0$ with random phases, producing no net transverse magnetization. However, slightly more of the nuclei are oriented toward the field than away from it, giving rise to a small net longitudinal magnetization, $\mathbf{M}_0$.

can be explained on the basis of energy considerations. The energy of a magnetic moment depends on its orientation in the magnetic field, through the equation:

$$E = -\boldsymbol{\mu} \cdot \mathbf{B}_0. \tag{3}$$

The more closely the magnetic moment is aligned to the field, the lower its energy. As we will see in **Subheading 1.3.3.**, it turns out the energy savings is tiny compared with the available thermal energy. Nevertheless, the nuclei exhibit a slight preference for being tilted toward the external field (up) rather than away from it (down). At equilibrium, therefore, slightly more of the nuclei are oriented upwards than downwards (**Fig. 3**). The small excess of nuclei pointing upwards gives rise to the equilibrium magnetization $\mathbf{M}_0$.

1.2.2. RF Excitation

By applying a transverse oscillating magnetic field to the tissue at exactly the Larmor frequency ω_L, the nuclear magnetization can be tipped away from the longitudinal axis, producing a finite component in the transverse plane. The excess nuclei that had been pointing upwards at equilibrium then precess in synchrony, emitting a detectable signal. The process is one of resonant excitation, and is similar to the mechanism involved in pushing a child's swing.

The equilibrium state of a swing is that in which it rests at the lowest point of its arc. Energy can be transferred to the swing by pushing it at its natural or

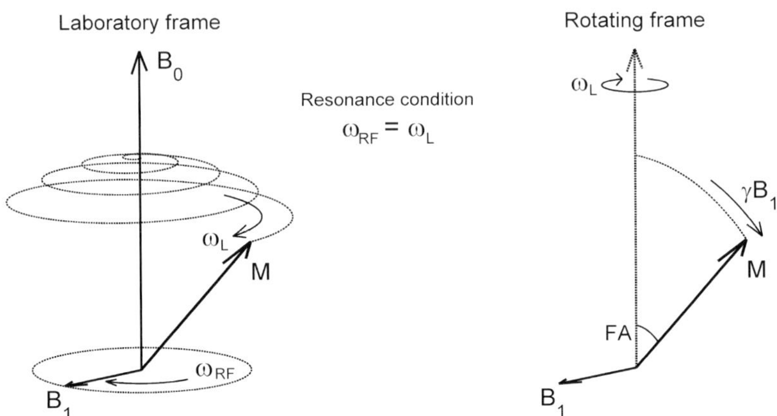

Fig. 4. When a radio frequency (RF) field $\mathbf{B}_1$ is applied at a frequency that exactly matches the Larmor frequency of the nuclei, $\omega_{RF} = \omega_L$, the net magnetization is tipped away from the longitudinal direction. In a frame rotating at the Larmor frequency, the $\mathbf{B}_1$ field appears stationary and the motion can be interpreted as a secondary precession of the nuclei about $\mathbf{B}_1$.

resonant frequency. As the swing gains energy it begins to oscillate back and forth, and its amplitude of motion gradually increases. The resonant frequency of the swing is identical to the frequency at which it will oscillate by itself when the driving force is stopped.

Just as the swing can be made to oscillate by applying a periodic force, the nuclei in a sample of tissue can be made to precess in synchrony by applying a rotating magnetic field in the transverse plane. The applied field is denoted $\mathbf{B}_1(t)$, and its frequency of rotation must exactly match the Larmor frequency of the nuclei to satisfy the resonance condition. Because the Larmor frequency falls in the RF regime, the process is described as RF excitation, and the resonance condition is written $\omega_{RF} = \omega_L$. As the $\mathbf{B}_1(t)$ field transfers energy to the nuclei, the amplitude of their transverse magnetization gradually increases (**Fig. 4**).

When the $\mathbf{B}_1(t)$ field is switched off, the transverse magnetization continues to rotate at the Larmor frequency, producing an oscillating magnetic field that can be detected by the RF receiver coil. Eventually, however, the transverse magnetization will decay back to zero and the signal will disappear.

1.2.3. The Rotating Frame

To understand the process of RF excitation, it is helpful to visualize the effect of the $\mathbf{B}_1$ field in a reference frame rotating at the Larmor frequency ω_L. In this frame, the static magnetic field $\mathbf{B}_0$ can be ignored, because its effect is already accounted for in the rotation of the reference frame itself. Spins that were precessing about $\mathbf{B}_0$ in the laboratory frame appear stationary in the rotating frame, as if the $\mathbf{B}_0$ field had disappeared. The RF field $\mathbf{B}_1$ will also appear stationary in the rotating frame, provided its frequency exactly matches the Larmor frequency of the spins, $\omega_{RF} = \omega_L$. Within this frame, it produces a secondary precession of the spins, analogous to the precession about $\mathbf{B}_0$ in the laboratory frame, but at a rate equal to γB_1, where B_1 denotes its amplitude. This secondary precession tips the net magnetization $\mathbf{M}$ away from the longitudinal axis, producing a measurable component in the transverse plane. The $\mathbf{B}_1$ field is applied in a short intense burst, known as an RF pulse, which is tailored to produce the desired degree of excitation. The excitation is quantified by the flip angle (FA) through which the net magnetization is tipped away from the longitudinal axis. For a so-called 'hard' pulse, of constant amplitude B_1 and exactly on resonance, the FA is proportional to B_1 and the pulse duration τ:

$$FA = \gamma B_1 \tau. \tag{4}$$

1.2.4. Limits on Signal Amplitude

Assuming the magnetization is at equilibrium before RF excitation, the maximum achievable signal is obtained with a FA of 90°, which transfers all the longitudinal magnetization into the transverse plane. The amplitude of the signal is then limited only by the magnitude of the equilibrium magnetization $\mathbf{M}_0$. This, in turn, is determined by the strength of the static magnetic field $\mathbf{B}_0$; the stronger the magnetic field, the greater the tendency for spins to align in its direction, and the larger the equilibrium magnetization. Using stronger fields, therefore, increases the signal-to-noise ratio (SNR), allowing MR measurements to be made on smaller samples or with higher resolution.

In certain circumstances, a further increase in signal can be achieved by 'hyperpolarizing' the spins, that is, by artificially increasing the fraction aligned in the direction of the magnetic field. The noble gases xenon and helium-3 can be hyperpolarized by means of optical pumping with circularly polarized light *(8)*. Hyperpolarized gases have found applications in ventilation imaging of the lungs (*see* Chapter 13).

1.2.5. Summary

- The MR signal arises from the transverse component of the nuclear magnetization, which rotates at the Larmor frequency.
- At equilibrium, there is no net transverse magnetization, and hence no signal. However, there is a small net longitudinal magnetization, $\mathbf{M}_0$.
- By applying an RF field $\mathbf{B}_1(t)$ at the Larmor frequency, the magnetization is tipped away from the longitudinal axis, to produce a finite transverse component and a detectable signal.

1.3. Quantum Mechanical Description

The preceding discussion of MR has been conducted entirely in terms of classical physics. Because the number of nuclei in a macroscopic sample is extremely large, such a description is adequate for explaining many aspects of their collective behavior. In particular, this description is sufficient for understanding most of the techniques used in imaging. Individual nuclei, however, obey the laws of quantum mechanics, and this is manifested in certain aspects of their MR spectra. The present section describes the rules of quantization, and the quantum mechanical description of RF excitation and signal emission. Although an acquaintance with these concepts provides a more complete picture of MR physics, a detailed understanding is not necessary for gaining a working knowledge of MR techniques.

1.3.1. Quantization

According to quantum mechanics, neither matter nor energy can be divided indefinitely into ever-smaller parts; on a sufficiently tiny scale one encounters fundamental units or "quanta" that cannot be further divided. Electromagnetic energy, such as X-rays, light, and radio waves, exists in discrete energy packets, called photons. The energy of an individual photon is proportional to the frequency, ω, of the electromagnetic wave:

$$E_{\mathrm{photon}} = \hbar\omega. \qquad [5]$$

The parameter $\hbar$ is a fundamental constant known as Planck's constant, with the value $\hbar = 1.0546 \times 10^{-34}$ J.s.

Whenever an atom or nucleus absorbs or emits electromagnetic waves, an entire photon is consumed or created. To conserve the total energy of the system, the atom or nucleus must simultaneously undergo a 'quantum jump' to a state of different energy. A nucleus has only a few different states available to it, however, because of a separate quantization condition governing angular momentum. This restricts the possible frequencies of the electromagnetic waves that it can absorb or emit.

Angular momentum is a vector quantity, whose direction is determined by the axis of rotation. The quantization condition for angular momentum stipulates that its component along any given measurement axis may adopt only certain discrete values, equal to integer or half-integer multiples of $\hbar$. Because nuclear spin **I** is a form of angular momentum, this rule applies to the component of spin along the longitudinal axis, conventionally denoted I_z. So-called spin-$\frac{1}{2}$ nuclei, such as hydrogen, have only two possible values, namely: $I_z = \pm\frac{1}{2}\hbar$. Spin-1 nuclei, such as deuterium (^{2}H), have three possible values, $I_z = 0, \pm\hbar$, and spin-$\frac{3}{2}$ nuclei, such as sodium, have four, $I_z = \pm\frac{1}{2}\hbar, \pm\frac{3}{2}\hbar$ (**Fig. 5**). Note that, in each case, the difference in the z-component of spin between adjacent states is $\Delta I_z = \hbar$.

Quantization of nuclear spin

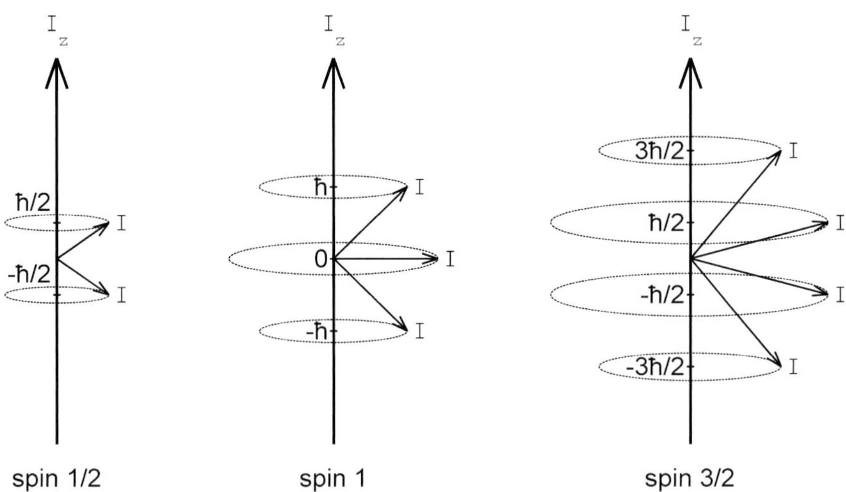

Fig. 5. According to quantum mechanics, the total spin **I** of a nucleus has fixed magnitude, and its component along any direction (for example, the z-axis) can adopt only discrete values. The difference in I_z between adjacent states is $\Delta I_z = \hbar$.

When the nucleus is subjected to an external magnetic field, the energies of the states also differ, and the energy differences among them can be used to derive the resonance condition governing RF excitation and signal emission.

1.3.2. Absorption and Emission of RF Energy

As discussed in **Subheading 1.2.1.**, the energy of a nucleus depends on the orientation of its magnetic moment with respect to the external magnetic field, as given in **Eq. [3]**. However, because the magnetic moment is parallel to the spin, through **Eq. [1]**, the energy of the nucleus varies with the spin direction according to:

$$E = -\gamma \mathbf{I} \cdot \mathbf{B}_0. \tag{6}$$

The energy is thus proportional to the component of spin in the longitudinal direction,

$$E = -\gamma I_z B_0. \tag{7}$$

This relation shows that states with different I_z values have different energies when subjected to an external magnetic field. Because the angular momentum differs between adjacent spin-states by $\Delta I_z = \hbar$, the energy separation between the states is equal to:

$$\Delta E = \hbar \gamma B_0. \tag{8}$$

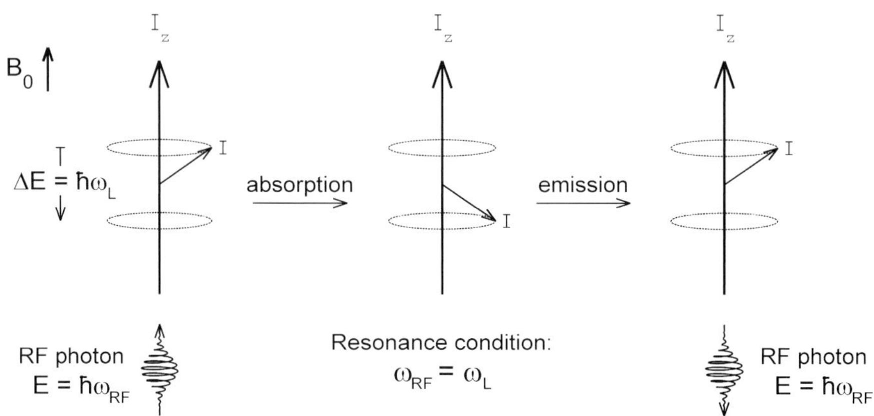

Fig. 6. The energy difference between adjacent spin states of a nucleus is given by $\Delta E = \hbar\omega_L$, where ω_L is the Larmor frequency. Excitation occurs when the nucleus absorbs a radio frequency (RF) photon whose frequency ω_{RF} exactly equals the Larmor frequency of the nucleus. When the nucleus subsequently decays back to its initial state, it emits a photon of the same frequency, which contributes to the MR signal.

The product γB_0, however, equals the Larmor frequency, ω_L, through **Eq. [2]**. The energy difference can therefore be written as:

$$\Delta E = \hbar\omega_L. \tag{9}$$

To excite the nucleus to the next energy level requires the absorption of a photon whose energy equals this energy difference,

$$E_{photon} = \Delta E. \tag{10}$$

By substituting **Eqs. [9]** and **[5]** into **[10]**, we find that the frequency of the photon must, therefore, exactly match the Larmor frequency, ω_L, of the nucleus. Because the value of the Larmor frequency is typically on the order of MHz, the photon represents an RF wave of frequency:

$$\omega_{RF} = \omega_L. \tag{11}$$

This is the resonance condition, which was explained earlier using classical arguments, but which is derived here using the law of energy conservation, together with the rules of quantization.

The quantum mechanical interpretation of NMR is that a photon at the Larmor frequency excites the nucleus to a higher energy state (**Fig. 6**). The excited nucleus may lose its energy through frictional processes to the environment, or it may decay back to its initial state, releasing a photon of the same frequency, which contributes to the observed MR signal.

1.3.3. Population Distribution

The signal in an MR experiment is limited by the amplitude of the equilibrium magnetization, $\mathbf{M}_0$. Because $\mathbf{M}_0$ is given by the vector sum of the nuclear magnetic moments, it is proportional to the population difference between the spin states. At equilibrium, the relative populations of the states are determined by their energy separation, ΔE, relative to the available thermal energy. The thermal energy equals kT, where T is the absolute temperature of the sample in Kelvin (approx 310 K for body temperature), and k is a fundamental constant known as Boltzmann's constant, with the value $k = 1.381 \times 10^{-23}$ J/K. In a system of spin-$\frac{1}{2}$ nuclei, such as hydrogen, the relative populations of the up and down states are:

$$\frac{N_\downarrow}{N_\uparrow} = \exp\left(-\frac{\Delta E}{kT}\right), \qquad [12]$$

where ΔE is given in **Eq. [8]**. For the magnetic field strengths typically used in MR systems, ΔE is only a very tiny fraction of the thermal energy kT. In fact, at 1.5 T (a typical field strength for clinical scanners) the ratio $\Delta E/kT$ is around 10^{-5}. Under such conditions, **Eq. [12]** can be expanded as:

$$\frac{N_\downarrow}{N_\uparrow} \approx 1 - \frac{\Delta E}{kT}. \qquad [13]$$

The fractional population difference thus equals $\Delta E/kT$, or about 1 in 100,000 nuclei at 1.5 T. Because the population difference is so low, the equilibrium magnetization, $\mathbf{M}_0$, is very small. MR is, therefore, an inherently insensitive technique.

The sensitivity can, however, be improved by using higher magnetic field strengths. This is demonstrated by substituting **Eq. [8]** for ΔE into **Eq. [13]**, to give:

$$\frac{N_\downarrow}{N_\uparrow} \approx 1 - \frac{\hbar\gamma B_0}{kT}. \qquad [14]$$

Thus, the fractional population difference increases with field strength, producing a corresponding increase in the equilibrium magnetization, $\mathbf{M}_0$, and an enhancement of the MR signal. When the available tissue volume is very limited, as in studies of small animals or ex vivo samples, an extremely strong $\mathbf{B}_0$ field is required to obtain adequate SNR.

1.3.4. Summary

- The states of a nucleus are discrete, and differ in energy by $\Delta E = \hbar\omega_L$, where ω_L is the Larmor frequency.
- Electromagnetic energy, including radio waves, exists in discrete bundles called photons. The energy of each photon is related to the frequency, ω, of the electromagnetic wave through $E_{photon} = \hbar\omega$.
- To reach a higher energy state, the nucleus must absorb an RF photon whose frequency equals the Larmor frequency, $\omega_{RF} = \omega_L$. The MR signal is produced when nuclei decay back to their initial states, emitting photons of the same frequency.

1.4. Spin Relaxation

Excitation of nuclei by means of an RF pulse makes a macroscopic number of spins precess in synchrony, producing a rotating magnetic field that can be detected with an RF coil. The signal will not persist indefinitely, however, because of inter-nuclear and inter-molecular forces, which cause a loss of phase coherence among the spins and a corresponding attenuation of the transverse magnetization. The nuclei simultaneously lose energy to their surroundings, resulting in a recovery of the longitudinal magnetization to its equilibrium value. These processes are termed transverse and longitudinal relaxation, respectively. Relaxation processes limit the available acquisition time, and broaden the spectroscopic linewidths. However, because their rates depend on the molecular environment of the nuclei, they can be exploited to produce signal contrast among different tissues in MR imaging. The present section provides a brief discussion of the physical mechanisms underlying relaxation processes, and the means by which they can be harnessed to produce signal contrast. (A more detailed exposition can be found in Chapter 3 of **ref. 2**.)

1.4.1. Longitudinal Relaxation (Loss of Energy)

Excitation by an RF pulse $\mathbf{B}_1(t)$ increases the net energy of the nuclei above its equilibrium value. The nuclei will eventually lose that additional energy through interactions with neighboring nuclei and molecules, and the system will return to equilibrium (**Fig. 7**). Because the net energy of the system is related to the longitudinal nuclear magnetization, the processes that cause energy loss are collectively termed longitudinal relaxation. The timescale on which longitudinal relaxation occurs is denoted T_1, and defined as the reciprocal of the rate of energy loss. Because longitudinal relaxation is caused by interactions between the nuclei and their environment, the value of T_1 varies according to the molecule in which the nucleus is bound and the type of tissue in which it is present. For example, the T_1 of tissue water tends to be longer in body fluids, such as blood and cerebrospinal fluid, than in more solid tissues, such as the white matter of the brain. Intensity differences between these tis-

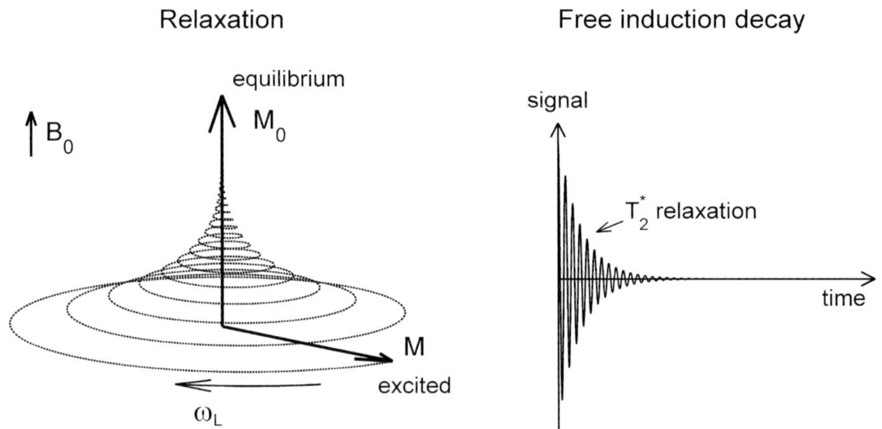

Fig. 7. When the excitation field $\mathbf{B}_1$ is turned off, the net magnetization, $\mathbf{M}$, continues to rotate about $\mathbf{B}_0$ at the Larmor frequency, producing an oscillating magnetic field that can be detected with a radio frequency coil. However, the magnetization also undergoes transverse relaxation, causing a gradual attenuation of the signal, known as a free induction decay. The nuclei simultaneously lose energy to the environment, resulting in longitudinal relaxation of the magnetization toward its equilibrium value, $\mathbf{M}_0$.

sues can be achieved on an MR image by tailoring the acquisition so that it is sensitive to T_1.

Longitudinal relaxation arises from fluctuations in the local magnetic field at the site of each nucleus. The local magnetic field is a sum of the applied field $\mathbf{B}_0$ and the smaller secondary fields generated by the surrounding electrons, neighboring nuclei, and nearby molecules. As the host molecule moves and tumbles within the medium, the position of each nucleus varies randomly with respect to adjacent nuclei and molecules. As a result, the nucleus experiences a fluctuating magnetic field. If the fluctuations have frequency components equal to the Larmor frequency, they can induce transitions between nuclear energy states. Excited nuclei will, on average, lose energy to their surroundings. The energy loss continues until the nuclei reach thermal equilibrium with their environment and the magnetization returns to its equilibrium value, $\mathbf{M}_0$. The recovery of the longitudinal magnetization follows an exponential curve:

$$M_{\parallel}(t) = M_0 + \left[M_{\parallel}(0) - M_0 \right] e^{-t/T_1} , \qquad [15]$$

where $M_{\parallel}$ denotes the longitudinal magnetization and t is the time following the RF excitation. The value of $M_{\parallel}(0)$ is determined by the longitudinal magnetization available before the excitation and by the FA of the RF pulse.

Longitudinal relaxation occurs most efficiently when the molecular tumbling rate is near the Larmor frequency. The value of T_1, therefore, depends on the mobility of the host molecule, which, in turn, varies with molecular weight and tissue type. It turns out that the tumbling rate is closest to the Larmor frequency for medium-sized molecules, such as lipids. Fat, therefore, has a relatively short T_1 (on the order of 250 ms at 1.5 T). By contrast, the free water in body fluids has a relatively long T_1 (greater than 1 s at similar field strengths), because its molecular tumbling rate is much faster than the Larmor frequency. The T_1 of water is shortened, however, in solid tissues, where its motion is more restricted.

T_1 differences among tissues are exploited to produce signal contrast on MR images. As we will see in **Subheading 3.**, MRI involves the collection of a large amount of spatial information. This requires the process of excitation and signal acquisition to be repeated many times in succession. The repetition time, TR, between successive excitations is important in determining the signal amplitude from a given tissue type. If the TR is short with respect to the T_1 of the tissue, the longitudinal magnetization will not have fully recovered to its equilibrium value, M_0, before the next excitation. Because the magnetization remains partially saturated, the signal from the tissue is reduced accordingly. By comparison, a tissue with a faster relaxation rate will be less saturated and will exhibit a relatively higher signal. In general, the degree of magnetization recovery depends on the factor $\exp(-TR/T_1)$. If TR is chosen to be sufficiently short that the signal from each tissue depends heavily on its T_1 value, the resulting image is described as being 'T_1-weighted.'

1.4.2. Transverse Relaxation (Loss of Phase Coherence)

The MR signal is produced by the transverse component of the magnetization, whose amplitude depends on the degree of phase coherence among the nuclei. The transverse magnetization is zero at equilibrium, and attains a finite value only through RF excitation by the $\mathbf{B}_1(t)$ field. After excitation, its amplitude gradually decays back to zero. The signal must, therefore, be acquired during the short period after the excitation pulse but before the transverse magnetization has disappeared. Transverse relaxation occurs more rapidly than longitudinal relaxation, because it involves additional mechanisms. These are related to dephasing among the spins, and originate from a variety of processes, both microscopic and mesoscopic. The component caused by microscopic processes depends on intrinsic factors, such as molecular size and tissue type, and occurs on a timescale denoted T_2. Dephasing over a larger scale is a result of effects such as magnetic field inhomogeneity. This further shortens the coherence time of the transverse magnetization within a given volume of tissue, to a value denoted T_2^*. Tissue-dependent differences in both T_2 and T_2^* can be exploited to produce signal contrast on MR images.

Variations in the local magnetic field strength cause dephasing among the spins by making them precess at slightly different rates. On a microscopic scale, the variations are caused by the presence of neighboring nuclei and molecules, which produce their own tiny magnetic fields. Dephasing also arises when energy is exchanged between identical nuclei. Both these processes contribute to T_2 relaxation, and occur most efficiently if the molecular tumbling rate is low. Rapid motion tends to inhibit T_2 relaxation by averaging out the effects of microscopic interactions over time. Free water in body fluids, for example, relaxes relatively slowly (on the order of 1 s), because its molecules are in constant rotation. By comparison, molecules that are very large or bound to cell membranes have very short T_2 values (on the order of microseconds), because of their relative immobility. Macromolecules, such as proteins and DNA, are, therefore, not directly detectable in vivo by MRI or MRS, because their transverse magnetization relaxes too quickly to permit signal acquisition.

Dephasing also results from larger-scale variations in magnetic field strength, which arise from inhomogeneities in the applied field and differences in magnetic susceptibility among the tissues themselves. These effects contribute to T_2* relaxation. Magnetic susceptibility refers to the tendency of a material to become magnetized[†] in the presence of an external magnetic field. This alters the strength of the field both within the material itself and in its immediate neighborhood. Ferromagnetic materials, such as iron, have very high susceptibility, and cause substantial distortions in the local magnetic field. Air, by contrast, has almost zero susceptibility. Most biological materials are diamagnetic, meaning that they have a small negative susceptibility. A few biological substances, mostly blood proteins, such as deoxyhemoglobin and hemosiderin, are paramagnetic and have a small positive susceptibility. Whenever a sample contains tissues of different susceptibility, the strength of the magnetic field changes across their boundaries, causing spin dephasing and shortening the T_2* value. This occurs around air-filled cavities, such as the sinuses and petrous bones in the head, and in tissue containing deoxygenated blood or byproducts of hemorrhage.

1.4.3. The Free Induction Decay and the Spin Echo

The attenuation of the transverse magnetization following RF excitation is known as the free induction decay (FID) (**Fig. 7**). It results from both microscopic interactions and larger-scale field variations, and occurs on a timescale T_2*. The value of T_2* varies according to the host molecule and tissue type, but, in each case, the transverse magnetization follows an exponential decay:

[†]The bulk magnetization that determines a material's susceptibility is primarily a result of its electrons, and should not be confused with the nuclear magnetization.

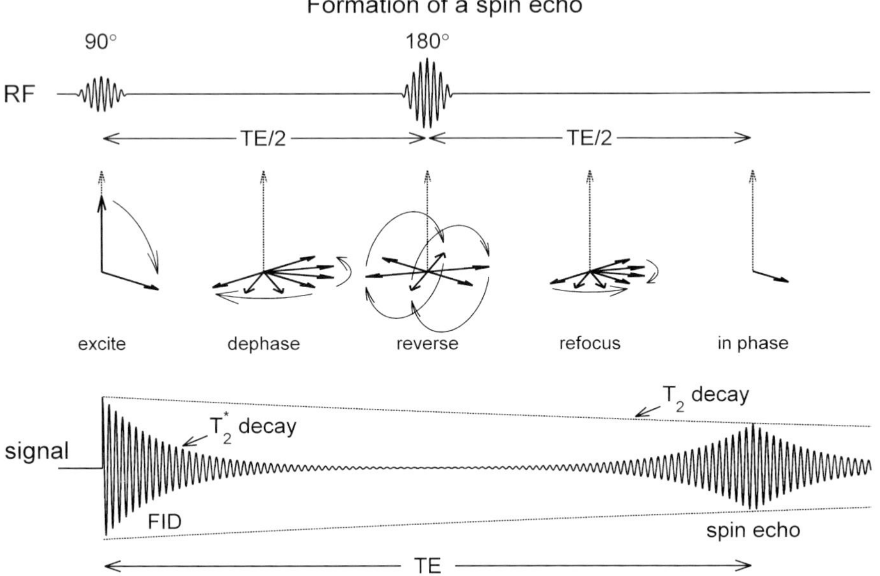

Fig. 8. Dephasing caused by magnetic field inhomogeneities can be reversed by means of a refocusing pulse, resulting in the formation of a spin echo. The amplitude of the spin echo is determined by the amount of T_2 relaxation that has occurred during the echo time TE. Because T_2 relaxation is caused by microscopic interactions and diffusion, it cannot be reversed.

$$M_\perp(t) = M_\perp(0)e^{-t/T_2^*}.$$ [16]

Here, $M_\perp$ is the amplitude of the transverse magnetization and t is the time following the RF excitation. The value of $M_\perp(0)$ is determined by the longitudinal magnetization available before the excitation and by the FA of the RF pulse.

The dephasing caused by macroscopic and mesoscopic field inhomogeneities is considered reversible, because it can be undone using a simple refocusing procedure. The technique relies on the use of a 180° RF pulse (the refocusing pulse) to reverse the phase differences that have accumulated among the spins. The refocusing pulse effectively resets the phase evolution, giving the faster spins a handicap and the slower spins a head start. As the spins continue to precess under the influence of the same field inhomogeneities, they gradually come back into phase, producing a brief signal recovery known as a spin echo (**Fig. 8**). The time taken for the spins to rephase exactly equals the time during which they were allowed to dephase, and the total is known as the echo time, TE.

The procedure is only able to compensate for magnetic field inhomogeneities on a mesoscopic and macroscopic scale, which remain relatively constant with time. Microscopic interactions, which vary as the molecules rotate and diffuse, produce irreversible dephasing that cannot be undone by the refocusing procedure. The amplitude of the spin echo is therefore attenuated by T_2 relaxation, and equals:

$$M_\perp(\text{TE}) = M_\perp(0)e^{-\text{TE}/T_2}. \qquad [17]$$

Both spin-echo and FID acquisition techniques are used in imaging and spectroscopy. In imaging, they offer alternative types of signal contrast among tissues. Spin-echo acquisitions provide T_2 weighting, whereas FID acquisitions provide T_2^* weighting. The degree of T_2 or T_2^* weighting depends on the time delay between RF excitation and signal acquisition. A longer delay allows more time for transverse relaxation, so that tissues with short T_2 or T_2^* will appear darker than those with longer relaxation times. Note that to obtain pure T_2 weighting, the signal must be acquired during the spin echo. The TE can, however, be controlled via the timing of the refocusing pulse.

1.4.4. Summary

- Longitudinal relaxation describes loss of energy from the nuclei and recovery of the equilibrium magnetization, $\mathbf{M}_0$, which occur on a time-scale denoted T_1.
- Transverse relaxation describes loss of phase coherence among the nuclei and decay of the signal. It is characterized by two time-scales, denoted T_2 and T_2^*, which govern the amplitudes of the spin echo and FID, respectively.
- The values of the longitudinal and transverse relaxation times depend on the host molecule and tissue type. Differences in relaxation times are used to produce signal contrast on MR images.

2. Magnetic Resonance in Practice

The use of MR as a probe for biological research dictates certain important aspects of experimental design. In particular, the presence of extremely strong magnetic fields precludes the use of any ferromagnetic materials and most electronic devices in the vicinity of the scanner. The choice of RF coil is also an important consideration in any experiment, because the coil must be adapted to the anatomy under consideration, and be designed to resonate at the Larmor frequency, which depends on the nucleus and the field strength. The purpose of the present section is to describe the instrumentation used in an MR scanner and the basic steps and safety precautions involved in planning and performing an MR scan.

2.1. Instrumentation

The central component of an MR scanner is the primary magnet, which produces the $\mathbf{B}_0$ field. The scanner also incorporates gradient coils and higher-order shim coils to adjust the spatial variations in $\mathbf{B}_0$. RF coils and related circuitry are required for RF transmission and signal reception, and a computer system is used to control the acquisition and process the results.

2.1.1. Primary Magnet

The amplitude of the MR signal is ultimately limited by the magnitude of the equilibrium magnetization, M_0, which is proportional to the strength of the static magnetic field, B_0. To obtain adequate SNR requires an extremely strong magnetic field, especially for studies on small animals or ex vivo samples, in which signal must be acquired from tiny volumes of tissue.

Magnetic field strength is measured in gauss (G) or tesla, where 1 T = 10,000 G. Gauss is the more natural unit for the magnetic fields typically encountered in everyday situations; the earth's own magnetic field for example is about 0.5 G (5×10^{-5} T). The fields used in MR scanners, however, are of an order 10,000 to 100,000 times stronger, and are specified in tesla. Most clinical MR scanners in current use have field strengths of 1.5 T or 3.0 T, whereas the ultrahigh field systems used for animal studies have field strengths attaining approx 14 T.

In addition to being extremely strong, the magnetic field in an MR system must be very stable, to prevent the Larmor frequency from drifting over time. The field is normally produced by an electromagnet made from coils of niobium–titanium wire, which become superconducting at about 10 K (–263°C). Immersed in a bath of liquid helium (4 K), the coils carry large electrical currents with negligible resistance, producing a magnetic field that is both strong and stable. The most common configuration is a solenoidal (cylindrical or donut) geometry, as shown in **Figs. 9** and **10**. During the scan, the subject or sample is positioned at the center of the solenoid, where the field is strongest and most homogeneous.

2.1.2. Gradient and Shim Coils

Homogeneity of the $\mathbf{B}_0$ field is very important in minimizing spin dephasing. This is particularly critical in spectroscopy, because any inhomogeneity will broaden the spectral lines. Inhomogeneities result from manufacturing imperfections in the primary magnet and from metallic structures in the building where the scanner is housed. Susceptibility differences within the sample itself also introduce spatial variations in $\mathbf{B}_0$, so the field must be shimmed dynamically at the beginning of each scan.

The MR system incorporates shim coils that produce compensatory magnetic fields to correct for spatial variations in the main magnetic field. Gradient coils are used to adjust for linear variations, and higher-order shim coils provide compensation for quadratic variations. The gradient coils serve a dual purpose in the MR system because they are also used in imaging and localized spectroscopy to provide volume selectivity and to encode spatial information into the signal. These techniques will be discussed further in **Subheadings 3.** and **4.**

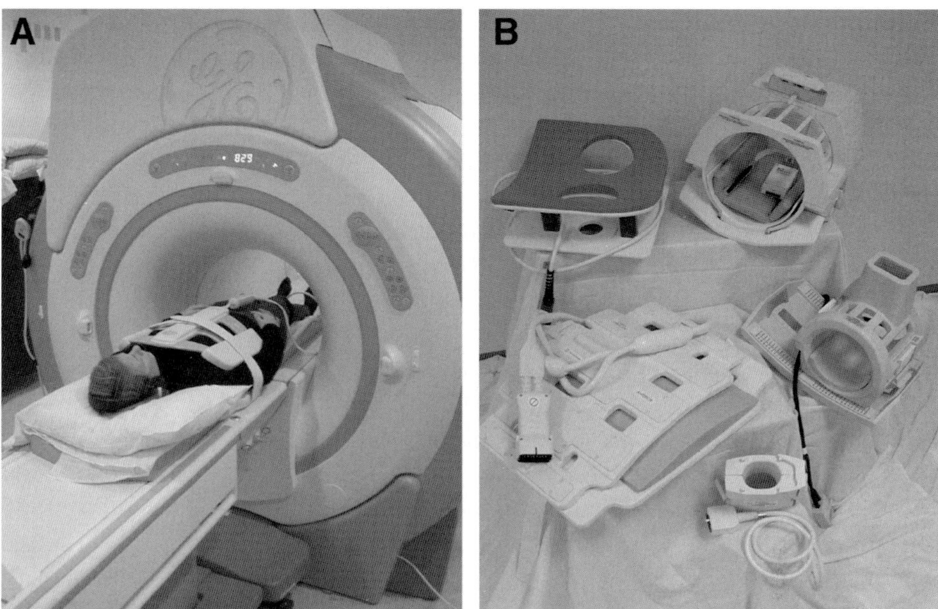

Fig. 9. **(A)** A 1.5 T whole body clinical MRI scanner (GE Healthcare, Milwaukee, WI). A torso phased-array coil has been placed over the subject's chest for localized signal reception. **(B)** Examples of other coils used in clinical MRI. Clockwise from top left: a breast coil, head coil, extremity coil (for knee, ankle, and foot imaging), wrist coil, and torso coil.

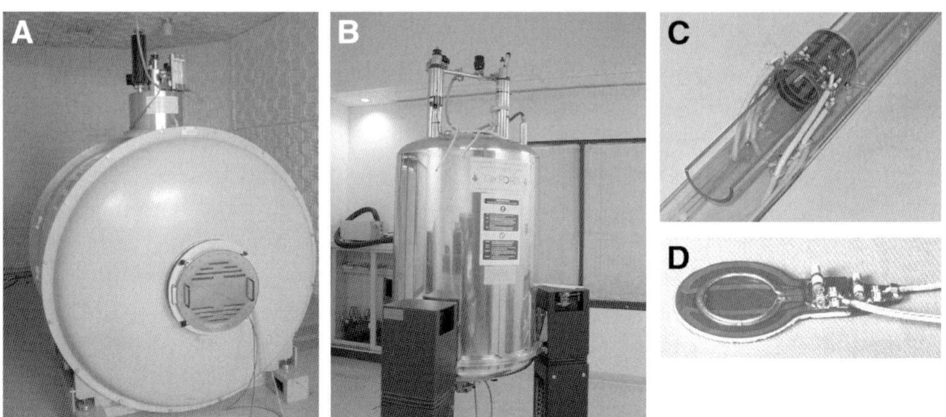

Fig. 10. A 4.7-T horizontal bore scanner **(A)** and a 9.4-T vertical bore system **(B)** used for imaging and spectroscopic studies of small animals. (Reprinted with permission of Alice Wyrwicz, Ph.D.) **(C,D)** Examples of small volume and surface coils respectively (Doty Scientific, Columbia, SC).

An MR system contains three gradient coils, which produce magnetic fields that vary linearly in strength along each of three orthogonal directions *X*, *Y*, and *Z*. They can be used in combination to produce magnetic field gradients in any direction. As we will describe later, this allows images to be acquired in arbitrary oblique planes. The coils used in whole-body clinical systems are typically capable of producing magnetic field gradients of around 40 mT/m (millitesla per meter), whereas those in small-bore scanners have maximum amplitudes in the range of 100 to 3000 mT/m. The higher gradient strengths allow finer spatial resolution, which is important in imaging small animals and samples.

2.1.3. RF Coils

The MR system includes RF transmitter coils and related circuitry to produce the $\mathbf{B}_1(t)$ field for RF excitation. It also incorporates receiver coils and data acquisition boards to detect and process the signal emitted by the excited nuclei. Separate coils may be used for transmission and reception, or a single coil may serve both purposes. RF coils are equivalent to radio antennae and are produced in a variety of geometries (*see* **Figs. 9** and **10**). They are generally classified as volume or surface coils (*see* Chapter 2). Volume coils enclose the tissue of interest, and are designed to have roughly uniform sensitivity inside. Surface coils are placed over the region of interest, and have a penetration depth on the order of the coil radius. Surface coils are very useful for detecting signal from a relatively superficial region of interest. As transmitters, however, they produce a $\mathbf{B}_1(t)$ field whose amplitude diminishes with distance from the tissue surface, resulting in a nonuniform FA (**Eq. [4]**).

To maximize SNR, the coil should match the size and shape of the anatomy. This is because signal is generally acquired only from a thin slice or small volume of tissue, whereas noise is detected from all of the tissue within the coil's range of sensitivity. The coil must also be resonant at the Larmor frequency, which depends (through **Eq. [2]**) on both the field strength, B_0 (e.g., 1.5 T or 3.0 T), and the nucleus under study (e.g., hydrogen or phosphorus). Because coils can be tuned only within a limited frequency range, it is necessary to design specific coils for each field strength and each nucleus. For spectroscopic applications in which signal must be acquired both from protons and from another nucleus, it is possible to purchase double-tuned coils, which resonate at the Larmor frequencies of both nuclei.

2.1.4. Computer System

To facilitate the acquisition process and automate the reconstruction of images or spectra, the scanner is interfaced to a computer system. The investigator uses the console to input the desired acquisition parameters and to display the results. In an imaging experiment, for example, the input parameters may include such variables as the imaging plane, field of view (FOV), and spatial resolution (discussed further in **Subheading 3.2.4.**). The resulting images are displayed to the screen, and can be used to prescribe slices for later acquisitions.

2.1.5. Summary

- The central component of an MR scanner is the primary magnet, which is typically a superconducting electromagnet, producing a field in the range of 1.5 to 14 T.
- The MR system incorporates gradient and shim coils to maintain the homogeneity of the B_0 field, and to provide volume selectivity and spatial encoding for imaging and localized spectroscopy.
- RF coils are required for excitation and signal detection. They must be designed to resonate at the Larmor frequency, which depends on the nucleus and the field strength.

2.2. Safety

Provided that elementary safety precautions are observed, MR imaging and spectroscopy are believed to pose no risk to people, animals, or biological samples. Violation of the safety precautions, however, can lead to injury or even death. The principal hazards of which the user must be aware involve ferromagnetic materials and electronic devices. There is also a potential risk of excessive RF power deposition or nerve stimulation, but this is minimized by inbuilt safeguards. Finally, certain studies may involve administration of MR contrast agents or anesthetics, and these, like any drugs, should be used with care.

2.2.1. Ferromagnetic Materials and Electronic Devices

The superconducting magnets used in MR systems are extraordinarily strong, and are always on, even when the scanner console has been shut off. If a ferromagnetic object, such as a pair of scissors, is taken inadvertently into the vicinity of the scanner, it can be torn out of a person's grasp, and turned into a lethal projectile. The strong magnetic fields can also disrupt the operation of delicate electronic devices, such as pacemakers. Consequently, anyone using the scanner or being scanned should first be screened for contraindications, which include metallic or electronic implants.

The magnetic field extends well outside the bore of the scanner, and potentially hazardous items should be kept beyond the so-called 5-G line (the line at which the field falls to 5 G, or 0.0005 T). In a research environment, this line may be marked on the floor, but in a clinical MR suite, all hazardous objects should be kept outside the scanner room.

Hazardous objects include anything that contains ferromagnetic materials. Such materials become strongly magnetized in the presence of a magnetic field, and are drawn into the scanner with extremely high force. Not all metals are ferromagnetic, but it is prudent to avoid taking any metallic items into the vicinity of the scanner. Those that are not ferromagnetic may still heat up when exposed to an RF field and can cause burning on contact. In addition to their safety risks, metal objects can also spoil the homogeneity of the magnetic field and compromise data quality.

The dangers posed by ferromagnetic materials place severe restrictions on the equipment that can be used in an MR study. Many companies now sell MR-compatible devices, including infusers, ventilators, and physiological monitoring devices, which can safely be used near an MR scanner without risk to human or animal subjects, or to scanner operation.

2.2.2. RF Power and Gradient Switching

It is well to be aware of additional safety issues, including RF power deposition and nerve stimulation, although these are usually of less practical concern to the investigator because of inbuilt safeguards. RF quanta have extremely low energy (as given in **Eq. [5]**) and cannot cause tissue damage through ionization. However, they can produce heating if their intensity is sufficiently high. The RF power deposition, known as the specific absorption rate (SAR), can be calculated from the FA and the TR of the acquisition. Clinical scanners are programmed to reject any choice of acquisition parameters that might cause the SAR to exceed regulatory limits.

MRI and localized spectroscopy require the use of pulsed magnetic field gradients to provide volume selectivity and spatial encoding. The gradient switching, however, induces small transitory voltages within the tissue, which, if large enough, can cause nerve stimulation. Clinical scanners have internal constraints on the gradient ramping rates to keep them within physiological limits.

2.2.3. Contrast Agents

MRI is often performed with an injected contrast agent, a substance that enhances the signal contrast between various tissues via its effect on longitudinal or transverse relaxation times. The clinically approved gadolinium chelates are well tolerated and very safe *(9–11)*. Adverse reactions, although uncommon, may include nausea, vomiting, and urticaria (hives). Cases of anaphylactic shock have been reported but are extremely rare.

There is enormous interest in the development of new contrast materials with more specific biodistribution characteristics. Most of these agents are based on alternative gadolinium complexes or superparamagnetic iron oxide (SPIO) particles, and many are currently undergoing clinical trials. Manganese chloride also has powerful MR properties, and has been used extensively in animal experiments (*see* Chapter 15). However, it has not been applied to human studies because of concerns about acute cardiovascular toxicity *(12)*.

2.2.4. Summary

- The primary magnet in an MR system is always on.
- Metal objects and electronic devices should not be taken into the vicinity of the scanner.
- MR scanning has the potential to cause heating or nerve stimulation.

2.3. Planning and Conducting an MR Study

The most important considerations in planning an MR study are the physiological stability and monitoring of the subject, the use of MR-compatible equipment, and the choice of RF coil. The scan itself involves several steps, and can take anywhere between half an hour and several hours, depending on the purpose of the study and the size of the subject or sample.

2.3.1. MR Compatibility

For a device to be MR compatible, it must be MR safe (*see* **Subheading 2.2.**), and it must not interfere with the measurement process. Many electronic devices, for example, contain CPUs (central processing units) that emit electromagnetic waves in the megahertz range. Radiative emissions that contain frequencies within the bandwidth of the MR signal can introduce errors or artifacts into the data. It may be necessary to purchase or construct special MR-compatible equipment, or to adapt existing equipment so that it can be operated at a safe distance from the scanner.

2.3.2. Subject Preparation and Monitoring

Scanning a person usually requires a minimum of half an hour, whereas studies of small animals and ex vivo samples can take several hours to achieve similar SNR levels. During this time, the subject must be kept immobile and physiologically stable. To minimize motion in human studies, it is usually sufficient to provide comfortable cushioning. Sedation may be required for disoriented patients and young children. Animal experiments should be performed using inhaled or injected anesthetics. If the experiment is to be conducted on a small-bore MR system, a cradle is required to support the animal at the isocenter of the bore (**Fig. 10C**). The cradle may incorporate a tooth-bar to keep the animal's head immobile, and a nose cone or chamber into which isoflurane can be administered. It may also contain hollow cavities or tubing through which warm water may be circulated to maintain body temperature. Physiological monitoring is required for all animal experiments, and for studies involving very ill patients. Temperature probes, pulse oxymeters, and electrocardiogram (ECG) leads must all be MR compatible. The ECG trace may also be used for cardiac-triggered data acquisition to obtain images of the heart or any other organ that exhibits pulsatile motion or flow.

2.3.3. Choice of RF Coil

To maximize the SNR it is important to use an RF coil that is matched to the size and shape of the sample or anatomical region under investigation. A variety of coils are available for human studies, including volume coils designed to fit the head or extremities, and surface coils adapted for the spine, thorax, or breasts (**Fig. 9B**). For animal experiments, it is common to build or purchase a dedicated coil for each project (**Figs. 10C,D**). The coils must resonate at the Larmor frequency, which depends on both the magnetic field strength, B_0, and the nucleus under study. In spectroscopic studies using nuclei other than hydrogen, signal must be acquired both from protons (for shimming and localization) and from the nucleus of interest (for spectral analysis). The signals can be acquired either with separate coils or by using double-tuned coils that resonate at the frequencies of both nuclei.

2.3.4. Basic Steps in Scanning

Subject preparation includes setting up any required anesthesia equipment, physiological probes, and intravenous lines, and placing the RF coil around the anatomy of interest. The subject should then be positioned in the scanner so that the region of interest lies at the isocenter of the bore, where the magnetic field is strongest and most homogeneous. Before scanning, the RF coil must be tuned to the Larmor frequency. The RF transmitter amplitude and receiver gain must then be calibrated and the static magnetic field shimmed. On clinical MR scanners, these tasks are performed automatically as part of a prescan procedure, whereas, on research systems, some or all of them may require operator input.

The purpose of the transmitter calibration is to determine how much current has to be passed through the RF transmitter coil to produce a $\mathbf{B}_1(t)$ field of the desired amplitude. The calibration must be repeated for each subject, because the field depends on coil loading. It involves adjusting the current until the signal reaches a maximum, corresponding to a FA of exactly 90°. The current required for any other FA can then be calculated.

The receiver gain must be calibrated to ensure adequate dynamic range for signal acquisition. If the gain is too low, the digitizer may not distinguish between signals that are very close in amplitude, whereas, if it is too high, overflow errors may occur.

Shimming is performed to maximize the homogeneity of the $\mathbf{B}_0$ field. The homogeneity is assessed either by measuring the linewidth of the FID, or by analyzing the phase variations in the signal across the region of interest. Adjustments are then made to the currents through the shim coils[†], until the homogeneity is optimized.

[†]On many clinical systems, only the gradient coils allow for dynamic current adjustments.

After tuning, calibration, and shimming, the first scan is usually a three-plane localizer or 'scout,' which produces images in axial, sagittal, and coronal planes. These allow visualization of the anatomy, and can be used to prescribe slices in arbitrary orientations through the organs of interest.

2.3.5. Summary

- The subject must be kept immobile and physiologically stable throughout the scan.
- Any equipment used in the vicinity of the scanner must be MR compatible.
- RF coils should be chosen to match the size and shape of the anatomy under investigation.

3. Imaging

Although all nuclei with nonzero spin exhibit MR, imaging is usually performed with hydrogen, because of its excellent MR sensitivity and its high concentration in biological tissues. The signal originates predominantly from water and fat; contributions from other hydrogen-containing species are negligible by comparison, either because of low concentration or because of molecular immobility, which causes extremely rapid T_2 relaxation. To reconstruct an image, the signal from each point within the tissue must be correctly identified and mapped onto the corresponding point within the image. This is achieved with the use of magnetic field gradients, which alter the Larmor frequency of the nuclei in a spatially dependent manner. The signal contrast between different tissues can be controlled via the timing and amplitude of the RF excitation pulses and through the use of exogenous (injected) contrast agents.

3.1. Formation of an Image

Imaging can be performed using 2D or 3D acquisitions, which involve the excitation of nuclei in a specified slice or slab of tissue, respectively. Once excited, all of the tissue within the slice or slab emits signal simultaneously. To produce images, it is, therefore, necessary to identify the contribution from each point. This is achieved by encoding spatial information into the phase and frequency of the signal. Both slice-selective excitation and spatial encoding involve the use of magnetic field gradients.

3.1.1. Slice-Selective Excitation

Nuclei can absorb energy from the RF field $\mathbf{B}_1(t)$ only if their Larmor frequency exactly matches the frequency of the RF field. Slice-selective excitation is achieved by applying the RF field in the presence of a magnetic field gradient. The gradient introduces a small spatial variation into the strength of the $\mathbf{B}_0$ field, producing a corresponding variation in the Larmor frequency (**Fig. 11**). Only those nuclei whose Larmor frequency ω_L equals the frequency of the applied RF field ω_{RF} will be excited. The condition $\omega_L = \omega_{RF}$ is satisfied for

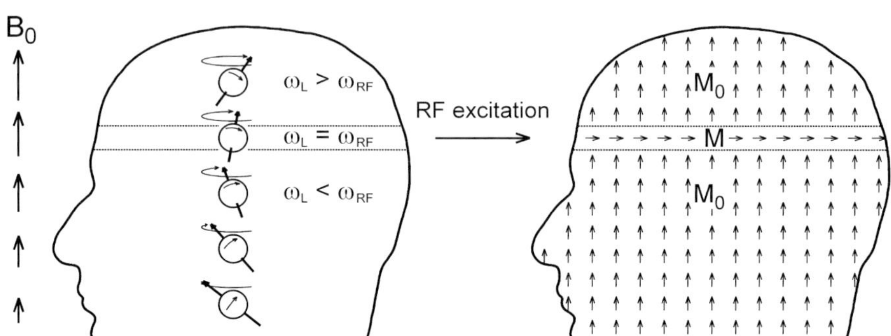

Fig. 11. To acquire an image of a particular slice of tissue, the scanner must excite the nuclear magnetization only within that slice. Slice-selective excitation is achieved by applying a radio frequency (RF) pulse in the presence of a magnetic field gradient. The gradient produces a linear variation in the strength of the static field, $\mathbf{B}_0$, which gives rise to a spatial variation in the value of the Larmor frequency. Only those spins whose Larmor frequency, ω_L, exactly matches the frequency of the applied RF field, ω_{RF}, will be excited.

nuclei lying in a particular slice of tissue perpendicular to the magnetic field gradient. The thickness of the slice is determined by the bandwidth of the RF pulse and the amplitude of the gradient, each of which can be selected independently. Thin slices are chosen for 2D imaging, and thicker slabs for 3D imaging. The location of each slice along the direction of the gradient is controlled via the frequency of the RF field. Increasing the RF frequency will excite nuclei in a slice of tissue where the Larmor frequency is correspondingly higher. Finally, the orientation of the slice is determined by the direction of the magnetic field gradient. The gradient coils can be used singly or in combination to excite a slice in any oblique plane.

3.1.2. Spatial Encoding

Because the RF pulse excites all of the tissue in the selected slice, the emitted signal is a sum of contributions from all of the spins within that slice. To identify the contribution from each tissue element, spatial information is encoded into the signal by means of magnetic field gradients that are applied after the RF excitation.

By applying a magnetic field gradient during data acquisition, position information is encoded into the frequency of the signal (**Fig. 12**). Tissue located at points where the $\mathbf{B}_0$ field is slightly stronger will emit signal at a fractionally higher frequency than tissue located at points where it is weaker. Because the

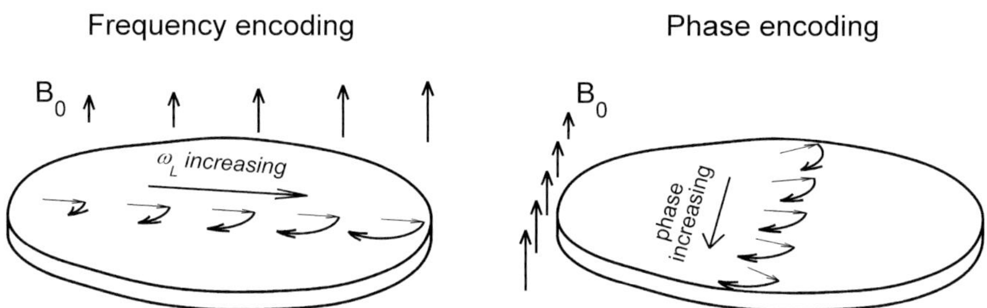

Fig. 12. Having excited the nuclear magnetization within a desired slice of tissue, the position of the spins within the imaging plane must be determined. This is achieved using frequency encoding in one direction and phase encoding in the perpendicular direction. In frequency encoding, a magnetic field gradient is applied during signal acquisition. The position of the spins along the direction of the gradient can then be identified by the frequency of their emitted signals. In phase encoding, a magnetic field gradient is applied as a brief pulse before data acquisition. This introduces a phase variation among the spins, which is imprinted on their signals. To extract position information from the phase, the process must be repeated many times with phase-encoding gradients of incrementally different amplitudes.

detected signal comes from the entire slice, it will contain a range of different frequencies, corresponding to contributions from different tissue elements. The amplitude of each component indicates how much signal came from each position along the direction of the gradient. The technique is known as frequency encoding, because the origin of the signal can be identified by its frequency. Frequency encoding is not sufficient by itself to reconstruct an image, however, because it provides position information in only one direction.

Position information in the perpendicular direction is obtained through a mechanism known as phase encoding, which is used in combination with frequency encoding to produce an image in 2D. A gradient pulse is applied in the phase-encoding direction before signal acquisition. The gradient pulse alters the Larmor frequency of the spins, but only for a brief period, resulting in a relative phase shift among the spins (**Fig. 12**). The detected signal, therefore, contains components with different phases, which originate from different positions along the direction of the gradient. To extract the amplitude of each component, the entire process of excitation and signal acquisition must be repeated many times, with gradient pulses of incrementally different strengths. The change in phase between successive acquisitions uniquely identifies the position of the tissue along the direction of the gradient. Phase encoding is, in fact, mathematically equivalent to frequency encoding, except that the data are acquired in a discrete rather than continuous manner.

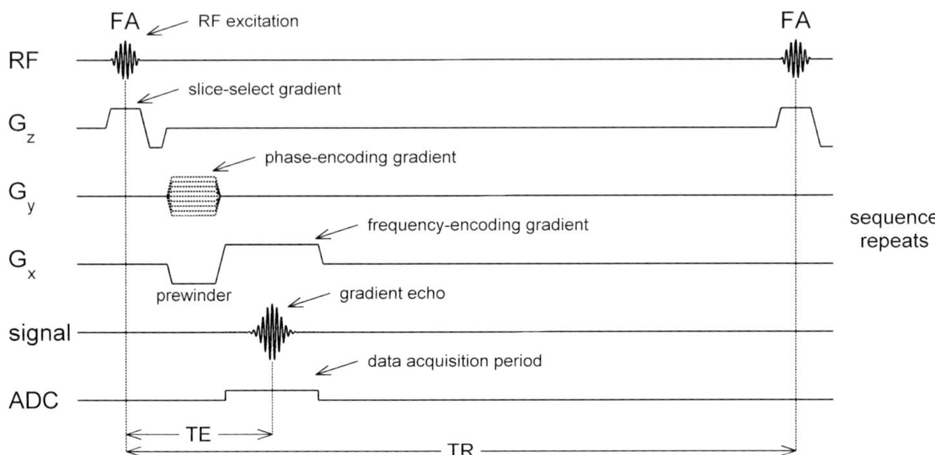

Fig. 13. A simple pulse sequence illustrating the implementation of slice selection and spatial encoding. The presentation of a pulse sequence is analogous to an orchestral score, with time increasing from left to right, and the various parts played by the hardware instrumentation displayed one above the other. The top line illustrates the radio frequency pulses produced by the transmitter, which have flip angle, FA. The lines marked G_z, G_y, and G_x indicate the magnetic field gradients in the slice-select, phase-encoding, and frequency-encoding directions, respectively. The label ADC denotes the analog-to-digital converter, which is turned on during signal acquisition.

3.1.3. Image Reconstruction

Frequency and phase encoding are used in combination to produce an image in 2D. The directions of frequency and phase encoding are conventionally denoted x and y, respectively, and the through-slice direction is denoted z. These labels are completely arbitrary, however, and are not connected with the physical axes of the scanner or the gradient coils. In fact, the gradient coils can be used in combination to image the tissue in any oblique plane.

To produce an image, the same slice of tissue is excited repeatedly, and the signal is sampled as a function of time after each excitation. The amplitude of the frequency-encoding gradient remains constant with each repetition, whereas that of the phase-encoding gradient is incremented from one repetition to the next (**Fig. 13**). The resulting data are recorded as a series of lines in a 2D array known as k-space (**Fig. 14**). By applying a 2D Fourier transform to the k-space data, the spatial distribution of the signal is recovered. The phase information is usually discarded at that stage, leaving a map of the signal amplitude, which constitutes the image.

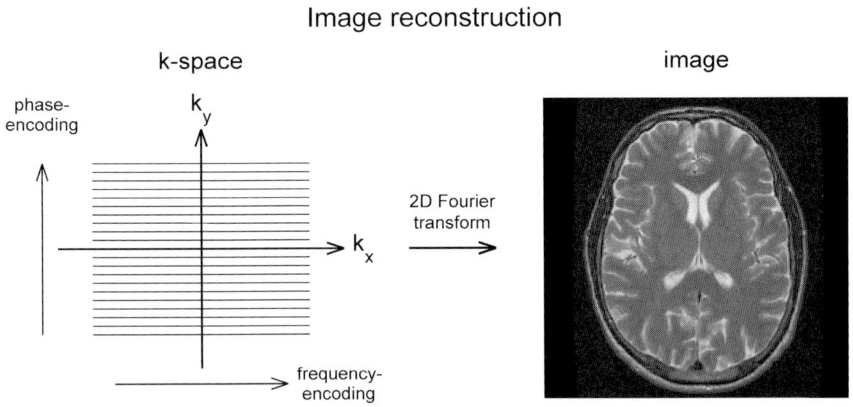

Image reconstruction

k-space

image

Fig. 14. After each excitation, the magnetic resonance signal is acquired as a function of time and recorded as a row of numbers in a data array known as k-space. The process is repeated with phase-encoding gradients of incrementally different amplitudes, and each time the signal is recorded as an adjacent line in k-space. After all of the k-space data have been collected, the image is extracted by means of a 2D fast Fourier transform. Note that, in accordance with convention, the image is oriented so that the anterior of the head appears at the top.

The resolution of the image in the phase-encoding direction is determined by the number of k-space lines collected. An image with a resolution of 256 pixels in the phase-encoding direction for example requires the acquisition of 256 k-space lines. Resolution in the frequency-encoding direction is determined by the amplitude of the frequency-encoding gradient and the duration of the acquisition period.

For 3D acquisitions, phase encoding is used in the through-slab direction as well as one of the in-plane dimensions. This produces a 3D set of k-space data, which can be reconstructed into a 3D map of the tissue by means of a 3D Fourier transform. The results are typically displayed as a stack of 2D images but can be reformatted along any plane.

It is useful to note that data in k-space can be interpreted as spatial-frequency components of the image. Data near the center of k-space ($\mathbf{k} = 0$) correspond to low spatial-frequency components and represent the large-scale or coarse spatial structure in the image. Data near the outer edges of k-space correspond to high spatial-frequency components, and represent the fine structure in the image.

3.1.4. Summary

- MR imaging involves the selective excitation of a slice or slab of tissue. This is achieved by applying an RF pulse in the presence of a magnetic field gradient.

- Spatial information within the slice or slab is encoded into the phase and frequency of the emitted signal, by applying magnetic field gradients to the excited tissue after the RF pulse.
- The raw data are recorded as lines in k-space, from which images are reconstructed using a Fourier transform.

3.2. Pulse Sequences

The acquisition of an MR image requires repeated RF pulses and signal acquisitions, each of which must be coordinated with magnetic field gradients. The entire process is known as a pulse sequence, and can be tailored to provide optimal signal contrast for each application *(1–5)*. Among the most commonly used pulse sequences are the so-called gradient-echo and spin-echo sequences, and variants thereof.

3.2.1. Gradient-Echo Sequences

In a gradient-echo sequence, a single RF pulse is applied during each TR period, and data are acquired during the subsequent FID. The term gradient echo refers to the resurgence of signal that occurs at the center of the acquisition period (**Fig. 13**). It arises because the frequency-encoding gradient dephases the spins in a spatially dependent manner, and this gradient-induced dephasing is minimized at the center of the acquisition period. The fact that it occurs at the center of the acquisition rather than the beginning results from the presence of a preparatory gradient pulse, which prewinds the spins (**Fig. 13**).

The term TE is used in the context of gradient-echo sequences to denote the interval between RF excitation and the center of the gradient echo. The value of TE is important in determining the signal contrast of the image. Because the transverse magnetization is subject to T_2^* dephasing during the FID, regions of tissue whose T_2^* value is short compared with TE will exhibit greatly attenuated signal. By contrast, regions with longer T_2^* will have relatively higher signal. The degree of T_2^*-weighting in the image depends on the value of TE, which for gradient-echo sequences is usually a few milliseconds.

Gradient-echo sequences often employ very short TR values (on the order of several milliseconds), with the result that the images also exhibit T_1-weighting. Tissues with short T_1 appear brighter than those with long T_1 because their longitudinal magnetization is less easily saturated. The degree of T_1-weighting also increases with the FA, because a high FA causes greater saturation. The FAs typically used in gradient-echo sequences range from approx 10° to approx 40°.

3.2.2. Spin-Echo Sequences

In a spin-echo sequence, two RF pulses are applied during each TR period, namely a 90° excitation pulse and a 180° refocusing pulse (as discussed in

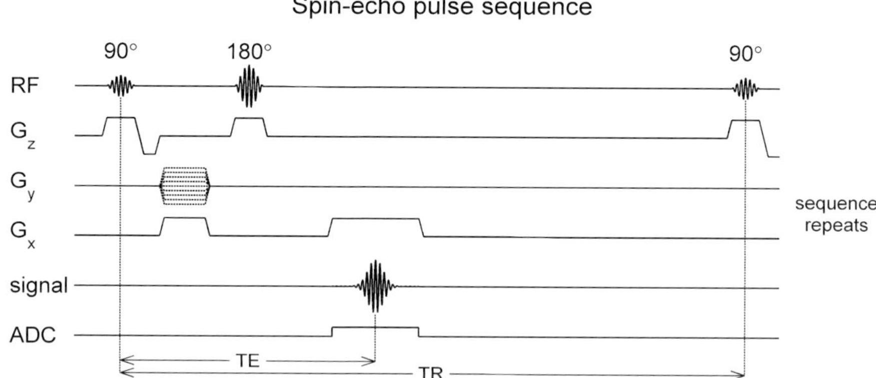

Fig. 15. A spin-echo imaging sequence. Note that it is similar to the gradient-echo pulse sequence of **Fig. 13**, except that it employs two radio frequency pulses per repetition time (TR). The initial pulse (the excitation) has a flip angle (FA) of 90°, whereas the second (the refocusing pulse) has a FA of 180°. Data are collected during the spin echo, which occurs at an echo time (TE) equal to twice the interval between the excitation and refocusing pulses (c.f., **Fig. 8**). The data acquisition is performed in the presence of a frequency-encoding gradient, and is preceded by a phase-encoding gradient pulse, whose amplitude changes from one TR period to the next.

Subheading 1.4.3.). Both are applied in the presence of a slice-selection gradient (**Fig. 15**). Data are acquired during the subsequent spin echo, when the spins are refocused. Because the amplitude of the spin echo is affected by T_2 relaxation, the resulting images are T_2-weighted. The degree of T_2-weighting is determined by the value of TE, which for a spin-echo sequence may range from a few milliseconds to hundreds of milliseconds.

Because spin-echo sequences employ large FAs, they require long TRs to allow adequate recovery of the longitudinal magnetization. Typical TR values range from hundreds of milliseconds to several seconds, the shorter values producing greater degrees of T_1-weighting. Because the total scan time depends on the product of the TR and the number of k-space lines, spin-echo sequences can be very lengthy to run. Their efficiency can, however, be improved by acquiring multiple lines of data during each TR period. This is achieved by inserting additional refocusing pulses after each excitation, thereby generating a train of spin echoes, each of which is used to acquire an additional line of data. This variant is known as a fast spin-echo (FSE) sequence.

3.2.3. Inversion and Saturation Recovery

Both gradient-echo and spin-ccho sequences produce T_1-weighting if the TR is relatively short. An alternative way to introduce T_1-weighting is to pre-

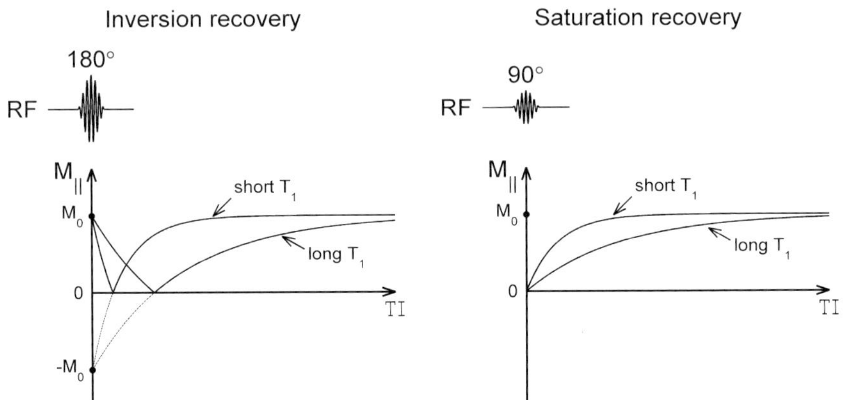

Fig. 16. Strong T_1-weighting can be achieved using an inversion- or saturation-recovery technique. In the first case, the acquisition sequence is preceded by a 180° radio frequency (RF) pulse, which inverts the longitudinal magnetization. Signal is acquired at a chosen inversion time (TI) after the inversion pulse, as the longitudinal magnetization, $M_\parallel$, recovers toward its equilibrium value, M_0. The graph shows how the amplitude of the signal varies with TI for tissues with two different T_1 values. Note that magnetic resonance images display only the magnitude of the signal, which is proportional to the absolute value of the magnetization (solid line). In saturation-recovery techniques, the acquisition sequence is preceded by a 90° RF pulse, which nulls the longitudinal magnetization.

cede the initial excitation by a 180° inversion pulse (**Fig. 16**). This is known as an inversion-recovery technique, because data are acquired during the recovery of the longitudinal magnetization toward its equilibrium value, M_0. The interval between the inversion pulse and the first excitation of the acquisition sequence is called the inversion time, TI. The value of the longitudinal magnetization at this time determines the amplitude of the signal. It can be calculated from **Eq. [15]** by substituting $t = $ TI and setting $M_\parallel(0) = -M_0$. Because the rate of recovery is inversely proportional to T_1, the resulting images are T_1-weighted. The signal contrast, however, depends on the value of TI. If TI is sufficiently short that the longitudinal magnetization has not passed zero for any of the tissues, then those with shorter T_1 will appear darker than those with longer T_1. This is called a short-TI inversion recovery, or STIR technique. If TI is beyond the so-called null point, the signal contrast will be reversed.

In a variant known as saturation-recovery, the 180° inversion pulse is replaced with a 90° saturation pulse and a strong dephasing gradient, which null both the longitudinal and transverse magnetization. Data are acquired during the recovery of the longitudinal magnetization toward its equilibrium value.

3.2.4. Imaging Parameters

For any given type of pulse sequence, there are many different parameters under the user's control, and these provide much of the versatility of MR imaging. The timing parameters and FA govern the signal contrast; the spatial parameters determine the resolution, and the number of signal averages affects the overall SNR. The timing parameters include TR, TE, and, for inversion-recovery techniques, TI. The values of TR and FA determine the degree of T_1-weighting, whereas the value of TE determines the amount of T_2-weighting for spin-echo sequences, or T_2^*-weighting for gradient-echo sequences.

The spatial parameters include the FOV, slice thickness, and matrix size. The matrix size specifies the dimensions of the raw data set in k-space and determines the number of pixels in the image (in the absence of interpolation). Each pixel represents a volume element (voxel) of the tissue, and the dimensions of each voxel indicate the resolution of the image. The in-plane resolution is determined by the matrix size and the FOV, whereas the through-plane resolution is equal to the slice thickness. Typical matrix sizes range from 64 × 64 to 512 × 512, whereas the FOV is chosen according to the size of the subject. The FOV cannot be reduced arbitrarily in an effort to improve resolution, because any tissue extending outside the FOV in the phase-encoding direction will cause 'wraparound' artifacts *(1)*.

Internally, the slice thickness is controlled by the amplitude of the slice-select gradient, whereas the FOV is determined by the amplitudes of the phase- and frequency-encoding gradients. Thinner slices and smaller FOVs require stronger gradients. They also produce lower SNR, because the volume of tissue within each voxel is correspondingly smaller. For these reasons, studies of small animals and ex vivo samples are typically performed on ultrahigh-field scanners equipped with high-performance gradient coils. Further discussion is provided in Chapter 2 on MR microscopy.

The SNR of the images is influenced by the FA, timing parameters, and spatial resolution of the acquisition. It can also be controlled independently of these parameters by changing the number of signal averages or NEX (literally, the number of excitations). Increasing the number of averages improves the SNR but also lengthens the scan time.

The scan time is proportional to the TR, the NEX, and the number of phase-encoding steps, N_y (which is identical to the matrix size in the y direction). In a simple gradient-echo or spin-echo sequence, a single line of k-space data is acquired per TR period, bringing the total scan time for a 2D image to:

$$N_y \cdot \text{NEX} \cdot \text{TR}. \qquad [18]$$

If TR is only a few milliseconds (as is common for gradient-echo sequences) an entire image can be obtained in a fraction of a second. However, if TR is on the order of a second or more (as is common for spin-echo sequences) the scan time can be very lengthy. For example, a TR of 3 s with a matrix size of 256 × 256 and a NEX of only 1 gives a scan time of almost 13 min. It is possible in this situation, however, to acquire several 2D images simultaneously by interleaving the acquisitions from different slices. This involves exciting a new slice and acquiring a line of data from that slice while the spins in the other slices are relaxing. By circulating among the various slices, several 2D images can be acquired in the same time that it would take to obtain just one image. A further increase in efficiency can be achieved by using FSE sequences (discussed in **Subheading 3.2.2.**).

For 3D acquisitions, the scan time in **Eq. [18]** is multiplied by an additional factor, N_z, equal to the number of slices in the slab. It is not possible to interleave the slices in this case, because the entire slab is excited with each RF pulse. To keep the scan time within reasonable limits, 3D imaging is usually implemented using a gradient-echo sequence with short TR.

3.2.5. Summary

- Gradient-echo and spin-echo sequences provide T_2^*- and T_2-weighting, respectively. They may also provide T_1-weighting, depending on their TR value.
- In images acquired with long TE, the signal amplitude is higher for tissues with long T_2 or T_2^*.
- In images acquired with short TR, the signal amplitude is higher for tissues with short T_1.

3.3. Endogenous Sources of Signal Contrast

Differences in relaxation rates among tissues provide an important source of signal contrast in MR imaging. The degree of T_1-, T_2-, or T_2^*-weighting can be controlled via the choice of pulse sequence and the values of TR and TE. The amplitude of the MR signal is sensitive not only to relaxation times, however, but also to a vast array of other tissue-dependent factors, such as flow and diffusion. The pulse sequence can be tailored to enhance the effect of a selected factor, thereby increasing the conspicuity of certain structures or lesions. The tissue parameters to which the MR signal is sensitive are known as endogenous sources of signal contrast.

3.3.1. Relaxation Rates

Biological fluids, such as blood and cerebrospinal fluid, tend to have long T_1 and T_2 times, because of the relatively unrestricted motion of their water molecules. By comparison, solid tissues, such as muscle and liver, tend to have

Types of signal contrast in MRI

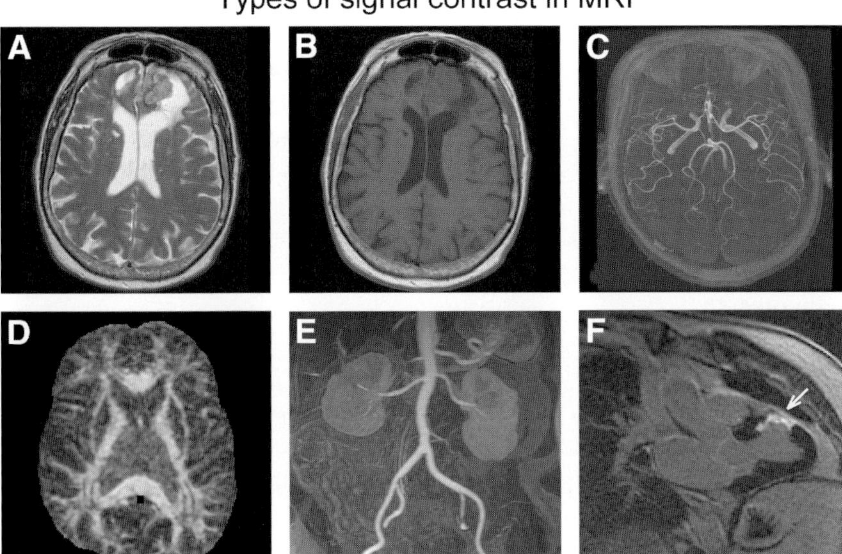

Fig. 17. Example images demonstrating a few of the many different sources of signal contrast available in magnetic resonance imaging. **(A)** A T_2-weighted brain image from a patient with an inferior frontal meningioma. **(B)** A T_1-weighted image from the same patient. **(C)** A maximum intensity projection of a 3D time-of-flight magnetic resonance angiogram (MRA) in the brain. **(D)** A diffusion anisotropy map showing myelinated white matter tracts. **(E)** A maximum intensity projection of a 3D contrast-enhanced MRA of the abdomen. **(F)** A delayed enhancement image from a patient with a myocardial infarct (arrow).

shorter relaxation times, because the water they contain is in frequent contact with macromolecules. Continual binding to the macromolecules decreases the average tumbling rate of the water, thereby promoting relaxation processes and shortening the relaxation times.

Sufficient signal contrast is produced by the differences in relaxation rates to obtain exquisite morphological depiction. In the brain, for example, cerebrospinal fluid has a longer T_2 than gray matter, which, in turn, has a longer T_2 than white matter. On a T_2-weighted image, therefore, the ventricles appear brighter than the cortex, which, in turn, is brighter than the white matter. The various structures can thereby be clearly distinguished. T_2-weighted images are useful in identifying brain tumors, which usually appear hyperintense because of the presence of edema (**Fig. 17A**). On a T_1-weighted image, the signal contrast among the tissues is reversed, with the ventricles appearing darker than the brain parenchyma (**Fig. 17B**).

Functional imaging (fMRI) of brain activity exploits the sensitivity of T_2* to blood oxygenation levels *(13,14)*. The relationship between T_2* and oxygenation arises from the fact that deoxyhemoglobin is paramagnetic, and, therefore, causes dephasing among water protons in its immediate neighborhood (*see* Chapter 7). When a particular region of the brain is active, blood flow to that area is augmented, resulting in higher oxygenation, a lower concentration of deoxyhemoglobin, and a longer T_2*. Brain activity can thereby be mapped using a pulse sequence that is sensitive to T_2*. Blood oxygenation level-dependent imaging has also been used to detect blood flow changes in the kidney (*see* Chapter 8).

3.3.2. Flow

By using a gradient-echo sequence with high FA and short TR, the magnetization of stationary spins can be saturated, without affecting the signal from fresh spins flowing into the imaging slice. This produces signal contrast between vessel lumens and surrounding tissue, providing a means to generate angiograms without the use of exogenous contrast material (**Fig. 17C**). Various ways to alter the magnetization of inflowing spins, collectively known as arterial spin labeling (*see* Chapter 6), have also been used to map perfusion *(15)*.

3.3.3. Diffusion

Diffusion refers to the random motion of molecules associated with their thermal energy. In intact tissue, diffusion is restricted by the presence of cell membranes. Increased diffusivity is, therefore, a signature of membrane disruption, and can be used to identify certain types of lesions and degenerative changes. Preferential diffusion of water along a particular direction indicates the presence of tissue fibers and can be used to assess myelination of white matter tracts (*see* Chapter 5).

Diffusion of tissue water can be mapped using a pulse sequence that incorporates pairs of strong magnetic field gradients between the RF excitation and data acquisition *(16)*. Stationary spins remain unaffected by the gradients, whereas spins moving randomly along the gradient direction become dephased, causing signal loss in regions where the diffusion coefficient is high. By repeating the acquisition with gradients in different directions, it is possible to determine, on a pixel-by-pixel basis, the mean diffusivity and the diffusion anisotropy (a measure of its directionality). The diffusion anisotropy is high along myelinated white matter tracts (**Fig. 17D**).

3.3.4. Magnetization Transfer

Another endogenous contrast mechanism exploited in MRI is magnetization transfer *(17)*. This refers to the exchange of longitudinal magnetization between the protons in water and those in macromolecules, such as proteins. Protons in macromolecules do not contribute directly to the MR signal because their T_2 times are too short. However, they can alter the signal amplitude indirectly via magnetization transfer. One of the ways to observe this effect is by adding a strong preparatory RF pulse whose frequency is offset from the water resonance. Because the macromolecules have a very short T_2, their resonance peak is much broader than that of water. An RF pulse that is shifted from the water resonance will, therefore, saturate some of the protons in the macromolecules without directly affecting the water protons. However, in regions where water is in close contact with macromolecules, longitudinal magnetization can be transferred between them, causing an attenuation of the water signal. The effect can be used to suppress background tissue signal in MR angiograms and to quantify tissue damage in white matter diseases *(18)*.

3.3.5. Summary

- T_1- and T_2-weighted imaging provide excellent depiction of soft-tissue morphology, including lesions.
- Changes in blood oxygenation can be monitored using T_2*-weighted imaging, and form the basis of fMRI.
- MR angiography and perfusion imaging can be realized by exploiting inflow effects.
- Diffusion of tissue water can be mapped with the aid of strong magnetic field gradients that dephase moving spins.

3.4. Exogenous Contrast Agents

Further scope for modifying signal contrast in MRI is provided by the use of exogenous contrast materials. MR contrast agents do not contribute to the signal directly; rather, they alter the signal of surrounding water protons via their effect on relaxation rates. The present section outlines the various types of agents and their biodistribution. (A more detailed discussion of their mechanisms of action can be found in Chapter 12 of **ref. 2**.)

3.4.1. Types of Contrast Agents

The contrast agents currently in clinical or laboratory use can be roughly divided into two types: those incorporating paramagnetic ions, such as gadolinium or manganese, and those containing SPIO particles.

Paramagnetic ions are typically chelated to organic ligands or bound to macromolecules, such as albumin. This minimizes their toxicity and reduces their tumbling rates, thereby increasing their effectiveness or 'relaxivity.' When water molecules bind to the agent and tumble with it in solution, they experience randomly oscillating magnetic fields that stimulate longitudinal relaxation, thereby shortening T_1. Although only a small fraction of the water can bind to the agent at any one time, the bound fraction is in continual exchange with the free water, so that the T_1-shortening effect is distributed throughout the bulk fluid. This results in an enhancement of signal on T_1-weighted images.

SPIO particles *(19)* have much stronger magnetic moments than individual paramagnetic ions, and, therefore, alter the magnetic field over a much longer range. They induce rapid dephasing of water protons, causing strong signal attenuation on T_2- and T_2*-weighted images. Although SPIO particles are primarily T_2 agents, they also shorten T_1 relaxation times and can be used to produce enhancement on T_1-weighted images. In such applications, the concentration of the agent and the TE of the sequence must be chosen to minimize T_2 and T_2* effects, so that they do not counteract the T_1-related signal enhancement.

3.4.2. Biodistribution

The range of applications of exogenous contrast agents is determined largely by their biodistribution and pharmacokinetics. Contrast agents are typically injected intravenously, and, depending on their chemical structure, may remain in the vasculature, enter the interstitial space, or be taken up by cells. The standard gadolinium chelates are described as 'extracellular agents.' They remain in the vasculature long enough to perform first-pass angiography (**Fig. 17E**), and are also widely used in perfusion imaging, particularly for the assessment of tumors *(20,21)* and myocardial ischemia *(22)*. However, they gradually diffuse into the interstitial space over time. This property has been exploited for imaging infarcts *(22,23)*, which have slower distribution kinetics and a larger extracellular volume than viable tissue. Gadolinium chelates remain in infarcted tissue longer than in viable tissue, producing so-called delayed enhancement on T_1-weighted images (**Fig. 17F**).

Free manganese is an intracellular agent. It behaves as a calcium analog in vivo and is taken up into cells through voltage-gated calcium channels. Manganese-enhanced MRI *(24)* can therefore be used to image cellular viability and activity (*see* Chapter 15).

Macromolecular and particulate contrast agents are considered intravascular agents and are well suited to quantitative imaging of perfusion and vascular volume (*see* Chapter 11). SPIO particles are eliminated via the reticuloendothelial system and are, therefore, also useful for imaging the liver *(25)*, evaluating lymph node function *(26)*, and visualizing macrophage activity within atherosclerotic plaque *(27)*. Because of their long-range T_2* effect, SPIO particles have found further applications in labeling and in vivo tracking of stem cells and monocytes (*see* Chapter 18).

One of the latest avenues of research in MRI is the development of so-called 'targeted' and 'smart' contrast agents *(28,29)*. Targeted agents (*see* Chapter 16) incorporate ligands, such as antibodies, that bind to specific molecular markers in the tissue, whereas smart agents (*see* Chapter 17) are activated by the presence of specific ions or enzymes. These agents open the way to visualization of gene expression in vivo, an emerging field known as molecular imaging *(30)*.

3.4.3. Summary

- Compounds containing paramagnetic ions, such as gadolinium and manganese, primarily shorten T_1 relaxation times, producing enhancement on T_1-weighted images.
- Superparamagnetic particles primarily shorten T_2 and T_2^* relaxation times, producing attenuation on T_2- and T_2^*-weighted images.
- Most contrast agents can be classified as extracellular, intracellular, or intravascular.
- Visualization of gene expression in vivo is becoming possible with the advent of targeted and smart contrast agents.

4. Spectroscopy

Whereas MRI uses the strong proton signals from water and fat to achieve high-resolution anatomical depiction, spectroscopy employs the MR signals from a variety of other chemical species to probe tissue metabolism. Signals can be detected from any molecule containing nuclei with nonzero spin (**Table 1**), provided the molecule is sufficiently mobile that its transverse nuclear magnetization is not lost through rapid T_2 relaxation before data acquisition. Proton spectroscopy, for example, is used to detect hydrogen-containing metabolites, such as *N*-acetylaspartate and choline, whereas phosphorus spectroscopy is used to monitor levels of phosphorus-containing compounds, such as adenosine triphosphate (ATP) and phosphocreatine. For a given resonant nucleus, the signals from different metabolites can be identified by virtue of their distinct chemical shifts. The amplitude of each component can then be used to infer metabolite concentrations. Because the concentrations of most metabolites are 10,000 to 100,000 times lower than that of water, their signals are too weak to permit high spatial resolution, even with substantial averaging (i.e., large NEX). In some applications, the only spatial localization is that provided by the sensitivity profile of the RF coil.

4.1. MR Spectra

Different metabolites containing a given resonant nucleus emit signals at slightly different frequencies, because of the effect of chemical shift. The signals appear as distinct peaks on an MR spectrum. The areas of the peaks are proportional to metabolite concentration but also depend on factors such as coil sensitivity and relaxation times. The spectral data are acquired using techniques similar to those employed in MRI, but without frequency-encoding gradients. This is because frequency is used in spectroscopy to extract chemical information and cannot also be used for spatial encoding.

4.1.1. Chemical Shift

The chemical shift is the fractional amount by which the Larmor frequency of a nucleus is altered as a result of its chemical environment. The shift is caused by the effect of orbital electrons on the magnetic field at the site of the nucleus.

In the presence of an external magnetic field, $\mathbf{B}_0$, the motion of the orbital electrons in a molecule is modified to induce tiny electronic currents. The currents, in turn, generate small secondary magnetic fields, proportional to $\mathbf{B}_0$, which alter the strength of the net field at the site of the nucleus. The resultant effective field can be written as:

$$\mathbf{B}_{\mathrm{eff}} = \mathbf{B}_0(1-\sigma), \qquad [19]$$

where σ denotes the so-called shielding constant. Because the Larmor frequency is proportional to the net magnetic field strength at the nucleus, it also is shifted by an amount proportional to σ,

$$\omega_{\mathrm{L}} = \gamma B_0(1-\sigma). \qquad [20]$$

The shielding constant depends on the electron density around the nucleus. Because the electron density is a function of the bonding structure within the molecule, the magnitude of the frequency shift varies among different types of molecules, and among distinct chemical groups within the same molecule. After RF excitation, the nuclei in these different chemical environments emit signals at their own characteristic frequencies, which appear as peaks on an MR spectrum. A given metabolite typically produces multiple spectral peaks, according to the number of resonant nuclei it contains in distinct chemical groups. In proton spectroscopy, for example, creatine produces a peak at 3.02 ppm, corresponding to signal from its CH_3 group, and another peak at 3.94 ppm from its CH_2 group (**Fig. 18**). Because the frequencies of the peaks reflect the molecular environments of the resonant nuclei, they provide a characteristic signature for each metabolite. By analyzing the frequency spectrum of the MR tissue signal, it is possible to determine which metabolites are present, and in what concentration. In practice, however, some peaks may not be easily distinguishable because of spectral overlap. An example is the proton signal from lactate, which overlaps with that from lipids.

As shown in **Eq. [20]**, the frequency shift is proportional not only to the shielding constant but also to the strength of the applied magnetic field, B_0. The frequency separation, therefore, increases with field strength, making the peaks easier to resolve at higher fields (*31*). To facilitate comparisons among

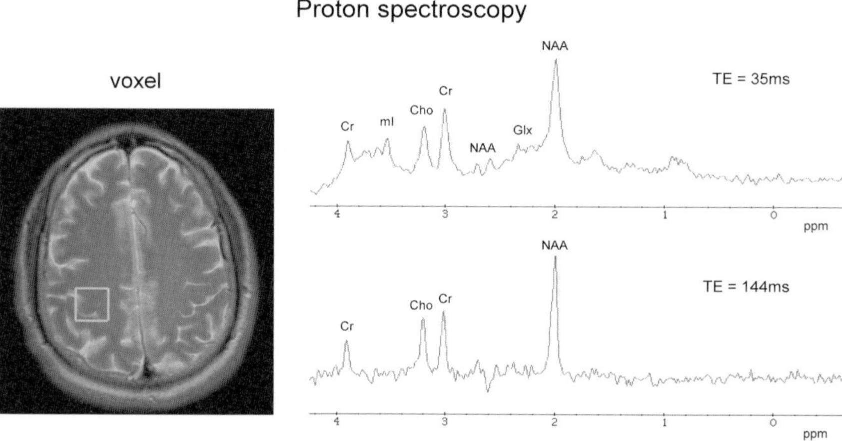

Fig. 18. Examples of single-voxel spectra acquired from the brain of a healthy adult. The resonances at 2.02 ppm and 2.6 ppm arise from *N*-acetylaspartate (NAA). Those at 3.02 ppm and 3.94 ppm represent total creatine (Cr), a combination of creatine and phosphocreatine. Choline-containing compounds (Cho) produce a peak at 3.22 ppm. Myoinositol (mI) is visible at 3.56 ppm, but only on the short echo time (TE) spectrum. Also on the short TE spectrum is a set of complex overlapping multiplets between 2.2 ppm and 2.6 ppm (Glx) produced by glutamine, glutamate, γ-aminobutyric acid (GABA) and aspartate.

data acquired at different field strengths, the chemical shift is usually expressed in dimensionless units of parts per million. Furthermore, for practical reasons, it is conventionally calculated relative to the Larmor frequency of a convenient reference solution rather than that of the bare nucleus.

4.1.2. Acquisition and Reconstruction

The acquisition techniques used in MRS are similar in many ways to those used in MRI. After RF excitation, the signal is recorded as a function of time and decomposed into its constituent frequency components by means of a Fourier transform. However, whereas MRI uses the frequency information to deduce the spatial profile of the tissue, MRS uses it for identification of tissue metabolites. Spectral data, unlike imaging data, must therefore be acquired in the absence of frequency-encoding gradients. In fact, because the magnitudes of the chemical shifts are so small (on the order of parts per million) MRS requires an extremely homogeneous magnetic field to resolve the spectral peaks. Any inhomogeneity in the field over the excitation volume will broaden the peaks and may render them indistinguishable from neighboring peaks or background noise.

Careful shimming is, therefore, of critical importance in MRS. It is performed using the strong proton signal from water and requires RF coils tuned to the Larmor frequency of hydrogen. If the spectra are to be acquired from a different nucleus, such as phosphorus, it is necessary to have an additional coil, or to use a double-tuned coil that resonates at the frequencies of both nuclei.

The widths of the spectral peaks are inversely proportional to T_2^* and thus depend not only on magnetic field inhomogeneities, but also on the intrinsic relaxation processes of the molecular environment. Molecules such as lipids that have short T_2 values produce broad resonances, which may appear on short TE spectra as variations in the baseline rather than as distinct peaks.

4.1.3. Metabolite Concentrations

Metabolite concentrations in vivo provide valuable physiological and pathological information. The concentrations can, in principle, be deduced from the MR spectra, because the areas of the spectral peaks are proportional to the numbers of nuclei that produced them. In practice, however, the calculation is not so simple, because the peak areas depend on an array of additional factors. Some, like coil sensitivity, affect the overall amplitude of the spectrum, whereas others, such as relaxation effects, modulate the relative areas of the peaks.

MR spectra, like MR images, are influenced by T_1- and T_2-weighting. The values of T_1 and T_2 are determined by the molecular environments of the nuclei, whereas the degree of weighting depends on the sequence and timing parameters. T_1-weighting arises from the finite TR of the sequence, whereas T_2-weighting occurs in spin-echo acquisitions. Because the relaxation times vary among different metabolites and different tissue types, T_1- and T_2-weighting alter the relative areas of the peaks. Signals from metabolites with relatively short T_2, for example, are attenuated in spectra acquired with long TE. This is demonstrated in **Fig. 18**, in which the peaks corresponding to myoinositol and glutamate are clearly visible at TE = 35 ms, but not at TE = 144 ms. Because of the difficulty of accounting for relaxation effects and coil sensitivity, it is common in clinical spectroscopy not to calculate absolute metabolite concentrations at all, but to base diagnostic interpretation instead on the differences in peak-area ratios between the lesion and a region of unaffected tissue in the same organ.

Accurate determination of the peak areas is not in itself entirely trivial, however, owing to spectral overlap between the metabolites and variations in baseline across the spectrum. The baseline contains small random fluctuations, which derive from noise, as well as larger variations, which represent the broad resonances of molecules with very short T_2. These broad resonances can be suppressed using a spin-echo sequence with long TE (**Fig. 18**). This flattens the baseline, but also reduces the information content of the spectrum, by attenuating contributions from metabolites with intermediate T_2 values.

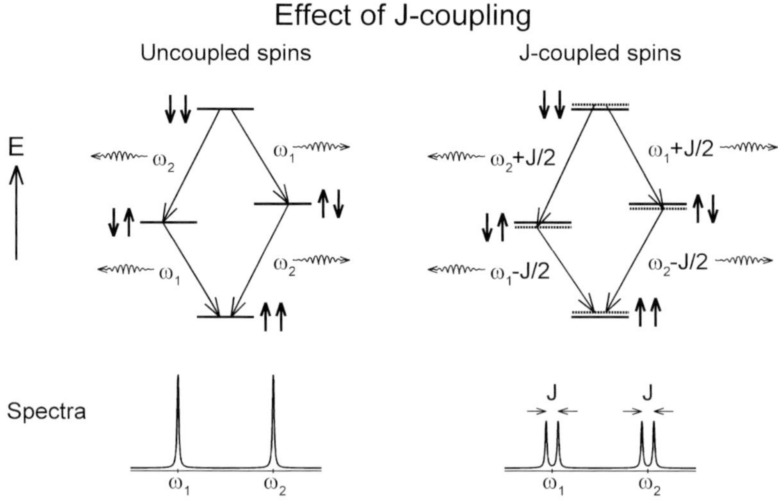

Fig. 19. An illustration of the effect of spin–spin or J coupling on the spectrum. The combined energy levels (top) and resulting spectra (bottom) are illustrated for two nuclei with different chemical shifts. The total energy is lowest if both nuclei are pointing up (along $\mathbf{B}_0$) and highest if both are pointing down (opposite $\mathbf{B}_0$). When a nucleus makes a transition from its spin-down state to its spin-up state, it releases a photon, whose frequency is proportional to the energy difference between the states. In the absence of J coupling (left), this energy difference is independent of the spin state of the other nucleus, and depends only on chemical shift. Each nucleus, therefore, produces a single spectral line. If the two nuclei are coupled (right), the energy levels are displaced up or down (dashed lines), according to the relative orientation of the nuclei. The coupling splits each spectral line into a doublet.

The areas of the peaks are commonly estimated by integrating the spectrum over suitable frequency ranges. This method, however, inevitably truncates the tails of the spectral lines, which contain a significant portion of their area. Estimates that are more accurate can be obtained using peak-fitting routines. Such approaches also have their limitations, however, because they rely on assumptions about line shape that may not be entirely valid, owing to the influence of magnetic field inhomogeneity and spin–spin coupling (discussed in **Subheading 4.1.4.**).

4.1.4. Spin–Spin Coupling

The Larmor frequency of a nucleus is affected not only by orbital electrons, which produce the chemical shift, but also by other nuclei within the same molecule, which can split the spectral lines into doublets or multiplets (**Fig. 19**). Bound nuclei interact with each other via a mechanism known as spin–

spin coupling, or J coupling, which is mediated through the electronic bonds. The energies of the coupled nuclei vary according to the relative orientation of their magnetic moments. In the case of two coupled spin-$\frac{1}{2}$ nuclei, subjected to a strong external magnetic field, both nuclei may be oriented spin-up, both may be spin-down, or one nucleus may be spin-up while the other is spin-down. By virtue of their spin–spin coupling, the total energy of each configuration depends not only on the orientation of each nucleus with respect to the external field, but also on their orientation relative to each other. This causes a shift in the energy levels, as illustrated in **Fig. 19**. When a nucleus makes a transition from the spin-down to the spin-up state, the change in its energy depends on the spin state of the second nucleus at the time of the transition. The frequency of the emitted RF photon will accordingly be shifted up or down by an amount proportional to the coupling strength. This causes the spectral peak to be split into two components, collectively called a doublet. The frequency splitting reflects the coupling strength, denoted J, and is independent of the magnitude of the external magnetic field, B_0. In cases in which a nucleus is coupled to two or more other nuclei, its spectral line may be split into multiple components, called a multiplet.

Spin–spin coupling among nuclei in a molecule can complicate the spectrum considerably and reduce its SNR. This can be particularly problematic in carbon-13 and phosphorus spectroscopy, in which the resonant nuclei may be coupled to protons within the same molecule. It is possible, however, to simplify ^{13}C and ^{31}P spectra through a mechanism known as proton decoupling. A strong RF field is applied at the resonant frequency of the protons during the signal acquisition. The RF field induces rapid transitions of the protons between their two energy states, thereby alternating the sign of the coupling and averaging out its effect. This removes the frequency splitting, thereby collapsing the multiplets into single lines and improving their SNR.

4.1.5. Summary

- MR spectra display the signals from various metabolites as a function of their chemical shift.
- The areas of the peaks are proportional to metabolite concentration but also depend on factors such as coil sensitivity and relaxation rates.
- The peaks may be split into doublets or multiplets by spin–spin or J coupling.

4.2. Localization

Spectroscopic information cannot be obtained with high spatial resolution in vivo because of the low concentrations of the metabolites and the inherently poor sensitivity of the MR technique. However, a number of methods exist to provide some degree of spatial localization. The simplest is to use a surface coil with limited depth penetration. Surface coils are useful for studying super-

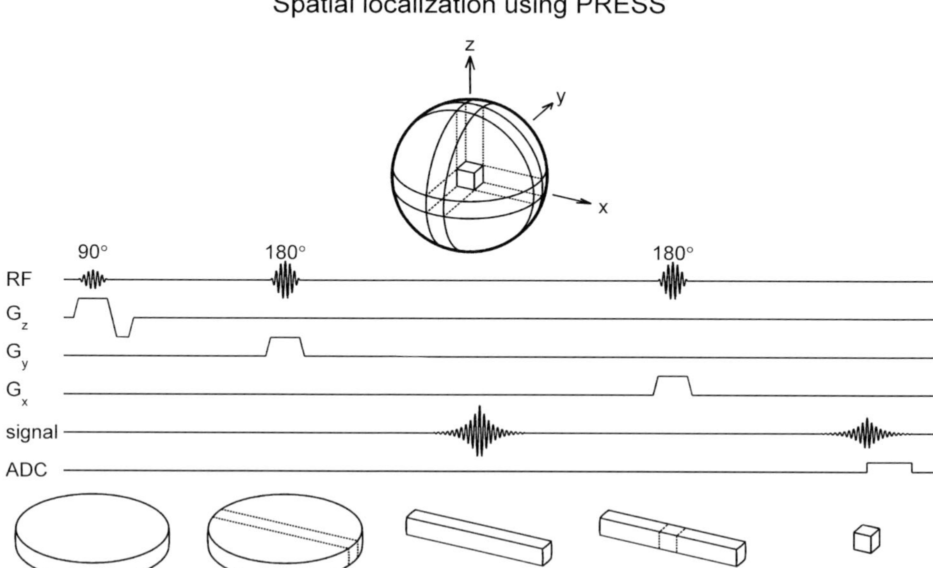

Fig. 20. An illustration of point-resolved spectroscopy (PRESS), which is used to obtain signal from a localized 3D volume of tissue. The technique employs a 90° excitation pulse followed by two 180° refocusing pulses, each of which provides spatial selectivity along a different direction. The initial 90° pulse excites tissue within a given slab along the z direction, whereas the subsequent 180° pulse refocuses only the magnetization lying within a certain slab along the y direction. The final 180° pulse refocuses the magnetization again, but only in tissue lying within a given slab in the x direction. The spin echo following the second refocusing pulse represents signal from the intersection of the three slabs. Spectral data is acquired during the latter half of this spin echo.

ficial tissues but do not provide well defined or easily controllable spatial selectivity. Improved localization can be achieved using volume-selective and phase-encoding techniques, similar to those used in imaging.

4.2.1. Single-Voxel Techniques

Single-voxel techniques use magnetic field gradients to excite and refocus only those spins lying within a certain prescribed volume of tissue. One such technique, based on a spin-echo pulse sequence, is known by the acronym PRESS (point-resolved spectroscopy). It involves a 90° excitation pulse followed by two 180° refocusing pulses, each of which provides spatial selectivity along a different direction (**Fig. 20**). The spectrum is acquired during the latter half of the second spin echo and represents signal from the intersection of the three slabs. The thickness of the slabs can be tailored to produce a voxel of the desired size, which is positioned over the region of interest (such as a tumor). The voxel is prescribed from images acquired using standard proton MRI, as shown in **Fig. 18**.

Another single-voxel localization technique is STEAM (stimulated echo acquisition mode). STEAM is similar to PRESS, except that the FAs of the RF pulses are all 90°. The initial 90° pulse excites the spins as before, whereas the second 90° pulse transfers some of the magnetization from the transverse plane to the longitudinal axis, where it is preserved from further dephasing. The final pulse returns the stored magnetization to the transverse plane, where it is rephased at a later time. The result is a stimulated echo, which has lower amplitude than a spin echo because less of the magnetization is refocused.

Because of the time required between the three RF pulses, neither PRESS nor STEAM is suited to detection of metabolites with very short T_2, such as those of interest in phosphorus spectroscopy. An alternative technique, which is more appropriate for fast-decaying metabolites, is ISIS (image-selected in vivo spectroscopy). In contrast to PRESS and STEAM, ISIS does not involve echo formation but instead uses the signal of the FID. The signal is first acquired from an FID produced by a nonselective 90° excitation pulse. The process is then repeated with the addition of a slice-selective inversion pulse immediately before the 90° excitation. This inverts the signal from within the slice but leaves the signal from outside unaffected. By subtracting the two FIDs, the contributions from outside the slice cancel out, leaving only the signal from within the slice. The method can be extended to two or three dimensions by incorporating extra slice-selective inversion pulses in various combinations.

4.2.2. Multivoxel Techniques

Each of the localization techniques described above allows signal to be acquired from a single volume of interest. To make comparisons among different regions, the measurement must be repeated at different positions. An alternative approach is to apply the method of phase encoding used in imaging, to allow simultaneous acquisition of spectra from multiple voxels.

Phase encoding can be used either with a simple FID acquisition or in combination with volume-selective methods, such as PRESS or STEAM. The result is a hybrid of spectroscopic and imaging techniques, known by the names multivoxel spectroscopy, chemical shift imaging (CSI), or magnetic resonance spectroscopic imaging (MRSI). Because frequency encoding is not possible in spectroscopy, phase encoding must be applied in each of the directions in which spatial information is required, namely two directions for 2D chemical shift imaging, or three directions for 3D CSI. Given that each phase-encoding step requires a separate TR period, the scan time increases as N^2 for 2D or N^3 for 3D CSI, where N is the number of voxels in each direction. Because the scan time

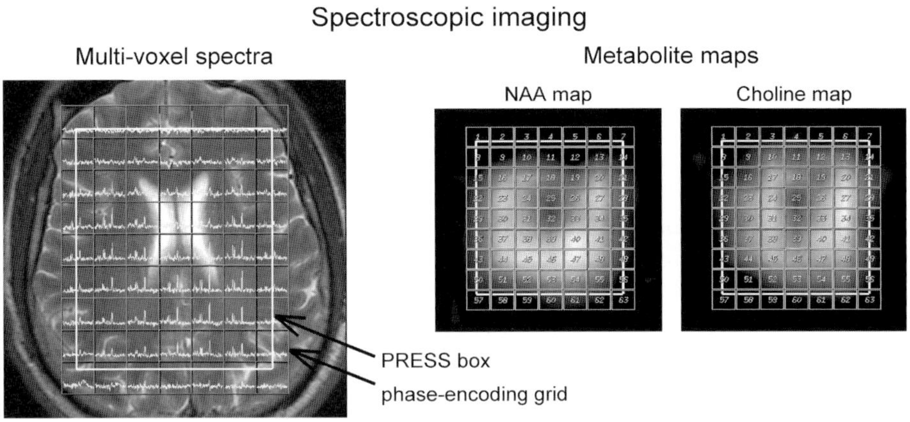

Spectroscopic imaging

Multi-voxel spectra   **Metabolite maps**

PRESS box

phase-encoding grid

Fig. 21. Multivoxel proton spectroscopy in a healthy adult brain. The volume delineated by the heavy white line is selectively excited using PRESS, and tissue within it is divided into a coarse grid of voxels using 2D phase encoding. The resulting data can be represented as an array of spectra or as a set of metabolite maps. The maps in this case do not represent metabolite concentrations in absolute units, but only the integrated areas of the respective peaks.

increases so rapidly with N, this imposes a further constraint on the possible spatial resolution. In multivoxel proton spectroscopy, typical in-plane resolutions are on the order of 1 to 2 cm. In phosphorus spectroscopy, even lower resolutions are used, because of the poorer sensitivity of the ^{31}P nucleus.

The information collected in a multivoxel acquisition may be presented either as an array of spectra or as a set of metabolite concentration maps (**Fig. 21**). The metabolite maps can be displayed in color and overlaid on an MR image of the same slice.

4.2.3. Summary

- Spatial resolution is inherently limited in MR spectroscopy because of the low concentration of the metabolites.
- Spectra can be obtained from a chosen region of tissue using volume-selective methods, such as PRESS and STEAM.
- Spectra can be obtained from multiple voxels simultaneously by incorporating phase encoding into the data acquisition.

4.3. In Vivo Applications

In vivo spectroscopic studies are performed primarily with hydrogen, phosphorus, carbon-13, and fluorine *(32–34)*. Of these, the most extensively used are hydrogen, because of its high sensitivity, and phosphorus, because of its importance in energy metabolism. Studies involving carbon-13 and fluorine are usually performed using injectable markers, because of their low endogenous concentrations.

4.3.1. Proton Spectroscopy

Proton (^{1}H) spectroscopy is commonly used in investigations of the brain *(35–38)*, and can detect a wide range of metabolites, including *N*-acetylaspartate, creatine/phosphocreatine, choline-containing compounds, and lactate. *N*-acetylaspartate is an amino acid found only in the central nervous system, and is considered a marker of neuron density and viability. It produces a peak at 2.02 ppm and a second smaller peak at 2.6 ppm, which arise from its methyl (CH_3) and methylene (CH_2) groups, respectively (**Fig. 18**). Creatine and phosphocreatine are involved in the regulation of cellular energy metabolism, and together produce a prominent peak at 3.02 ppm and a second peak at 3.94 ppm. The total creatine concentration is considered relatively stable, and is frequently used as an internal reference, although studies have shown that it may vary under certain pathological conditions. The peak at 3.22 ppm arises from choline, as well as other compounds containing the N-$(CH_3)_3$ group, such as phosphorylcholine, glycerophosphorylcholine, and betaine. Choline-containing compounds are involved in a wide range of metabolic functions, including synthesis of cell membranes and transport of lipids. Elevated choline levels may indicate myelin degeneration or cell proliferation associated with tumor growth. Myoinositol, together with myoinositol monophosphate and glycine, produce a peak at 3.56 ppm on short TE spectra. Myoinositol is high in the normal neonate brain but declines during the first few months of life. Lactate, when present, produces a doublet centered at 1.32 ppm. It is the end product of anaerobic glycolysis, and is increased in hypoxia, stroke, and diseases of oxidative metabolism. Lipids produce broad peaks at 0.9 ppm and 1.3 ppm, which can obscure signal from lactate.

Because the metabolites of interest occur in much lower concentrations than water, their signals can be detected and quantified only if the dominant water signal is suppressed. This can be achieved by applying chemical shift selective saturation (CHESS) pulses at the water resonance (4.7 ppm) before acquisition of the spectrum. Lipids also produce a strong signal, but because the lipid resonances overlap some of the peaks of interest (such as those of lactate), it is preferable to use spatial selectivity to eliminate the fat signal. The excitation volume in a PRESS or STEAM acquisition, for example, should be chosen to exclude fatty tissues. In addition, spatial saturation bands can be applied over subcutaneous fat and bone marrow. Because lipids have short T_2, their signal can be further suppressed by using a long TE acquisition.

4.3.2. Phosphorus Spectroscopy

Phosphorus-31 is the naturally occurring isotope of phosphorus and is used extensively for studies of energy metabolism and phosphorus-containing markers of disease *(39–44)*. Although the phosphorus nucleus has a smaller gyromagnetic ratio than hydrogen, and hence a lower MR sensitivity, its chemical shift range is larger (approx 30 ppm) and its spectrum is simpler.

The principal metabolites contributing to the phosphorus spectrum are ATP, phosphocreatine, inorganic phosphate, phosphodiesters, and phosphomonoesters. Other phosphorus-containing biological molecules, such as membrane phospholipids, are highly immobile and either invisible by MR or represented by broad signals underlying the metabolite peaks. ATP has three peaks, labeled α-, β- and γ-ATP, corresponding to its three phosphorus nuclei. Adenosine diphosphate occurs in much lower concentration and has two peaks, but these coincide with the α and γ resonances of the ATP spectrum. The areas of the ATP, phosphocreatine, and inorganic phosphate peaks reveal information about cellular energy metabolism and exhibit characteristic changes in response to muscle fatigue *(40)* and certain disease processes *(41,42)*. The chemical shift of the inorganic phosphate resonance varies with tissue pH and is useful in assessing renal acidosis and alkalosis, and in characterizing tumors (*see* Chapter 14). The phosphodiester and phosphomonoester compounds, which include phosphorylcholine, are involved in cell membrane synthesis and degradation. Their concentrations may be modified under certain pathological conditions, such as cancer, that involve a change in the rate of membrane turnover *(42–44)*.

Phosphorus spectroscopy requires pulse sequences with short TE (less than ~10 ms) because of the rapid T_2 relaxation of its resonances. The spectrum may be acquired during the FID or a short-TE spin echo. Spatial localization is commonly provided by a surface coil or through use of the ISIS technique.

4.3.3. Carbon-13 Spectroscopy

The most abundant isotope of carbon is ^{12}C, which is not detectable by MR because it has no net spin. Carbon-13 exhibits MR but has a natural abundance of only 1.1% and, therefore, very low concentration in vivo. The low endogenous concentration can, however, be exploited in studies of metabolic pathways *(45–50)* by injecting ^{13}C-labeled tracers, such as ^{13}C-enriched glucose. For example, incorporation of glucose into glycogen, for storage in liver and muscle cells, can be monitored using serial measurements of ^{13}C-labeled glycogen concentration *(47)*. Breakdown of carbohydrates for energy production via glycolysis and the citric acid cycle can also be investigated by tracking the ^{13}C-label through intermediary metabolites, such as glutamate *(48)*.

The ^{13}C spectrum exhibits a broad range of chemical shifts (~200 ppm) but is fairly complex because of the large number of carbon-containing metabolites. Its complexity is further increased because of strong J coupling between carbon and hydrogen nuclei, which splits the spectral peaks into multiplets. Proton decoupling is commonly used to identify the peaks, and to simplify the spectra and improve SNR. The heights of the peaks can also be amplified via the nuclear Overhauser effect. This exploits dipole–dipole interactions between the hydrogen and carbon nuclei to enhance the magnetization of the carbon nuclei through saturation of the protons. The result is an approximately three-fold increase in the amplitude of the ^{13}C signal.

4.3.4. Fluorine Spectroscopy

Fluorine-19 is the naturally occurring isotope of fluorine but is not present endogenously in the body, except in the teeth, where it is highly immobile and effectively MR invisible. Fluorine-19 spectroscopy can, therefore, be used to monitor the biodistribution and pharmacokinetics of exogenous fluorine-containing compounds, such as the chemotherapeutic drug, 5-fluorouracil *(51,52)*. pH-sensitive fluorinated probes have also been used for noninvasive measurements of intracellular and extracellular pH (*see* Chapter 14).

4.3.5. Summary

- Proton spectroscopy is commonly used in the brain and provides information about the concentrations of N-acetylaspartate, creatine/phosphocreatine, choline-containing compounds, and lactate. The dominant signals from water and fat must be suppressed.
- Phosphorus spectroscopy is used to study energy metabolism and cell membrane turnover and allows quantification of ATP, phosphocreatine, inorganic phosphate, phosphodiesters, and phosphomonoesters.
- Spectroscopy of ^{13}C and fluorine are generally performed using injectable markers because of their low endogenous concentrations.

Acknowledgments

I am grateful to Belinda Li, Ph.D., and Wei Li, M.D., for their assistance.

References

1. Edelman, R. R., Hesselink, J. R., and Zlatkin, M. B., eds. (2005) *Clinical Magnetic Resonance Imaging.* Elsevier (Saunders), New York, NY.
2. Stark, D. D. and Bradley, W. G., eds. (1999) *Magnetic Resonance Imaging.* Mosby, New York, NY.
3. Haacke, E.M., Brown, R.W., Thompson, M.R., and Venkatcsen, R. (1999) *Magnetic Resonance Imaging: Physical Principles and Sequence Design.* John Wiley and Sons, New York, NY.

4. Kuperman, V. (2000) *Magnetic Resonance Imaging: Physical Principles and Applications*. Academic Press, San Diego, CA.

5. Vlaardingerbroek, M. T. and Den Boer, J. A. (2003) *Magnetic Resonance Imaging*, Springer-Verlag, Berlin, Germany.

6. Salibi, N. and Brown, M. A. (1998) *Clinical MR Spectroscopy: First Principles*. Wiley-Liss, New York, NY.

7. Gadian, D. G. (1995) *NMR and its Applications to Living Systems*. Oxford University Press, Oxford, UK.

8. Moller, H. E., Chen, X. J., Saam, B., et al. (2002) MRI of the lungs using hyperpolarized noble gases. *Magn. Reson. Med.* **47,** 1029–1051.

9. Goyen, M. and Debatin, J. F. (2004) Gadopentetate dimeglumine-enhanced three-dimensional MR-angiography: dosing, safety, and efficacy. *J. Magn. Reson. Imaging* **19,** 261–273

10. De Ridder, F., De Maeseneer, M., Stadnik, T., Luypaert, R., and Osteaux, M. (2001) Severe adverse reactions with contrast agents for magnetic resonance: clinical experience in 30,000 MR examinations. *JBR-BTR* **84,** 150–152.

11. Okada, S., Katagiri, K., Kumazaki, T., and Yokoyama, H. (2001) Safety of gadolinium contrast agent in hemodialysis patients. *Acta Radiol.* **42,** 339–341.

12. Wolf, G.L. and Baum, L. (1983) Cardiovascular toxicity and tissue proton T1 response to manganese injection in the dog and rabbit. *Am. J. Roentgenol.* **141,** 193–197.

13. Buxton, R. (2002) *Introduction to Functional Magnetic Resonance Imaging: Principles and Techniques*. Cambridge University Press, Cambridge, UK.

14. Huettel, S.A., Song A. W., and McCarthy, G. (2004) *Functional Magnetic Resonance Imaging*. Sinauer Associates, Sunderland, MA.

15. Golay, X., Hendrikse, J., and Lim, T. C. (2004) Perfusion imaging using arterial spin labeling. *Top Magn. Reson. Imaging* **15,** 10–27.

16. Van Zijl, P. C. and Le Bihan, D., eds. (2002) Special issue: diffusion tensor imaging and axonal mapping–state of the art. *NMR Biomed.* **15,** Issue 7–8.

17. Henkelman, R. M., Stanisz, G. J., and Graham, S. J. (2001) Magnetization transfer in MRI: a review. *NMR Biomed.* **14,** 57–64.

18. Filippi, M. and Rocca, M. A. (2004) Magnetization transfer magnetic resonance imaging in the assessment of neurological diseases. *J. Neuroimaging* **14,** 303–313.

19. Jensen, J. H. and Helpern, J. A., eds. (2004) Special issue: iron-fortified MRI: effects and applications of iron-induced NMR relaxation in biological tissues. *NMR Biomed.* **17,** Issue 7.

20. Cha, S. (2004) Perfusion MR imaging of brain tumors. *Top. Magn. Reson. Imaging* **15,** 279–289.

21. Kuhl, C. K. and Schild, H. H. (2000) Dynamic image interpretation of MRI of the breast. *J. Magn. Reson. Imaging* **12,** 965–974.

22. Edelman, R. R. (2004) Contrast-enhanced MR imaging of the heart: overview of the literature. *Radiology* **232,** 653–668.

23. Kim, R. J., Shah, D. J., and Judd, R. M. (2003) How we perform delayed enhancement imaging. *J. Cardiovasc. Magn. Reson.* **5,** 505–514.

24. Silva, A. C. and Koretsky, A. P., eds. (2004) Special issue: manganese-enhanced magnetic resonance imaging (MEMRI). *NMR Biomed.* **17,** Issue 8.
25. Semelka, R. C. and Helmberger, T. K. (2001) Contrast agents for MR imaging of the liver. *Radiology* **218,** 27–38.
26. Anzai, Y. (2004) Superparamagnetic iron oxide nanoparticles: nodal metastases and beyond. *Top. Magn. Reson. Imaging* **15,** 103–111.
27. Quick, H. H., Debatin, J. F., and Ladd, M. E. (2002) MR imaging of the vessel wall. *Eur. Radiol.* **12,** 889–900.
28. Artemov, D. (2003) Molecular magnetic resonance imaging with targeted contrast agents. *J. Cell. Biochem.* **90,** 518–524.
29. Meade, T. J., Taylor, A. K., and Bull, S. R. (2003) New magnetic resonance contrast agents as biochemical reporters. *Curr. Opin. Neurobiol.* **13,** 597–602.
30. Dzik-Jurasz, A. S. K., ed. (2003) Special issue: molecular imaging. *Br. J. Radiol.* **76,** Spec. No. 2.
31. Di Costanzo, A., Trojsi, F., Tosetti, M., et al. (2003) High-field proton MRS of human brain. *Eur. J. Radiol.* **48,** 146–153.
32. Golder, W. (2004) Magnetic resonance spectroscopy in clinical oncology. *Onkologie* **27,** 304–309.
33. Dobbins, R. L. and Malloy, C. R. (2003) Measuring in vivo metabolism using nuclear magnetic resonance. *Curr. Opin. Clin. Nutr. Metab. Care* **6,** 501–509.
34. Ross, B. and Bluml, S. (2001) Magnetic resonance spectroscopy of the human brain. *Anat. Rec.* **265,** 54–84.
35. Cecil, K.M. and Jones, B.V. (2001) Magnetic resonance spectroscopy of the pediatric brain. *Top. Magn. Reson. Imaging* **12,** 435–452.
36. Burtscher, I. M. and Holtas, S. (2001) Proton MR spectroscopy in clinical routine. *J. Magn. Reson. Imaging* **13,** 560–567.
37. McKnight, T. R. (2004) Proton magnetic resonance spectroscopic evaluation of brain tumor metabolism. *Semin. Oncol.* **31,** 605–617.
38. Howe, F. A. and Opstad, K. S. (2003) 1H MR spectroscopy of brain tumours and masses. *NMR Biomed.* **16,** 123–131.
39. Mattei, J. P., Bendahan, D., and Cozzone, P. (2004) P-31 magnetic resonance spectroscopy. A tool for diagnostic purposes and pathophysiological insights in muscle diseases. *Reumatismo* **56,** 9–14.
40. Bendahan, D., Giannesini, B., and Cozzone, P. J. (2004) Functional investigations of exercising muscle: a noninvasive magnetic resonance spectroscopy-magnetic resonance imaging approach. *Cell. Mol. Life Sci.* **61,** 1001–1015.
41. Stanley, J. A. (2002) In vivo magnetic resonance spectroscopy and its application to neuropsychiatric disorders. *Can. J. Psychiatry* **47,** 315–326.
42. Schaefer, S. (2000) Magnetic resonance spectroscopy in human cardiomyopathies. *J. Cardiovasc. Magn. Reson.* **2,** 151–157.
43. Arias-Mendoza, F. and Brown, T. R. (2003–2004) In vivo measurement of phosphorous markers of disease. *Dis. Markers* **19,** 49–68.
44. Taylor-Robinson, S. D. (2001) Applications of magnetic resonance spectroscopy to chronic liver disease. *Clin. Med.* **1,** 54–60.

45. Roden, M. (2001) Non-invasive studies of glycogen metabolism in human skeletal muscle using nuclear magnetic resonance spectroscopy. *Curr. Opin. Clin. Nutr. Metab. Care* **4,** 261–266.

46. Baverel, G., Conjard, A., Chauvin, M. F., et al. (2003) Carbon 13 NMR spectroscopy: a powerful tool for studying renal metabolism. *Biochimie.* **85,** 863–871.

47. Landau, B. R. (2001) Methods for measuring glycogen cycling. *Am. J. Physiol. Endocrinol. Metab.* **281,** E413–419.

48. Cerdán, S., ed. (2003) Special issue: 13C NMR studies of cerebral metabolism. *NMR Biomed.* **16,** Issue 6–7.

49. Garcia-Espinosa, M. A., Rodrigues, T. B., Sierra, A., et al. (2004) Cerebral glucose metabolism and the glutamine cycle as detected by in vivo and in vitro 13C NMR spectroscopy. *Neurochem. Int.* **45,** 297–303.

50. Portais, J. C. and Delort, A. M. (2002) Carbohydrate cycling in micro-organisms: what can (13)C-NMR tell us? *FEMS Microbiol. Rev.* **26,** 375–402.

51. Martino, R., Malet-Martino, M., and Gilard, V. (2000) Fluorine nuclear magnetic resonance, a privileged tool for metabolic studies of fluoropyrimidine drugs. *Curr. Drug Metab.* **1,** 271–303.

52. Wolf, W., Presant, C. A., and Waluch, V. (2000) 19F-MRS studies of fluorinated drugs in humans. *Adv. Drug Deliv. Rev.* **41,** 55–74.

2

Magnetic Resonance Microscopy

Concepts, Challenges, and State-of-the-Art

Barjor Gimi

Summary

Recent strides in targeted therapy and regenerative medicine have created a need to identify molecules and metabolic pathways implicated in a disease and its treatment. These molecules and pathways must be discerned at the cellular level to meaningfully reveal the biochemical underpinnings of the disease and to identify key molecular targets for therapy. Magnetic resonance (MR) techniques are well suited for molecular and functional imaging because of their noninvasive nature and their versatility in extracting physiological, biochemical, and functional information over time. However, MR is an insensitive technique; MR microscopy seeks to increase detection sensitivity, thereby localizing biochemical and functional information at the level of single cells or small cellular clusters. Here, we discuss some of the challenges facing MR microscopy and the technical and phenomenological strategies used to overcome these challenges. Some of the applications of MR microscopy are highlighted in this chapter.

Key Words: Magnetic resonance; Microimaging; Microcoil; Scroll coil; Microscopy; RF sensitivity; Signal-to-noise ratio (SNR).

1. Introduction

Advances in genetics and bioengineering have inspired therapeutic approaches targeted at the cellular and molecular levels. Investigating how cellular pathways and manipulated cells interact with their environment in vitro and in vivo, their response to drugs and immune attack, and their viability over time requires tools that allow for long-term and noninvasive assessment. Magnetic resonance (MR) spatially correlates biochemical information, providing a context in which these issues may be addressed. Refinement of microfabrication and nanofabrication techniques, electronic circuitry, and pulse sequences has propelled MR toward the realm of microscopy. High-resolution in vitro and in vivo information on a biological system is instructive in study-

From: *Methods in Molecular Medicine, Vol. 124*
Magnetic Resonance Imaging: Methods and Biologic Applications
Edited by: P. V. Prasad © Humana Press Inc., Totowa, NJ

ing disease progression, regression, and aggressiveness, as well as the pH, oxygen tension, and energy status of cellular systems, metabolite levels, changes in their distribution in regions-of-interest, drug delivery, and the outcome of treatment.

The term 'MR microscopy' is loosely defined in the scientific literature. Traditionally, for in vitro systems, microscopy refers to voxels whose dimensions are on the order of tens of microns. In vivo systems entail a lower operating frequency, smaller magnetic gradients, and a less-sensitive detection system. Therefore, for in vivo systems, the term 'microscopy' applies to voxels whose dimensions are on the order of hundreds of microns. This nomenclature is not very revelatory. Assuming all observations are performed at a given field strength, the attainable voxel resolution depends on the time taken to acquire the signal. An insensitive system can provide high spatial resolution if the acquisition is long, whereas a comparatively sensitive system may provide lower spatial resolution if the acquisition is effectuated in a shorter time period. MR resolution is also a function of the nucleus/molecule being observed. Nuclei with higher magnetic receptivity (gyromagnetic ratio) will produce more signal; the more nuclei a given voxel contains, the higher the attainable signal from that voxel. To complicate matters further, MR observation is dependent on experimental parameters (e.g., pulse sequence and type of encoding system). Different pulse sequences and encoding systems tailored to observe specific phenomena, such as diffusion, perfusion, and compartmentalization, will yield different resolution. Thus, in light of these caveats, how one defines microscopy depends on what one wants to observe.

Although most principles governing conventional MR and MR microscopy are analogous, there are certain challenges distinct to microscopy. This chapter introduces the reader to microscopy—its salient concepts, its challenges, and its applications. The body of the chapter is divided into four sections. The first section deals with obtaining high-resolution data. The second examines phenomenological issues, classified as 'broadening effects,' which impede on or can be exploited in microscopy. Biological applications of microscopy are addressed in the third section. The final section explores future directions.

2. Challenges Facing MR Microscopy

Three major components of an MRI acquisition system influence the image quality, namely signal-to-noise ratio (SNR), spatial resolution, and contrast. The field strength of the scanner, of course, is a crucial determinant of the signal strength. However, once field strength is fixed by choice of a scanner, the only other component available for the user to optimize further is the radio frequency (RF) excitation and receiver chain. Spatial resolution is determined by the gradient system. This section will review the primary issues and strategies usually employed to address those issues. Also included is a discussion on different contrast mechanisms available.

2.1. Technical Strategies: RF Excitation and Reception

A principal impediment in MR is low detection sensitivity, which is directly related to the signal strength and SNR. The objective in optimizing MRI sensitivity is to increase the signal strength while minimizing the noise contributions.

2.1.1. Improving Signal Strength

MR is an insensitive technique because its signal depends on the population difference of nuclear spins in two energy states, which is on the order of mere parts per million. For instance, at room temperature and in a magnetic field of 1 T, only 6 of approx 2 million ^{1}H nuclei contribute to the MR signal. The impediment of low signal is exacerbated at higher spatial resolution because a smaller voxel will contain proportionately fewer nuclear spins. Furthermore, acquisition time varies inversely with SNR^2. For a given detection sensitivity, improving spatial resolution by an order of magnitude in each Cartesian axis while keeping SNR the constant requires an acquisition time that is 1 million times longer. The task of improving resolution is daunting for ^{1}H, which has high biological abundance and high magnetic receptivity, but when observing nuclei that are less abundant in the body and have low signal receptivity, such as ^{13}C and ^{31}P, the task becomes inordinately difficult. Therefore, technical efforts in MR microscopy are directed toward enhancing signal amplitude, reducing noise, and increasing detection sensitivity.

Signal amplitude may be increased by increasing the nuclear spin population differential between two energy states, one where the nucleus is parallel to the applied magnetic field and one where the nucleus is antiparallel to the applied magnetic field. An increase in this population difference can be achieved by increasing the strength of the applied static magnetic field, or by polarizing the sample. MR at high magnetic field strengths is desirable despite the significant expense and increased static field inhomogeneity associated with it. However, although SNR increases roughly linearly with static magnetic field strength, microscopy requires several orders of magnitude improvement in SNR over conventional MR. Signal enhancement is also achieved by polarizing the sample, which, in turn, increases the relative population of nuclear spins that contribute to the signal. The hyperpolarization technique is sometimes used in imaging airways and blood volume, but is often not physiologically possible or appropriate. However, recent studies show that hyperpolarized ^{13}C can be used in medical applications, such as contrast-enhanced MR angiography (*1*).

2.1.2. Minimizing Noise Contributions

Another approach to increasing SNR is to decrease noise from both the spectrometer and the sample. Noise arising from the spectrometer can be reduced or eliminated using cryocooled probes and preamplifiers or high-temperature superconducting (HTS) RF coils *(2–4)*. HTS coils appear to be the obvious choice for reducing the thermal noise, and have been used in loop transmission line and Helmholtz configurations, but they have a low usable bandwidth. Neglecting sample loading, HTS coils can achieve a Q-factor (i.e., the quality of a resonant system, defined as the resonant frequency divided by the bandwidth) increase of two to three orders of magnitude, at liquid nitrogen temperatures:

$$\left(SNR \propto \sqrt{Q} \right).$$

However, at temperatures where the sample becomes the dominant source of noise, supercooled conventional coils can yield SNR gains approaching those of HTS coils *(5)*. Therefore, cooling conventional copper coils may be preferred from the standpoint of simplicity and cost. Although these noise reduction techniques have potential, they have yet to be refined to the point of implementation for widespread application. At present, engineering efforts to increase SNR are directed principally toward increasing RF sensitivity at room temperature by miniaturizing the RF coil.

2.1.3. Improving RF Sensitivity by Dedicated RF Coils

Designing a good RF circuit (**Fig. 1**) involves manufacturing a suitable RF coil, ensuring that signal emanating from the coil's electrical leads does not interfere with the image or spectrum quality, ensuring that no capacitors or other circuit elements resonate at the operating frequency, minimizing energy losses in the circuit, and impedance matching the sample–coil construct to the preamplifier for a continuous wave transmission to ensure maximum power transfer at resonance. The goal is to maximize SNR.

SNR is directly proportional to RF sensitivity and can be expressed as *(6,7)*:

$$SNR \propto \frac{\omega_0^2 \cdot \left(\dfrac{B_1}{i}\right) \cdot V_s}{\sqrt{R_{noise}}},$$

where ω_0 is the resonance frequency, B_1/i is the coil sensitivity and is defined as the transverse magnetic field generated by the coil per unit current, V_s is the sample volume, and R_{noise} is the noise resistance from the sample and the coil. Sample resistive losses are negligible in the microcoil regime, and the total resistance is dominated by the coil resistance and $R_{noise} \cong R_{microcoil}$ *(8,9)*.

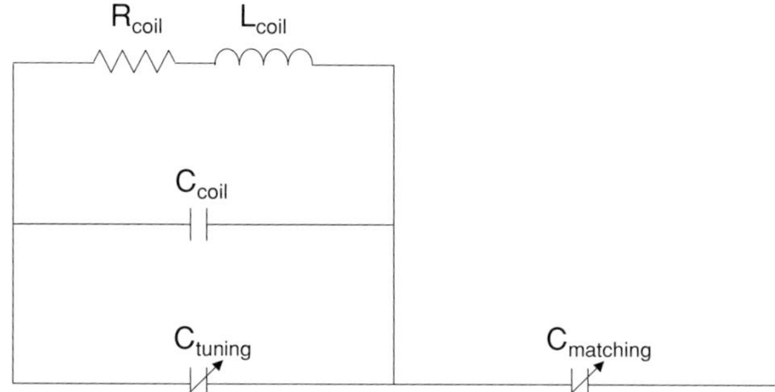

Fig. 1. A schematic of the radio frequency circuit. The coil can be modeled as a capacitor in parallel with an inductor and resistor. A capacitor in parallel with the coil is used for tuning the circuit, whereas a capacitor in series is used for impedance matching.

SNR can be increased by increasing the static field strength (thereby increasing ω_0^2), increasing the sample volume, increasing the coil sensitivity, and decreasing the noise. For a volume-limited sample, V_s cannot be altered but the effective sample volume can be increased by increasing the coil's filling factor such that the sample occupies most of the sensing region of the coil. For a given field strength, SNR increase is most expediently and effectively achieved by decreasing the coil size to match the sample size, thereby increasing the effective volume and the sensitivity. SNR improvements result in significant reduction in acquisition time and permit observation of physiological processes, and avoid prolonged anesthesia in in vivo studies. Therefore, coil miniaturization and geometric optimization are the foci of RF coil design for MR microscopy.

To address the sensitivity requirements of microscopy, a new generation of coils called 'microcoils' has been developed *(10–14)*. Microcoils are loosely defined as coils whose sensing volume is less than 10 µL *(15)*. Microcoils have distinct challenges related to scalability issues. The coils must be mechanically stable, capable of incorporating the sample within their sensing volume, able to carry large currents, and able to dissipate heat without adverse effects on the sample.

As the conductor thickness and inter-turn separation (in the case of multiturn microcoils) are reduced, eddy currents in the wire reduce its effective cross-section through skin effects and proximity effects. A high frequency alternating current (AC) generates eddy currents at the center of the wire, and the conductive current concentrates toward the wire perimeter, in a region characterized by skin depth, δ. This results in losses beyond the resistive direct current (DC) losses. For multiturn microcoils, each turn of the microcoil generates eddy currents in neighboring turns, resulting in an additional AC loss mechanism called 'proximity loss.' When the wire radius is equal to the skin depth, the cross-sectional current distribution is uniform, and closely approximates the DC case. Therefore, although one would ideally design microcoils with conductors several times thicker than the skin depth, limitations in fabrication techniques constrain conductor thickness to be close to the skin depth. In such a case, fabricating microcoils with a conductor thickness equal to twice the skin depth provides better performance than slightly thicker conductors, with a few provisos that are beyond the scope of this chapter *(7)*.

Thus, there are competing geometry requirements for high microcoil performance. As the microcoil dimension decreases, inter-turn separation must decrease to provide a strong and homogeneous field. The reduced separation between turns results in additional proximity losses. We address these competing design requirements in our ensuing discussing of microcoil design. It should be noted that the microcoils discussed in this chapter are transceivers, i.e., the same microcoil is used to transmit power and receive signal. Therefore, better field characteristics in the microcoil's transmission mode will result in increased sensitivity in its reception mode.

2.1.3.1. VOLUME MICROCOILS

Volume coils are best suited for applications requiring high field homogeneity and for sample geometry that is primarily three-dimensional. Saddle, birdcage, and solenoid coils are typical (**Fig. 2**). This section will focus on the solenoid, a well studied and widely used microcoil, and the novel multilayered scroll microcoil that can increase SNR by incorporating several sensing layers.

Solenoid microcoils have been routinely fabricated by winding thin wire on a small-diameter capillary. A method for constructing solenoid microcoils is detailed below. A small-diameter, polyimide-coated, fused silica capillary is held in a pin vise, and a polyurethane-coated copper wire loop with a preload at both ends is suspended from the capillary and glued onto it with cyanoacrylate. The capillary should be free of contaminants and the adhesive must be used sparingly to avoid field distortions arising from susceptibility effects. Once the adhesive is bound, the preload at one end is removed and the coil is wound by rotating the pin vise to achieve the necessary solenoid. The wire at the other end of the solenoid is then glued, and the preload removed. The polyurethane coating is chemically etched or mechanically removed from the leads, the coil-capillary construct is mounted between two struts on a printed circuit board, and the leads are soldered to the necessary circuitry. In the case of solenoids with a stipulated inter-turn separation, the capillary may be replaced by a threaded former of appropriate pitch, and the wire wound in the threads. Alternatively, wire spacing may be maintained by simultaneously winding two wires

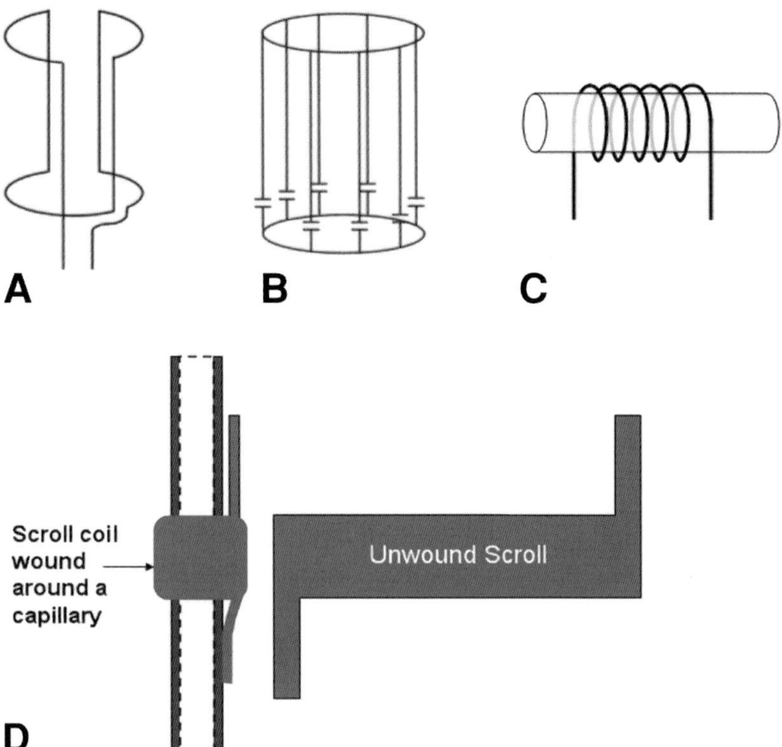

Fig. 2. Schematic drawings showing various configurations of radio frequency volume coils: **(A)** a saddle coil, **(B)** a birdcage coil, **(C)** a solenoid, and **(D)** the novel scroll geometry.

on the capillary and then unfurling one wire whose cross-sectional dimension is equal to the desired inter-turn spacing. Solenoid microcoils have been fabricated by winding thin wire on a micropipette tip while using a geared translational driver to achieve the necessary winding *(16,17)*. Although the separation between the windings is difficult to control and reproduce, it is a critical factor in microcoil performance *(18)*.

The performance of a single-layered solenoid is a function of the wire diameter, number of turns, inter-turn spacing, and aspect ratio (length:diameter). For the first approximation in the DC case, a solenoid's sensitivity at the center of the coil is:

$$\frac{B_1}{i} = \frac{\mu_0 \cdot n}{d \cdot \sqrt{1 + \left(\frac{l}{d}\right)^2}},$$

where μ_0 is the permeability of free space, n is the number of turns of the solenoid, d is the coil's diameter, and l is its length. The coil sensitivity increases inversely with d. However, in the microcoil regime, skin-effect losses play a dominant role in coil performance, and SNR improves inversely with $d^{1/2}$ *(7)*. B_1 field homogeneity can be improved by winding a solenoid on a former that is nonuniform in its cross-section, or by varying the inter-turn spacing, thereby reducing field distortion from edge effects *(19)*. Solenoid microcoils suffer from scalability and difficulty in fabrication. Wire thickness is a limiting factor in coil miniaturization, and multilayered solenoids are very difficult to wind. Scroll microcoils were developed to overcome these limitations *(20,21)*

A scroll microcoil (**Fig. 2**) is a conductor ribbon, laminated with a dielectric, and wound on itself to generate several sensing layers. Scroll microcoils can be fabricated from conductor sheets of thickness equal to twice the skin depth, and their dielectric layer makes them robust and easy to wind. A method for constructing scroll microcoils is detailed here. First, aluminum-backed copper sheets are laminated on the copper side with a dielectric polymer using vapor deposition. The aluminum backing is etched with sodium hydroxide and the copper–dielectric bilayer is used for patterning the microcoil and two leads with standard photolithography techniques. All subsequent steps of microcoil construction are similar to those described for the solenoid. Additional sensing layers of the scroll intensify the field and increase reception sensitivity up to a point, beyond which, the added resistance from incremental sensing layers outweighs the sensitivity gains, resulting in a drop in SNR.

SNR improvements of scrolls over solenoids were reported in a preliminary study by Gimi et al. *(20)*. Although these SNR improvements are overestimated because the scroll design incorporated a sensing lead that contributed to signal, the basic approach is valid.

A major advantage of the scroll microcoil is that the B_1 field homogeneity can be increased by varying the conductor pattern across the length of the microcoil to minimize edge effects, thereby eliminating the need to use a nonuniform capillary or former to achieve a similar effect, as is the case with the solenoid.

2.1.3.1.1. Susceptibility Matching

The difference in magnetic susceptibility of the microcoil conductor and the surrounding air induces field distortion artefacts in the sample. To achieve high sensitivity, the filling factor must be maximized. A thin-walled capillary will allow sample proximity to the microcoil conductor, but makes the construct mechanically fragile and increases the penetration of susceptibility distortions into the sample. In imaging applications, the resultant line broadening may not be detrimental to signal quality, but for high-resolution spectroscopy, a compromise must be made between sensitivity and resolution. To minimize these susceptibility artefacts, the conductor is surrounded by a material whose susceptibility closely matches that of the conductor.

2.1.3.2. Surface Microcoils

The surface coil is the coil of choice for principally planar sample geometry because of high localized SNR in a plane proximal to the coil. The use of small samples in MR microscopy makes it very difficult to accurately place the sample within the sensing region of a volume microcoil. A surface microcoil provides ample space for sample placement and greater access to the sample for perfusion, manipulation, and replacement.

The spiral geometry is most commonly used in surface microcoils. As is the case with the scroll microcoil, additional turns of the spiral intensify the field generated, but as the number of conductor turns increases beyond an optimum number, the resistive losses from the additional turns overcome their contribution to SNR gain. Furthermore, with an augmenting spiral, the distance between the outer conductor trace and the sample region increases, progressively diminishing the outer turn's contribution to field strength. A plot of SNR per unit volume vs the number of spiral turns shows the optimal number of turns for a range of axial distance to starting radius ratios (**Fig. 3A**).

Taking advantage of photolithography and microfabrication techniques, the geometric parameters of a surface microcoil can be controlled with submicron resolution, and several microcoils can be fabricated on a single substrate. This section details two techniques used in fabricating surface microcoils, one that involves an easy approach to generating spiral microcoils with a starting radius upward of 750 μm, and another that is more involved and robust and can be used for sub-500 μm microcoils.

First, we discuss a straightforward method used to fabricate large spiral microcoils with starting radii upward of 750 μm *(22)*. Here, a double-sided, copper-clad Teflon substrate serves as a foundation for the microcoil, but the procedure can be easily adapted for any conductor and MR-compatible substrate. The spiral microcoil and main leads are patterned on one side using photolithography. The outer turn of the spiral is directly connected to one main lead. The inner turn of the spiral and the second lead are connected through a trace on the reverse side, using via holes to electroplate them to the trace. A strong electroplated connection through the via holes is critical, because this is a potential weak point in the circuit when delivering large currents to the microcoil. The assembly is laminated on 500 μm Teflon for mechanical stability, and the microcoil is coated with a polymeric isolation layer. Such surface microcoils have been used in high-resolution imaging of implantable

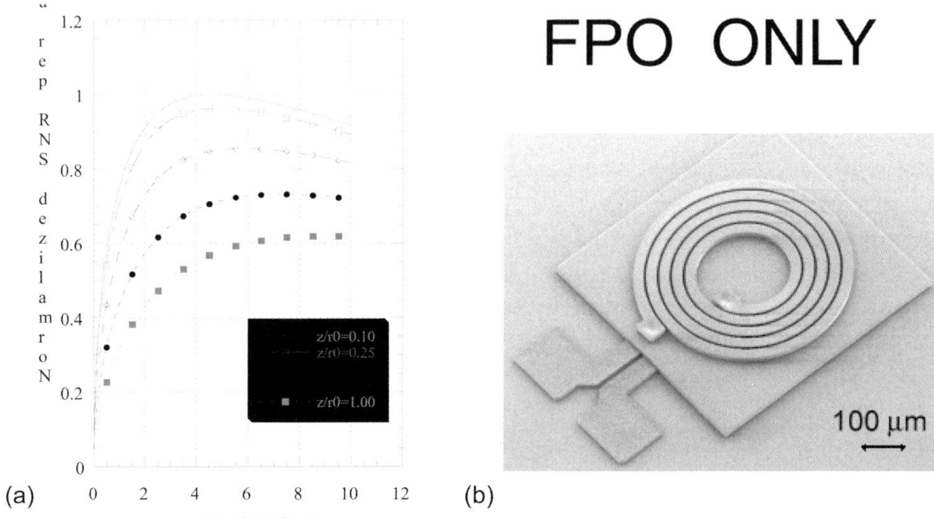

Fig. 3. **(A)** Normalized signal-to-noise ratio (SNR) per unit volume vs number of turns for a spiral coil with starting radius of 750 μm; trace width and inter-turn spacing, 100 μm; and trace width, 20 μm. The figure shows that SNR increases with the number of turns of the spiral, up to a point, beyond which, the electrical losses in the circuit surmount the SNR gains from the additional turns. (Reproduced with permission from **ref. 22**.) **(B)** A scanning electron micrograph of spiral surface microcoil mold, showing the spiral conductor and the leads. (Reproduced with permission from **ref. 25**. © 2003 IEEE.)

biocapsules *(23)*. The high-resolution images allow for investigating intracapsule cell distribution, viability, and diffusion and transport of nutrients and waste products. Surface microcoils have also been used in high-resolution imaging of intact pancreatic islets and *Xenopus laevis* oocytes *(23)* (**Fig. 4**). Easy replacement of the sample allows for the investigation of comparisons.

Another method used to generate a family of sub-500 μm spiral microcoils involves electroplating copper into an SU-8 photoresist mold *(24)* (**Fig. 3B**). Copper leads are electroplated on a glass substrate and a 10-μm–patterned SU-8 isolation layer is deposited to separate the leads from the microcoil. An additional seed layer is patterned, proceeded by the deposition of a 55-μm SU-8 mold. The microcoil spiral is constructed by depositing copper into the SU-8 mold. The leads are wire bonded to a printed circuit board on the RF probe, and embedded in epoxy for protection. Such microcoils were used to obtain high-resolution imaging of pancreatic islets and *Xenopus laevis* oocytes *(25)*.

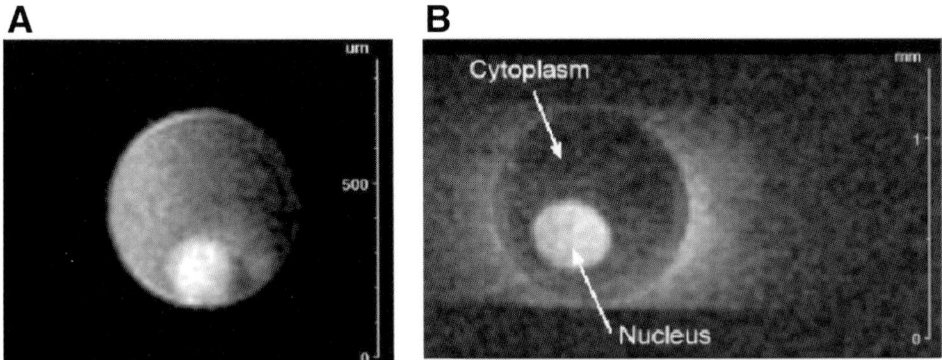

Fig. 4. **(A)** Image of a single islet of Langerhans with 14 μm × 14 μm, in-plane resolution on a 100-μm slice. The standard spin-echo image was acquired with TE = 11.56 ms and TR = 1200 ms. **(B)** An image of an *Xenopus laevis* oocyte showing clear delineation between the nucleus and cytoplasm; gradient-echo image with TR = 300 ms, TE = 6.8 ms, 16 × 23 × 100 μm³ resolution, over a 1 h and 30 min acquisition. (Reproduced from **ref. 25** with permission. © 2003 IEEE.)

Although there can be no direct comparison between the sensitivity of volume coils and surface coils because surface coils have an ill-defined sensing volume, some broad comparisons are instructive in selecting a suitable coil for an experiment. Surface coils provide very high localized SNR, although their SNR advantage over volume coils decreases rapidly with increasing imaging distance from the plane of the coil *(23)*. Surface coils generate radiant, inhomogeneous magnetic fields, resulting in spectral broadening. This obstacle can be avoided by imaging in a thin plane where the field is relatively homogeneous, correcting for B_1 inhomogeneity during postprocessing, or using a Helmholtz configuration to increase the sensing region and RF homogeneity. To achieve high local SNR when imaging a large field-of-view, several surface microcoils may be used in a phased array *(26)*. Parallel imaging techniques *(27)*, such as sensitivity encoding (SENSE) *(28)* and simultaneous acquisition of spatial harmonics (SMASH) *(29)*, are frequently employed in such applications *(30,31)*. Chieh-Lin et al. *(32)* have shown that if the sample volume is fixed, an array of coils is preferred a single coil; whereas, if the sample can be scaled with the coil dimension, a single coil is preferred.

2.2. Technical Strategies: Gradients

The role of gradients in microscopy must be discussed in the context of diffusion, magnetic susceptibility, and the imaging sequence, all of which will be addressed in **Subheading 2.3.** In this section, we briefly discuss gradient function, the need for strong gradients in microscopy, and hardware requirements and technical strategies to achieve efficient gradient operation. Sweeping through space with a magnetic field gradient results in spins at different points in space experiencing different local magnetic fields, which affects their precession frequency, which, in turn, reveals their spatial location. The stronger the gradient, the more accurate the spatial encoding, resulting in a direct correlation between gradient strength and spatial resolution. In addition, at high resolution, stronger and faster-switching gradients are required in MR microscopy to overcome signal degradation from broadening induced by susceptibility effects and molecular diffusion.

Effective gradients require high power, rapid switching, field homogeneity, and active shielding to prevent eddy current losses. The power requirements of strong gradients are achieved through very large pulsed currents with a high duty cycle; this sometimes requires custom-built power supplies to meet the current requirements and frequently requires external cooling. Overcoming signal loss through molecular diffusion requires rapid gradient switching. Seeber et al. *(33)* have achieved switching times as short as 10 μs.

Gradient linearity, required for linear spatial encoding, is difficult to achieve over a large spatial region. Fortunately, microscopy requires gradient linearity over a small region of interest.

The changing magnetic flux from gradients generates eddy currents in other conducting structures, such as the magnetic bore, degrading SNR. Eddy currents may be reduced by actively shielded gradients or by using small gradient coils far from the magnetic bore.

Several approaches have been used to tackle these requirements and challenges of gradient design. Botwell and Robyrr *(34)* propose multilayered gradients with up to 650 W power dissipation. Zhang and Cory *(35)* demonstrate how fast-switching gradients of 600 T/m can be used in solid-state diffusion applications. Seeber et al. *(36)* have designed triple-axis gradients, as high as 50 T/m in one axis, capable of achieving approx 1 to 2 μm resolution. As is evident from the proceeding sections, there are competing requirements on gradient strength and performance based on susceptibility and diffusion effects, involving trade-offs between resolution, SNR, and acquisition time (*see* **ref.** *37* for further details).

2.3. Phenomenological Strategies

Resolving biological systems at the level of single cells and cellular clusters is critical to understanding the cellular response to perturbation and to discerning microscopic biochemical heterogeneity. The issue is not just that of resolution but also of information content. Contrast from cellular/subcellular boundaries and changes in relaxation times of the environment play a role in providing information about the biological system. MR signal and contrast depends on the pulse sequence used to excite the sample and acquire the signal. Pulse sequences can be tailored to observe or highlight different physiological and functional phenomena, such as the structure and permeability of boundaries and interfaces, and molecular diffusion.

Several techniques are used to sensitize MR to tissue properties or tissue changes and are employed in microscopy. Cellular activation–based T_1 weighting has been recently used in microscopy to study the function and viability of pancreatic β-cells, with paramagnetic Mn^{2+} as a T_1 contrast agent *(38,39)*. T_2-weighted microscopy exploits susceptibility effects to track stem-cell migration *(40)* and to observe immune responses in the central nervous system *(41)*. Cobalt labeling has also been used in T_2-weighted microscopy to track nerve cell pathways *(42)*. Fast spin-echo, high-field imaging has been developed for microscopy to increase imaging efficiency by reducing diffusion losses *(43)*. Diffusion-weighted MR microscopy has shed light on compartmentalization of single neurons *(44)* and diffusion tensor imaging microscopy has been used to image the internal gray matter structure of the hippocampus, the thalamus, and the cortex *(45)*. Chemical shift imaging techniques have tracked the metabolism of invading cells in cancer *(46)*. Constant time imaging improves SNR when the gradient switching time is longer than T_2 *(47)*. The use of q-space imaging reveals cellular dimensions *(48)*. Here, we accord susceptibility and diffusion effects more attention because they are salient to microscopy.

2.3.1. Susceptibility

MR spectral linewidth is defined as the full-width half maximum of a Lorentzian function, and is equal to:

$$\frac{1}{\pi \cdot T_2^*} .$$

Susceptibility mismatches create local field inhomogeneity and increase linewidth, resulting in signal attenuation from line broadening.

These susceptibility effects can be undesirable and can lead to poor image quality, or they can provide a valuable signature of the sample. Field distortions arising from cellular boundaries can be distinguished in gradient-echo experiments, providing a useful tool for microscopy of cell and tissue constructs.

2.3.1.1. TECHNICAL STRATEGIES TO MINIMIZE SUSCEPTIBILITY-RELATED EFFECTS

For a given pixel, if the field variation caused by susceptibility is less than the variation caused by the gradient, susceptibility does not have an effect on image quality. Therefore, susceptibility effects are overcome by using large gradients, such that:

$$\frac{\Delta B_0}{\Delta r} << G \, ,$$

where ΔB_0 is the local variation in the magnetic field over a pixel of dimension Δr, and G is the strength of the gradient along that direction.

In the absence of diffusion effects, and only as a result of T_2 and T_2^*:

$$\Delta r = \frac{1}{\gamma \cdot G \cdot \pi \cdot T_2^*} \, ,$$

where $r \cdot \gamma \cdot G$ is the bandwidth.

Thus, increasing G will increase resolution, but SNR will decrease because of line broadening. It should be noted that there is a limit on resolution that is imposed by the bandwidth, expressed as:

$$\left(\Delta r \right)_{BW} = \frac{\Delta \phi^{min}}{\gamma \cdot G \cdot T} \, ,$$

where ϕ^{min} is the minimum detectable phase and T is the signal acquisition time or the time of the applied phase encoding gradient *(49)*. The minimum detectable phase is a function of the reconstruction algorithm and is equal to π for half-echo data in Fourier imaging. The above equation shows that bandwidth-limited resolution can be improved by increasing the signal acquisition time. Longer acquisition times are often undesirable because they involve loss of signal from molecular mobility, long breath holds, and prolonged anesthesia. Therefore, increasing the gradient strength helps improve bandwidth-limited resolution.

When using phase-encoding sequences, longer echo times are required to allow for longer phase-encoding times, resulting in T_2 signal loss. For a given reconstruction method, the bandwidth-limited resolution may be increased by increasing the gradient strength.

Susceptibility artefacts are rendered negligible by using several pulse sequences, for instance by employing a spin-echo sequence and acquiring images at the center of k space, where the refocusing of pixel distortion occurs. The gradient-echo sequence, on the other hand, will highlight contrast because of susceptibility effects.

2.3.1.2. SUSCEPTIBILITY AS A CONTRAST MECHANISM

Signal destruction by T_2 and T_2^* effects creates hypointensity in weighted images.

Labeling cells with particles that induce susceptibility contrast is useful in tracking cell migration, homing, and biodistribution *(50)*. MR detection of single cells is possible at low resolution by using large iron oxide particles to enhance susceptibility effects. Uptake of large iron oxide particles in mesenchymal stem cells and hematopoietic $CD34^+$ cells has exhibited very good T_2^* contrast *(51)*. Microscopy can detect single cells at high resolution, potentially reducing the doses of contrast agents.

Superparamagnetic monocrystalline iron oxide nanoparticles (MIONs) have been recently used to track stem cells and exhibit potential for sharp delineation of tumor borders. The rate of MION endocytosis in tumor cells exceeds that of normal cells, especially for cells at the tumor border, thus sharpening the tumor border in MR images. These MIONs have been used to image tumor cell endocytosis in vivo and ex vivo with microscopic resolution *(52)*. Tumor border delineation has a potential application in the accurate estimation of tumor volume and in minimally invasive surgery. Therefore, susceptibility effects can deteriorate image quality or be used to track cells and image boundaries.

2.3.2. Diffusion

As is the case with susceptibility effects, signal loss caused by diffusion, blurring, and boundary artefacts are major challenges in microscopy, but signal loss and boundary artefacts can also be used to measure and deduce important biological information.

2.3.2.1. TECHNICAL STRATEGIES TO MINIMIZE DIFFUSION-RELATED EFFECTS

Random Brownian motion results in some spins dispersing outside the voxel of interest. When spins disperse outside the voxel within the time of an acquisition they do not contribute to signal, resulting in low SNR. The diffusion-limited resolution is expressed as:

$$\Delta r_D = \sqrt{\frac{2}{3} D T_{acq}} \, ,$$

where Δr_D is the diffusion-limited spatial resolution, D is the coefficient of diffusion of the observed molecule, and T_{acq} is the acquisition time *(49)*. Therefore, diffusion from random-phase fluctuation impedes on resolution only when the diffused distance is greater than the voxel dimension. Strong gradients can be applied to overcome phase dispersion and signal loss from diffusion.

Because time-varying signal attenuation has the effect of line broadening, resolution is adversely affected if the line broadening exceeds the voxel dimensions. This line-broadening effect is another limit on resolution because of diffusion. For a given resolution and diffusion coefficient, the optimum acquisition time for maximum SNR is *(53)*:

$$T_D^{opt} = \frac{3\Delta r^2}{2\pi^2 D}.$$

In both frequency- and phase-encoding sequences, large gradients are required to overcome diffusive attenuation, but in the phase-encoding case, the gradient strength does not adversely affect bandwidth. When diffusive attenuation in the read direction is a significant factor, T_2 cannot be accurately measured by varying the echo time, TE. A Carr-Purcell-Meiboom-Gill pulse train is used to precede the echo sequence, providing T_2 weighting. Other modified pulse sequences have been used to eliminate diffusion losses in microscopy *(54)*.

2.3.2.2. Diffusion as a Contrast Mechanism

In some applications, diffusion effects must be compensated for, and, in others, diffusion effects can be used to provide a signature of the sample. For instance, diffusion near cell walls is limited, and manifests as boundary hyperintensity in the read direction. Fast and slow compartmental exchange are used to estimate cell size, membrane permeability, intracellular and extracellular volume fractions, and nuclear vs cytoplasmic signal contributions *(55–57)*. Diffusion influences oxygen and nutrient gradients and bears on intercellular communication *(58)*, making it a useful tool for the study of cellular microenvironment changes to local perturbation. Diffusion rates depend on the molecular environment as well as on restrictions that are either impermeable or partially permeable, and help distinguish physical and chemical domains.

The effective T_2 relaxation time is a function of the true T_2 relaxation time, as well as the b value, which, in turn, is a function of compartmentalization. The scenario is complicated by compartmentalization. Slow exchange will yield distinct values of T_2 and the diffusion coefficient for each compartment, whereas fast exchange will yield a single value for the two parameters that is a weighted average of the components. These slow and fast exchange components can quantify membrane permeability, cell swelling and shrinkage, and the proliferation, destruction, and repopulation of cells in a tumor.

3. Applications

The effort toward MR microscopy is driven by the need to noninvasively detect molecular events, and to do so with high spatial localization and sufficient sensitivity to characterize low concentrations of metabolites. Investigators have used MR microscopy for high-resolution spectroscopy *(11,13,59)* and localized spectroscopy *(60)*, as well as for microscopic imaging of cell and

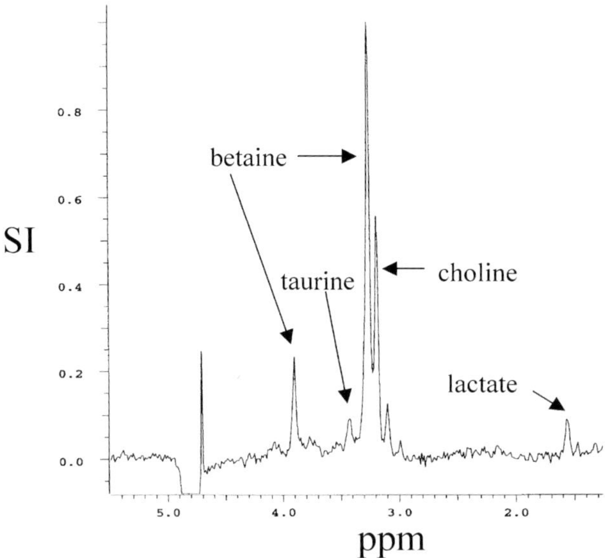

Fig. 5. [1]H spectrum from a single neuron, averaged over 1 h and 40 m, shows betaine, taurine, and choline peaks, along with an emerging lactate peak. The spectrum was obtained from a 220 × 220 × 220 μm^3 voxel. The spectrum was acquired at 14 T, from a 220 μm × 220 μm × 220 μm voxel. (From **ref. *60***. Copyright ©, 2000 Wiley InterScience. Reprinted by permission of Wiley-Liss, Inc., a subsidiary of John Wiley & Sons, Inc.)

tissue structures *(61)* and large single cells *(10)*. Headway in cell tracking, single cell detection, and compartmental diffusion provides avenues to noninvasively study the molecular mechanism of disease onset and progression, and the response of cells and cellular structures to immune attack, gene therapy, and other perturbation.

3.1. Spectroscopy

With localized spectroscopy, NMR spectra of osmolytes and metabolites have been obtained from single neurons in concentrations on the order of tens of millimolar. **Figure 5** shows spectra from the L7 neuron of *Aplysia californica* taken every 8 min and averaged over 1 h and 40 min *(60)*. These spectra were obtained from nanoliter volumes (220 μm isotropic voxel) using the stimulated echo acquisition mode (STEAM) sequence, and show betaine, taurine, and choline peaks, with the emergence of a lactate peak. Combined with single neuron microscopy in perfused systems *(62)*, localized spectroscopy can be a potent tool in understanding the neuronal response to change in tonicity and other physiological perturbations.

3.2. Cellular Imaging and Compartmental Diffusion

MR microscopy is particularly well suited for imaging *Xenopus laevis* oocytes and embryos because light scattering from yolk inclusions severely impede optical imaging. Furthermore, intrinsic MR contrast can be used to identify the blastocoel (which has a higher water content than the rest of the embryo), and distinguishing the animal pole and the vegetal pole, the latter containing more fat. Sehy et al. *(63)* obtained high-resolution images of *Xenopus laevis* oocytes, measuring T_1, T_2, and apparent diffusion coefficient (ADC) values. They measured ADC in the nucleus, the animal pole, and the vegetal pole of the oocyte, showing a higher ADC value in the animal pole compared with the vegetal pole, the latter containing less free water and more fat.

Schoeniger et al. *(64)* obtained proton density, T_1, and T_2 images of single neurons of *Aplysia californica*. They also obtained diffusion coefficients from the nucleus and the cytoplasm, showing that proton diffusion in the nucleus was faster than in the cytoplasm. Similarly, Grant et al. *(44)* showed a higher ADC for the nucleus compared with the cytoplasm, using diffusion-weighted images.

3.3. Cellular Function

The noninvasive evaluation of tissue implants and transplants has emerged as a requisite for periodic evaluation of their function. To optimize implant and transplant function, one must thoroughly understand cellular response to drugs, immune attack, and other physiological perturbation. Transplanted pancreatic islets have emerged as a promising therapy for patients with type I diabetes. Given that a patient can be normoglycemic with as few as 2% of the native islets being functional, there is a clinical need to assess in vivo islet function to monitor and improve diabetes treatment. Manganese-enhanced MR microscopy of islet function was proposed by Gimi et al. *(38,39)* as an approach for the noninvasive in vivo scoring of islet activity. The islet microimaging study achieved 14 × 14 µm in-plane resolution on a 100-µm slice over a 1 h and 36 min acquisition, with a standard spin-echo sequence. The study also performed MR microscopy on implantable biocapsules that encapsulate insulin-secreting β-cells. Although these high-resolution images are of value in studying the transplanted islets and implantable biocapsule, the system was designed to observe islet and β-cell activation maps. Much higher resolution is possible with further optimization of sample placement, using a more appropriate pulse sequence, and employing stronger gradients.

3.4. Embryonic Development and Multidimensional Animal Atlases

To gain insights into embryonic development and cell lineage, MR microscopy of single cells and cellular clusters must be evaluated in the context of the entire biological system. A multidimensional atlas of the embryo can identify the genetic and molecular factors involved in embryonic development, and correlate morphological data to region-specific gene expression and biochemical data. (*see* **ref. 65** for a review). MR microscopy has a prominent role to play in the development of such atlases.

Jacobs and Fraser *(66)* longitudinally tracked cell motion and lineage of *Xenopus* embryos; Smith et al. *(67)* imaged fixed mouse embryos at different stages of development. MR microscopy was also employed in 3D angiography of fixed mouse embryos *(68)*. Recently, Louie et al. *(69)* imaged gene expression in the *Xenopus* tadpole with a contrast agent that was enzymatically activated by removing its sugar cap from a water-coordinating site. Some of this work will be detailed later in the book.

3.5. Imaging Organ Microstructure and Function

High-resolution MR has been employed in studying microscopic structure and function of the brain using standard imaging methods and contrast agents *(70,71)*. Brain pathologies, including stroke, atrophy, dementia, hydrocephalus, and tumors have also been explored with MR microscopy (*see* **ref. 72** for an excellent review). Zhang et al. *(45)* have obtained high-resolution diffusion tensor images of the hippocampus, which is implicated in developmental and aging disorders, such as Down syndrome and Alzheimer's disease, respectively. Discovering microscopic anomalies and changes in neuronal architecture in the hippocampus will greatly aid in the understanding and early detection of these diseases. Although diffusion tensor microscopy does not achieve the resolution obtained through histology, the modality is less labor intensive than a three-dimensional histological reconstruction of the entire brain, and largely avoids sectioning artefacts, such as tissue deformation and loss. Therefore, diffusion tensor microscopy is not an alternative to histology but can be viewed as a noninvasive complementary technique that can be employed for rapid screening.

As mentioned previously, sample polarization enhances signal amplitude but is not always physiologically appropriate or possible. A notable exception is the use of hyperpolarized inert gas to image pulmonary microstructure and function, including pulmonary gas exchange, diffusion, and perfusion. Johnson et al. *(73)* have used the technique to discern airways down to the 7th branch.

4. Future

4.1. Combining Optical Microscopy With MR

Still within the realm of conventional MR microscopy, investigators have merged MR with optical microscopy to create an overlay of MR and optical images *(74,75)*. Glover et al. *(74)* were the first to merge these two imaging modalities, imaging onion epidermal cells with 4.5-μm in-plane resolution.

Wind et al. *(75)* used the technique to spatially register diffusion data from MR with organelle positions obtained from confocal images, showing a reduced diffusion rate in the region of mitochondrial clusters in a *Xenopus laevis* oocyte. Advances in integrated MR/optical systems will simultaneously yield high-resolution spatial resolution with high-resolution biochemical information.

4.2. Magnetic Resonance Force Microscopy

Although technical improvements will incrementally increase resolution, new approaches may drastically change the landscape of MR microscopy. An emerging technique called magnetic resonance force microscopy (MRFM) uses force-detection MR instead of induction-detection MR; MRFM combines MR with conventional probe microscopy such as atomic force microscopy and scanning tunnel microscopy, and is capable of achieving atomic resolution on the order of 1 to 1000 Å *(76,77)*.

The MR force microscope usually involves a cantilever with a ferromagnetic tip (magnetic field source) in close proximity to the sample. When an RF field is applied to the sample, the resulting magnetic moment in a small ensemble of spins generates a force on the cantilever, causing it to deflect. Resonance in the cantilever is achieved by modulating the RF field around the Larmor frequency, at the resonance frequency of the cantilever. The cantilever deflection is detected by an optical interferometer (**Fig. 6**).

In the system described above, natural field gradients (on the order of 10 G/nm) are generated by the ferromagnetic tip that is attached to the free end of the cantilever. In some cases, the sample is placed on the cantilever, with the ferromagnetic magnetic source is in close proximity to it. An alternate Better observation of magnetization, enhanced resolution, and no gradient (BOOMERANG) configuration places the detector magnet on the cantilever beam, with the sample being polarized. Here, the gradient is provided by the sample field, and the entire sample can be used for signal detection.]

Comparative studies show that MRFM provides sensitivity gains over conventional MR microscopy for small samples, such as membrane proteins, that are in close proximity to the cantilever *(32)*. This sensitivity advantage increases as the nucleus gyromagnetic ratio decreases, further adding to the desirability of the technique. Even so, increasing distance from the cantilever results in loss of both sensitivity and gradient strength; for cell-sized samples, conventional MR microscopy is preferable to MRFM.

In conclusion, technological advances in microfabrication and nanofabrication; improved contrast techniques, such as targeted molecular probes and enzymatically amplified contrast; and the emergence of new technologies, such as MRFM and the integrated optical microscope/MR microscopes, are likely to carry microscopy into the realm where subcellular

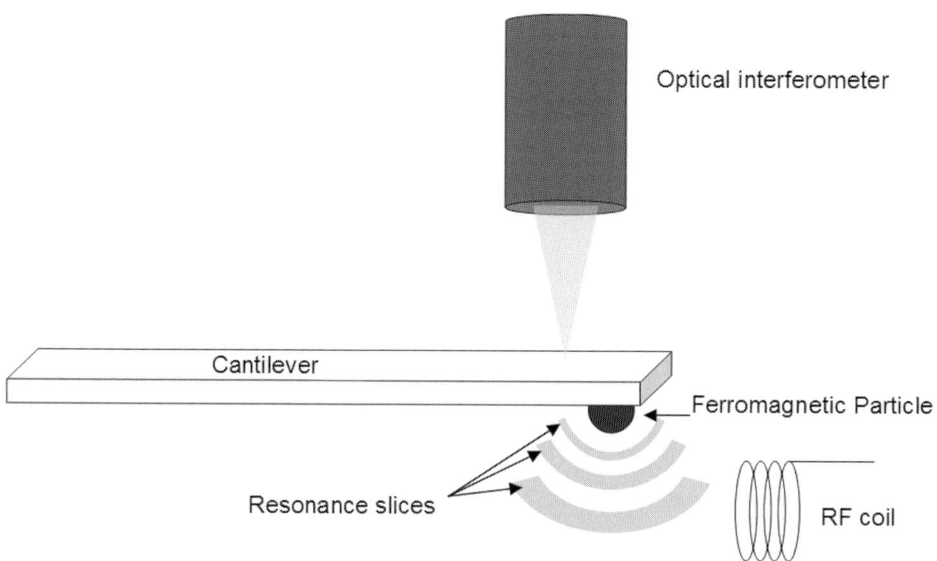

Fig. 6. A schematic of a magnetic resonance force microscope. The ferromagnetic particle generates magnetic field and a natural gradient. As the distance from the ferromagnetic particle increases, the magnetic gradient decreases and the resonance slice becomes thicker. Cantilever resonance is achieved by modulating the RF field around the Larmor frequency, at the resonant frequency of the cantilever. The interferometer measures the cantilever motion.

detection is routine. With developments in therapeutic implants and regenerative medicine, a greater push toward implantable coils is foreseeable for high-resolution, in vivo imaging. Integrating microfluidics with MR systems will prolong sample viability and provide the capability for dynamic perturbation of cellular and subcellular systems.

Acknowledgments

I gratefully acknowledge Dr. Andrew Webb, Dr. Dmitri Artemov, Dr. Richard L. Magin, and Dr. Zaver Bhujwalla for important insights and support.

References

1. Svensson, J., Mansson, S., Johansson, E., Petersson, J. S., and Olsson, L. E. (2003) Hyperpolarized 13C MR angiography using trueFISP. *Magn. Reson. Med.* **50,** 256–262.
2. Black, R. D., Early, T. A., Roemer, P. B., et al. (1993) A high-temperature superconducting receiver for nuclear magnetic resonance microscopy. *Science* **259,** 793–795.

3. Ginefri, J. C., Darrasse, L., and Crozat, P. (2001) High-temperature supercon-
    ducting surface coil for in vivo microimaging of the human skin. *Magn. Reson.
    Med.* **45,** 376–382.
4. Hurlston, S. E., Brey, W. W., Suddarth, S. A., and Johnson, G. A. (1999) A high-
    temperature superconducting Helmholtz probe for microscopy at 9.4 T. *Magn.
    Reson. Med.* **41,** 1032–1038.
5. Wright, A. C., Song, H. K., and Wehrli, F. W. (2000) In vivo MR micro imaging with
    conventional radiofrequency coils cooled to 77K. *Mag. Reson. Med.* **43,** 163–169.
6. Hoult, D. I. and Richards, R. E. (1976) Signal-to-noise ratio of the nuclear mag-
    netic-resonance experiment. *J. Magn. Reson.* **24,** 71–85.
7. Peck, T. L., Magin, R. L., and Lauterbur, P. C. (1995) Design and analysis of
    microcoils for NMR microscopy. *J. Magn. Reson. B* **108,** 114–124.
8. Hoult, D. I. and Lauterbur, P. C. (1979) The sensitivity of the zeugmatographic
    experiment involving human samples. *J. Magn. Reson.* **34,** 425–433.
9. Cho, Z. H., Ahn, C. B., Juh, S. C., et al. (1988) Nuclear magnetic resonance
    microscopy with 4-um resolution: theoretical study and experimental results. *Med.
    Phys.* **15,** 815.
10. Aguayo, J. B., Blackband, S. J., Schoeniger, J., Mattingly, M. A., and Hintermann, M.
    (1986) Nuclear magnetic resonance imaging of a single cell. *Nature* **322,** 190–191.
11. Olson, D. L., Peck, T. L., Webb, A. G., Magin, R. L., and Sweedler, J. V. (1995)
    High-resolution microcoil 1H-NMR for mass-limited, nanoliter-volume samples.
    Science **270,** 1967–1970.
12. Subramanian, R., Lam, M. M., and Webb, A. G. (1998) RF microcoil design for
    practical NMR of mass-limited samples. *J. Magn. Reson.* **133,** 227–231.
13. Subramanian, R. and Webb, A. G. (1998) Design of solenoidal microcoils for
    high-resolution 13C NMR spectroscopy. *Anal. Chem.* **70,** 2454–2458.
14. Lee, S. C., Kim, K., Kim, J., et al. (2001) One micrometer resolution NMR
    microscopy. *J. Magn. Reson.* **150,** 207–213.
15. Webb, A. G. (1997) Radiofrequency microcoils in magnetic resonance. *Progress
    in Nuclear Magnetic Resonance Spectroscopy* **31,** 1–42.
16. Seeber, D. A., Cooper, R. L., Ciobanu, L., and Pennington, C. H. (2001) Design
    and testing of high sensitivity micro-receiver coil apparatus for nuclear magnetic
    resonance imaging. *Rev. Sci. Instrum.* **72,** 2171–2179.
17. Ciobanu, L., Seeber, D. A., and Pennington, C. H. (2002) 3D MR microscopy
    with resolution 3.7 micron by 3.3 micron by 3.3 micron. *J. Magn. Reson.* **158,**
    178–182.
18. Peck, T. L. (1992) Ph.D. dissertation. University of Illinois at Urbana/Champaign,
    IL. 19. Idziak, S. and Haeberlen, U. (1982) *J. Magn. Reson.* **50,** 281.
20. Gimi, B., Grant, S. C., Magin, R. L., Fienerman, A., Frolova, E., and Friedman,
    G. (2000) SNR improvements for RF scroll microcoils. *Experimental Nuclear
    Magnetic Resonance Conference.* Asilomar, CA. April 2000.
21. Gimi, B., Grant, S. C., Magin, R. L., and Friedman, G. (2000) Investigation of
    NMR signal-to-noise for RF scroll microcoils. *Proceedings of 1st Annual Inter-
    national IEEE-EMBS Special Topics Conference on Microtechnologies in Medi-
    cine & Biology.* Oct. 2000,. Lyons, France.

22. Eroglu, S., Gimi, B., Roman, B., Friedman, G., and Magin, R. L. (2003) NMR spiral surface microcoils: field characteristics and applications. *Concepts in Magnetic Resonance Imaging Part B,* **17B**(1), 1–10.
23. Gimi, B., Eroglu, S., Leoni, L., Desai, T. A., Magin, R. L., and Roman, B. (2003) NMR spiral surface microcoils: applications. *Concepts in Magnetic Resonance Imaging Part B,* **18B**(1), 189–200.
24. Massin, C., Boero, G., Vincent, F., Abenhaim, J., Besse, P.-A., and Popovic, R. S. (2002) High-Q factor RF planar microcoils for micro-scale NMR spectroscopy. *Sens. Actuators A Phys.* **97–98,** 280–288.
25. Massin, C., Eroglu, S., Vincent, F., et al. (2003) Planar microcoil-based magnetic resonance imaging of cells. Proceedings of *Transducers '03*, Boston, MA, June, 2003, 967–970.
26. Roemer, P. B., Edelstein, W. A., Hayes, C. E., Souza, S. P., and Mueller, O. M. (1990) The NMR phased array. *Magn. Reson. Med.* **16,** 192–225.
27. Sodickson, D. K. and McKenzie, C. A. (2001) A generalized approach to parallel magnetic resonance imaging. *Med. Phys.* **28,** 1629–1643.
28. Wright, S. M., Magin, R. L., and Kelton, J. R. (1991) Arrays of mutually coupled receiver coils: theory and application. *Magn. Reson. Med.* **17,** 252–268.
29. Sodickson, D. K. and Manning, W. J. (1997) Simultaneous acquisition of spatial harmonics (SMASH): fast imaging with radiofrequency coil arrays. *Magn. Reson. Med.* **38,** 591–603.
30. Pruessmann, K. P., Weiger, M., Scheidegger, M. B., and Boesiger, P. (1999) SENSE: sensitivity encoding for fast MRI. *Magn. Reson. Med.* **42,** 952–962.
31. Sodickson, D. K., McKenzie, C. A., Ohliger, M. A., Yeh, E. N., and Price, M. D. (2002) Recent advances in image reconstruction, coil sensitivity calibration, and coil array design for SMASH and generalized parallel MRI. *Magma* **13,** 158–163.
32. Lin, W.-C. and Fedder, G. K. (2001) *A Comparison of Induction-Detection NMR and Force-Detection NMR on Micro-NMR Device Design.* The Robotics Institute of Computer Science, Carnegie Mellon University, Pittsburgh, PA.
33. Seeber, D. A., Hoftiezer, J. H., and Pennington, C. H. (2002) Pulsed current gradient power supply for microcoil magnetic resonance imaging. *Concepts in Magnetic Resonance Imaging Part B* **15,** 189.
34. Bowtell, R. and Robyr, P. (1998) *J. Magn. Reson.* **131,** 286–294.
35. Zhang, H. and Cory, D. G. (1998) Pulsed gradient NMR probes for solid state studies. *J. Magn. Reson.* **132,** 144–149.
36. Seeber, D. A., Hoftiezer, J. H., Daniel, W. B., Rutgers, M. A., and Pennington, C. H. (2000) Triaxial magnetic field gradient system for microcoil magnetic resonance imaging. *Rev. Sci. Instrum.* **71,** 4263–4272.
37. Glover, P. M. and Mansfield, P. (2002) Limits to magnetic resonance microscopy. *Rep. Prog. Phys.* **65,** 1489–1511.
38. Gimi, B., Leoni, L., Braun, M., Eroglu, S., Magin, R. L., and Roman, B. (2003) Non-invasive functional microimaging of pancreatic islets using manganese enhanced MRI. *The Society for Molecular Imaging, Second Annual Meeting.* San Francisco, CA, Aug, 2003.

39. Gimi, B., Leoni, L., Eroglu, S., Desai, T. A., Magin, R. L., and Roman, B. (2002) Non-invasive monitoring of encapsulated beta cell function using Mn2+-enhanced magnetic resonance imaging. *Second Annual Diabetes Technology Meeting, Atlanta, GA*, Oct.–Nov., 2002.

40. Bulte, J. W., Douglas, T., Witwer, B., et al. (2001) Magnetodendrimers allow endosomal magnetic labeling and in vivo tracking of stem cells. *Nat. Biotechnol.* **19**, 1141–1147.

41. Dousset, V., Delalande, C., Ballarino, L., et al. (1999) In vivo macrophage activity imaging in the central nervous system detected by magnetic resonance. *Magn. Reson. Med.* **41**, 329–333.

42. Quast, M. J., Neumeister, H., Ezell, E. L., and Budelmann, B. U. (2001) MR microscopy of cobalt-labeled nerve cells and pathways in an invertebrate brain (Sepia officinalis, Cephalopoda). *Magn. Reson. Med.* **45**, 575–579.

43. Zhou, X., Cofer, G. P., Suddarth, S. A., and Johnson, G. A. (1993) High-field MR microscopy using fast spin-echoes. *Magn. Reson. Med.* **30**, 60–67.

44. Grant, S. C., Buckley, D. L., Gibbs, S., Webb, A. G., and Blackband, S. J. (2001) MR microscopy of multicomponent diffusion in single neurons. *Magn. Reson. Med.* **46**, 1107–1112.

45. Zhang, J., van Zijl, P. C., and Mori, S. (2002) Three-dimensional diffusion tensor magnetic resonance microimaging of adult mouse brain and hippocampus. *Neuroimage* **15**, 892–901.

46. Artemov, D., Pilatus, U., Chu, S., Mori, N., Nelson, J. B., and Bhujwalla, Z. M. (1999) Dynamics of prostate cancer cell invasion studied in vitro by NMR microscopy. *Magn. Reson. Med.* **42**, 277–282.

47. Gravina, S. and Cory, D. G. (1994) Sensitivity and resolution of constant-time imaging. *J. Magn. Reson. Series B* **104**, 53–61.

48. Cohen, Y. and Assaf, Y. (2002) High b-value q-space analyzed diffusion-weighted MRS and MRI in neuronal tissues—a technical review. *NMR Biomed.* **15**, 516–542.

49. Cho, Z. H., Lee, S. C., and Cho, M. H. *NMR Microscopy: Resolution, in: Methods in Biomedical Magnetic Resonance Imaging and Spectroscopy* (Young, I., ed.), John Wiley & Sons, pp. 433–439.

50. Gimi, B., Mori, N., Ackerstaff, E., Frost, E. E., Bulte, J. W. M., and Bhujwalla, Z. M. (2004) MR imaging of superparamagnetically labeled endothelial cells revealed directed migration in response to factors secreted by human breast cancer cells. *The Third Annual Meeting of the Society for Molecular Imaging*. St. Louis, MO., Sept. 2004.

51. Hinds, K. A., Hill, J. M., Shapiro, et al. (2003) Highly efficient endosomal labeling of progenitor and stem cells with large magnetic particles allows magnetic resonance imaging of single cells. *Blood* **102**, 867–872.

52. Zimmer, C., Wright, S. C., Jr., Engelhardt, R. T., et al. (1997) Tumor cell endocytosis imaging facilitates delineation of the glioma-brain interface. *Exp. Neurol.* **143**, 61–69.

53. Cho, Z. H., Ahn, C. B., Juh, S. C., et al. (1988) Nuclear magnetic resonance microscopy with 4-microns resolution: theoretical study and experimental results. *Med. Phys.* **15**, 815–824.

54. Hsu, E. W., Schoeniger, J. S., Bowtell, R., Aiken, N. R., Horsman, A., and Blackband, S. J. (1995) A modified imaging sequence for accurate T2 measurements using NMR microscopy. *J. Magn. Reson. B* **109,** 66–69.

55. Duong, T. Q., Sehy, J. V., Yablonskiy, D. A., Snider, B. J., Ackerman, J. J., and Neil, J. J. (2001) Extracellular apparent diffusion in rat brain. *Magn. Reson. Med.* **45,** 801–810.

56. Sehy, J. V., Banks, A. A., Ackerman, J. J., and Neil, J. J. (2002) Importance of intracellular water apparent diffusion to the measurement of membrane permeability. *Biophys. J.* **83,** 2856–2863.

57. Sehy, J. V., Ackerman, J. J., and Neil, J. J. (2002) Evidence that both fast and slow water ADC components arise from intracellular space. *Magn. Reson. Med.* **48,** 765–770.

58. Francis, K. and Palsson, B. O. (1997) Effective intercellular communication distances are determined by the relative time constants for cyto/chemokine secretion and diffusion. *Proc. Natl. Acad. Sci. USA* **94,** 12,258–12,262.

59. Minard, K. R. and Wind, R. A. (2002) Picoliter (1)H NMR spectroscopy. *J. Magn. Reson.* **154,** 336–343.

60. Grant, S. C., Aiken, N. R., Plant, H. D., et al. (2000) NMR spectroscopy of single neurons. *Mag. Reson. Med.* **44,** 19–22.

61. Cho, Z. H., Ahn, C. B., Juh, S. C., et al. (1990) Recent progress in NMR microscopy toward cellular imaging. *Trans. Royal Soc. London* **333,** 469–475.

62. Hsu, E. W., Aiken, N. R., and Blackband, S. J. (1996) Nuclear magnetic resonance microscopy of single neurons under hypotonic perturbation. *Am. J. Physiol.* **271,** C1895–C1900.

63. Sehy, J. V., Ackerman, J. J., and Neil, J. J. (2001) Water and lipid MRI of the Xenopus oocyte. *Magn. Reson. Med.* 46, 900–906.

64. Schoeniger, J. S., Aiken, N., Hsu, E., and Blackband, S. J. (1994) Relaxation-time and diffusion NMR microscopy of single neurons. *J. Magn. Reson. B* **103,** 261–273.

65. Jacobs, R. E., Papan, C., Ruffins, S., Tyszka, J. M., and Fraser, S. E. (2003) MRI: volumetric imaging for vital imaging and atlas construction. *Nat. Rev. Mol. Cell. Biol.* **4** (**Suppl**). SS10–SS16.

66. Jacobs, R. E. and Fraser, S. E. (1994) Magnetic resonance microscopy of embryonic cell lineages and movements. *Science* **263,** 681–684.

67. Smith, B. R., Linney, E., Huff, D. S., and Johnson, G. A. (1996) Magnetic resonance microscopy of embryos. *Comput. Med. Imaging Graph.* **20,** 483–490.

68. Smith, B. R., Johnson, G. A., Groman, E. V., and Linney, E. (1994) Magnetic resonance microscopy of mouse embryos. *Proc. Natl. Acad. Sci. USA* **91,** 3530–3533.

69. Louie, A. Y., Huber, M. M., Ahrens, E. T., et al. (2000) In vivo visualization of gene expression using magnetic resonance imaging. *Nat. Biotechnol.* **18,** 321–325.

70. Johnson, G. A., Benveniste, H., Engelhardt, R. T., Qiu, H., and Hedlund, L. W. (1997) Magnetic resonance microscopy in basic studies of brain structure and function. *Ann. N. Y. Acad. Sci.* **820,** 139–147; discussion 147–148.

71. Ahrens, E. T., Laidlaw, D. H., Readhead, C., Brosnan, C. F., Fraser, S. E., and Jacobs, R. E. (1998) MR microscopy of transgenic mice that spontaneously acquire experimental allergic encephalomyelitis. *Magn. Reson. Med.* **40,** 119–132.

72. Benveniste, H. and Blackband, S. (2002) MR microscopy and high resolution small animal MRI: applications in neuroscience research. *Prog. Neurobiol.* **67,** 393–420.
73. Johnson, G. A., Cofer, G. P., Hedlund, L. W., Maronport, R. R., and Suddarth, S. A. (2001) Registered H-1 and He-3 magnetic resonance microscopy of the lung. *Mag. Reson. Med.* **45,** 365–370.
74. Glover, P. M., Bowtell, R. W., Brown, G. D., and Mansfield, P. (1994) A microscope slide probe for high resolution imaging at 11.7 Tesla. *Magn. Reson. Med.* **31,** 423–428.
75. Wind, R. A., Minard, K. R., Holtom, G. R., et al. (2000) An integrated confocal and magnetic resonance microscope for cellular research. *J. Magn. Reson.* **147,** 371–377.
76. Sidles, J. A. and Rugar, D. (1993) Signal-to-noise ratios in inductive and mechanical detection of magnetic resonance. *Phys. Rev. Lett* **70,** 3506–3509.
77. Schaff, A. and Veeman, W. S. (1997) Mechanically detected nuclear magnetic resonance at room temperature and normal pressure. *J. Magn. Reson.* **126,** 200–206.

II

ANATOMY

3

Magnetic Resonance Imaging of Embryonic and Fetal Development in Model Systems

Eric T. Ahrens, Mangala Srinivas, Saverio Capuano,
Hyagriv N. Simhan, and Gerald P. Schatten

Summary

We give an overview of the applications and methods of high-resolution anatomical magnetic resonance imaging (MRI) in the study of embryonic and fetal development in animal models. Challenges associated with performing *in utero* studies are described. Recent *in utero* images in mouse and in nonhuman primates are presented. Results using magnetic resonance microscopy in fixed mouse embryos and in amphibian embryos in vivo are reviewed. We discuss how studies of pregnancy in animal models aid in the translation of innovative new MRI techniques to clinical applications.

Key Words: *In utero* MRI; embryo; fetus; primate; developmental biology.

1. Introduction

The study of embryonic and fetal development in animal models is an application well suited to the multitude of capabilities offered by magnetic resonance imaging (MRI). High-resolution 3D MRI can noninvasively resolve fine details of body axis formation and organogenesis. Longitudinal studies can be used to visualize dynamic processes, such as morphological changes. Quantitative imaging methods, such as diffusion tensor imaging (DTI), can provide information about developmental changes at the cellular and microstructural level. Exogenous contrast agents can be employed to highlight specific tissues and patterns of cell migration, and possibly to visualize molecular developmental processes, such as patterns of gene expression.

The proliferation of valuable genetically manipulated animals, particularly mice, provides a strong rationale for developing noninvasive imaging techniques to monitor fetal development. Often, these genetic manipulations do not yield any viable embryos, produce embryos that become reabsorbed

From: *Methods in Molecular Medicine, Vol. 124*
Magnetic Resonance Imaging: Methods and Biologic Applications
Edited by: P. V. Prasad © Humana Press Inc., Totowa, NJ

preterm, or cause defects in extraembryonic tissues, such as the placenta; high-resolution MRI can be invaluable for rapidly assessing these phenotypes. Structural studies can be performed either *in utero* or in fixed specimens. In fixed subjects, extremely high field magnetic resonance microscopy (MRM) can be used to visualize the 3D embryo anatomy at near cellular isotropic resolution *(1–6)*.

Nonhuman primates (NHPs) are another high-value model system in which MRI can have great utility, although, to date, few developmental studies using MRI have been reported in NHPs *(7)*. NHPs are used as a model for abnormal pregnancies and fetal development. In rhesus macaques, oocyte collection, in vitro fertilization by assisted reproductive technologies, and embryo culture is well established *(8)*. The feasibility of generating transgenic NHPs has also been demonstrated *(9)*. Transgenic NHPs open up new possibilities for using genetic approaches to generate human disease models, and provide a pathway for the reliable and efficient study of critical gaps in our knowledge of early pregnancy outcomes in humans.

Recently, there has been intense interest in reproductive cloning technologies in animal models, such as by using somatic cell nuclear transfer techniques *(10,11)*. With cloned fetuses, an early high-resolution anatomical assessment of the fetal development will be an invaluable future application of MRI.

In this article, we give a brief overview of the applications and methods of high-resolution anatomical MRI applied to embryonic and fetal developmental studies in animal models. We describe some of the experimental challenges associated with performing *in utero* studies. Experiments in mice and in NHPs are described in detail, followed by a brief discussion of results in amphibians.

2. *In Utero* MRI: Technical Challenges

The most vexing challenge associated with *in utero* fetal MRI is minimizing motion image artifacts. The first line of defense is immobilization of the dam in a humane fashion by using anesthesia and physical restraints. Even in anesthetized subjects, motion artifacts can arise from both maternal and fetal sources. The dominant maternal motion sources affecting the uterus are from respiration, cardiac motion, blood flow, peristalsis, and bladder filling and emptying. Motion of the fetus represents another set of challenges, especially with the onset of cardiac activity and quickening. To minimize motional ghosts from all of these compounding sources, a multipronged approach is best. Strategies for treating subject displacements during the repetition time (TR) period have been reviewed by several authors (for example, *see* **refs.** *12* and *13*). A partial list of approaches include respiratory/cardiac triggering *(14–16)*, rapid imaging, retrospective gating *(17)*, signal averaging, and adaptive correction using navigator echoes *(18–21)*. In the uterus, the largest displacements are from maternal breathing motion. Artifacts from this can be minimized by triggering each radio frequency (RF) excitation of the pulse sequence at the same place in the respiratory cycle. It is preferable to use a mechanical ventilator to maintain the physiological stability of the anesthetized subject, and a trigger pulse can be conveniently generated by the ventilator during each cycle. Furthermore, the electrocardiogram signal from magnet-compatible chest electrodes can be used as a trigger source for cardiac gating. Dealing with embryo motion is more problematic. Anesthesia tends to attenuate large fetus displacements, but fetal cardiac motion must be handled with postprocessing approaches *(17–21)*. Rapid imaging sequences (e.g., single-shot echo planar imaging, EPI) that are fast enough to freeze fetal motion are only feasible at lower field strengths. At the extremely high field strengths used in many MRI and MRM systems, implementation of high-resolution, single-shot EPI is problematic; there is an increase in the ratio of T_1/T_2 as the magnetic field strength is increased, and imaging time increases monotonically with the parameter T_1/T_2 *(22,23)*. Additionally, at extreme fields, magnetic susceptibility mismatches among tissues in abdominal areas can significantly degrade magnetic field homogeneity and image quality of single-shot EPI.

Before MRI, subjects must be given general anesthesia to eliminate motion artifacts and to maintain proper positioning. A variety of injectable agents, such as dissociatives (ketamine, tiletamine), benzodiazepines (valium, zolazepam), α-2-adrenergic agonists (medetomidine, xylazine), barbiturates (pentobarbital), and hypnotics (propofol) are available for the sedation of rodents and NHPs before the induction of general anesthesia with inhalant agents (halothane, isoflurane, or sevoflurane). Ketamine is generally the agent of choice for preinhalant sedation of NHPs. Volatile anesthetic agents, such as isoflurane, are commonly used in human obstetrical anesthesia, especially for caesarian deliveries. Although all volatile inhalant anesthetics induce generalized CNS depression and freely cross the placenta *(24)*, isoflurane produces minimal cardiovascular effects in animals *(25)*. Furthermore, during inhalant anesthesia, an increase in the maternal inspired oxygen level can actually result in increased oxygen delivery to the fetus *(26)*.

Administration of inhalant anesthesia to a dam for an extended period (1–2 h) results in anesthesia of the fetus as well. Therefore, multiple steps must be taken to ensure the respiratory, cardiovascular, and thermoregulatory status of the dam and fetus during an imaging procedure. In NHPs, dams should be intubated with a cuffed endotracheal tube to maintain a patent airway and to protect against accidental aspiration of gastric contents. Additionally, an MRI-compatible pulse oximeter should be used to obtain continuous readings of the dam's oxygen saturation. The dam should also be instrumented with a large bore venous catheter in a readily accessible vessel (e.g., saphenous, or radial). This catheter will permit the administration of intravenous fluids for the purpose of blood pressure and hydration maintenance and can also serve as ready access for the administration of emergency drugs in the event of any adverse anesthetic reaction. Finally, an MRI-compatible heat source surrounding the dam must be used to prevent hypothermia and the accompanying hypotension that could affect blood flow to the placenta.

Other considerations include the possible adverse effects of the magnetic field and heating caused by RF power deposition. Widespread use of human MRI, with increasingly strong magnetic field strengths, is actively driving research in the safety aspects of MRI. There have been no teratological studies in humans, although several inconclusive epidemiological studies on children born to parents exposed to RF radiation have been carried out *(27)*.

The effect of static magnetic fields on embryogenesis has been studied in several model organisms, including chick *(28)*, frog *(29)*, mouse *(30)*, and rat *(31)*. The results of these studies are often contradictory; therefore it is still unclear whether the magnetic field has any effect *(32)*. Importantly, these studies involve long, continuous exposure and thus may not be relevant to typical MRI scans. In vitro studies on proteins have shown that large aggregates can experience a significant magnetic torque because of anisotropic diamagnetism *(33)*; however, the relevance of such studies to in vivo conditions remains unclear.

Several groups have shown that tissue heating from high levels of RF deposition can be harmful to developing embryos *(27)*. Raising maternal temperature in rats was found to increase birth defects in a dose-dependent manner *(34)*. Furthermore, fluids in the lens of the eye, and possibly also amniotic fluid, are poor at heat dissipation. However, no definite genotoxic or oncogenic effects have ever been identified from the RF absorption rates used in typical MRI protocols (reviewed in **ref.** *12*). One study directly measured the heating effect in amniotic fluid, fetal brain, and abdomen in pregnant pigs using fiber optic thermoprobes during the MRI scan *(35)*. A high RF duty factor imaging sequence was used (half-Fourier acquisition single shot turbo spin-echo [HASTE]), with 72 refocusing RF pulses, and it was found that temperature changes were minimal *(35)*. Thus, it seems unlikely that MRI, especially with low specific absorption rate (SAR), will have any adverse effects on the fetus.

3. Imaging Examples in Mice

Genetically altered mice are a major tool in the study of the molecular basis of development and serve as a model for human developmental disorders. MRI can be used to phenotype mouse embryos *in utero*. In addition, there are extraordinary technologies available for creating mouse models of contraception and infertility. The mouse is easily maintained and has short generation times, both of which provide strong justification for using lower mammals for modeling human pregnancy outcomes. Because MRI is noninvasive, one can image the same embryo repeatedly over the course of the pregnancy. Alternatively, at

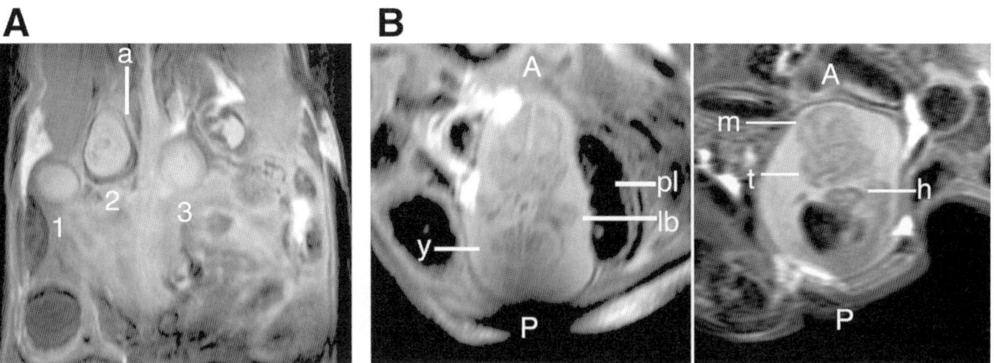

Fig. 1. In vivo images of the same pregnant mouse at two time-points; **(A)** shows 10.5-d *postcoitum* (dpc) embryos and **(B)** shows a 13-dpc embryo in two different orientations. In **(A)**, three embryos are numbered; a indicates uterus. In **(B)**, A and P indicate anterior and posterior; y, yolk sac cavity; pl, placenta; lb, limb bud; m, midbrain; t, telencephalon; and h, heart. Data were acquired at 11.7 T using a 2D Fourier transform spin-echo imaging sequence with repetition time (TR) / echo time (TE) = 1500/30 ms. Multiple contiguous slices were obtained with 110 × 80 μm in-plane resolution and 750-μm-thick slices. Respiratory gating was used to minimize image motional artifacts.

the experimental end point, one can use MRM to record a high-resolution digital 3D atlas of the intact, fixed embryo. If needed, one can perform traditional histological or histochemical analysis on the same embryo studied in vivo or with MRM.

Figure 1 shows an example of a pregnant C57Bl/6J mouse longitudinally imaged in vivo at two time points, at approx 10.5 d *postcoitum* (dpc) and 13 dpc. By 13 dpc, numerous anatomical features are clearly identifiable, such as the limb buds, midbrain, telencephalon, and two chambers of the developing heart. The imaging procedure was not harmful to the mother or embryo. From these types of data, one can assess embryo number, viability, developmental stage, as well as quantitatively assess phenotypic differences of the fetus and placenta during the pregnancy. These data were acquired in approx 20 min using a multislice 2D Fourier transform (2DFT) spin-echo imaging sequence on an 11.7 T MRM system. To limit motion-induced artifacts, the mouse was anesthetized using 1.25% isoflurane in 70% O_2 and 30% N_2O. The animal was then intubated and placed on a mechanical ventilator that produced a synchronized trigger signal to acquire each line in k-space.

An alternative approach to visualize the 3D embryo anatomy is by performing "virtual histology" *(36,37)* in fixed specimens using MRM. Standard histological methods involve extreme tissue manipulations, including fixation,

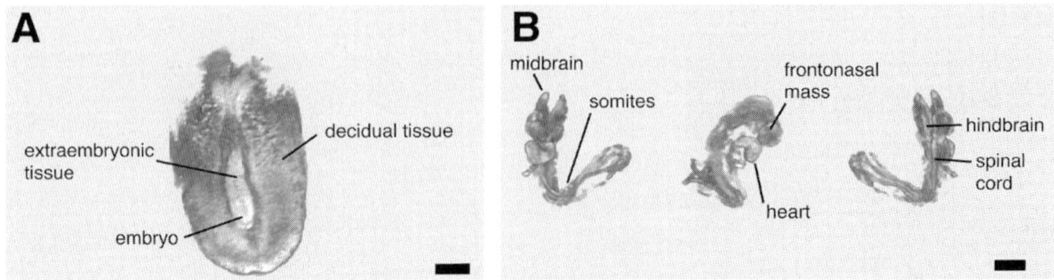

Fig. 2. Minimally annotated semitransparent volume renderings of fixed mouse embryos at 6.5 d *postcoitum* (dpc) (**A**) and 8.5 dpc (**B**). Three views of the 8.5-dpc embryo are shown: left, ventral; middle, side; and right, dorsal. Isotropic voxel resolution is 20 μm in both images. Data were acquired at 11.7 T using a 3D Fourier transform spin-echo imaging sequence with repetition time (TR) / echo time (TE) = 800/10 ms. Timed pregnancies between C57Bl/6J females and DBA/2J males were used to generate embryos at various stages. Pregnant females were euthanized and the embryos were excised and fixed by immersion in paraformaldehyde, then washed in PBS. For imaging, the fixed specimen was immersed in magnetite-doped agarose. Scale bar, 1 mm. Data are taken from Jacobs et al. *(4)*.

dehydrating, sectioning, and staining. The 3D fetus must be viewed as a series of digitized 2D sections. For a given embryo, the section orientation is fixed, and following complex 3D structures through multiple sections is problematic, as are comparisons among specimens. Furthermore, histologically prepared tissues undergo dehydration, which introduces substantial differential shrinkage artifacts and degrades the accuracy of morphometric analysis. With 3D MRM data, digitally sectioning the embryo at arbitrary angles, 3D segmentation, and morphometrics of complex structures are feasible.

Figures 2 and **3** show examples of fixed mouse embryos imaged in 3D with isotropic voxels using 11.7 T MRM instrumentation *(4,5)*. Embryos were excised at 6.5 dpc, 8.5 dpc, and 14.5 dpc and immersed in fixative (4% paraformaldehyde). In the 6.5-dpc embryo (**Fig. 2A**), the decidua was left intact and a cut-away view of the 3D data is shown *(4)*; T_2-weighted image contrast can be seen between embryonic and extraembryonic tissues. The 8.5-dpc embryo (**Fig. 2B**) has the extraembryonic tissue removed and shows three perspectives of a semitransparent surface rendering of the intact embryo *(4)*. The surface morphologies of several structures, such as the heart, somites, midbrain, hindbrain, and spinal cord, are apparent. **Fig. 3** shows a 14.5-dpc embryo; a semitransparent rendering reveals many clearly identifiable internal structures.

Although the tissue preparation method used in the examples shown in **Figs. 2** and **3** yields excellent and reproducible intrinsic MRI contrast, all fixation protocols produce some distortion from the homeostatic physiological state.

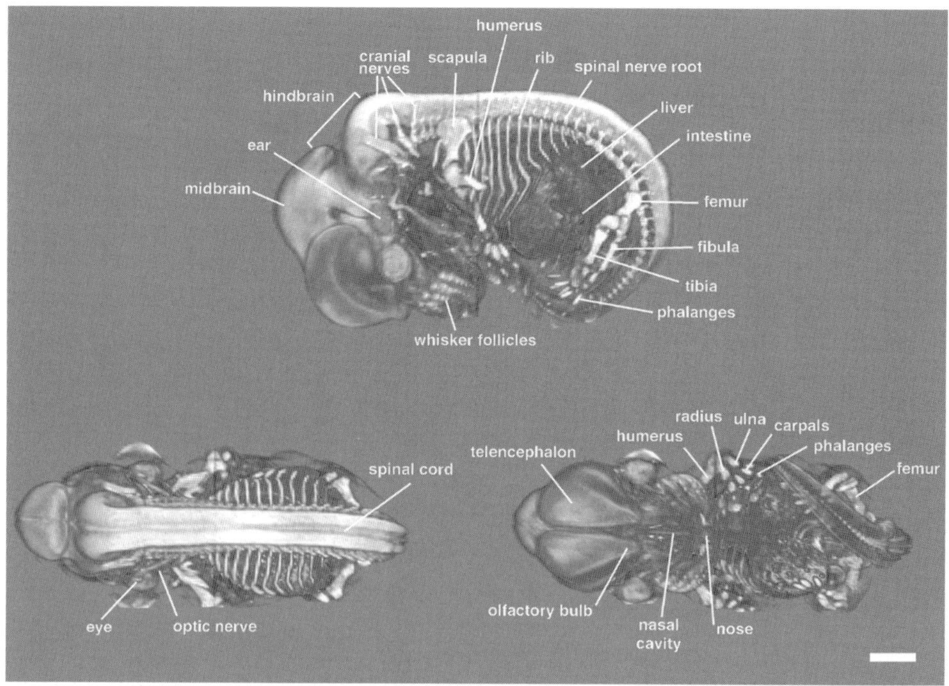

Fig. 3. Minimally annotated volume rendering of a 14.5-d *postcoitum* (dpc) fixed mouse embryo. In this semitransparent rendering, a large number of features are identifiable, not all of which are labeled. For example, the heart, somites, brachial arches, forming limbs, and digits are all apparent. Note the similar intensities of large nerves (e.g., cranial nerves) and the not-yet ossified skeletal system (e.g., scapula). Nonisotropic voxel size is 27 × 46 × 46 μm. Similar embryo preparation methods and MR acquisition parameters were used as in **Fig. 1**. Scale bar, 1 mm. Data are taken from Ahrens et al. *(5)*.

Nonetheless, this approach yields a more accurate quantitative representation of structure size than well-accepted histological analyses that use frozen, plastic, or wax-embedded sections, all of which undergo dehydration that introduces substantial structural artifacts. Thus, these types of data provide a valuable high-throughput alternative to histology for phenotyping normal and abnormal embryonic development.

MRM of fixed mouse embryos has been used in numerous studies. Progress toward construction of a mouse embryo atlas from normal fixed specimens at various embryonic stages has been described by several groups *(1,2,4–6,38–40)*. Novel methods for elucidating 3D angiography in fixed mouse embryos have been reported *(1,2)*; in these experiments the entire vasculature was rendered hyperintense via a gelatinous gadolinium-based contrast media that was perfused throughout the embryo through the umbilical vein. In studies of trisomy-16 mice, a model system for human Down syndrome, MRM was used to investigate fixed d-17 embryos exhibiting abnormal cerebellum development *(41)*.

Visualizing axonal fiber connectivity in embryos has long been a goal of developmental neurobiologists. Microscopic DTI is effective in elucidating the location and directionality of white matter fiber pathways in the brain *(3–5,42–44)*. Pathways are identified on the basis of their diffusion anisotropy of mobile water; other components of the CNS (e.g., gray matter or ventricles) exhibit essentially isotropic diffusion. Ahrens et al. *(5)* described visualizations of premyelinated fiber pathways using DTI methods in the spinal cord of a fixed 12.5-dpc mouse embryo. A more detailed DTI study of mouse embryos was reported by Zhang et al. *(44)*, which also compared Netrin-1 mutants with wild type. Although the image resolution is limited when compared with classical histological methods, the nondestructive nature of MRM makes it ideal for rapidly phenotyping the 3D embryonic anatomy at near cellular resolution.

4. Nonhuman Primates

Pregnancy studies in NHPs are invaluable in bridging the gap between rodent models and human clinical research. To date, biomedical researchers have only begun to consider MRI as a tool to study pregnancies in these important animal models *(7)*. MRI can noninvasively monitor the 3D embryonic development at a resolution far exceeding any other noninvasive technique, particularly ultrasound imaging, which currently is the most accepted approach. We are currently performing longitudinal MRI studies of fetal development in rhesus macaques. Initial studies are focusing on confirming that the same subject can be repeatedly anesthetized and imaged without any adverse effects on the pregnancy outcome. Secondarily, these studies show that maternal–fetal displacement artifacts can be managed to obtain quality MR images in a high-field scanner. Conventional ultrasound imaging is also performed in parallel with the MRI studies. Typical results are shown in **Fig. 4A–C. Figure 4A** is 40 to 44-d gestation; a differentiated tissue mass is apparent and shows the body axis, limb buds, developing brain, and liver. By 60 to 65-d gestation (**Fig. 4B**), the developing brain and many internal organs are apparent (e.g., heart, liver, spleen, intestines, bladder, and so on). The placenta is clearly seen in both images.

For comparative purposes, **Fig. 4C** shows a typical ultrasonogram of a 63 to 68-d rhesus macaque fetus. In veterinary medicine, ultrasonography remains the modality of choice for fetal imaging because of its speed, low cost, and portability. However, despite its usefulness for biometrics, determination of fetal sex, and screening for structural abnormalities, ultrasonography of the fetus is fraught with technical difficulties. Oligohydramnios, maternal obesity,

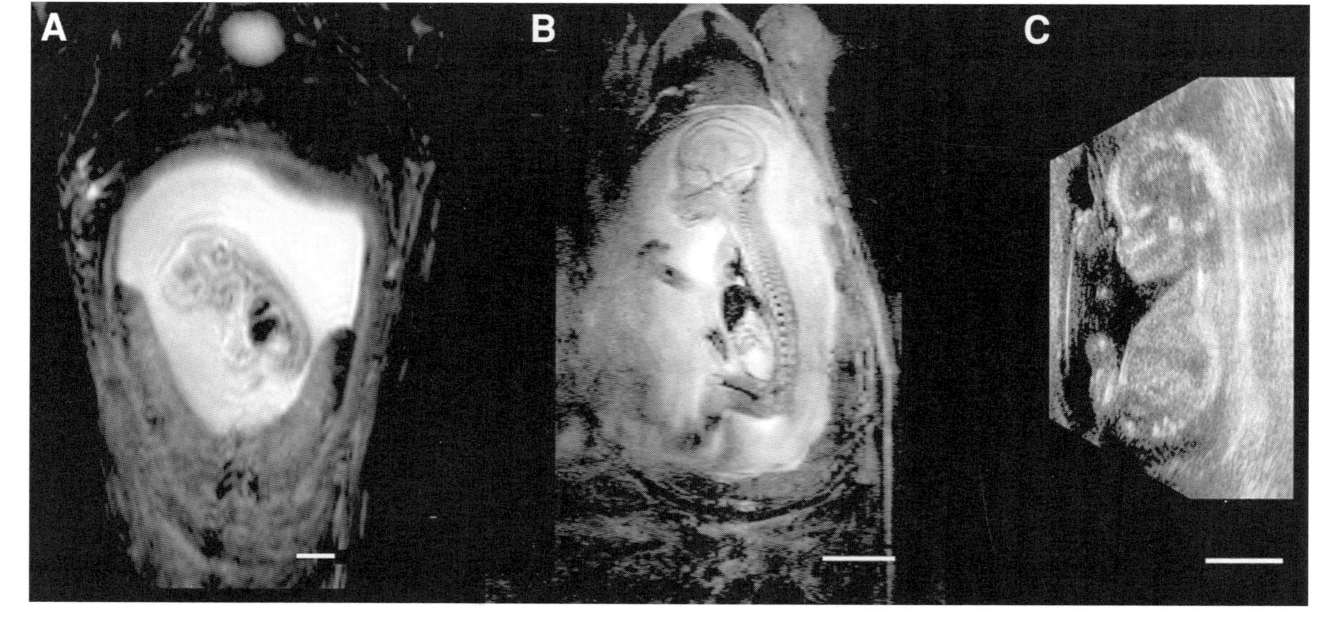

Fig. 4. *In utero* magnetic resonance imaging (MRI) of fetal development in Chinese rhesus macaque. (**A**) Shows a fetus at 40 to 44-d gestation and (**B**) at 60 to 65-d gestation. (**C**) Shows a typical ultrasonogram of a 63 to 68-d gestation of a macaque of Indian origin. Magnetic resonance images were acquired in anesthetized animals using a 4.7 T / 40 cm instrument using a T_2-weighted rapid acquisition with relaxation enhancement (RARE) spin-echo imaging technique, with eight lines of k-space per excitation. The in-plane resolution was approx 200 and 500 µm, for (**A**) and (**B**), respectively. The slice thickness was 1 and 3 mm for (**A**) and (**B**), respectively. The ultrasonogram was taken using a Siemens Sonoline Antares instrument. The scale bar represents 0.5 cm, 1 cm, and 2 cm for (**A**) to (**C**), respectively.

fetal head position, and fetal skull sonic interference have all been identified as factors that diminish image quality *(45)*. Furthermore, ultrasonograms of the fetal CNS often cannot detect structural anomalies and frequently are unable to detect subtle parenchymal abnormalities *(46)*.

In our MRI studies, the subject is anesthetized using an intramuscular injection of ketamine, intubated, placed on a mechanical ventilator, and kept under gaseous isoflurane anesthesia in oxygen for the duration of the experiment. The animal is placed in a laboratory-built cradle incorporating temperature-regulated heating pads, and a rectal thermometer records the core temperature. Blood oxygen levels and heart rate are monitored continuously during the experiment using an MRI-compatible optical sensor. The bladder is catheterized and a saline drip is connected for hydration. Typical imaging sessions last for 1.5 to 2 h. Images are acquired using a Bruker AVANCE DRX 4.7 T / 40-cm instrument equipped with a 30-cm, actively shielded gradient set and a 20-cm RF volume coil. MR images are acquired using a T_2-weighted RARE rapid spin-echo imaging technique, with eight lines of k-space per excitation. Multiple contiguous slices are acquired through the uterus. To limit breathing motion artifacts, each excitation of the imaging sequence is triggered by a logic pulse synchronized with the ventilator. The in-plane resolution is approx 200 and 500 μm for **Figs. 4A** and **B**, respectively. The imaging time is approx 20 min per data set. To date, there does not appear to be any detectable alteration in fetal development caused by any of our procedures. These studies will set the foundation for future studies investigating abnormal pregnancies and monitoring of cellular and molecular processes during development.

5. Amphibians

Amphibians are a widely studied model system in vertebrate development and are ideal subjects for in vivo MRM. *Xenopus laevis* (African clawed frog) embryos have been widely studied with both molecular and grafting approaches, are readily cultured, develop rapidly, and have large cells at early embryonic stages. *Xenopus laevis* were the subject of one of the first studies demonstrating microscopic MRI at a resolution of $10 \times 13 \times 250$ μm *(47)*. The work of Jacobs and Fraser *(48)* used MRM to follow cell lineages and cell movements over time in developing *Xenopus* embryos. A targeted cell from a 16-cell embryo was labeled intracellularly with a gadolinium (Gd)–DTPA–dextran agent using single-cell microinjection. Three-dimensional volumetric images were acquired every few hours, resulting in a time-lapse view of the lineage and movements of the labeled cells. Using MRM, it was possible to track the positions of both surface ectodermal and deep mesodermal cells *(48)* that would normally be inaccessible using optical probes in the intact embryo. *Xenopus* embryos and oocytes have also been used as a test-bed for in vivo studies of MRI contrast agents and novel cellular MRI approaches *(49–55)*. For example, Louie et al. *(49)* used MRI of *Xenopus* tadpoles to demonstrate the effectiveness of a novel class of contrast agents that can visualize gene expression in vivo.

6. Future Directions

There is a vast array of emerging MRI methodologies that have benefited from advances in instrumentation, software, new contrast agents, and pulse sequences that have yet to be applied to fetal imaging. Using commercially available MRM instrumentation, it is now feasible to obtain 10 to 100-μm-resolution 3D images of embryos in a reasonable acquisition time, and this should bring this once esoteric methodology into the imaging mainstream. For *in utero* studies, there are many potential avenues for improving the signal-to-noise ratio and image resolution, such as by using phased array coils *(56)* or by using surgically implantable surface coils *(57,58)*. New MRI contrast agents that report on cellular–molecular events during the course of the pregnancy will further expand the usefulness of MRI for developmental studies. For example, there has been significant progress in developing imaging agents that can track inflammatory cells in vivo with MRI, such as by using intracellular superparamagnetic iron-oxide nanoparticles *(59,60)*. These cellular imaging approaches may advance the understanding of the leukocyte invasion and the inflammatory response associated with physiological and pathological labor. Complementary imaging modalities, such as PET and bioluminescence, can be used to image monocyte activity and transgene expression in the developing embryo *(7,61–63)*. By amalgamating high-resolution anatomical MRI with data from PET or photonic reporters in the same subject, it is feasible to visualize a range of cellular–molecular information in its anatomical context.

Interdisciplinary approaches to solve clinical problems during pregnancy have been challenged by the appropriate limitations on experimental investigations using pregnant women. Challenges also arise in determining the appropriate mammalian animal model as well as their availability. In addition, there is the seemingly insurmountable problem of garnering quantitative spatial and temporal measures on fetal and placental normalcy without jeopardizing the pregnancy itself. In the United States, the generally accepted medical practice is that fetal MRI is restricted to circumstances in which high-resolution anatomic evaluation of the fetus is critical before delivery and in which ultrasound provides inadequate images. Many new MRI methodologies tested in model systems will eventually make their way into the clinical realm, perhaps even for routine obstetrics. Innovative techniques and application of protocols for investigating the genetic and environmental origins of pregnancy outcomes can first be applied to rodents in a timely and cost-effective manner, and, once this technology is perfected, it can be translated to the more precious NHP that closely mimics events in humans. Thus, there is a strong rationale for evaluating new MRI methodologies in model systems as a stepping-stone toward the clinical application of new MRI methodologies.

Acknowledgments

We thank Joyce Horner and Dr. Kevin Hitchens for their assistance. This work was funded in part by the National Institutes of Health (P50-ES012359 and P41-EB001977).

References

1. Smith, B. R., Johnson, G. A., Groman, E. V., and Linney, E. (1994) Magnetic-resonance microscopy of mouse embryos. *Proc. Natl. Acad. Sci. USA* **91,** 3530–3533.
2. Smith, B. R. (1999) Magnetic resonance microscopy for developmental biology. *Dev. Biol.* **210,** 222–222.
3. Jacobs, R. E., Ahrens, E. T., Meade, T. J., and Fraser, S. E. (1999) Looking deeper into vertebrate development. *Trends Cell Biol.* **9,** 73–76.
4. Jacobs, R. E., Ahrens, E. T., Dickinson, M. E., and Laidlaw, D. (1999) Towards a microMRI atlas of mouse development. *Comput. Med. Imaging Graph.* **23,** 15–24.
5. Ahrens, E. T., Blumenthal, J., Jacobs, R. E., and Giedd, J. N. (2000) Imaging brain development, in: *Brain Mapping: The Systems* (Toga, A. W. and Mazziotta, J. C., eds.), Academic, San Diego, CA, pp. 561–589.
6. Dhenain, M., Ruffins, S. W., and Jacobs, R. E. (2001) Three-dimensional digital mouse atlas using high-resolution MRI. *Dev. Biol.* **232,** 458–470.
7. Benveniste, H., Fowler, J. S., Rooney, W. D., et al. (2003) Maternal-fetal in vivo imaging: a combined PET and MRI study. *J. Nucl. Med.* **44,** 1522–1530.
8. Schatten, G., Hewitson, L., Simerly, C., Sutovsky, P., and Huszar, G. (1998) Cell and molecular biological challenges of ICSI: ART before science? *Law Med. Ethics* **26,** 29–37.5
9. Chan, A. W. S., Chong, K. Y., Martinovich, C., Simerly, C., and Schatten, G. (2001) Transgenic monkeys produced by retroviral gene transfer into mature oocytes. *Science* **291,** 309–312.
10. Wilmut, I., Schnieke, A. E., McWhir, J., Kind, A. J., and Campbell, K. H. S. (1997) Viable offspring derived from fetal and adult mammalian cells. *Nature* **385,** 810–813.
11. Campbell, K. H. S., McWhir, J., Ritchie, W. A., and Wilmut, I. (1996) Sheep cloned by nuclear transfer from a cultured cell line. *Nature* **380,** 64–66.
12. Stark, D. D. and Bradley Jr., W. G., eds. (1992) *Magnetic Resonance Imaging.* 2nd ed., vols. 1 and 2, Mosby-Year Book, St. Louis, MO.
13. Liang, Z. P. and Lauterbur, P. C. (2000) *Principles of Magnetic Resonance Imaging: A Signal Processing Perspective.* IEEE, Piscataway, NJ.
14. Cassidy, P. J., Schneider, J. E., Grieve, S. M., Lygate, C., Neubauer, S., and Clarke, K. (2004) Assessment of motion gating strategies for mouse magnetic resonance at high magnetic fields. *J. Magn. Reson. Imaging* **19,** 229–237.

15. Wiesmann, F., Szimtenings, M., Frydrychowicz, A., et al. (2003) High-resolution MRI with cardiac and respiratory gating allows for accurate in vivo atherosclerotic plaque visualization in the murine aortic arch. *Magn. Reson. Med.* **50,** 69–74.

16. Hofman, M. B. M., Paschal, C. B., Li, D. B., Haacke, E. M., Vanrossum, A. C., and Sprenger, M. (1995) MRI of coronary arteries—2D breath-hold vs 3D respiratory-gated acquisition. *J. Comput. Assist. Tomogr.* **19,** 56–62.

17. Lenz, G. W., Haacke, E. M., and White, R. D. (1989) Retrospective cardiac gating—a review of technical aspects and future-directions. *Magn. Reson. Imaging* **7,** 445–455.

18. Korin, H. W., Felmlee, J. P., Riederer, S. J., and Ehman, R. L. (1995) Spatial-frequency-tuned markers and adaptive correction for rotational motion. *Magn. Reson. Med.* **33,** 663–669.

19. Wood, M. L., Shivji, M. J., and Stanchev, P. L. (1995) Planar-motion correction with use of k-space data acquired in Fourier MR-imaging. *J. Magn. Reson. Imaging* **5,** 57–64.

20. Hedley, M. and Yan, H. (1992) Motion artifact suppression—a review of post-processing techniques. *Magn. Reson. Imaging* **10,** 627–635.

21. Ehman, R. L. and Felmlee, J. P. (1989) Adaptive technique for high-definition MR imaging of moving structures. *Radiology* **173,** 255–263.

22. Callaghan, P. T. (1991) *Principles of Nuclear Magnetic Resonance Microscopy,* Oxford University Press, New York, NY.

23. Ahrens, E. T. and Dubowitz, D. J. (2001) Peripheral somatosensory fMRI in mouse at 11.7 T. *NMR Biomed.* **14,** 318–324.

24. Dwyer, R., Fee, J. P., and Moore, J. (1995) Uptake of halothane and isoflurane by mother and baby during caesarean section. *Br. J. Anaesth.* **74,** 379–383.

25. Muir, W., Hubbell, J., and Skarda, R. (1989) *Handbook of Veterinary Anesthesia.* Mosby, St. Louis, MO, pp. 95–107.

26. Ramanathan, S., Gandhi, S., Arismendy, J., Chalon, J., and Turndorf, H. (1982) Oxygen transfer from mother to fetus during cesarean section under epidural anesthesia. *Anesth. Analg.* **61,** 576–581.

27. Heynick, L. and Merritt, J. (2003) Radiofrequency fields and teratogenesis. *Bioelectromagnetics* **Suppl 6,** S174–S186.

28. Espinar, A., Piera, V., Carmona, A., and Guerrero, J. (1997) Histological changes during development of the cerebellum in the chick embryo exposed to a static magnetic field. *Bioelectromagnetics* **18,** 36–46.

29. Denegre, J., Valles, J., Lin, K., Jordan, W., and Mowry, K. (1998) Cleavage planes in frog eggs are altered by strong magnetic fields. *Proc. Natl. Acad. Sci. USA* **95,** 14,729–14,732.

30. Narra, V. R., Howell, R. W., Goddu, S. M., Rao, D. V. (1996) Effects of a 1.5-Tesla static magnetic field on spermatogenesis and embryogenesis in mice. *Invest. Radiol.* **31,** 586–590.

31. Canedo, L., Cantu, R., and Hernandez, J. (2003) Magnetic field exposure during gestation: pineal and cerebral cortex serotonin in the rat. *Int. J. Dev. Neurosci.* **52,** 263.

32. Allahyar, K. and Robitaille, P. (2000) Biological effects and health implications in magnetic resonance imaging. *Concepts Magnetic Res.* **15**, 321–359.
33. Iwasaka, M., Ueno, S, and Tsuda, H. (1994) Effects of magnetic fields on fibrinolysis. *J. Appl. Phys.* **75,** 7162–7164.
34. Lary, J. M., Conover, D. L., Johnson, P. H., and Hornung, R. W. (1986) Dose-response relationship between body-temperature and birth defects in radio frequency-irradiated rats. *Bioelectromagnetics* **7,** 141–149.
35. Levine, D., Zuo, C., Faro, C., and Chen, Q. (2001) Potential heating effect in the gravid uterus during MR HASTE imaging. *J. Magn. Reson. Imaging* **13**, 856–861.
36. Johnson, G. A., Benveniste, H., Black, R. D., Hedlund, L. W., Maronpot, R. R., and Smith, B. R. (1993) Histology by magnetic resonance microscopy. *Magn. Reson. Q.* **9,** 1–30.
37. Johnson, G. A., Cofer, G. P., Gewalt, S. L., and Hedlund, L. W. (2002) Morphologic phenotyping with MR microscopy: the visible mouse. *Radiology* **222,** 789–793.
38. Smith, B. R., Linney, E., Huff, D. S., and Johnson, G. A. (1996) Magnetic resonance microscopy of embryos. *Comput. Med. Imaging Graph.* **20,** 483–490.
39. Schneider, J. E., Bamforth, S. D., Grieve, S. M., Clarke, K., Bhattacharya, S., and Neubauer, S. (2003) High-resolution, high-throughput magnetic resonance imaging of mouse embryonic anatomy using a fast gradient-echo sequence. *MAGMA* **16,** 43–51.
40. Chapon, C., Franconi, F., Roux, J., Marescaux, L., Le Jeune, J. J., and Lemaire, L. (2002) In utero time-course assessment of mouse embryo development using high resolution magnetic resonance imaging. *Anat. Embryol.* **206,** 131–137.
41. Kornguth, S., Bersu, E., Anderson, M., and Markley, J. (1992) Correlation of increased levels of class-I MHC H-2K(k) in the placenta of murine trisomy-16 conceptuses with structural abnormalities revealed by magnetic resonance microscopy. *Teratology* **45**, 383–391.
42. Basser, P. J. and Pierpaoli, C. (1996) Microstructural and physiological features of tissues elucidated by quantitative-diffusion-tensor MRI. *J. Magn. Reson. B* **111,** 209–219.
43. Ahrens, E. T., Narasimhan, P. T., Nakada, T., and Jacobs, R. E. (2002) Small animal neuroimaging using magnetic resonance microscopy. *Prog. Nucl. Mag. Res.* **40,** 275–306.
44. Zhang, J. Y., Richards, L. J., Yarowsky, P., Huang, H., van Zijl, P. C. M., and Mori, S. (2003) Three-dimensional anatomical characterization of the developing mouse brain by diffusion tensor microimaging. *Neuroimage* **20,** 1639–1648
45. Glastonbury, C. M. and Kennedy, A. M. (2002) Ultrafast MRI of the fetus *Australas. Radiol.* **46,** 22–32.
46. Levine, D. (2001) Ultrasound versus magnetic resonance imaging in fetal evaluation. *Top. Magn. Reson. Imaging* **12,** 25–38.
47. Aguayo, J. B., Blackband, S. J., Schoeniger, J., Mattingly, M. A., and Hintermann, M. (1986) NMR imaging of a single cell. *Nature* **322,** 190–191.
48. Jacobs, R. E. and Fraser, S. E. (1994) Magnetic resonance microscopy of embryonic cell lineages and movement. *Science* **263,** 681–684.

49. Louie, A. Y., Huber, M. M., Ahrens, E. T., et al. (2000) In vivo visualization of gene expression using magnetic resonance imaging. *Nat. Biotechnol.* **18,** 321–325.
50. Ahrens, E. T., Rothbacher, U., Jacobs, R. E., and Fraser, S. E. (1998) A model for MRI contrast enhancement using T1 agents. *Proc. Natl. Acad. Sci. USA* **95,** 8443–8448.
51. Huber, M. M., Staubli, A. B., Kustedjo, K., et al. (1998) Fluorescently detectable magnetic resonance imaging agents. *Bioconjugate Chem.* **9,** 242–249.
52. Pauser, S., Keller, K., Zschunke, A., and Mugge, C. (1993) Study of the membrane premeability of a paramagnetic metal complex on single cells by NMR microscopy. *Magn. Reson. Imaging* **11,** 419–424.
53. Sehy, J. V., Ackerman, J. J. H., and Neil, J. J. (2002) Apparent diffusion of water, ions, and small molecules in the Xenopus oocyte is consistent with Brownian displacement. *Magn. Reson. Med.* **48,** 42–51.
54. Sehy, J. V., Ackerman, J. J. H., and Neil, J. J. (2001) Water and lipid MRI of the Xenopus oocyte. *Magn. Reson. Med.* **46,** 900–906.
55. Pascolo, L., Cupelli, F., Anelli, P. L., et al. (1999) Molecular mechanisms for the hepatic uptake of magnetic resonance imaging contrast agents. *Biochem. Biophys. Res. Commun.* **257,** 746–752.
56. Wald, L. L., Carvajal, L., Moyher, S. E., et al. (1995) Phased-array detectors and an automated intensity-correction algorithm for high-resolution MR-imaging of the human brain. *Magn. Reson. Med.* **34,** 433–439.
57. Fenyes, D. A. and Narayana, P. A. (1998) In vivo echo-planar imaging of rat spinal cord. *Magn. Reson. Imaging* **16,** 1249–1255.
58. Arnder, L. L., Shattuck, M. D., and Black, R. D. (1996) Signal-to-noise ratio comparison between surface coils and implanted coils. *Magn. Reson. Med.* **35,** 727–733.
59. Ahrens, E. T., Feili-Hariri, M., Xu, H., Genove, G., and Morel, P. A. (2003) Receptor-mediated endocytosis of iron-oxide particles provides efficient labeling of dendritic cells for in vivo MR imaging. *Magn. Reson. Med.* **49,** 1006–1013.
60. Weissleder, R., Cheng, H. C., Bogdanova, A., and Bogdanov, A. (1997) Magnetically labeled cells can be detected by MR imaging. *J. Magn. Reson. Imaging* **7,** 258–263.
61. Contag, C. H. and Bachmann, M. H. (2002) Advances in vivo bioluminescence imaging of gene expression. *Annu. Rev. Biomed. Eng.* **4,** 235–260.
62. Costa, G. L., Sandora, M. R., Nakajima, A., et al. (2001) Adoptive immunotherapy of experimental autoimmune encephalomyelitis via T cell delivery of the IL-12 p40 subunit. *J. Immunol.* **167,** 2379–2387.
63. Gambhir, S. S., Barrio, J. R., Phelps, M. E., et al. (1999) Imaging adenoviral-directed reporter gene expression in living animals with positron emission tomography. *Proc. Natl. Acad. Sci. USA* **96,** 2333–2338.

4

Mouse Morphological Phenotyping
With Magnetic Resonance Imaging

X. Josette Chen

Summary

The field of mouse phenotyping with magnetic resonance imaging (MRI) is rapidly growing, with both MRI physicists and biologists starting to use MRI to identify mouse models of human disease. The purpose of this chapter is to provide details of the animal handling necessary for routine and robust in vivo imaging with particular emphasis on multiple-mouse imaging. In addition, techniques for perfusion-fixation for postmortem imaging of specimens and whole mice are given.

Key Words: MRI; magnetic resonance imaging; mouse; phenotyping; random mutagenesis; anesthesia; mouse handling; monitoring; central nervous system; cardiac; whole-body perfusion; excised organs.

1. Introduction

The mouse was the first live animal to be imaged using magnetic resonance imaging (MRI) *(1)*, but it has not been used extensively in small animal imaging experiments. Historically, rats and guinea pigs have been better studied because of their larger size, which allows for easier manipulation and more signal available for imaging. However, because both the draft sequences of the human and mouse genome have been completed in the last few years, the field of murine MRI is rapidly growing as biologists need new tools to discover models of human disease.

Although some diseases are associated with a specific gene (e.g., cystic fibrosis, Huntington's disease, and sickle-cell anemia) we can hardly expect this to be true of most diseases. It is probable that many functional disorders arise from a combination of failed genes or maybe even subtle mutations within genes. Toward the end of understanding the genome, there is now a worldwide effort to discover new mouse models of human disease by studying both genotype and phenotype—the physical and biochemical manifestation of a given genotype.

From: *Methods in Molecular Medicine, Vol. 124*
Magnetic Resonance Imaging: Methods and Biologic Applications
Edited by: P. V. Prasad © Humana Press Inc., Totowa, NJ

There are three complementary methods of creating new mouse models: targeted, gene-trap, and random mutagenesis *(2)*. The basic premise of these techniques is to engineer a subtle, genetically modified mouse and to study the resulting phenotype. If an interesting heritable mutant is found, genotyping is performed to fully characterize the genetics of the disease. With these methods, the rate-limiting factor is not the creation of the new mutant; rather, the time-consuming step is the phenotyping to hunt for useful disease models. This is where MRI could potentially play an essential role.

After creation of a new disease model, the model is characterized by looking for changes in anatomy, physiology, behavior, and function. Many of these tests can be done in vivo, but the final step is to perform histopathology to look for organ and biochemical abnormalities. This is not a desirable end point if there is only one mouse, and it is required for reproduction. Additionally, given the enormous numbers of mouse mutants produced, it is difficult for mouse pathologists to characterize each mouse in depth. By adapting the techniques and tools of MRI, which is inherently noninvasive, detailed images of the inside of a mouse can be taken without conventional "slicing and dicing." This way, one is able to make anatomical, physiological, and functional measurements in the same living mouse.

The field of mouse phenotyping with MRI is rapidly growing. Early approaches used fairly simple MRI techniques in conjunction with other phenotyping tests *(3–5)*. More recently, MRI physicists have started to develop methodologies to enhance mouse phenotyping *(6–12)*.

In this chapter, we will discuss how the mechanics of MRI has to change to phenotype mice; what sort of animal handling is required for in vivo imaging; what special considerations are required for focusing on different organ systems; considerations for postmortem imaging; and, finally, we will describe image analysis tools, with the concept of a digital atlas introduced as an automated tool to look for anatomical variants.

Typically, easy entry into this field is gained by using available clinical scanners and associated hardware and software. However, this chapter will focus primarily on using higher field magnets—specifically 7 T—for higher-resolution studies. The descriptions of animal handling and imaging applications are independent of the magnet choice, except where noted.

1.1. MRI Requirements to Phenotype Mice

1.1.1. Hardware

As discussed in more detail in Chapter 2, MRI uses a static magnet field, nonionizing radio frequency (RF) pulses, and magnetic gradients to give exquisite images of soft tissues. In the clinic, MRI is essential in both research and routine diagnosis. To scale the technology down to small animals—ranging in size from 25 to 40 g—requires a number of changes. Because there is less signal in mice, higher magnetic field strengths are better suited as useful signal scales with field strength; 7, 9.4, and 11.7 T are usual field strengths, as compared with 1.5 or 3 T for clinical MRIs. For comparison, the earth's magnetic field is only 0.5×10^{-4} T. Correspondingly, the RF also increases, as do the gradient field strengths, to obtain higher resolutions. The net result is the ability to image less than a hundred micrometers, instead of the usual millimeter resolution on clinical scanners. In general, two types of RF coils are used: volume and surface coils. Volume coils (either solenoid or birdcage coils) are used to excite and receive signal evenly over a large area. Solenoid coils are perpendicular to the main magnetic field and are typically used for imaging specimens. In contrast, birdcage coils are coaxial with the magnetic field, which makes them suited for in vivo studies in horizontally oriented magnets. Surface coils are more sensitive and excite a more localized area, but usually with a nonuniform profile. Hence, they are used to image regions close to the surface of the body, such as superficial tumors.

1.1.2. Pulse Sequences

A pulse sequence is a series of user-controllable commands that drives the gradients and the RF to obtain images. Different pulse sequences can exploit varying contrast mechanisms highlighting different anatomy *(13)*. For high fields, pulse sequences typically used are T_2-weighted or T_1-weighted with a contrast agent (*see* **Note 1**). The key thing to keep in mind when performing a phenotyping project is to maintain the same type of imaging from subject to subject for consistency.

Another factor that also results in increased imaging time is the fact that phenotyping requires full 3D images as opposed to a few 2D slices. Most importantly, it is only with 3D imaging that true volumes of structures can be measured. This also leads to the ability to digitally "slice and dice" in any direction, even at oblique angles. The use of 3D also allows the viewer to see the relationship of organ systems in real 3D space.

1.1.3. Increasing Throughput

When performing research in a biological research setting, the ability to find conclusive results requires studying multiple subjects—on the order of dozens—to improve the statistics of the experiment. From another point of view, random mutagenesis programs can create upwards of thousands of mice per year. With such numbers, using MRI as a phenotyping tool becomes problematic because imaging times for one mouse can be on the order of hours.

To overcome this problem, a number of groups have begun to investigate various methods to image multiple mice, thereby increasing throughput *(6,14–*

16) (*see* **Note 2**). Imaging mice four at a time in a cancer screen has been accomplished in our laboratory *(17)*. Prototypical four-mouse imaging systems are now commercially available (Varian NMR, Palo Alto, CA). We have more recently increased our throughput to 7 live mice and 16 fixed mice.

2. Materials

2.1. Animal Preparation for In Vivo Imaging

1. Anesthetic (e.g., isoflurane).
2. Oxygen.
3. Heat source (e.g., forced air or recirculating water bath).
4. Electrocardiograph (ECG) connectors (pads, tape, and needles).
5. ECG gel.
6. Temperature probe.
7. Respiratory bellows.
8. Animal monitoring system.
9. Saline ($\frac{1}{2}$ mL) and syringe.
10. Depilatory and electric razor.
11. Gloves and goggles.

2.2. Considerations for Multiple Mice

Everything from **Subheading 2.1.** and the following:
1. Custom-built loading array.
2. Large induction chamber.
3. Custom-built "sleds" with embedded ECG pads and temperature probe.
4. Centrifuge tubes with holes drilled into the tips.

2.3. Imaging Specific Organs

1. Motion restraints (e.g., Velcro or tape).
2. Triggering system for cardiac and/or respiratory gating.
3. Contrast agent (e.g., 1 mM/kg gadopentetate dimeglumine; Magnevist, Berlex, Wayne, NJ).

2.4. Postmortem Imaging (Excised Organs)

1. Injection anesthetic (e.g., Avertin).
2. Syringe and needle.
3. Scalpel.
4. Heparin (10 U/mL).
5. Saline.
6. Contrast agent (optional, e.g., 1 mM gadopentetate dimeglumine).
7. Fixative (formalin).
8. Proton-free susceptibility matching fluid (e.g., Fluorinert).
9. Nuclear magnetic resonance (NMR) sample tube that fits sample.
10. Gloves and goggles.

2.5. Postmortem Imaging (Whole Body)

1. Injection anesthetic (e.g., 100 mg/kg ketamine and 20 mg/kg xylazine).
2. Medical tape.
3. Custom-built mold for mouse.
4. Depilatory.
5. Ultrasound gel.
6. Ultrasound biomicroscope (Vevo 660, VisualSonics Inc., Toronto, Canada).
7. Intravenous catheter (0.62 mm outside diameter) with needle (24 gage, 0.75").
8. Peristaltic pump.
9. Saline.
10. Heparin (10 U/mL).
11. Contrast agent (e.g., 1 mM gadopentetate dimeglumine).
12. Food coloring (any color except red).
13. Fixative (e.g., 10% buffered formalin phosphate).
14. Gloves and goggles.

3. Animal Preparation for In Vivo Imaging

One of the advantages of MRI is the ability to image the living organism, which allows for longitudinal studies in the same subject. In other words, instead of performing histology on different mice at different time points, progress of disease or tumor in the same animal can be followed over time. The survival of the animal is especially important when studying valuable mutants that can be "one of a kind" as well as being expensive and difficult to produce.

3.1. Anesthesia and Monitoring

To perform in vivo imaging requires maintaining and monitoring the physiology of the mouse during imaging sessions. Anesthesia affords more control over the subject and a recent review discusses usage of different anesthetics for MRI *(18)*. In general, inhalation anesthetics, such as isoflurane and halothane, are employed because they are easy to control and are fairly gentle to the animal (*see* **Note 3**). Induction of the mouse is typically done at 3 to 4%, whereas maintenance is at 1% isoflurane in 100% oxygen. After induction, mice are injected intraperitoneally with saline to prevent dehydration. Because anesthesia causes the animal's temperature to drop, a heating system is necessary; in fact, Hedlund et al. have demonstrated that image quality improves with tighter temperature control *(19)*, though a few degrees of control is generally sufficient. Heating is usually done with forced, heated air or circulating water baths with feedback control (*see* **Note 4**).

Monitoring of the physiological state can involve any or all of the following: ECG, temperature, ventilation, exhaled CO_2, and blood pressure. However, more interfaces with the mouse require more preparation time. In general, the first two measurements are usually sufficient to observe the status of the mouse. Because the monitoring of the mouse will take place inside a magnetic field, all connections need to be nonmagnetic. Furthermore, to prevent interference from the gradients, either fiberoptic connections *(20)* or analog filters are necessary.

ECG connections can be made with copper tape, ECG pads, or silver needle electrodes. If using tape or pads, hair from the contact points (chest or limbs) must be removed. Applying ECG gel helps improve electrical contact. The internal temperature of the mouse can be monitored with a rectal probe.

Beyond simple monitoring of the mouse, some experiments require gating on either or both of the cardiac and respiratory signals (*see* **Subheading 5.**). With the ECG connections arranged across the mouse's chest, the respiratory signal can usually be seen superimposed with the cardiac signal. The two signals can be separated electronically but for a "cleaner" signal, a respiratory bellows system can be used to measure the breathing separately.

Although most of the monitoring equipment can be developed in-house with basic electronics equipment, commercial packages are available. Two of the most popular vendors that provide MR-compatible animal monitoring equipment are SA Instruments (Stony Brook, NY) and Rapid Biomedical (Wuerzburg, Germany).

3.2. Considerations for Multiple Mice

Animal handling is exacerbated when dealing with multiple mice. Because it is important to minimize the time the mouse is under anesthesia (*see* **Note 5**), every attempt should be made to streamline the process of preparing the individual mice. This is so that the first mice are not under anesthesia for too long while the other mice are being prepared. In our laboratory, we have devised several practical shortcuts to reduce preparation of seven mice to less than half an hour *(21)*. The MRI we use is a 7-T, 40-cm, clear bore magnet (Magnex, Oxford, UK) driven by a UnityINOVA console (Varian NMR) with four parallel receivers. The steps can be broken down into three categories described below (**Subheadings 3.2.1.–3.2.3.**).

3.2.1. The Mouse Loading System

The mouse loading system consists of two major parts: the "mouse hive" and the "loading array" (**Fig. 1**). The mouse hive's main function is to position up to 19 Millipede RF coils *(12)* in a hexagonal array inside the magnet bore. The loading array is designed to hold and transport multiple mice housed in 50-mL centrifuge tubes with holes drilled through their tips to allow entry of anesthetic gas. After the mice are anesthetized in the vicinity of the magnet, they are inserted into the modified centrifuge tubes and mounted onto the load-

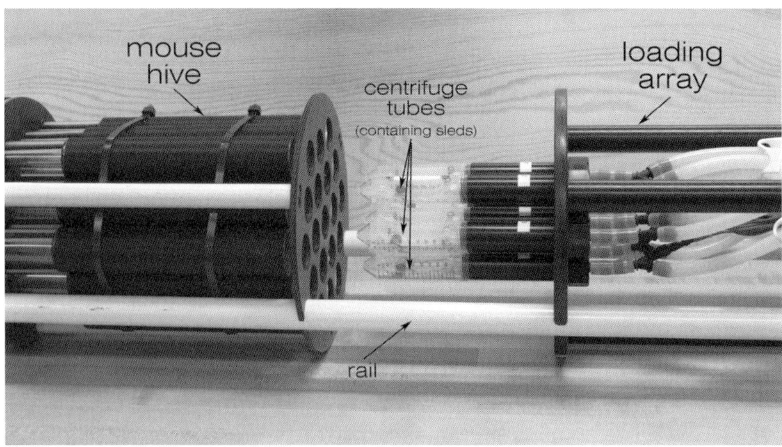

Fig. 1. The mouse loading system. The loading array and mouse hive are connected with a common fiberglass rail system. (Magnetic Resonance in Medicine copyright 2004 Wiley-Liss, Inc.)

ing array. After all mice are mounted, the loading array is transported and inserted into the magnet, where it is positioned on a rail system, which allows the array to couple with the mouse hive when pushed down bore of the magnet.

When fully inserted into the magnet, the centrifuge tubes dock onto the anesthetic delivery system within the RF coils (**Fig. 2**; *see* **Note 6**). Isoflurane mixed with oxygen is supplied from the mouse hive end to the specimen through a tube along the axis of each individual coil. This anesthetic gas mixture flows into the tubes, past the mice, and is collected by a passive scavenging unit attached to the back of the loading array.

3.2.2. The Induction Chamber

The custom induction chamber creates a single environment for both induction and handling of multiple mice (**Fig. 3**). Constructed from clear acrylic, the induction chamber features self-closing silicone iris ports to minimize anesthetic leakage and allows the user to access the internal environment without the need for special gloves. Compared with conventional mask and circuits for a single mouse, the induction chamber is large enough to house up to 20 mice and allows for free manipulation of the mice without the attachment of cumbersome tubes and masks. The unit is supplied with a constant flow of anesthetic gas, which is collected using a passive scavenging system. Resistive heating elements are used to heat the floor of the chamber to maintain the animals' body temperature during preparation (*see* **Note 7**).

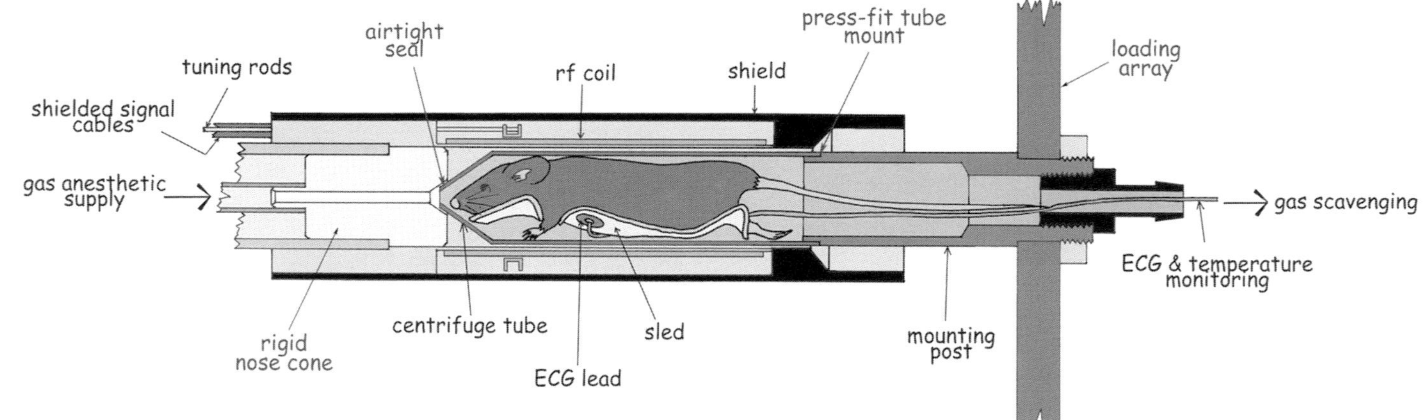

Fig. 2. Cross-sectional diagram illustrating the integration between the loading array and mouse hive. (Magnetic Resonance in Medicine © 2004 Wiley-Liss, Inc.)

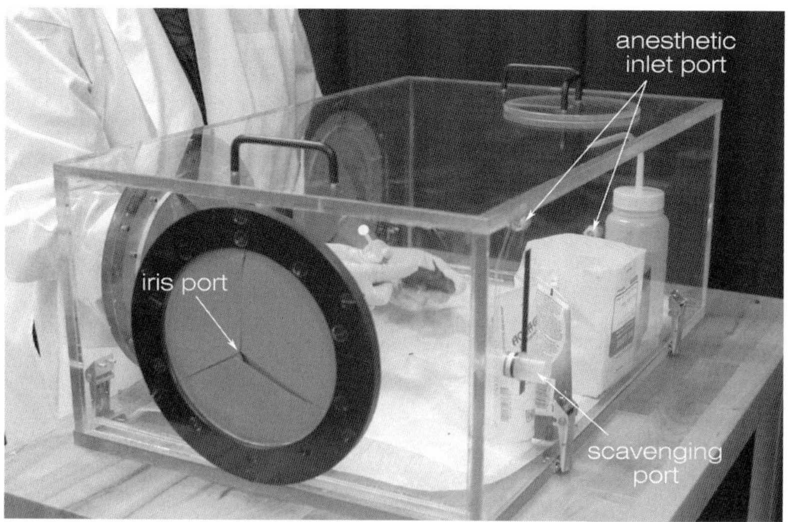

Fig. 3. The induction chamber. (Magnetic Resonance in Medicine copyright 2004 Wiley-Liss, Inc.)

3.2.3. The Sled

One of the most awkward and time-consuming aspects of preparing mice for the MRI are the application of ECG electrodes and rectal temperature probes. In addition, many of the conventional electrodes, such as cuff and needle electrodes, can distort the animal's posture, making it difficult to standardize positioning. Therefore, we devised a custom form-fitted positioning platform with embedded ECG and temperature probes called the sled (**Fig. 4**) (patent pending).

The sled was constructed by generating a precise physiological plaster facsimile of a representative specimen in a favorable position (*see* **Note 8**). Polypropylene sheets were then vacuum formed and cut around the plaster facsimile to create thin, lightweight, autoclavable sleds. Nonmagnetic neonatal/pediatric ECG electrodes were embedded into the sled to contact the chest, and a thermocouple was mounted in a similar fashion to measure skin temperature at the abdomen. A nonmagnetic electrical connector mounted on each sled allows for easy sensor connection to the loading system. Motion restraints made from Velcro fasteners are used to limit movement of the head.

After removing the hair from a mouse's chest (*see* **Note 9**), the mouse is positioned on a sled (**Fig. 4B**) and loaded into a modified 50-mL centrifuge tube. The sleds are electrically connected the monitoring system. Once the mice are all loaded, the loading array can be docked into the RF coils within the magnet bore.

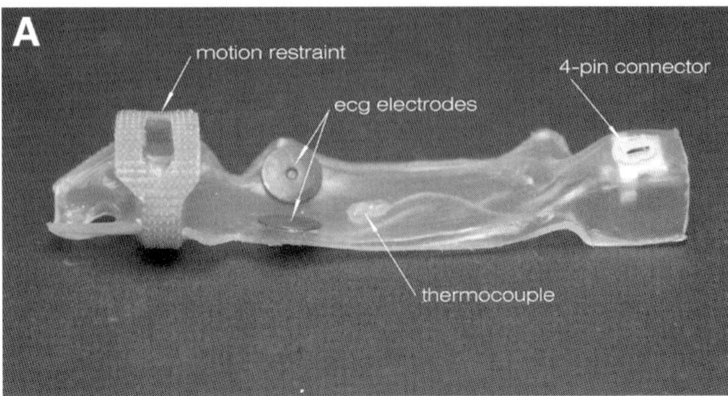

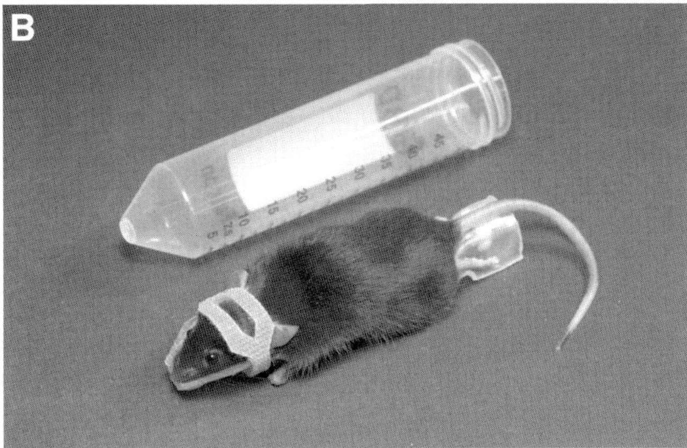

Fig. 4. **(A)** The sled, showing embedded monitoring sensors and head restraint. **(B)** An anesthetized mouse on a sled with the head restraint attached. The sled assembly easily slides into the centrifuge tube. (Magnetic Resonance in Medicine copyright 2004 Wiley-Liss, Inc.)

An added benefit in using the sled is that the position of the animal is standardized, making it easier for comparisons, either by observer or with postprocessing algorithms (*see* **Subheading 3.5.**).

3.2.4. Results

Figure 5 shows seven mice imaged at the same time arranged in the same configuration as in mouse loading array. The full 3D data sets are volume rendered, and cutaways show a single slice from each brain. MR parameters: 48 h before imaging, these mice were injected with $MnCl_2$ (*see* **Note 10**). Spin-echo sequence; repetition time (TR) = 300 ms; echo time (TE) = 7.7 ms; number of excitations (NEX) = 2; field of view (FOV) = (20 × 20 × 40) mm; matrix = 128 × 128 × 256; for a resolution of (156 µm)^3 and an imaging time of 2.75 h.

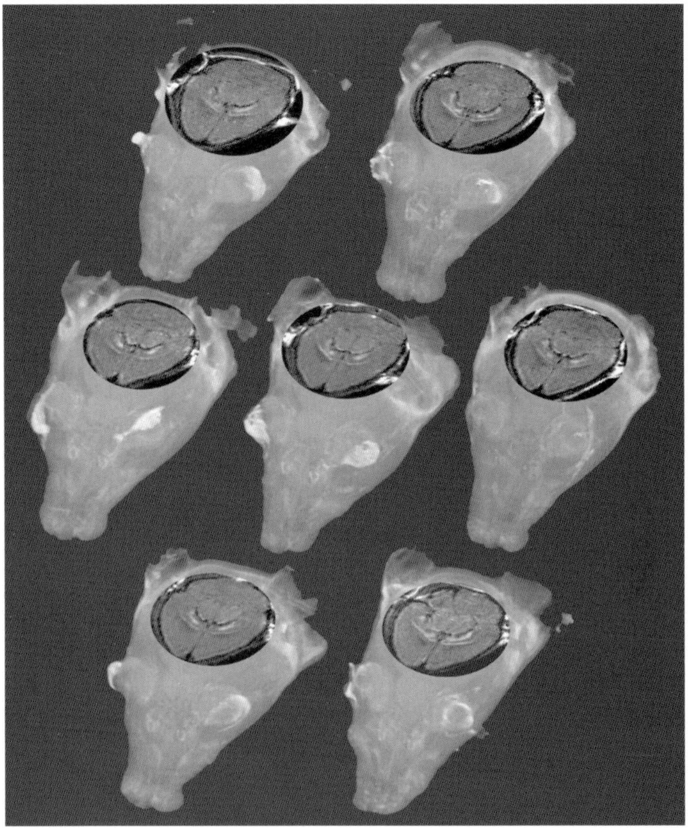

Fig. 5. Seven live mice imaged simultaneously. The full 3D data is volume rendered, with a horizontal slice shown in the cutaway.

3.3. Imaging Specific Organs

In many phenotyping experiments—especially targeted mutations—the anatomical region of interest is known, therefore, imaging can focus on that area. Currently, major developments have been for the brain and heart, although other organ systems are studied as well.

3.3.1. Brain

When the mouse is anesthetized, the head still moves, especially with inhalation anesthetics. Typically, most groups employ stereotaxic holders to fix the head position in place *(10,22,23)*. This type of approach is best when using surface coils or sufficiently large volume coils. Because we use birdcage coils that optimize filling factor, more form-fitting head restraints are used (**Fig. 4B**).

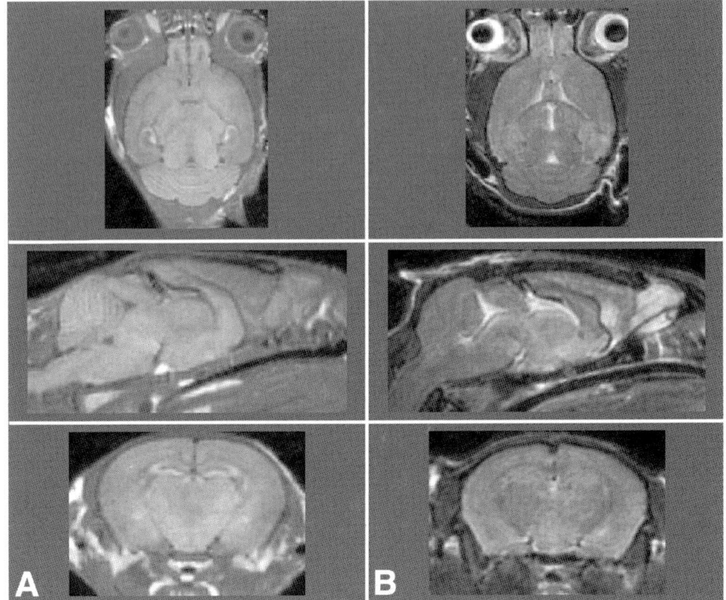

Fig. 6. Two examples of different contrast weighting in the brains of two different live mice. Three orthogonal views are shown for each mouse. (**A**) 48 h after ip injection of $MnCl_2$, this mouse was imaged with T_1 weighting and resolution of $(156 \ \mu m)^3$. (**B**) T_2-weighting with a fast spin-echo sequence and a resolution of $(115 \times 115 \times 104)$ μm^3. Please *see* **Subheading 3.3.2.** for further details.

Successful use of MRI to help phenotype mouse models of human disease include Alzheimer's disease *(24)*, Caravans disease *(25)*, megencephaly *(26)*, hydrocephalous *(27,28)*, as well as other CNS mutations *(29,30)*.

Mouse brain phenotyping has been recently used to follow growth of brain tumors *(17,31–35)*. Because these studies involve following a growth progression, careful attention must be paid to ensure reproducibility of position and imaging sequence in all scans.

3.3.2. Results

Figure 6 shows two examples of different contrast weighting in a live mouse. MR parameters for T_1-weighted image: 48 h before imaging, these mice were injected with $MnCl_2$ (*see* **Note 10**). Spin-echo sequence; TR = 300 ms; TE = 7.7 ms; NEX = 2; FOV = $(20 \times 20 \times 40)$ mm; matrix = $128 \times 128 \times 256$; for a resolution of $(156 \ \mu m)^3$ and an imaging time of 2.75 h. MR parameters for T_2-weighted image: fast spin-echo sequence; 40° flip angle; TR = 900 ms; eight echoes; effective TE = 36 ms (single echo TE = 12 ms); NEX = 2; FOV =

(24 × 24 × 40) mm; matrix = 208 × 208 × 384; for a resolution of (115 × 115 × 104) μm^3 and an imaging time of 2.7 h.

3.3.3. Heart

Because the mouse heart rate is between 300 and 500 beats per minute, accounting for motion is necessary to prevent artifacts in the images. Recently, several groups have investigated various gating strategies—in which the ECG signal generated from the mouse is used to trigger the MRI acquisition—and imaging paradigms *(36–39)*.

3.3.4. Other Organs

Organs that are in the vicinity of the thorax typically require respiratory gating; this motion is from the superior–inferior motion of the diaphragm. For example, studies of the liver and diaphragm require such gating *(39,40)*, whereas kidney and hindlimb studies only need securing of the region of interest with tape *(41–43)*.

As mentioned in **Note 1**, a consequence of imaging at high fields means that relaxation times (T_1) can be on the order of seconds. By lowering these times with a contrast agent, scans can be accomplished in a shorter amount of time. The most popular form of contrast agent is a chelated gadolinium compound, such as gadopentetate dimeglumine. To lower T_1 across almost all tissues (*see* **Note 10**), an ip injection of contrast agent is given 20 min before imaging (*see* **Note 11**).

3.3.5. Whole-Body Imaging

The ultimate goal in phenotyping with MRI is to image the whole body of a mouse. Because gene expression can occur in a number of organ systems, imaging the entire mouse is highly desirable. To our knowledge, no one has been able to image a whole mouse in vivo yet. Current work in our lab indicates that a fast spin echo is required along with motion compensation.

3.4. Postmortem Imaging

Without a doubt, in vivo imaging is an extremely useful aspect of MRI. However, MR images can approach microscopic resolutions when obtained postmortem. This is because animal motion and imaging time are no longer issues. Because the scan times can approach tens of hours, it is necessary to fix the mice because tissue degradation occurs during the first few hours after death.

3.4.1. Excised Organs

To image individual organs such as the brain, kidneys, and liver, the mouse is first fixed by conventional perfusion, which involves a midline incision fol-

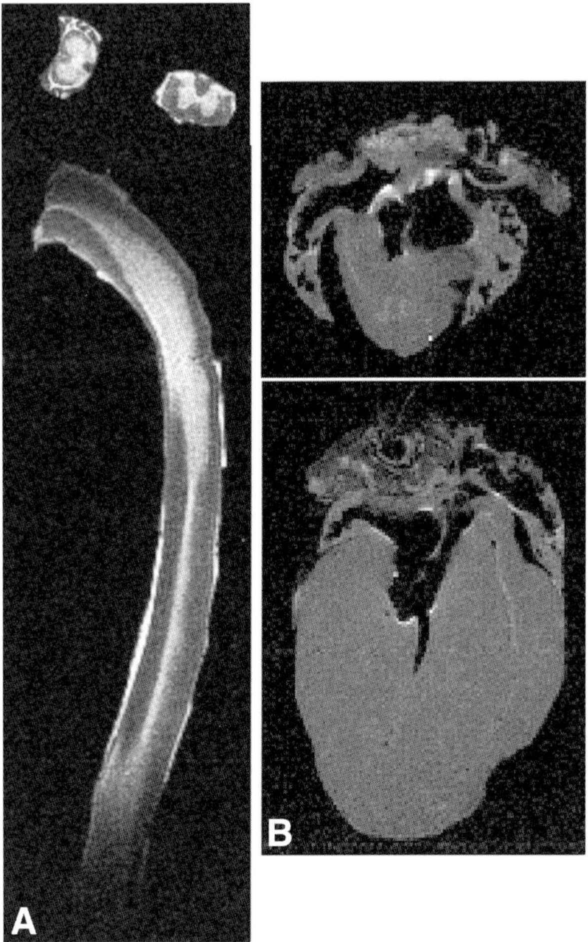

Fig. 7. Two examples of fixed specimens. (**A**) Cross-sectional views and the side view (bottom) of a fixed spine. (**B**) Short-axis view (top) and long-axis view (bottom) through a fixed heart.

lowed by a left ventricular puncture and drainage through the right atrium. A contrast agent can be mixed with the fixative solution to reduce imaging time (*see* **Note 12**). The organ of interest is then excised, immersed in a proton-free, susceptibility-matching fluid and imaged. The benefit of excision is that it allows use of smaller RF coils, which give better sensitivity. **Figure 7** shows examples of a fixed heart and spine. MR parameters for spine: spin-echo sequence; TR = 1600 ms; TE = 35 ms; NEX = 1; FOV = (6 × 13.8 × 13.8) mm; matrix = 100 × 230 × 230; for a resolution of (60 μm)^3 and an imaging time of 10.2 h. The spine was excised and cut into two pieces so it could fit into an

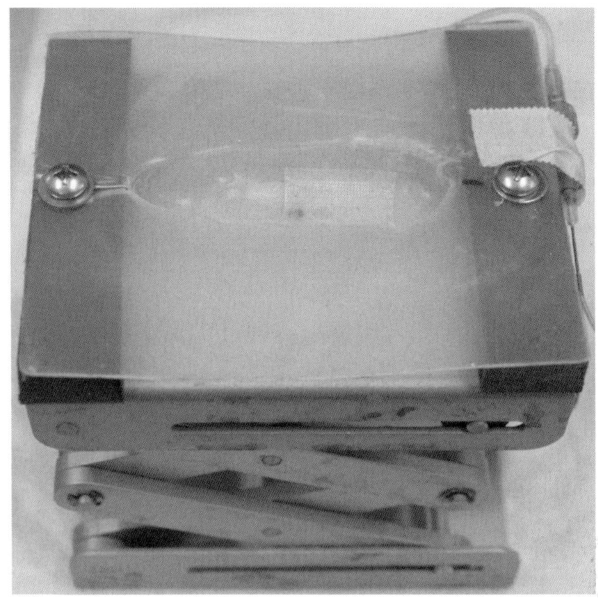

Fig. 8. The custom-built mold to preserve the shape of the mouse after whole-body perfusion and fixation.

existing coil. MR parameters for heart: spin-echo sequence; TR = 300 ms; TE = 9.2 ms; NEX = 1; FOV = (2.8 × 2.8 × 12) mm; matrix = 420 × 420 × 1800; for a resolution of (67 μm)^3 and an imaging time of 14.7 h.

3.4.2. Whole-Body Perfusion

Recently, there has been interest in preserving and imaging the entire mouse for phenotyping purposes *(9,44)*. The usual procedure to perfuse and fix the entire mouse is the same as in **Subheading 3.4.1.** However, the opening of the chest disturbs the integrity of the thoracic and abdominal cavity. To circumvent opening up the body, Johnson et al. use a multiple perfusion method that fixes all the organ systems with cannulations and drainages through various points in the body *(9,44)*. Alternatively, we have used an ultrasound-guided ventricular puncture and fixed the mouse via the beating heart *(45)*, which is described in the following paragraphs.

Mice are anesthetized using a mixture of ketamine/xylazine. When adequately anesthetized, the mouse is secured with tape in the supine position in a custom-built mold designed to maintain the mouse's natural body shape after fixation (**Fig. 8**). The hair on the chest wall is removed with a chemical hair remover. Ultrasound gel is spread over the precordial region and the ultrasound biomicroscope with a 30-MHz transducer is used to visualize the left

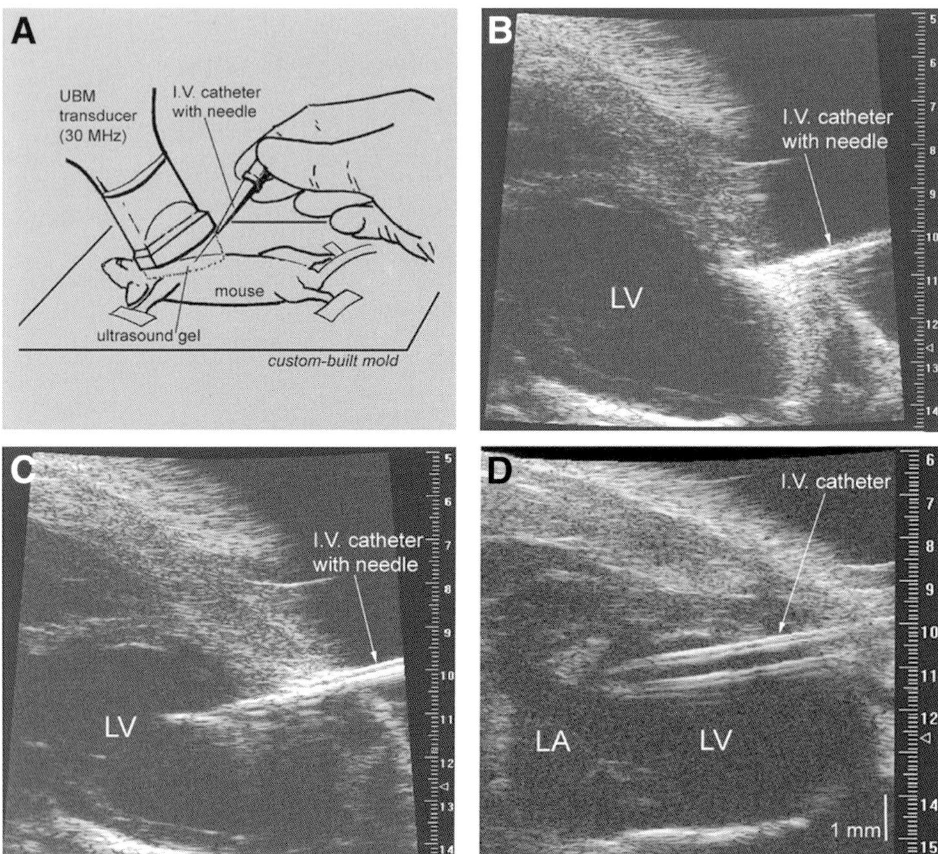

Fig. 9. Ultrasound-guided left ventricular catheterization of an anesthetized mouse. (**A**) Sketch showing the spatial relation among the mouse chest, ultrasound transducer, and the iv catheter with needle. (**B**) Two-dimensional ultrasound image showing the left ventricle (LV) and the tip of the needle on the surface of the chest. (**C**) Ultrasound image showing the needle punctured through the chest into the LV chamber. (**D**) Ultrasound image showing the catheter in the LV chamber after the needle was pulled out. (First published by the Nature Publishing Group, **ref. *45***).

ventricle (**Fig. 9A**). When the cross-section with the largest left ventricular chamber dimension is located, an iv catheter with needle is placed at the precordial area on the chest wall, with the longitudinal axis of the needle in the ultrasound imaging plane (**Fig. 9B**). Under real-time image guidance, the needle is punctured into the left ventricle (*see* **Note 13** and **Fig. 9C**). The needle is then removed and the catheter secured in place by tape (**Fig. 9D**) and connected to a peristaltic pump via a plastic tube. A mixture of saline, heparin, and

10 mM gadopentetate dimeglumine (Magnevist®, Berlex, Wayne, NJ) is perfused into the animal at a flow rate of 0.125 mL/min. This slow infusion with high concentration of the contrast agent is performed for about 5 min, to avoid rapid build-up of blood volume that could cause heart failure, and to ensure that the whole mouse is thoroughly perfused with contrast agent while the heart is beating. The jugular and femoral veins are cut to drain the blood and perfusate, and the mouse is flushed with a mixture of saline, heparin, 1 mM Magnevist, and blue dye (to monitor the progress of the perfusion) at a flow rate of 1.25 mL/min. Typically, the heart stops beating after 2 to 3 min with this faster perfusion procedure. When the drained fluid runs clear, a mixture of 10% buffered formalin phosphate, 1 mM Magnevist, and blue dye is pumped through at a flow rate of 1.25 mL/min for approx 15 min to fix the whole mouse. The perfusion and fixation procedure, from puncturing the left ventricle to the end of fixation, should take less than 30 min. During the perfusion, the proximal and distant ends of the right jugular vein and the right femoral vein are closed alternatively by hemostat to force the perfusate through the head, thorax, and abdomen.

3.4.3. Results

Figure 10 demonstrates a typical 3D data volume of a whole mouse MRI (**Fig. 10A**), and 2D cross-sections showing specific organs (**Fig. 10B–F**). The integrity of the thorax and the natural shape and spatial relation of the organs in the chest are well preserved (**Fig. 10B–D**), except for a small hole through the chest and the left ventricular wall because of the catheterization (**Fig. 10B**). MR parameters: spin-echo sequence; TR = 200 ms; TE = 10 ms; NEX = 1; FOV = (28 × 28 × 120) mm; matrix = 420 × 420 × 180; for a resolution of (67 μm)^3 and an imaging time of 9.8 h. Note that these parameters are specific to 7 T and the dosage of contrast agent. For higher fields, less contrast agent is used and the sequence timings will change *(46)*.

3.5. Image Analysis and Atlases

After acquisition of all of the images for a given study, the large amount of data must be analyzed. The most straightforward method is to use an image-processing package to segment the volumes of interest (*see* **Note 14**). This allows for quantitative comparisons between mutant and wild-type mice. **Figure 11** shows an example of a whole brain that has been segmented from a 3D image of a live mouse. Three internal structures have also been segmented and the volumes are easily calculated by voxel counting.

However, the image data contains much more information beyond simple volumetrics. A mutant can differ from a wild-type mouse through different shapes in structures or appearance of the tissue. This type of analysis requires

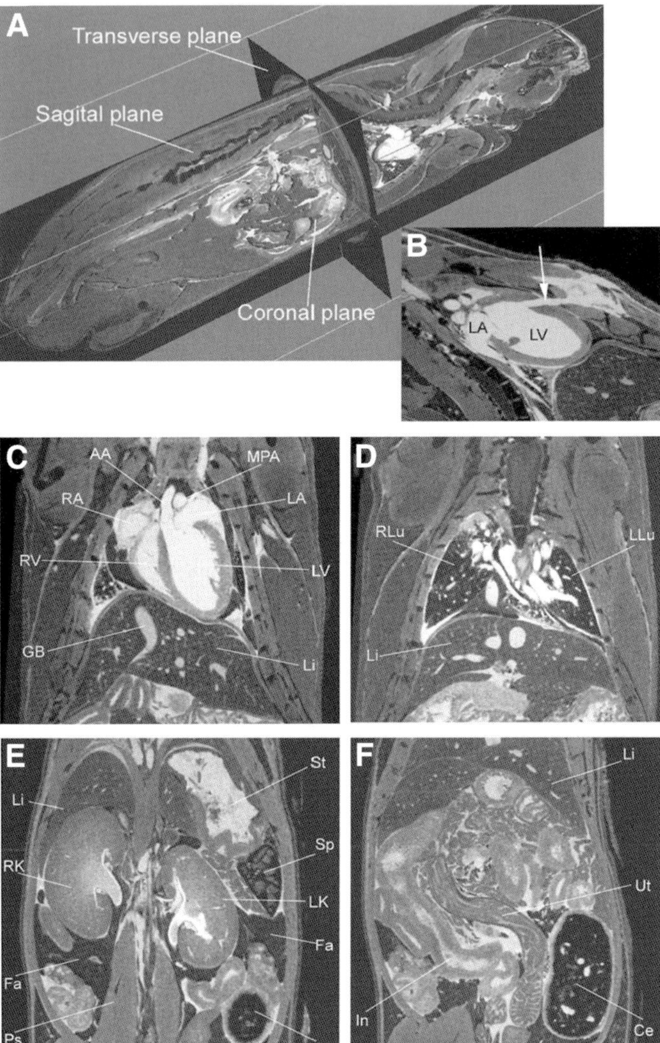

Fig. 10. Typical MR images of a mouse perfused with gadopentetate dimeglumine. (**A**) The 3D data volume of the whole-body MRI. (**B**) An oblique cross-section showing the left atrium (LA) and left ventricle (LV), and the hole (arrow) through the ventricular and the chest walls caused by the catheterization. (**C**) A coronal cross-section showing the cardiac structures, such as the LA, LV, ascending aorta (AA), right atrium (RA), right ventricle (RV), and main pulmonary artery (MPA) in the thoracic cavity, and the liver (Li) with gallbladder (GB). (**D**) A coronal cross-section showing the right lung (RLu) and left lung (LLu) and the pulmonary vasculature. (**E**) A coronal cross-section showing the right kidney (RK) and left kidney (LK), spleen (Sp), stomach (St), cecum (Ce), fat (Fa), and psoas (Ps) in the abdomen. (**F**) A slightly oblique coronal cross-section showing small and large intestines (In) and one horn of uterus (Ut). (First published by the Nature Publishing Group, **ref. 45**.)

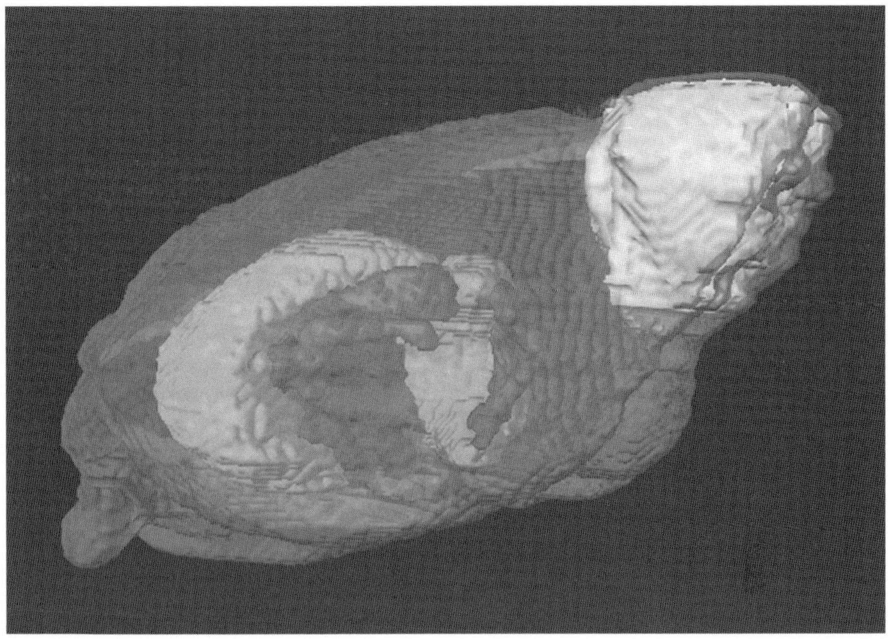

Fig. 11. Surface renderings of a wild-type brain and three internal structures: lateral ventricles, olfactory bulbs, and hippocampus.

more sophisticated image processing and leads to the concept of a "normal" mouse, as represented in an MR image. The idea of average or normal is relatively easy to comprehend when considering measurements such as heart rate or blood pressure; these are simple numbers that can be averaged across a sample of mice. However, this is not the case when dealing with anatomy in 3D space.

At the Mouse Imaging Centre, we are developing a variational atlas in which a number of normal age-, weight-, and sex-matched mice are imaged and then processed to give the variation from normalcy. A number of tools developed in human brain registration have been adapted for our purposes *(47,48)*. **Figure 12** shows our initial results from the averaging together of brains excised from nine 8-wk-old, male, inbred 129S1/SvImJ mice. We found the variability in this strain of mice to be low. For example, the mean volume and standard deviation of the cerebral cortex and corpus callosum were 109 ± 2 mm^3 and 13 ± 0.3 mm^3, respectively. Because the variability is so small, we believe that our variational atlas can serve as a metric against which mutants with anatomical anomalies can be measured. MR parameters: spin-echo sequence; TR = 1600 ms; TE = 35 ms; NEX = 1; FOV = $(12 \times 12 \times 24)$ mm; matrix = $200 \times 200 \times 400$; for a resolution of $(60 \ \mu m)^3$ and an imaging time of 18.5 h.

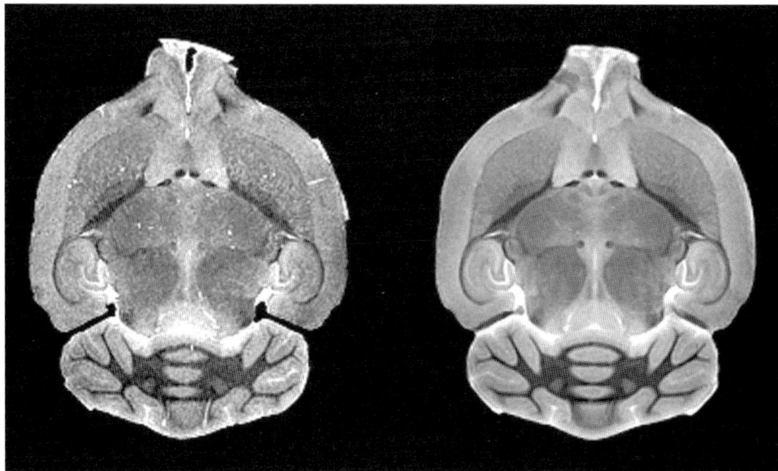

Fig. 12. Horizontal images from an individual excised brain (left) in comparison with the average atlas (right). The individual image suffers from artifacts, such as remnant fixative. The average brain shows overall improvement in the visibility and delineation of large anatomical structures but loss of definition in smaller structures, such as the blood vessels in the striatum.

4. Notes

1. A major ramification of imaging at high fields is that the T_1 (spin-lattice relaxation time) of tissues increases and converges to the same value. This results in increased imaging times and the lack of tissue contrast using T_1-weighted imaging unless a contrast agent is used. This means that T_2-weighted imaging is typically used. Another problem at high fields is an increased sensitivity to susceptibility differences, which makes gradient-echo techniques and fast-imaging techniques, such as spiral trajectories, difficult to use.

2. In general, there are two methods of multiple-mouse imaging, each having its own costs and benefits. The easier method involves placing several mice into clinical RF coils and using a clinical scanner. However, because the majority of clinical scanners are low field (1.5 and 3 T), the image resolution will be less than at high field. In addition, because the coil is so much bigger than the mouse, the so-called filling factor is low, leading to lower SNR. The more difficult method comprises using separate RF coils for each mouse in the same magnet. Although the implementation is more difficult, there is a significant gain in SNR. The theories behind these methods are fully discussed in **ref. 6**.

3. Injection anesthetics (e.g., ketamine/xylazine, or Avertin) can also be used because of their ease of use. However, it is cumbersome and disruptive to the image acquisition process to remove the mouse in the middle of an examination to check or maintain the anesthetic level. Alternatively, it is possible to maintain a catheter in the tail vein during the imaging session, but this adds a significant level of complication.

4. A water bath is usually not desirable because it is needs to be in close proximity to the mouse, thus necessitating a larger volume coil. This reduces the filling factor and, hence, the SNR. If a small, localized surface coil is used, then a water bath should have no impact on SNR.
5. A general rule to ensure recovery of the mouse is to only leave it under gas anesthetic for 3 h or less. Any longer runs the risk of compromising the health of the mouse.
6. To ensure an airtight seal with the anesthetic delivery system, two types of nose cones have been designed and fabricated: a rigid nose cone and a spring-loaded nose cone. The rigid nose cone is used only for the central position of the array and acts as a spacer to position the mice within the coils. The remaining positions in the array are all outfitted with spring-loaded nose cones to compensate for any geometrical discrepancies and create airtight seals with their respective centrifuge tubes.
7. Instead of custom building an induction chamber, a commercially available "glove box" can be modified to suit these purposes.
8. Our laboratory is currently in discussion with vendors who will be fabricating these sleds. Alternatively, it may be possible to cut down a centrifuge tube to serve as a platform for the mouse to lie in.
9. When imaging a large number of mice, we remove the hair from the mice the day before to save preparation time on the day of the scan.
10. The brain is difficult to perfuse with contrast agent because of the blood–brain barrier. Chapter 15 fully discusses the use of manganese as a novel brain contrast agent.
11. A popular method of getting contrast agent into the mouse is through a tail-vein injection. The benefit of doing so is that wash-in and wash-out curves can be made if the injection is done while the mouse is in the magnet. However, because tail-vein injections are labor intensive, we advocate using the ip method for rapid anatomical phenotyping.
12. As mentioned in **Note 10**, getting contrast into the brain is not easy. Current research in our lab is underway to investigate the use of mannitol to break the blood–brain barrier. The use of a nonchelated contrast agent ($GdCl_3$) has not been successful because the gadolinium precipitates out in formalin and paraformaldehyde.
13. It is critical to get the needle into the left ventricle on the first try because experience has proven that repeated punctures will kill the mouse.
14. One of the most popular "freeware" packages is NIH Image (http://rsb.info.nih.gov/nih-image/Default.html) for the Macintosh operating system. ImageJ is the java equivalent for all other environments and is found on the same webpage. Popular commercial software packages that offer more sophisticated segmentation algorithms and 3D rendering include Analyze (http://www.analyzedirect.com/) and Amira (http://www.amiravis.com/).

Acknowledgments

The author gratefully acknowledges the staff and students of the Mouse Imaging Centre. In particular, N. A. Bock, V. Bonn, L. Davidson, J. Dazai, Dr. R. M. Henkelman, Dr. N. Kovacevic, N. Lifshitz, B. J. Nieman, and Dr. Y. Q.

Zhou are thanked for providing figures and discussion. Also, the author thanks Drs. B. G. Bruneau and J. T. Henderson for providing samples.

This work is part of the Mouse Imaging Centre (MICe) at the Hospital for Sick Children and the University of Toronto. The infrastructure has been funded by the Canada Foundation for Innovation (CFI) and Ontario Innovation Trust (OIT). The research has been funded by an Ontario Research and Development Challenge Fund (ORDCF) grant to the Ontario Consortium for Small Animal Imaging (OCSAI).

References

1. Lauterbur, P. C. (1974) Magnetic resonance zeugmatography. *Pure Appl. Chem.* **40,** 149–157.
2. Bucan, M. and Abel, T. (2002) The mouse: genetics meets behaviour. *Nat. Rev. Genet.* **3,** 114–123.
3. Clapham, J. C., Arch, J. R., Chapman, H. et al. (2000) Mice overexpressing human uncoupling protein-3 in skeletal muscle are hyperphagic and lean. *Nature* **406,** 415–418.
4. Jalanko, A., Tenhunen, K., McKinney, C. E. et al. (1998) Mice with an aspartylglucosaminuria mutation similar to humans replicate the pathophysiology in patients. *Hum. Mol. Genet.* **7,** 265–272.
5. Jones, M. E., Thorburn, A. W., Britt, K. L. et al. (2000) Aromatase-deficient (ArKO) mice have a phenotype of increased adiposity. *Proc. Natl. Acad. Sci. USA* **97,** 12,735–12,740.
6. Bock, N. A., Konyer, N. B., and Henkelman, R. M. (2003) Multiple-mouse MRI. *Magn. Reson. Med.* **49,** 158–167.
7. Cha, S., Johnson, G., Wadghiri, Y. Z. et al. (2003) Dynamic, contrast-enhanced perfusion MRI in mouse gliomas: Correlation with histopathology. *Magn. Reson. Med.* **49,** 848–855.
8. Graf, H., Martirosian, P., Schick, F., Grieser, M., and Bellemann, M. E. (2003) Inductively coupled RF coils for examinations of small animals and objects in standard whole-body MR scanners. *Med. Phys.* **30,** 1241–1245.
9. Johnson, G. A., Cofer, G. P., Gewalt, S. L., and Hedlund, L. W. (2002) Morphologic phenotyping with MR microscopy: the visible mouse. *Radiology* **222,** 789–793.
10. Natt, O., Watanabe, T., Boretius, S., Radulovic, J., Frahm, J., and Michaelis, T. (2002) High-resolution 3D MRI of mouse brain reveals small cerebral structures in vivo. *J. Neurosci. Methods* **120,** 203–209.
11. Pautler, R. G. and Koretsky, A. P. (2002) Tracing odor-induced activation in the olfactory bulbs of mice using manganese-enhanced magnetic resonance imaging. *Neuroimage* **16,** 441–448.
12. Wong, W. H. and Sukumar, S. (2000) "Millipede" imaging coil design for high field micro imaging applications. Proceedings of the 8th Annual Meeting of ISMRM, Denver, CO, p. 1399.

13. Natt, O., Watanabe, T. Boretius, S., Frahm, J., and Michaelis, T. (2003) Magnetization transfer MRI of mouse brain reveals areas of high neural density. *Magn. Reson. Imaging* **21,** 1113–1120.
14. Matsuda, Y., Utsuzawa, S., Kurimoto, T. et al. (2003) Super-parallel MR microscope. *Magn. Reson. Med.* **50,** 183–189.
15. Schmiedl, U. P., Maravilla, K. R., and Nelson, J. A. (1991) Improved method for in vivo magnetic resonance contrast media research. *Invest. Radiol.* **26,** 65–70.
16. Xu, S., Gade, T. P., Matei, C., et al. (2003) In vivo multiple-mouse imaging at 1.5 T. *Magn. Reson. Med.* **49,** 551–557.
17. Bock, N. A., Zadeh, G., Davidson, L. M. et al. (2003) High-resolution longitudinal screening with magnetic resonance imaging in a murine brain cancer model. *Neoplasia* **5,** 546–554.
18. Lukasik, V. M. and Gillies, R. J. (2003) Animal anaesthesia for in vivo magnetic resonance. *NMR Biomed.* **16,** 459–467.
19. Qiu, H. H., Cofer, G. P., Hedlund, L. W. and Johnson, G. A. (1997) Automated feedback control of body temperature for small animal studies with MR microscopy. *I. E. E. E. Trans. Biomed. Eng.* **44,** 1107–1113.
20. Brau, A. C., Wheeler, C. T., Hedlund, L. W., and Johnson, G. A. (2002) Fiberoptic stethoscope: a cardiac monitoring and gating system for magnetic resonance microscopy. *Magn. Reson. Med.* **47,** 314–321.
21. Dazai, J., Davidson, L. M., Bock, N. A., Henkelman, R. M., and Chen, X. J. (2004) Multiple mouse biological loading and monitoring system for MRI. *Magn. Reson. Med.* **52,** 709–715.22. Benveniste, H., Kim, K, Zhang, L., and Johnson, G. A. (2000) Magnetic resonance microscopy of the C57BL mouse brain. *Neuroimage* **11,** 601–611.
23. Tada, T., Wendland, M., Kuriyama, N. et al. (2002) A head holder for magnetic resonance imaging that allows the stereotaxic alignment of spontaneously occurring intracranial mouse tumors. *J. Neurosci. Methods* **116,** 1–7.
24. Beckmann, N., Schuler, A., Mueggler, T. et al. (2003) Age-dependent cerebrovascular abnormalities and blood flow disturbances in APP23 mice modeling Alzheimer's disease. *J. Neurosci.* **23,** 8453–8459.
25. Matalon, R., Surendran, S., Rady, P. L. et al. (2003) Adeno-associated virus-mediated aspartoacylase gene transfer to the brain of knockout mouse for canavan disease. *Mol. Ther.* **7,** 580–587.
26. Diez, M., Schweinhardt, P., Petersson, S. et al. (2003) MRI and in situ hybridization reveal early disturbances in brain size and gene expression in the megencephalic (mceph/mceph) mouse. *Eur. J. Neurosci.* **18,** 3218–3230.
27. Cohen, A. R., Leifer, D. W., Zechel, M., Flaningan, D. P., Lewin, J. S., and Lust, W. D. (1999) Characterization of a model of hydrocephalus in transgenic mice. *J. Neurosurg.* **91,** 978–988.
28. Mueggler, T., Baumann, D. Rausch, M., Staufenbiel, M., and Rudin, M. (2003) Age-dependent impairment of somatosensory response in the amyloid precursor protein 23 transgenic mouse model of Alzheimer's disease. *J. Neurosci.* **23,** 8231–8236.

29. Xue, M., Balasubramaniam, J., Buist, R. J., Peeling, J., and Del Bigio, M. R. (2003) Periventricular/intraventricular hemorrhage in neonatal mouse cerebrum. *J. Neuropathol. Exp. Neurol.* **62,** 1154–1165.
30. Lin, T. Sandusky, S. B., Xue, H., et al. (2003) A central nervous system specific mouse model for thanatophoric dysplasia type II. *Hum. Mol. Genet.* **12,** 2863–2871.
31. Nelson, A. L., Algon, S. A., Munasinghe, J. et al. (2003) Magnetic resonance imaging of patched heterozygous and xenografted mouse brain tumors. *J. Neurooncol.* **62,** 259–267.
32. Moats, R. A., Velan-Mullan, S., Jacobs, R., et al. (2003) Micro-MRI at 11.7 T of a murine brain tumor model using delayed contrast enhancement. *Mol. Imaging* **2,** 150–158.
33. Rubin, J. B., Kung, A. L., Klein, R. S., et al. (2003) A small-molecule antagonist of CXCR4 inhibits intracranial growth of primary brain tumors. *Proc. Natl. Acad. Sci. USA* **100,** 13,513–13,518.
34. Weissfloch, L., Peller, M., Weber, J., et al. (2003) Comparison study of oxygen-induced MRI-signal changes and pO2 changes in murine tumors. *Adv. Exp. Med. Biol.* **530,** 461–465.
35. Yang, Y. S., Guccione, S., and Bednarski, M. D. (2003) Comparing genomic and histologic correlations to radiographic changes in tumors: a Murine SCC VII Model Study. *Acad. Radiol.* **10,** 1165–1175.
36. Nahrendorf, M., Hiller, K. H., Hu, K., Ertl, G., Haase, A., and Bauer, W. R. (2003) Cardiac magnetic resonance imaging in small animal models of human heart failure. *Med. Image Anal.* **7,** 369–375.
37. Schneider, J. E., Cassidy, P. J., Lygate, C., et al. (2003) Fast, high-resolution in vivo cine magnetic resonance imaging in normal and failing mouse hearts on a vertical 11.7 T system. *J. Magn. Reson. Imaging* **18,** 691–701.
38. Streif, J. U., Herold, V., Szimtenings, M., et al. (2003) In vivo time-resolved quantitative motion mapping of the murine myocardium with phase contrast MRI. *Magn. Reson. Med.* **49,** 315–321.
39. Cassidy, P. J., Schneider, J. E., Grieve, S. M., Lygate, C., Neubauer, S., and Clarke, K. (2004) Assessment of motion gating strategies for mouse magnetic resonance at high magnetic fields. *J. Magn. Reson. Imaging* **19,** 229–237.
40. Thomas, C. D., Chenu, E., Walczak, C., Plessis, M. J., Perin, F., and Volk, A. (2003) Morphological and carbogen-based functional MRI of a chemically induced liver tumor model in mice. *Magn. Reson. Med.* **50,** 522–530.
41. Checkley, D., Tessier, J. J., Wedge, S. R., et al. (2003) Dynamic contrast-enhanced MRI of vascular changes induced by the VEGF-signalling inhibitor ZD4190 in human tumour xenografts. *Magn. Reson. Imaging* **21,** 475–482.
42. Kostourou, V., Robinson, S. P., Whitley, G. S., and Griffiths, J. R. (2003) Effects of overexpression of dimethylarginine dimethylaminohydrolase on tumor angiogenesis assessed by susceptibility magnetic resonance imaging. *Cancer Res.* **63,** 4960–4966.
43. Raghunand, N., Howison, C., Sherry, A. D., Zhang, S., and Gillies, R. J. (2003) Renal and systemic pH imaging by contrast-enhanced MRI. *Magn. Reson. Med.* **49,** 249–257.

44. Johnson, G. A., Cofer, G. P., Fubara, B., Gewalt, S. L., Hedlund, L. W., and Maronpot, R. R. (2002) Magnetic resonance histology for morphologic phenotyping. *J. Magn. Reson. Imaging* **16**, 423–429.
45. Zhou, Y. Q., Davidson, L., Henkelman, R. M. et al. (2004) Ultrasound-guided left-ventricular catheterization: a novel method of whole mouse perfusion for microimaging. *Lab. Invest.* **84**, 385–389.
46. Nieman, B. J., Chen, X. J., Zhou, Y. Q., Davidson, L. M., Sled, J. G., and Henkelman, R. M. (2004) The relaxation effects of gadolinium concentration at 1.5 T and 7.0 T in fixed mice. Proceedings of the 11th Annual Meeting of ISMRM, Toronto, Canada, p. 808.
47. Collins, D. L. and Evans, A. C. (1997) Animal: validation and applications of nonlinear registration-based segmentation. *Int. J. Pattern Recogn.* **11**, 1271–1294.
48. Woods, R. P., Grafton, S. T., Watson, J. D., Sicotte, N. L., Mazziotta, J. C. (1998) Automated image registration: II. Intersubject validation of linear and nonlinear models. *J. Comput. Assist. Tomogr.* **22**, 153–165.

5

Magnetic Resonance Microscopy of Mouse Brain Development

Susumu Mori, Jiangyang Zhang, and Jeff W. M. Bulte

Summary

Magnetic resonance imaging (MRI) is increasingly becoming an important tool to study anatomy of rodent brains. Compared with histology, it has clear advantages because the entire 3D object can be captured as an image nondestructively. However, low imaging resolution and a small number of available contrast mechanisms are two critical disadvantages. In this article, the future potential of magnetic resonance (MR) microimaging is discussed, with special emphasis on diffusion tensor microimaging as an effective contrast mechanism for the developing central nervous system.

Key Words: Mouse; brain; MRI; microimaging; diffusion tensor imaging; DTI.

1. Introduction

Since the end of 1980s, it has become increasingly common to use high-field magnets (>9.4 T) to image small biological tissues samples, which can be as small as few millimeters (MR microscopy) *(1)*. MR microscopy can be applied to both in vivo and ex vivo samples. Although imaging living samples is one of the biggest advantages of MRI, living samples often pose significant limitations in pursuing higher resolutions. For example, high-resolution imaging requires rather long scanning times and prohibits motions larger than the pixel size. These issues can be significantly ameliorated by imaging tissue samples ex vivo (*see*, e.g., a publication by Johnson et al., **ref. 2**). One may argue the usefulness of MR microscopy for ex vivo samples because histology can provide thorough characterization with high in-plane resolution and numerous staining techniques. However, compared with traditional histology, MR microscopy allows a 3D characterization of tissue samples. It is nondestructive and, therefore, is free from sectioning-related artifacts and is often less labor intensive than histology. What it cannot measure up to with histology is the in-

From: *Methods in Molecular Medicine, Vol. 124*
Magnetic Resonance Imaging: Methods and Biologic Applications
Edited by: P. V. Prasad © Humana Press Inc., Totowa, NJ

plane imaging resolution and the variety of contrasts (histochemical staining) that histology commands. The resolution limitation of MR microscopy is believed to be approx 10 µm, which is dictated physically by the diffusion of water molecules between voxels and depends on available gradient strength *(2–7)*. The resolution of MRI is far less than histology (approx 1 µm for light microscope) and not high enough to examine morphology at the cellular level. However, the situation changes if one is interested in 3D examination of the sample. The thickness of a histology section is typically 10 to 20 µm, which the resolution of MR microscopy is approaching. In traditional histology, it is often practically impossible to obtain evenly spaced consecutive slices throughout the entire sample, something MR histology can easily achieve. Furthermore, because traditional histology usually samples only a limited area of tissues, MR and conventional histology are complementary to each other, that is, MR histology provides macroscopic characterization of tissue anatomy and traditional histology provides microscopic cellular characterization.

Probably the most significant limitation of MR microscopy stems from the lack of tissue contrast for delineation of various anatomical structures. Similar to the fact that unstained histological preparation is of limited value, the usefulness of MR images hinges on its power to provide contrast for differentiating various anatomical units. As long as MRI signal depends on the distribution of water molecules and their interactions with local environment, the only sources of contrast are subtle differences in the local physical and chemical environments in which these water molecules are located. If a biological event of interest does not alter the local environment significantly, it will be undetectable by MRI. Devising a new MR contrast method is, thus, an important research effort.

In this chapter, we will focus on the application of MR microscopy to the study of mouse brain anatomy and mouse brain development. Special emphasis will be placed on diffusion tensor imaging (DTI) because DTI often provides unmatched detail of cytoarchitecture of developing brains. We also confine the content to postmortem samples because of several limitations in current MR microscopy techniques, as mentioned previously. As long as we are imaging postmortem samples, we always have to ask ourselves what is the advantage of doing MRI over histology. This point will be highlighted in the following sections.

1.1. Diffusion Tensor Microimaging

MRI provides different contrast mechanisms and each contrast can be achieved on the same sample by appropriately adjusting image acquisition parameters. Most widely used contrast mechanisms are based on relaxation parameters of water molecules, such as T_1, T_2, and $T_2{}^*$. Previous studies have shown that these types of contrast can readily distinguish large brain structures, such as ventricles, white matter, and various gray matter structures. Therefore, the next target of MR microscopy is differentiation of smaller substructures within gray and white matter. For example, the cortex consists of multiple layers, which requires special staining techniques to examine individually, whereas white matter consists of various tracts with different orientations and paths. Unfortunately, conventional MR contrast mechanisms often fail to distinguish these substructures.

DTI is a new type of MRI that can provide unique image contrast called "diffusion anisotropy" *(8–10)*. Three important tissue-characterizing parameters can be obtained using DTI. First, the average extent of water diffusion (apparent diffusion constant) can be quantified, which provides information on restrictions and boundaries (e.g., higher packing density of cells) that water molecules encounter. If these obstacles have coherent alignment (e.g., axonal tracts), water, on average, tends to diffuse more along a certain axis (diffusion anisotropy). The degree of this diffusion anisotropy can be measured using DTI, which is the second important parameter. The anisotropy is higher when the density of the ordered structures (e.g., axonal fibers) is high *(11–14)*. Third, DTI can determine the orientation of such ordered structures *(10,15–18)*, which has recently been used for tract reconstruction *(19–23)*.

In **Fig. 1**, a process of DTI is shown using a schematic diagram. DTI measures the extent of water diffusion along many axes (**Fig. 1B**). From these measurements, orientations of the ordered structures, such as axonal tracts, are estimated (**Fig. 1C**) and several images with different contrast properties are calculated, such as anisotropy maps and orientation maps or a combination of the two (called color-coded orientation map or simply color map hereafter).

2. Applications of DTI

2.1. MR Microimaging of Adult Mouse Brains

The advent of gene engineering technologies has allowed the use of murine models for the study of involvement of specific genes in brain anatomy, pathology, and development. This generates a need for reliable methods for quick characterization of macroscopic anatomy to monitor possible phenotype changes *(24)*. As described in **Subheading 1.**, standard histological examination is often labor intensive and 3D macroscopic analysis is limited by tissue deformation and damage caused by sectioning processes. MR microscopy has been shown to have the potential to become a valuable option for phenotype-related brain characterization with high throughput and accuracy *(2,3,24)*. In **Subheadings 2.1.1.** and **2.1.2.**, usefulness of MRI to delineate detailed neural structures of adult mouse brains will be demonstrated.

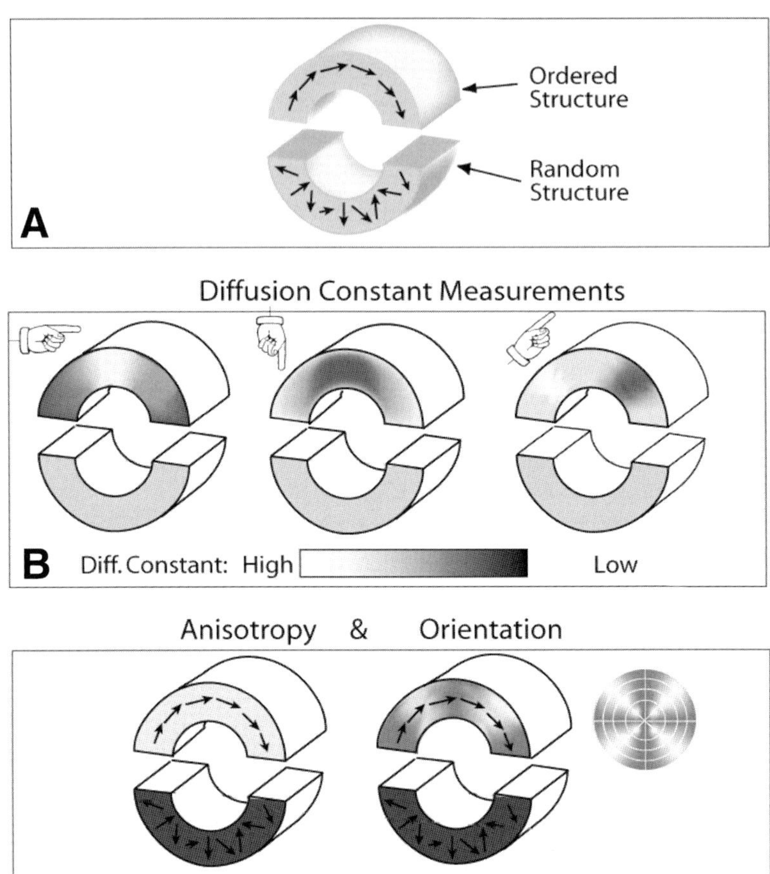

Fig. 1. Diffusion tensor imaging (DTI). (**A**) A schematic diagram of tissue structures. The upper region has an ordered structure caused by fibers running along the curved arrow. The lower region, although the shape of the structure is the same, has random fiber structure. (**B**) The results of diffusion measurement along three different axes are indicated by pointed fingers. The apparent diffusion constant becomes faster if the fiber orientation coincides with the measurement orientation and slower when they are perpendicular to each other. This results in different diffusion constants, which depend on the measurement orientation in the upper region, although the lower region is insensitive to measurement orientation. (**C**) Results of DTI. Anisotropy (diffusion directionality) of the upper region is high because the diffusion constant of this region depends on measurement orientation. When anisotropy is high, the fiber angle can be calculated based on the information in (**B**), which can be represented by vectors or by color. In this two-dimensional example, regions with fibers running horizontally are green and those running vertically are red. Transition areas become yellow, which is the mixture of green and red.

2.1.1. Information Obtained From Various Types of MR Contrasts

Figure 2 shows comparison of T_2-weighted, diffusion-weighted, and color map images. It can be seen that each contrast provides unique anatomical information. T_2 contrast (**Fig. 2B**) is heavily influenced by myelin content (the more myelin there is, the darker it appears) and provides a good gray matter–white matter contrast. A diffusion-weighted image (**Fig. 2C**) is suitable to define brain and ventricle shapes. A DTI-based color map carries rich information on the white matter and several gray matter structures with coherent axonal structures, such as thalamus and hippocampus. In **Fig. 3**, a comparison of histology and color maps is shown with anatomical assignments. Detailed assignments of colliculus and hippocampus are also shown in **Fig. 4**. These examples clearly demonstrate the usefulness of DTI to elucidate neuroanatomy.

2.1.2. DTI Study of Hippocampus

A striking landmark of the hippocampus is a dark arrow-like structure in Nissl staining (**Fig. 5A**), which corresponds to the stratum pyramidale (SP, the body of the arrow) and the stratum granulosum (SG, the arrow-head). We have investigated the hippocampal region of fixed C57BL/6J mouse brains using high resolution DTI and conventional T_2-weighted imaging and compared the results with published histological data.

Figure 5 shows coronal images of a histological slice (**Fig. 5A**), a T_2-weighted image (**Fig. 5B**), an isotropically diffusion-weighted image (iDWI) (**Fig. 5C**), an average apparent-diffusion coefficient map (ADCav) (**Fig. 5D**), a fractional anisotropy map (FA) (**Fig. 5E**), and a color map (**Fig. 5F**). The iDWI and ADCav maps clearly show the arrow-like structure. From comparison with histology, we tentatively assigned them the SP in the hippocampus and the V-shaped SG in the dentate gyrus. The SP/SG could be readily identified because of their low intensities in iDWI (**Fig. 5C**) and high intensities (55% higher than surrounding region) in ADCav images. This suggests high diffusion constants in these areas. Interestingly, the T_2-weighted image had lower intensity in regions that corresponded to SP defined in the iDWI, whereas the region corresponding to the SG layer did not show strong contrast with respect to surrounding tissue. The pattern of FA maps is much more complex, with no apparent correlation between these two layers and certain FA values. In the color map slice, we found that fibers in the stratum moleculare of the dentate gyrus and the stratum radiatum of the hippocampus run perpendicular to the surface of the SG and SP, respectively.

Once identified by MRI, 3D properties of these structures, such as their shapes and volumes, can be identified. **Fig. 6** shows an example of 3D analysis, which would be very time and labor intensive using conventional histology-based approaches (and could also be prone to artifacts during sectioning).

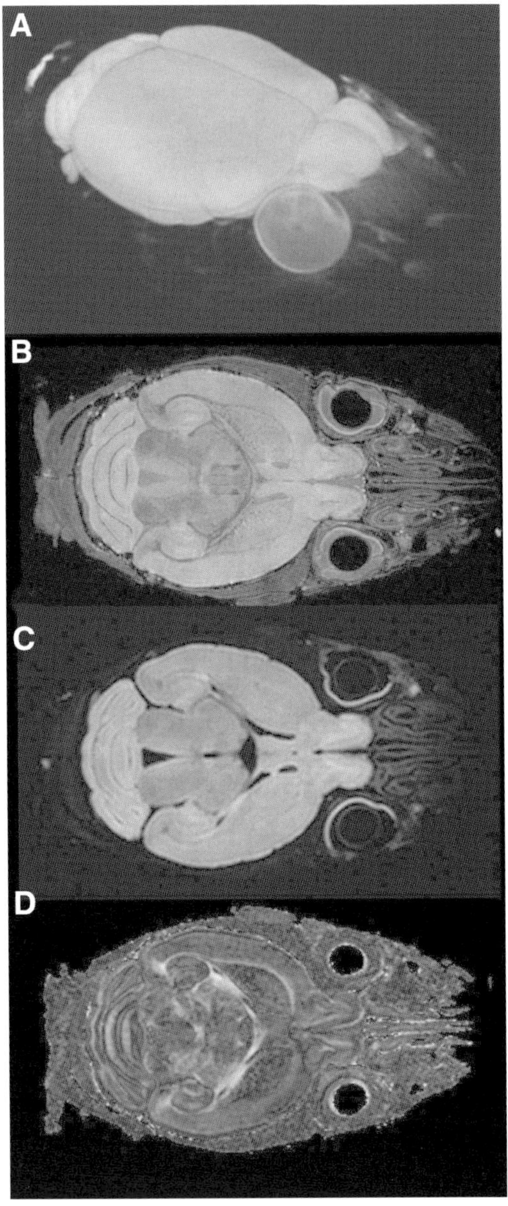

Fig. 2. Comparison of various magnetic resonance (MR) contrasts of a mouse brain. MR allows us to image a sample in 3D **(A)** with different types of contrast; **(B)** a T_2-weighted image; **(C)** a diffusion-weighted image; and **(D)** a color-coded orientation map. In **(D)**, red, green, and blue colors represent fibers running along anterior–posterior, right–left, and superior–inferior orientations, respectively. Images were acquired using an 11.7 T spectrometer (Bruker Biospin MRI, Inc., Billerica, MA). The mouse

2.2. Diffusion Tensor Microimaging of Developing Mouse Brains

Brain development consists of a cascade of complex, yet highly harmonized processes, of neuronal cell proliferation, migration, and differentiation. These processes have been studied mostly with optic- and electron-microscopy, which can provide cellular-level information, but spatially limited views. To study the dynamic process of 3D evolution of brain structures, the development of 3D-imaging techniques is essential. Although there are a number of techniques for obtaining 3D information about biological tissues *(2,6,25–30)*, it has not been possible to discretely identify early critical nervous structures, such as neuroepithelium (NE), cortical plate (CP), and axonal organization, without sectioning and/or staining processes. MR diffusion tensor microimaging allows rapid characterization of the 3D morphology of developing brains using their endogenous contrast and with minimum perturbation of the tissue.

Compared with conventional MRI, DTI is a breakthrough technology for imaging of the premyelinated central nervous system (CNS), because it provides a far superior contrast in delineating the neuroanatomy. This is demonstrated in **Fig. 7**. Conventional MRI is a useful technique to delineate the overall shape of CNS. However, it provides rather poor anatomical information for internal CNS structures. This is because conventional relaxation-based MR images, such as T_1 and T_2, rely on differences in chemical composition of tissues.

Fig. 2. *(continued)* brain sample was left in phosphate-buffered saline for 24 h and placed inside a custom-built, MR-compatible container filled with MR-inert fomblin (Fomblin Profludropolyether, Ausimont, Thorofare, NJ). A birdcage coil (20 mm in diameter) was used as radio frequency transmitter and receiver. The T_2-weighted image was acquired using a 3D fast spin-echo sequence with echo time (TE)/repetition time (TR) of 60/1200 ms with three signal averages. The field of view was 20.5 mm × 15.5 mm × 10 mm, and the matrix size was 512 × 256 × 256. The total imaging time was 8 h. Diffusion-weighted images were acquired using multiple spin-echo sequences with eight echoes, a TE/TR of 30/700 ms, and two signal averages. The field of view was 20.5 mm × 15.5 mm × 10 mm, and the matrix size was 128 × 88 × 80. Six diffusion weighted images with b value of 1200 mm²/s and two non–diffusion-weighted images were acquired. The total imaging time was 22 h. The diffusion tensor image (DTI) was calculated using a multivariate linear-fitting method and three pairs of eigenvalues and eigenvectors were calculated for each voxel *(37)*. The eigenvector associated with the largest eigenvalue was called the primary eigenvector. For the quantification of anisotropy, fractional anisotropy (FA) *(9)* was used. The color-coded orientation map was generated using the primary eigenvector data and FA. The red, green, and blue value of each pixel is defined by the orientation of the primary eigenvector and the intensity was proportional to the FA *(18)*. Red was assigned to the fiber orientation along anterior–posterior axis, green to the medial–lateral axis, and blue to the dorsal–ventral axis.

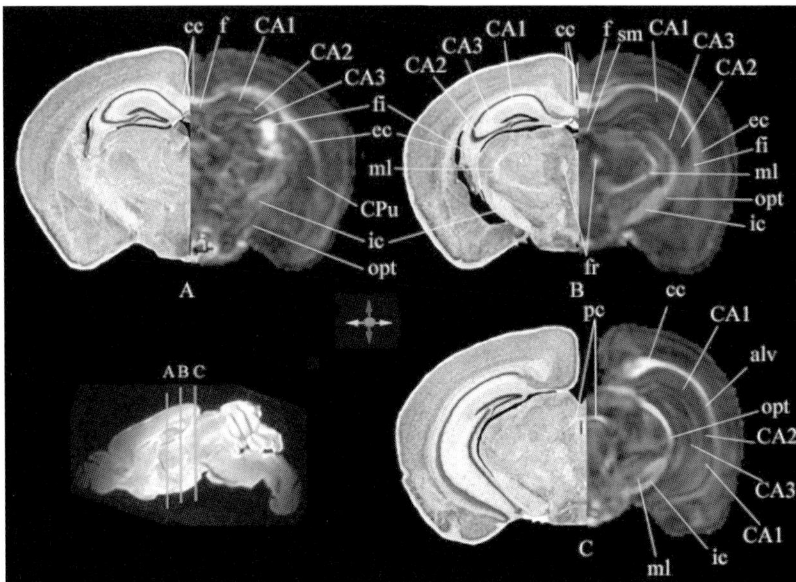

Fig. 3. Side-by-side comparison of three coronal slices from histology and diffusion tensor image (DTI) color mapping. Locations of the sections are shown in the sagittal plane in the lower left corner. Pixel color represents the dominant direction of diffusion within the pixel, as indicated by the arrow pattern in the center of this figure. Alv indicates alveus of the hippocampus; CA1, hippocampal field CA1; CA2, hippocampal field CA2; CA3, hippocampal field CA3; cc, corpus callosum; CPu, caudate putamen; ec, external capsule; f, fornix; fi, fimbria; fr, fasciculus retroflexus; ml, medial lemniscus; ic, internal capsule; opt, optical tract; pc, posterior commissure; and sm, stria medullaris of thalamus. The histology is from Dr. Sidman's 3D histology-based atlas (www.hms.harvard.edu/research/brain). (Images were reproduced with permission from Zhang et al., **ref. *32*.**)

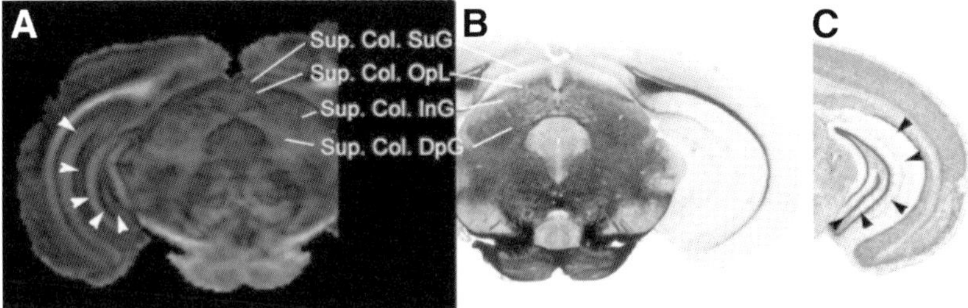

Fig. 4. Examples of assignment of magnetic resonance imaging (MRI)-visible structures from MRI-histology comparison. Images in **(A)**, **(B)**, and **(C)** show a diffusion tensor image (DTI)-based color map, myelin staining, and Nissl staining. Four layers of superior colliculus (SuG indicates superficial gray layer; OpL, optic nerve layer;

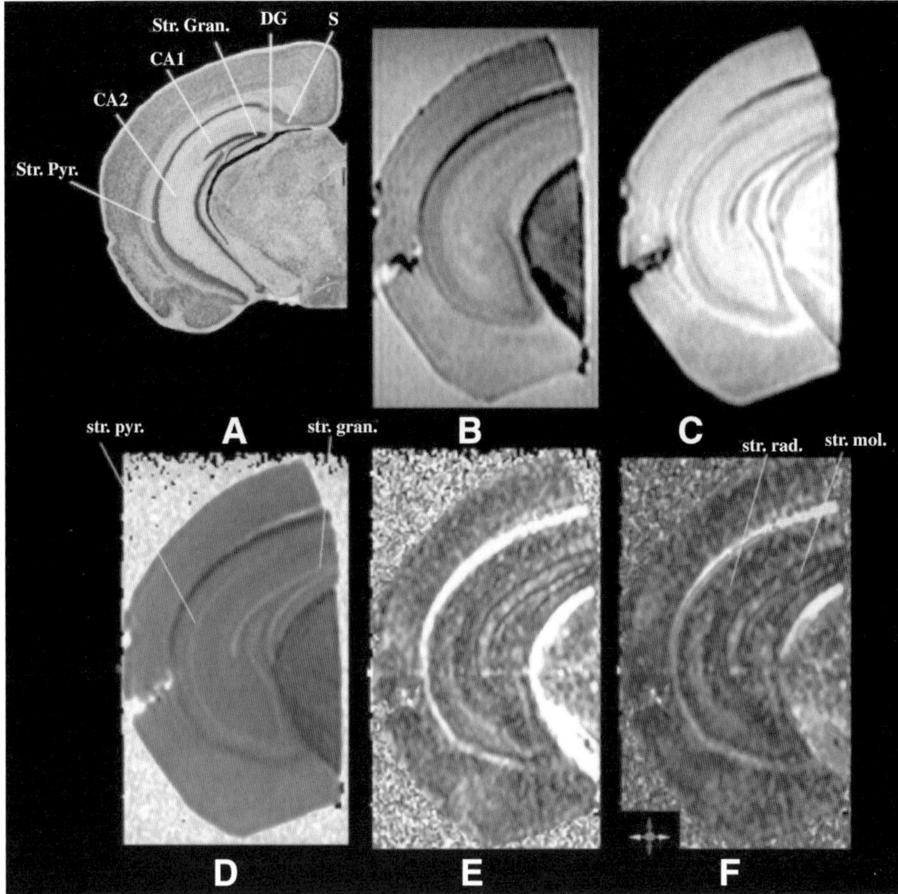

Fig. 5. Comparison of slices of isolated hippocampus from histology (**A**) with a T$_2$-weighted image (**B**), an isotropically diffusion-weighted image (iDWI) (**C**), an average apparent-diffusion coefficient map (ADCav) image (**D**), a fractional anisotropy map (FA) image (**E**), and a color map (**F**). In the histological slice, DG indicates dentate gyrus; S, subiculum. Notice the clear definition of the stratum pyramidale and stratum granulosum in the iDWI and ADCav images. (Images were reproduced with permission from Zhang et al., **ref. *32*.**)

Fig. 4. *(continued)* InG, intermediate gray layer; and DpG, deep gray layer) can be identified in the color map. Five visible layers in the hippocampus are also matched to Nissl-stained histology using arrowheads. These are, from lateral to medial regions, subiculum, CA1 (lacunosum molecular layer), dentate gyrus, granular layer, and polymorph layer. In addition, numerous white matter tracts and gray matter nuclei can be identified in the color map.

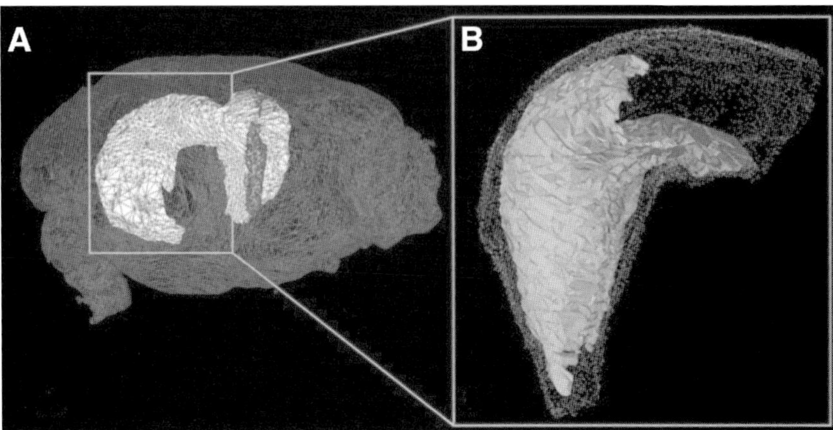

Fig. 6. Three-dimensional reconstructions of hippocampus, stratum granulosum, and stratum pyramidale in the ventral–temporal part of hippocampus. **(A)** Hippocampus (white surface) and brain surface (blue wire frame) rendered in 3D. **(B)** Stratum granulosum (light blue) and stratum pyramidale (light red) within the hippocampus (scattered white points), as taken out of the framed area in **(A)**, with a small rotation to enhance the view of the V-shaped stratum granulosum.

Myelination has an especially large impact on the T_1/T_2 contrast. As a result, unmyelinated younger brains have poor MR-detectable signatures. On the other hand, DTI is sensitive to "tissue orientation" and confirms that even prenatal brains are highly inhomogeneous in terms of the tissue orientation and can be differentiated. Several structures can be uniquely identified in the annotated color maps. **Figure 7** convincingly shows the superior power of DTI to identify various anatomical structures of developing brains in a noninvasive fashion.

Once it was believed that DTI would be useful to delineate only myelinated white matter tracts, which always have high anisotropy. However, recent studies in adult and embryo brains with high-resolution, high signal-to-noise ratio (SNR) imaging by our group *(31,32)* and others *(12,13,33)* have shown convincingly that many unmyelinated white and gray matter structures have coherent tissue organizations that can be uniquely delineated by DTI.

Fig. 7. *(opposite page)* Comparison between T_2 maps and diffusion tensor imaging (DTI)-based color maps at different developmental stages. Mid-sagittal levels of E15 to E18 brains are shown. Scout images are isotropically diffusion-weighted images (iDWI) and areas indicated by orange boxes are magnified to compare T_2 maps (upper boxes) with DTI-based color-orientation maps (CM, bottom boxes). The iDWIs are ideal for definition of the entire brain. The amount of anatomical information carried by the CM is far more than that of the T_2 maps, which provide rather uniform contrast

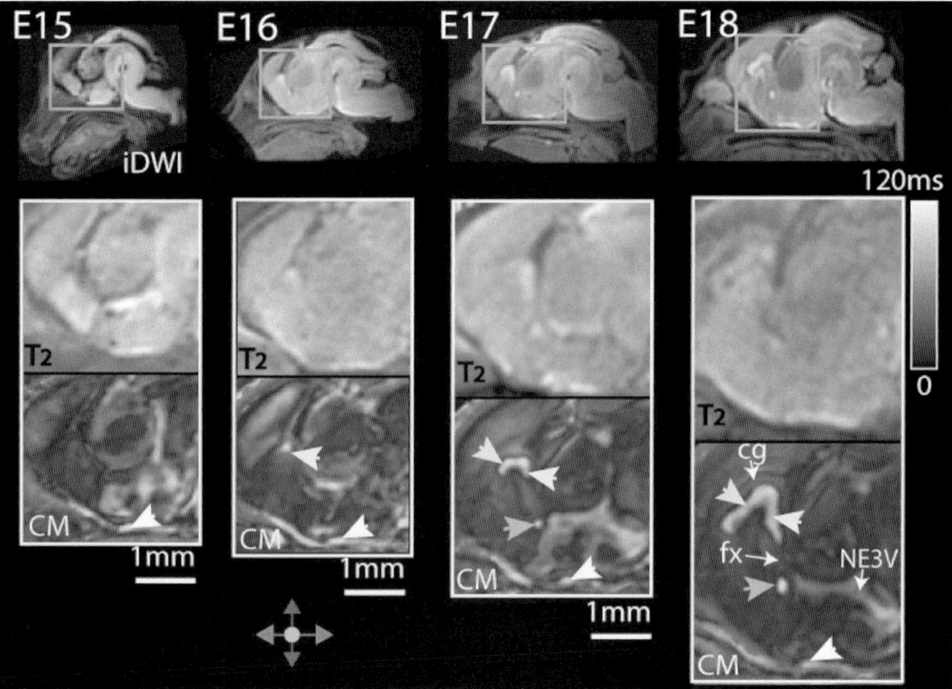

Fig. 7. *(continued)* within the brain. As examples, locations of commissural tracts (detected as green structures) are indicated by arrows; white indicates the optic chiasm; yellow, the hippocampal commissure; pink, the anterior commissure; and blue, the corpus callosum. Embryonic mouse brain specimens were fixed using 4% paraformaldehyde in phosphate-buffered saline and left in fixation solution for more than 1 mo. Before imaging, specimens were placed in phosphate-buffered saline for 24 h, and then transferred into home-built, MR-compatible tubes. The tubes were filled with fomblin to prevent dehydration. Imaging was performed using a GE Omega 400 (9.4 T) spectrometer. We used a custom-made solenoid volume coil as both the radio frequency signal transmitter and receiver. Both high-resolution T_2-weighted images and diffusion-weighted images were acquired with the same field of view (9.5 mm × 6 mm × 6 mm for the smallest sample, and 11 mm × 7.5 mm × 7.5 mm for the largest sample). The imaging matrix had a dimension of 128 × 70 × 72, which was zero-filled to 256 × 140 × 144 after the spectral data was apodized by a 10% trapezoidal function. Eight to fourteen diffusion-weighted images were acquired with different diffusion gradient directions and magnitudes. For diffusion-weighted images, a repetition time (TR) of 0.9 s, an echo time (TE) of 37 ms, and two echo acquisitions with two signal averages were used, for a total imaging time of 24 h. Four images were acquired with TR of 0.9 s and TEs of 30 ms, 60 ms, 80 ms, and 100 ms, with two signal averages, for a total imaging time of 8 h. T_2 images were generated from the four images using an exponential fitting method. We used the same procedures as described in the adult brain section to generate and process the diffusion tensor data.

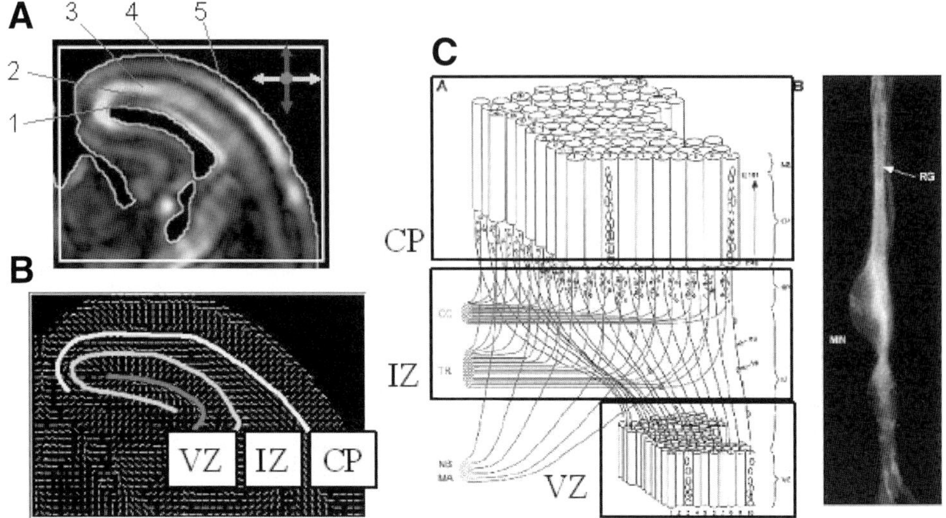

Fig. 8. **(A)** Identification of five layers in the early cortical formation (numbered 1 to 5) in a color-coded orientation map of E16 mouse brain. **(B)** Fiber orientations delineated by vector lines at the same image location of **(A)**. **(C)** Schematic diagram of cortical structures of the E16 stage of the brain *(38)*. Among the five identified layers in the image **(A)**, the three major layers (1, 3, and 5) are tentatively assigned to periventricular zone (vz), intermediate zone (iz), and cortical plate (cp), because their characteristic fiber orientations match those based on histology **(C)**.

2.2.1. Cortical Development Under Diffusion Tensor Microimaging

During CNS development, neurons are born in the NE surrounding the ventricle. They then differentiate and form axons to communicate with other neurons. As a result, many regions of the CNS have a neurons-inside (gray matter is closer to the ventricle)/axons-outside (white matter is closer to the pial surface of the CNS) configuration. One notable exception is the cerebral cortex, in which the gray matter lies outside the white matter. This gray matter/white matter inversion occurs during E12 to E18 in the mouse, when neurons born in the NE migrate outward along radial glia and detach to form the layers of the CP in an inside-out fashion *(34)*. **Figure 8** demonstrates how early cortical structures can be visualized by DTI. Among the embryonic structures, the periventricular zone and CP have been targets of extensive studies because these are the precursors of the cortex. Using DTI, five layers can be identified in the early cortical formation *(31,35)*. Among these layers, the No. 1, 3, and 5 layers are likely to be the periventricular zone (NE), intermediate zone (IZ), and CP, judging from their characteristic fiber orientations and histological correlation. **Figure 9** shows how these structures dynamically change during

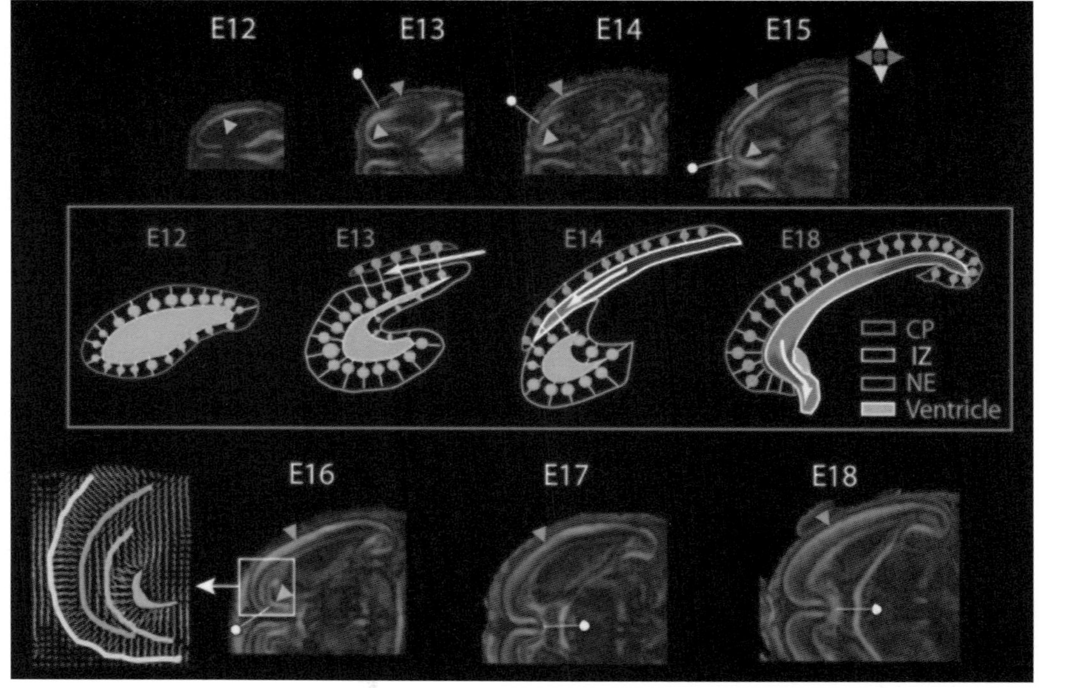

Fig. 9. Cortical development. Horizontal planes of color maps of E12 to E18 brains. Blue and pink arrowheads indicate locations of the neuroepithelium (NE) and cortical plate (CP). Yellow pins indicate the leading edge of the growing intermediate zone (IZ, axonal tracts) between the NE and CP. The inset diagram explains the cellular events during E12 to E18 based on radial migration theory. Blue circles indicate newly born neurons in the NE; white bars, migration scaffolds consisting of radial glia; pink circles, neurons in the CP; and yellow arrows, the growing axons. At E12, there is only one layer (NE), which has radial structures around the ventricle. At E13, the CP emerges and, simultaneously, afferent and efferent axons (IZ) arrive between the NE and CP layers, resulting in temporary three-layer structure. At E14 to E18, the CP formation progressively is completed, with concomitant loss of the NE layer and ventricle shrinkage, and the axons follow the leading edge of the CP. A portion of E16 brain (white box) is enlarged to show the fiber orientation in a vector picture. (From Zhang et al., **ref. 35**, with permission.)

development. The NE is the only structure with a high anisotropy at E12 (blue arrowhead in **Fig. 9**). At E13 to E14, two more structures with high anisotropy emerge; the CP and the IZ (axonal tracts). The CP (indicated by pink arrowheads in **Fig. 9**) arises first in the ventrolateral portion of the dorsal telencephalon and extends anteriorly and dorsomedially during development. It has the same fiber orientation (as indicated by the same color) as the NE and its appearance is followed by a drastic reduction in the NE below (*see* diagram and color maps in the inset of **Fig. 9**). The anterior and dorsomedial front of the emerging CP also coincides with the growing axonal tracts (IZ, its leading edge is indicated by yellow pins in **Fig. 9**). Unlike the NE and CP, which have fiber orientations perpendicular to the ventricular surface, the orientation of the IZ is always parallel to the surface, as can be seen from the color and vector maps shown at E16 (**Fig. 9**). By E17, medially projecting cortical axons within the IZ penetrate the midline, forming the corpus callosum. This inversion process can be easily viewed even within one single brain at E14 or E15 because of the lateral–medial developmental gradient.

2.2.2. Three-Dimensional Characterization of Brain Development

As mentioned previously, one of the benefits of scanning postmortem samples using MRI, rather than, or in addition to, histological processing, is that MRI provides an efficient and accurate means for 3D anatomical analyses. **Figure 10** shows the emerging CP, which originates at the lateral regions, extends toward the midline, and, by E16, covers the entire hemisphere; at the same time, becoming thicker from mid-anterior areas. Cortical thickness measurements cannot be easily achieved by 2D-based histology, because most predetermined slices contain cortical areas that are sliced obliquely, resulting in a thickness that seems artificially high.

Figure 11 shows another example of 3D segmentation, in which the entire E12 embryo was segmented. In the first step, the ventricle and the entire CNS can be delineated using conventional MRI, such as T_2-weighted images. The CNS can be further divided into the NE and differentiating field, based on DTI analysis.

2.3. Technical Considerations

2.3.1. Fixation

Because DTI is sensitive to axonal anatomy, fixation does not change its contrast significantly, as long as the anatomy is well preserved. Once the brain is properly fixed, it does not exhibit contrast change over a period of 6 mo and longer, in our experience. On the other hand, DTI is very sensitive to the fixation conditions. For example, if a brain is emersion fixed within a skull without

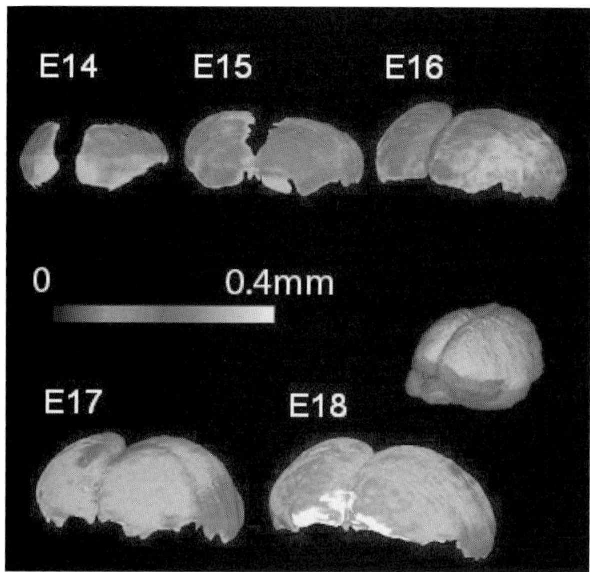

Fig. 10. Changes in 3D volumes and thickness of the cortical plate (CP) over the E14 to E18 period. The volumes were hand segmented, and the thickness of the volumes normal to the brain surface were measured.

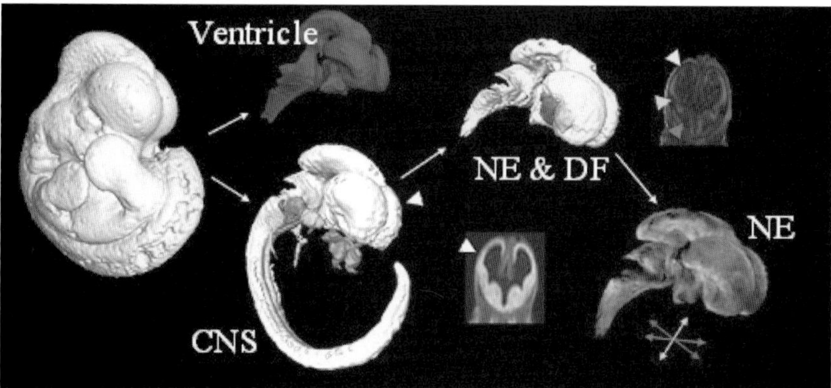

Fig. 11. Segmentation of the central nervous system (CNS) in an E12 embryo. The ventricle and CNS were segmented using conventional magnetic resonance imaging (MRI) microscopy. Several cranial nerves are also identified and colored brown (nasal nerve), blue (optic nerve), pink (cranial nerve V), red (cranial nerve VII), and green (cranial nerves IX and X). The neuroepithelium (NE, yellow) and differentiating field (DF, red and green) were segmented using the color map. The NE, with color presentation for the glial orientation, is also shown. (From Zhang et al., **ref. *35***, with permission.)

perfusion fixation, we often find the sample looses anisotropy, probably as a result of autolysis. Proper perfusion fixation is a key for successful sample preparation. Another important issue is that the fixative (4% paraformaldehyde) shortens the T_2 relaxation time and leads to a poor SNR. It is recommended that the fixative be replaced with buffer solution for at least 24 h before MR scans.

2.3.2. Scanner Requirement and Pulse Programs

Because of the small pixel sizes, high field magnets and strong magnetic field gradients are needed for microimaging. To achieve 100-μm resolution for DTI, approx 24 h are needed to obtain a good SNR using 9.4 and 11.7 T magnets. For example, if we acquire a 256 × 128 × 128 matrix, 16,384 scans are needed. With 0.8 s of repetition time, this is a 3.6-h scan. Because we need at least seven images, the total scanning time becomes 25.5 h. Apparently, rapid imaging techniques are in great need. Because of substantial susceptibility issues in high fields, echo planar imaging is not suitable for microimaging. Fast spin-echo (FSE)-based imaging is probably the best approach for the rapid imaging. However, the strong gradients required for the diffusion, readout, and phase-encoding gradient often produce a nonnegligible amount of Eddy current, and the Carr-Purcell-Meiboom-Gill conditions may break down. This issue needs to be addressed by instrumentation (better gradient performance), pulse programming (Eddy current cancellation and phase monitoring), and/or postprocessing phase correction *(36)*, which will be a major challenge to further pursue improvement of image resolution in the future.

3. Conclusions

In this chapter, we demonstrated the effectiveness of DTI in characterizing the global architecture of mouse neuroanatomy. Compared with other imaging modalities, the MR-based technique has two significant limitations; namely imaging resolution and contrast. We introduced an imaging resolution of up to 80 μm. In the future, because of the recent advent of microimaging techniques *(3,5)*, a resolution of 10 to 20 μm should be possible. Although this still cannot match the resolution of optical techniques and, therefore, imaging of cellular-level anatomy is difficult with this technique, MRI still has major advantages over conventional histological techniques. Conventional histology has a lower resolution along the slice orientation (typically 10–50 μm) and usually has information gaps unless hundreds of perfect and contiguous slices are obtained, which is painstaking and often not practical. In many cases, information about an entire brain is extrapolated from a limited number of histological slices for volumetric studies. As a result, histology-based studies do not always convey proficient resolution in 3D for the entire brain.

Compared with histological examination, MRI excels in surveying the entire brain in an unbiased fashion to detect abnormalities, which can arise because of gene alterations, pharmacological treatments, or induced lesions. Histology often requires assumptions about a possible phenotype before analysis, so that the optimal plane of section and the selection of appropriate stains or antibodies to visualize specific structures can be chosen. This need for *a priori* knowledge can cause some phenotypical changes to be overlooked, or require large numbers of mutant animals to analyze several possible phenotypes. Because DTI can examine the entire brain in an efficient and possibly more quantitative manner, it provides an excellent broad analysis of the phenotypeand can be followed by more detailed histological analyses of the appropriate regions. We foresee that the MR-based analyses of postmortem brain samples and DTI will be an important research effort to supplement conventional histology studies.

Acknowledgments

Studies presented in this article were supported by NIH grants, RO1AG020012 (SM), P41 RR15241-01 (SM), and NS45062 (JWMB).

References

1. Callaghan, P. T. (1991) Principles of Nuclear Magnetic Resonance Microscopy. Oxford University Press, Oxford, UK.
2. Johnson, G. A., Benveniste, H., Black, R. D., Hedlund, L. W., Maronpot, R. R., and Smith, B. R. (1993) Histology by magnetic resonance microscopy. *Magn. Reson. Q.* **9,** 1–30.
3. Johnson, G. A., Benveniste, H., Engelhardt, R. T., Qiu, H., and Hedlund, L. W. (1997) Magnetic resonance microscopy in basic studies of brain structure and function. *Ann. N. Y. Acad. Sci.* **820,** 139–147.
4. Ahrens, E. T., Laidlaw, D. H., Readhead, C., Brosnan, C. F., Fraser, S. E., and Jacobs, R. E. (1998) MR microscopy of transgenic mice that spontaneously acquire experimental allergic encephalomyelitis. *Magn. Reson. Med.* **40,** 119–132.
5. Jacobs, R. E., Ahrens, E. T., Dickinson, M. E., and Laidlaw, D. (1999) Towards a microMRI atlas of mouse development. *Comput. Med. Imaging Graph.* **23,** 15–24.
6. Jacobs, R. E., Ahrens, E. T., Meade, T. J., and Fraser, S. E. (1999) Looking deeper into vertebrate development. *Trends Cell. Biol.* **9,** 73–76.
7. Benveniste, H., Kim, K., Zhang, L., and Johnson, G. A. (2000) Magnetic resonance microscopy of the C57BL mouse brain. *Neuroimage* **11,** 601–611.
8. Basser, P. J., Mattiello, J., and Le Bihan, D. (1994) MR diffusion tensor spectroscopy and imaging. *Biophys. J.* **66,** 259–267.
9. Pierpaoli, C. and Basser, P. J. (1996) Toward a quantitative assessment of diffusion anisotropy. *Magn. Reson. Med.* **36,** 893–906.
10. Makris, N., Worth, A. J., Sorensen, A. G., et al. (1997) Morphometry of in vivo human white matter association pathways with diffusion weighted magnetic resonance imaging. *Ann. Neurol.* **42,** 951–962.

11. Moseley, M. E., Cohen, Y., Kucharczyk, J., et al. (1990) Diffusion-weighted MR imaging of anisotropic water diffusion in cat central nervous system. *Radiology* **176,** 439–445.
12. Beaulieu, C. and Allen, P. S. (1994) Determinants of anisotropic water diffusion in nerves. *Magn. Reson. Med.* **31,** 394–400.
13. Henkelman, R., Stanisz, G., Kim, J., and Bronskill, M. (1994) Anisotropy of NMR properties of tissues. *Magn. Reson. Med.* **32,** 592–601.
14. Pierpaoli, C., Jezzard, P., Basser, P. J., Barnett, A., and Di Chiro, G. (1996) Diffusion tensor MR imaging of human brain. *Radiology* **201,** 637–648.
15. Douek, P., Turner, R., Pekar, J., Patronas, N., and Le Bihan, D. (1991) MR color mapping of myelin fiber orientation. *J. Comput. Assist. Tomogr.* **15,** 923–929.
16. Coremans, J., Luypaert, R., Verhelle, F., Stadnik, T., and Osteaux, M. (1994) A method for myelin fiber orientation mapping using diffusion-weighted MR images. *Magn. Reson. Imaging* **12,** 443–454.
17. Nakada, T. and Matsuzawa, H. (1995) Three-dimensional anisotropy contrast magnetic resonance imaging of the rat nervous system: MR axonography. *Neurosci. Res.* **22,** 389–398.
18. Pajevic, S. and Pierpaoli, C. (1999) Color schemes to represent the orientation of anisotropic tissues from diffusion tensor data: application to white matter fiber tract mapping in the human brain. *Magn. Reson. Med.* **42,** 526–540.
19. Mori, S., Crain, B. J., Chacko, V. P., and van Zijl, P. C. M. (1999) Three-dimensional tracking of axonal projections in the brain by magnetic resonance imaging. *Ann. Neurol.* **45,** 265–269.
20. Xue, R., van Zijl, P. C. M., Crain, B. J., Solaiyappan, M., and Mori, S. (1999) In vivo three-dimensional reconstruction of rat brain axonal projections by diffusion tensor imaging. *Magn. Reson. Med.* **42,** 1123–1127.
21. Conturo, T. E., Lori, N. F., Cull, T. S., et al. (1999) Tracking neuronal fiber pathways in the living human brain. *Proc. Natl. Acad. Sci. USA* **96,** 10,422–10,427.
22. Basser, P. J., Pajevic, S., Pierpaoli, C., Duda, J., and Aldroubi, A. (2000) In vitro fiber tractography using DT-MRI data. *Magn. Reson. Med.* **44,** 625–632.
23. Poupon, C., Clark, C. A., Frouin, V., et al. (2000) Regularization of diffusion-based direction maps for the tracking of brain white matter fascicules. *Neuroimage* **12,** 184–195.
24. Bock, N. A., Konyer, N. B., and Henkelman, R. M. (2003) Multiple-mouse MRI. *Magn. Reson. Med.* **49,** 158–167.
25. Weninger, W. J. and Mohun, T. (2002) Phenotyping transgenic embryos: a rapid 3-D screening method based on episcopic fluorescence image capturing. *Nat. Genet.* **30,** 59–65.
26. Streicher, J., Donat, M. A., Strauss, B., Sporle, R., Schughart, K., and Muller, G. B. (2000) Computer-based three-dimensional visualization of developmental gene expression. *Nat. Genet.* **25,** 147–152.
27. Boppart, S. A., Bouma, B. E., Brezinski, M. E., Tearney, G. J., and Fujimoto, J. G. (1996) Imaging developing neural morphology using optical coherence tomography. *J. Neurosci. Methods* **70,** 65–72.

28. Jacobs, R. E. and Fraser, S. E. (1994) Imaging neuronal development with magnetic resonance imaging (NMR) microscopy. *J. Neurosci. Methods* **54,** 189–196.
29. Louie, A. Y., Huber, M. M., Ahrens, E. T., et al. (2000) In vivo visualization of gene expression using magnetic resonance imaging. *Nat. Biotechnol.* **18,** 321–325.
30. Sharpe, J., Ahlgren, U., Perry, P., et al. (2002) Optical projection tomography as a tool for 3D microscopy and gene expression studies. *Science* **296,** 541–545.
31. Mori, S., Itoh, R., Zhang, J., et al. (2001) Diffusion tensor imaging of the developing mouse brain. *Magn. Reson. Med.* **46,** 18–23.
32. Zhang, J., van Zijl, P. C., and Mori, S. (2002) Three dimensional diffusion tensor magnetic resonance micro-imaging of adult mouse brain and hippocampus. *Neuroimage* **15,** 892–901.
33. Neil, J., Shiran, S., McKinstry, R., et al. (1998) Normal brain in human newborns: apparent diffusion coefficient and diffusion anisotropy measured by using diffusion tensor MR imaging. *Radiology* **209,** 57–66.
34. Rakic, P. (1972) Mode of cell migration to the superficial layers of fetal monkey neocortex. *J. Comp. Neurol.* **145,** 61–83.
35. Zhang, J., Richards, L. J., Yarowsky, P., Huang, H., van Zijl, P. C., and Mori, S. (2003) Three-dimensional anatomical characterization of the developing mouse brain by diffusion tensor microimaging. *Neuroimage* **20,** 1639–1648.
36. Mori, S. and van Zijl, P. C. (1998) A motion correction scheme by twin-echo navigation for diffusion-weighted magnetic resonance imaging with multiple RF echo acquisition. *Magn. Reson. Med.* 40, 511–516.
37. Basser, P. J., Mattiello, J., and LeBihan, D. (1994) Estimation of the effective self-diffusion tensor from the NMR spin echo. *J. Magn. Reson. B* **103,** 247–254.
38. Raichle, M. E. (1998) Behind the scenes of functional brain imaging: a historical and physiological perspective. *Proc. Natl. Acad. Sci. USA* **95,** 765–772.

III

PHYSIOLOGY

6

Quantitative Perfusion Imaging Using Arterial Spin Labeling

Donald S. Williams

Summary

MRI-based perfusion imaging techniques can be classified into those that use exogenously administered contrast agents and those that use an endogenous material that reflects blood flow. This chapter focuses on the technique of arterial spin labeling (ASL), in which endogenous water is made a freely diffusible perfusion tracer by perturbing the magnetization of blood water in arteries prior to their entry into tissue of interest. The technique is totally noninvasive and allows repeated quantitative blood flow measurements in a time scale limited only by the spin lattice relaxation time (T_1). Absolute quantitation requires measurement of T_1, transit time, and labeling efficiency, as well as careful control for magnetization transfer effects. Two main variants of the ASL technique are in use: continuous ASL (CASL) and pulsed ASL (PASL). This chapter describes basic theory for CASL, and experimental and computational procedures for obtaining quantitative perfusion maps of the brain. Extension of the technique for renal perfusion imaging is outlined.

Key Words: Arterial spin labeling; ASL; perfusion; blood flow; MRI.

1. Introduction

Adequate blood flow is crucial to the supply of oxygen and nutrients and to the removal of waste from tissue; its measurement is a sensitive indicator of tissue function and viability. Since the pioneering experiments of Kety and Schmidt *(1)*, there has been much interest in the development of techniques for quantitative measurement of tissue perfusion *(2)*. The early work of Kety laid the foundation for many of the approaches to measurement of tissue perfusion used today *(3)*. These methods typically use the wash-in, wash-out kinetics of a freely diffusible tracer to measure tissue perfusion. A freely diffusible tracer is assumed to be one that diffuses from the vasculature and equilibrates with tissue rapidly compared with blood flow. Knowledge of wash-in, wash-out kinetics and input function of the tracer has allowed quantitation of perfusion in milliliters per minute per gram of tissue. Over the past two decades, there

From: *Methods in Molecular Medicine, Vol. 124*
Magnetic Resonance Imaging: Methods and Biologic Applications
Edited by: P. V. Prasad © Humana Press Inc., Totowa, NJ

has been a growing interest in the development of magnetic resonance imaging (MRI)-based techniques for measurement of perfusion *(4–6)*. The noninvasive nature of MRI, the high spatial resolution attainable, and the ability to manipulate the MRI signal intensity to reflect a variety of physical, biochemical, and physiological properties make these techniques attractive alternatives to many classical methods that have been in use. MRI-based perfusion techniques can be classified into two broad types: those that use exogenously administered contrast agents and those that use some endogenously available material that reflects blood flow. Perfusion imaging techniques relying on exogenously administered, freely diffusible tracers include measuring wash-in, wash-out kinetics of ^2H_2O by ^2H NMR *(7,8)*, measuring trifluoromethane by ^{19}F nuclear magnetic resonance (NMR) *(9)*, and measuring H_2O^{17} by ^{17}O NMR *(10)*. A second class of exogenous agents, the gadolinium chelates, has found widespread use in the brain. These agents remain in the vasculature as they pass through the brain, and monitoring the kinetics of their passage through the brain by measuring their influence on the ^1H MRI signal of surrounding tissue enables blood volume and mean transit time to be measured; perfusion is inferred from these measurements *(11,12)*. All of the perfusion imaging techniques that use exogenous agents suffer from limitations because of the toxicity and clearance times of the tracer. These limitations restrict the ability to carry out repeated measurements in the same subject. An attractive alternative is to use endogenous water as a blood-flow tracer. The high concentration of water protons in tissue (approx 100 *M*) and its high magnetic resonance (MR) sensitivity makes water an ideal candidate for imaging. Early attempts at using water to measure perfusion relied on MRI-determined diffusion coefficients of tissue water as an index of perfusion, but it was not clear whether changes in water diffusion coefficients directly correlated with changes in perfusion *(13)*. Another endogenous tracer that can be used to monitor changes in blood flow is hemoglobin. Deoxyhemoglobin is paramagnetic and causes local magnetic field susceptibility gradients, and the concentration of deoxyhemoglobin can be monitored by the signal reduction in imaging sequences sensitive to field inhomogeneities (T_2^*-weighted sequences) *(14)*. If changes in perfusion leads to a change in deoxyhemoglobin content, signal changes in a T_2^*-weighted sequence can be used to monitor changes in flow. This is the basis for functional MRI of task activation in the human brain *(15)*.

This chapter will focus on another approach that makes use of endogenous water as a freely diffusible perfusion tracer by perturbing the magnetization of blood water in arteries before their entry into tissue of interest *(16,17)*. For example, blood flowing into brain may be labeled by inverting the blood-water spins in the carotid arteries in the neck (**Fig. 1**). Labeled water will flow into tissue and exchange with tissue water, thereby altering its magnetization by an amount that is proportional to perfusion. A difference image computed be-

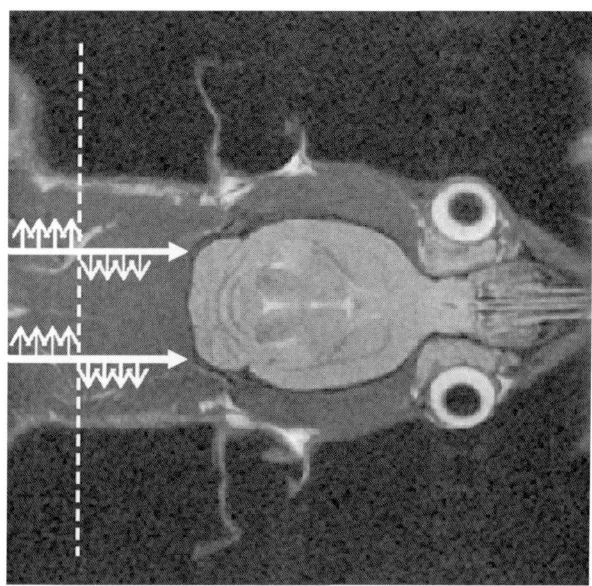

Fig. 1. Schematic description of arterial spin labeling applied to measurement of rat brain perfusion. A typical experiment will involve inverting proton spins in arterial blood water in the carotid arteries in the neck region. Labeled blood will flow into brain and exchange with brain tissue water, decreasing brain tissue water magnetization by an amount that depends on perfusion rate.

tween images with labeled and unlabeled water will provide a perfusion-weighted image depicting regional variations in perfusion in the slice. As detailed later, quantitative perfusion maps can be computed if other parameters, such as T_1, labeling efficiency, and so on, are known. This approach has led to a family of MR perfusion imaging methods, collectively known as arterial spin labeling (ASL) techniques, in which a variety of different ASL strategies have been used. ASL techniques fall under two broad categories, continuous ASL (CASL) and pulsed ASL (PASL).

1.1. Continuous ASL

CASL techniques require a continuous supply of labeled arterial water into tissue of interest. This labeled water freely diffuses into tissue and exchanges with tissue water leading to a steady-state tissue water Z-magnetization. Quantitation of perfusion by CASL requires the measurement of the steady-state Z-magnetization of tissue with and without ASL. Obtaining true measures of these magnetizations in an imaging mode has led to several variations of CASL methods with different labeling strategies, imaging sequences, and hardware. In the first ASL experiments, blood water entering the brain was labeled in a continuous manner by either repeated slab-selective saturation pulses *(16)* or adiabatic fast-passage inversion *(17)* applied in the neck region of a rat. This labeling module was applied during the entire repetition time (TR) in a 2D Fourier transform (2DFT) spin-warp, spin-echo imaging sequence to ensure that the Z-magnetization was maintained in the steady state throughout the imaging sequence. An alternate approach is to label blood until a steady state is reached and an image is acquired in a time short compared with tissue T_1 *(18,19)*.

1.1.1. Theory

1.1.1.1. LABELING BY FLOW-INDUCED ADIABATIC FAST-PASSAGE SPIN INVERSION

The most commonly used CASL technique involves inversion of the arterial spins using flow-induced adiabatic fast passage (AFP) *(17,20)*, and theory and experimental details will be described for this approach. The first ASL experiment used slab-selective 90° pulses to produce a continuous stream of saturated water *(16)*, but extending the same idea to inversion is difficult without the knowledge of the exact blood-flow velocity. An old theorem on AFP, relating to behavior of spins when the spins are swept through resonance has provided an elegant way of producing a continuous stream of inverted spins *(21)*. The theorem simply states that if low-power radio frequency (RF) of amplitude B_1 is applied continuously while the spins are swept through resonance at a rate of dB_0/dt (by sweeping the magnetic field or by sweeping the frequency of excitation RF), spins will undergo inversion if the AFP condition is satisfied:

$$\frac{1}{T_1}, \frac{1}{T_2} \ll \frac{1}{B_1}\frac{dB_0}{dt} \ll \gamma B_1 \qquad [1]$$

In the case in which spins flow in a blood vessel with a linear velocity, v, flowing spins may be swept through resonance by applying continuous RF in the presence of a magnetic field gradient, G, in the direction of flow. For flow-induced inversion, the AFP condition becomes *(20)*:

$$\frac{1}{T_1}, \frac{1}{T_2} \ll \frac{1}{B_1}Gv \ll \gamma B_1 \qquad [2]$$

T_1 and T_2 are the relaxation times of the water protons in blood. G and B_1 are chosen such that the condition in **Eq. [2]** is satisfied for the mean flow velocity of blood in the artery to be labeled. A major advantage of this technique of inversion is that the AFP condition is maintained over a range of blood-flow velocities, such that minor variation in flow velocities due to physiological conditions and pulsatile nature of blood flow are well tolerated *(17,22,23)*.

1.1.1.2. PERFUSION QUANTITATION USING CASL

Quantitation of perfusion using CASL involves tracer kinetics, the tracer in this case being labeled water in arterial blood. The quantity of tracer in the tissue is measured through its effect on the Z-magnetization of tissue water. The Z-magnetization for tissue water protons is influenced by T_1 relaxation, perfusion rate, and interaction of tissue water with the macromolecule pool present in the tissue. The Bloch equations for tissue magnetization can be written as a pair of coupled equations *(24)*:

$$\frac{dM_t}{dt} = \frac{\left(M_t^0 - M_t\right)}{T_{1t}} - k_{for} M_t + k_{rev} M_m + fM_a - fM_v \qquad [3]$$

$$\frac{dM_m}{dt} = \frac{M_m^0 - M_m}{T_{1m}} + k_{for} M_t - k_{rev} M_m, \qquad [4]$$

where M_t and M_m refer to Z-magnetization of tissue water and macromolecules per gram of tissue, respectively; M_t^0 and M_m^0 are the equilibrium values of M_t and M_m, respectively; M_a and M_v are the Z-magnetizations of arterial and venous water per mL of blood, respectively; k_{for} and k_{rev} are the forward and reverse magnetization transfer rate constants between tissue water and macromolecules, respectively; f is the perfusion rate in milliliters per gram per second; and T_{1t} is the longitudinal relaxation time for tissue water in the absence of perfusion.

If water is a freely diffusible tracer, it will distribute between tissue and blood according to the brain:blood partition coefficient, λ, defined as:

$$\lambda = \frac{mL \ of \ water \ / \ g \ tissue}{mL \ of \ water \ / \ mL \ of \ blood}.$$

Thus,

$$M_v = \frac{M_t}{\lambda} \qquad [5]$$

and

$$M_a^0 = \frac{M_t^0}{\lambda}. \qquad [6]$$

Let us now define the labeling efficiency, α as the extent to which arterial blood is labeled:

$$\alpha = \frac{M_a^0 - M_a}{2 M_a^0}.$$ [7]

For saturation, $\alpha = 0.5$, and for inversion, $\alpha = 1$. Substituting for M_a and M_t in **Eq. [3]** from **Eqs. [5]**, **[6]**, and **[7]**, we obtain:

$$\frac{dM_t}{dt} = \frac{M_t^0 - M_t}{T_{1t}} - k_{for} M_t + k_{rev} M_m - (2\alpha - 1)\frac{f}{\lambda} M_t^0 - \frac{f}{\lambda} M_t.$$ [8]

The solution to the coupled **Eqs. [4]** and **[8]** will describe how the Z-magnetization of tissue water relates to perfusion. There are two basic ways in which arterial spins can be labeled: using a single RF coil to carry out imaging as well as labeling of arterial blood, or using one coil to carry out imaging and a second smaller RF coil to label the blood. If a single RF coil is used for spin labeling as well as for imaging, the RF power used to label spins often saturates the macromolecule pool in the tissue ($M_m \to 0$). Under these circumstances, **Eqs. [4]** and **[8]** are uncoupled and **Eq. [8]** simplifies to:

$$\frac{dM_t}{dt} = \frac{M_t^0 - M_t}{T_{1t}} - k_{for} M_t - (2\alpha - 1)\frac{f}{\lambda} M_t^0 - \frac{f}{\lambda} M_t.$$ [9]

The solution to this equation, with $M_t = M_t^0$ at $t = 0$ is:

$$M_t(t) = T_{1app} M_t^0 \left[\left(\frac{1}{T_{1t}} - (2\alpha - 1)\frac{f}{\lambda} \right) + \left(k_{for} + 2\alpha \frac{f}{\lambda} \right) \exp\left(-t/T_{1app} \right) \right],$$ [10]

with

$$\frac{1}{T_{1app}} = \frac{1}{T_{1t}} + k_{for} + \frac{f}{\lambda}.$$ [11]

If a control experiment is carried out such that macromolecules are saturated but water spins are not labeled ($\alpha = 0$), the solution to **Eq. [9]** becomes:

$$M_t(t) = T_{1app} M_t^0 \left[\left(\frac{1}{T_{1t}} + \frac{f}{\lambda} \right) + k_{for} \exp\left(-t/T_{1app} \right) \right].$$ [12]

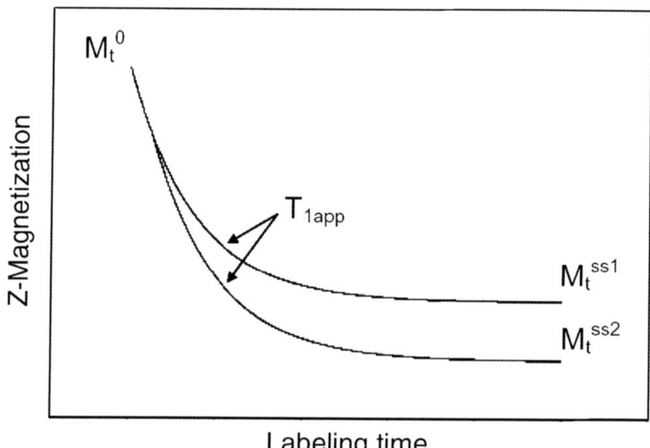

Fig. 2. Behavior of tissue water Z-magnetization according to **Eqs. [10]** and **[12]**, for control (upper curve) and labeling (lower curve) experiments, as a function of labeling time. Note that both curves coincide for short labeling times; the labeling time at which the magnetization for the labeling experiment starts to deviate signifies the arrival of labeled spins at the tissue site.

Figure 2 describes **Eqs. [10]** and **[12]**, the behavior of the tissue water Z-magnetization for the labeling and control experiments. As the duration of the labeling or control RF is increased, saturation of macromolecules causes the tissue water Z-magnetization to decrease exponentially to a steady state, M_t^{ss1} (control experiment), and saturation of macromolecules with ASL results in a lower steady-state value of M_t^{ss2} (labeling experiment), with:

$$M_t^{ss1} = T_{1app}\left(\frac{1}{T_{1t}} + \frac{f}{\lambda}\right) M_t^0 \tag{13}$$

and

$$M_t^{ss2} = \frac{\dfrac{1}{T_{1t}} - (2\alpha - 1)\dfrac{f}{\lambda}}{\dfrac{1}{T_{1t}} + \dfrac{f}{\lambda}} M_t^{ss1} \, . \tag{14}$$

T_{1t} is the longitudinal relaxation time of tissue water in the absence of perfusion and is difficult to measure. A practical form of **Eq. [14]** is:

$$ f = \frac{\lambda}{2\alpha T_{1obs}} \left(\frac{M_t^{ss1} - M_t^{ss2}}{M_t^{ss1}} \right) \qquad [15] $$

with

$$ \frac{1}{T_{1obs}} = \frac{1}{T_{1t}} + \frac{f}{\lambda}, \qquad [16] $$

where T_{1obs} as given in **Eq. [16]** is the longitudinal relaxation time measured in a slice-selective T_1 experiment (please note that in **refs. *16*** and ***17***, T_{1obs} was referred to as T_{1app}). In **Fig. 2**, note that both decay curves coincide for a time period, signifying the time taken for the label to travel from the labeling site to tissue (transit time, *see* in **Subheading 2.1.2.**). **Equation [15]** may be used only if the measured magnetizations are in steady state, i.e., labeling time $>>$ T_{1app}. If this condition is not satisfied, we may still use **Eqs. [10]** and **[12]** for any labeling time, t and write *(25)*:

$$ f = \frac{\Delta M_t}{M_t^0} \frac{\lambda}{2\alpha T_{1app}} \frac{1}{(1 - \exp(-t / T_{1app}))}, \qquad [17] $$

where ΔM_t is the difference in signal between label and control images, and t is the labeling duration. Quantifying perfusion using **Eq. [17]** requires the measurement of M_t^0, the magnetization without labeling or magnetization transfer, and T_{1app}, the T_1 relaxation time in the presence of flow and macromolecular saturation. In humans, RF power deposition, patient motion, etc., place restrictions on the imaging protocol, which sometimes makes achieving steady state difficult; in animal studies using research MR scanners, steady-state conditions may easily be achieved, and most animal studies have used **Eq. [15]** for quantitation.

Equation [15] is the fundamental equation of CASL describing how the Z-magnetization of tissue water relates to tissue perfusion when the water spins in the arterial blood supply are continuously labeled and the macromolecules are completely saturated. Note that the measured quantity in CASL experiments, the fractional change in signal intensity, i.e., $(M_t^{ss1} - M_t^{ss2})/M_t^{ss1}$, is small, and reliable measurement of this small change requires carefully controlled experiments. For example, in the rat brain, perfusion under normal conditions is approx 1 mL/g/min, and using typical values of $\lambda = 0.9$ mL/g, $\alpha = 1$, and $T_{1obs} = 1.6$ s in **Eq. [15]** predicts a fractional signal change of approx 6%. Experimental details for determination of each of the quantities in the right hand side of **Eq. [15]** for evaluating f will be described in **Subheading 2.**

1.2. Pulsed ASL

A generalization of the ASL concept is helpful in understanding some of the PASL techniques that have been proposed. Note that to render tissue magnetization flow sensitive, ASL techniques only require that tissue water and arterial water with different Z-magnetizations are allowed to mix in; allowing labeled blood water to flow into unperturbed tissue, or allowing unlabeled water to flow into Z-magnetization-perturbed tissue are both suitable. PASL techniques employing both approaches have been described in the literature. The main difference between CASL and PASL is the manner in which spins are labeled. In CASL techniques, continuously labeled arterial water flows into tissue and tissue-water Z-magnetization is measured after steady state is reached; in the approach of tissue-water Z-magnetization to steady state, arterial water enters tissue with a fixed labeling efficiency, α. In PASL techniques, water is labeled during a short time using a pulse, and the behavior of tissue-water magnetization is monitored after labeled and unlabeled water are allowed to mix; during this mixing period, labeled water relaxes according to the T_1 of blood, and α is a function of time. Because the label relaxes during the mixing time, in general, the theoretical signal difference predicted for PASL is less than that predicted for CASL with complete spin inversion. However, various limitations in CASL techniques, such as magnetization-transfer effects, transit time (*see* **Subheading 2.1.**), the requirement of a well-defined arterial input for labeling, etc., render CASL methods unsuitable in some situations; this has led to a search for alternate approaches. PASL techniques have been successful in overcoming some of these limitations.

In one of the earliest pulsed-labeling techniques proposed, the imaging slice was saturated and a slab of arterial water proximal to the tissue of interest was labeled using a single inversion pulse; labeled water was allowed to flow into the imaging slice and tissue-water magnetization in the imaging slice was measured after a mixing period, TI (*26*). A control image was acquired with the RF frequency for a slab-inversion pulse placed on the distal side of the detection slice, and the difference image was used for perfusion quantitation. Because the label relaxes during the mixing time, the difference between labeled and unlabeled images reaches a maximum at a mixing time approximately equal to tissue T_{1t} and approaches zero at longer mixing times. Maximum sensitivity is, therefore, obtained by measuring Z-magnetization after a period approximately equal to T_1 after application of the inversion slab; this maximum difference is less than the steady-state difference in CASL by a factor of $\exp(-TI/T_1)$.

A second group of PASL techniques takes advantage of the fact that mixing of labeled and unlabeled water causes the tissue water relaxation rate to increase linearly with the perfusion rate, according to **Eq. [16]**. This relationship has been verified by measuring slice-selective tissue T_1 in an isolated perfused heart preparation where flow can be varied over a wide range and independently validated using an in-line flow meter *(27)*. Dependence of tissue T_1 on flow was first used to monitor changes in perfusion using a T_1-weighted-imaging sequence in the human brain during functional activation *(28)*. Absolute perfusion quantitation requires T_{1t}, the tissue T1 without the effect of inflowing unlabeled water and may be measured using an inversion recovery sequence involving a nonselective inversion pulse. This is the basis of the flow-sensitive alternating inversion recovery (FAIR), in which the difference in magnetization between a slice selective and a non-slice selective inversion recovery sequence is used for flow quantitation *(29)*. These early approaches to PASL have led to the introduction of several PASL methods addressing various issues in the original protocols. A complete survey of PASL techniques, details of quantitation, and experimental details are beyond the scope of this chapter, and the reader is referred to the literature *(4,6,26,28–30)*.

2. Methods

2.1. The CASL Experiment

Measurement of perfusion in a transverse slice in the rat brain using a single coil for labeling as well as for detection is presented as an example. In this setup, it will be assumed that the macromolecules are saturated, and that labeling or control RF is applied for sufficiently long times, such that steady-state magnetizations are measured; perfusion is thus quantified by **Eq. [15]**. Almost any imaging sequence may be adapted for CASL, as long as the spin-labeling module is incorporated into the imaging sequence in such a way that steady-state magnetization is measured. This can be achieved in one of two ways. First, labeling can be applied for a sufficiently long time for magnetization to reach steady state (*see* **Fig. 2**, labeling time $\gg T_{1app}$) and the entire image acquired with a fast imaging sequence (imaging time $\ll T_{1obs}$). A centric phase-encoding approach will ensure that the image intensity closely corresponds to the Z-magnetization at the end of the labeling period. A second approach is to maintain the magnetization in its steady state during image acquisition by applying labeling or control RF during imaging. This can be achieved by applying the labeling RF during the entire TR period of the image. In this scheme, a condition of TR $\gg T_{1app}$ is not essential; TR is chosen to be sufficiently long, such that repeated application of labeling RF during image acquisition will cause the magnetization to reach steady state well before the middle of the k-space is acquired. Labeling blood in carotid arteries by AFP is achieved by applying a Z-gradient, G, together with RF power, B_1; the frequency of RF is set to the resonance of water spins in the neck. Optimal values for G and B_1 may be estimated according to **Eq. [2]**, if estimates of velocity and T_1 and T_2 of the blood are known. For AFP labeling in rat carotids, typical values of a blood velocity of 10 cm/s and T_1 and T_2 of 1.3 s and 100 ms, respectively (at 4.7 T) may be used. Previous studies in the rat have shown that a labeling gradient strength of 1 G/cm, and a B_1 field of 60 to 100 mG provide labeling efficiencies better than 0.8. MR scanner software often does not allow the input of a B_1 amplitude in gauss (or hertz) but are calibrated according to the B_1 amplitude needed for a fixed length 90° pulse. B_1 can be calculated conveniently using the equation:

$$B_1(Gauss) \approx \frac{60}{\text{length of } 90° \text{ square pulse } (\mu s)}. \qquad [18]$$

The frequency offset for the labeling RF is calculated as:

$$\Delta v(Hz) = \pm 4256 \cdot G(Gauss / cm) \cdot \Delta z_L (cm) \qquad [19]$$

where Δz_L is the distance of the labeling location from the isocenter of the gradients (magnet), and + or − is chosen to excite the region proximal to tissue of interest. Application of RF power in the presence of a gradient will define a resonance plane (**Fig. 3**), called the labeling plane, perpendicular to the gradient direction and located at Δz_L from the isocenter. Implications of magnetization transfer effects (MTC) brought about by the labeling RF power illustrated in **Fig. 4** will now be discussed. The application of labeling RF power for long durations causes a decrease in water signal in the detection slice. The labeling RF does not directly saturate the water signal in the detection slice because its frequency offset is much larger than the line width of water, but saturation of macromolecules (which have a much broader linewidth) does occur, and significant signal reduction in the water signal occurs through magnetization transfer *(31)*. It is essential that the experiment is performed in a way such that this signal reduction caused by MTC is maintained to be equal for the labeled (M_t^{ss2}) and unlabeled (M_t^{ss1}) images at all points in the image, so that MTC is eliminated from **Eq. [15]**. In practice, this is usually accomplished by acquiring the unlabeled, control image with the same labeling RF power as the labeled image but with a frequency offset placed symmetrically on the opposite side of the detection slice's water resonance. Because the labeling RF is applied in the presence of a labeling gradient, the frequency offset of the labeling RF from the tissue water resonance in the detection slice depends on the distance of the tissue from the labeling plane. It becomes immediately apparent that MTC can be controlled over the entire image only if the labeling plane, control plane, and detection planes are perpendicular to the labeling gradient, and that the labeling plane and the control plane are equidistant from the detection plane. The frequency offset for the control plane is thus set as:

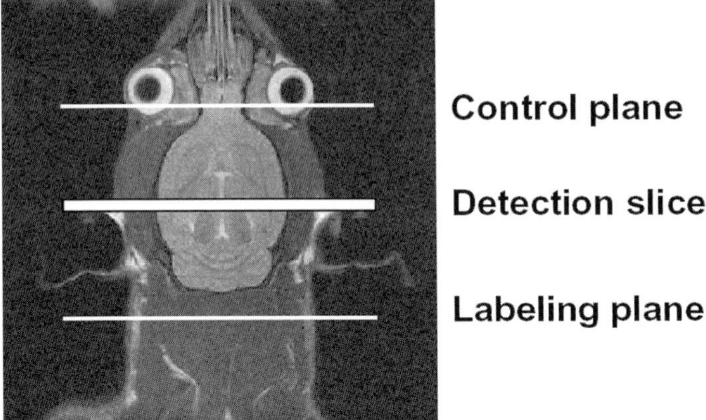

Fig. 3. Schematic of rat brain perfusion measurement in a coronal plane (detection slice) using flow-induced adiabatic fast passage inversion. Spins are labeled by applying continuous wave radio frequency (RF) in the presence of a gradient perpendicular to detection slice; this defines a resonance plane (labeling plane) at which flowing arterial spins are inverted. A control image is acquired by offsetting the frequency of continuous RF by the appropriate amount such that a resonance plane symmetrically distal to detection plane is excited.

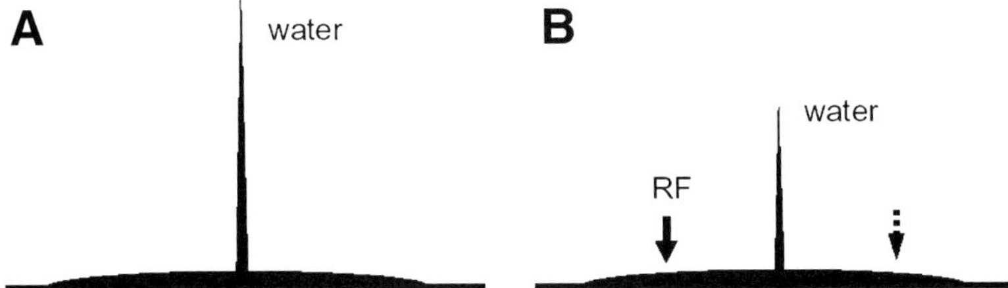

Fig. 4. **(A)** The proton spectrum of tissue consists of a narrow resonance for mobile water and a broad line representing macromolecules. **(B)** Radio frequency (RF) applied for labeling in a continuous arterial spin labeling experiment is offset in frequency such that it does not directly saturate the water resonance, but excitation of macromolecules results in reduced water resonance intensity through magnetization transfer effects (MTC). Reduction caused by MTC may be accounted for by acquiring a control image with RF placed on the symmetrically opposite side of the water resonance (dotted arrow).

$$\Delta v_c\,(Hz) = \mp 4256 \cdot G(Gauss\,/\,cm) \cdot \left(\Delta z_L\,(cm) - 2\Delta z_D\,(cm)\right), \qquad [20]$$

where Δz_D is the distance of the detection slice from the magnet isocenter. The presence of magnetization transfer (MT), and the need to control for it when a single coil is used for detection as well as labeling, imposes several restrictions on the experiment. First, the labeling and detection planes are required to be parallel and, in the case of rat brain perfusion imaging, this restricts images to the transverse plane (coronal for rat brain). Second, MT can be controlled for only one image at a time, therefore, multislice acquisitions in the same scan are not possible. Several modifications to overcome these limitations for 3D acquisitions of perfusion have been proposed and will be discussed in **Subheading 2.2.2.**

Another factor that needs to be considered is the signal from intravascular blood water in the detection slice. Perfusion by CASL is measured by changes in tissue water magnetization due to labeling, but pixel intensities in MR images often possess contributions from signal component from vascular water in blood vessels. Although venous blood magnetization is in equilibrium with tissue water and will not cause a major change to the overall signal intensity, pixels containing labeled arterial blood can significantly change the pixel intensity from that due to tissue water signal; thus, overestimating perfusion in these pixels. Signal from labeled vascular spins may be minimized by either crushing the signal from vascular spins using diffusion crusher gradients *(32)*, or by allowing a sufficient postlabeling time between labeling and imaging to allow the labeled spins in the arteries to flow out of the detection slice *(33)*.

2.1.1. Measurement of Labeling Efficiency, α

AFP inversion is a robust labeling technique and after it is optimized for a particular RF coil and animal combination, it often provides a reliable and reproducible labeling efficiency for subsequent measurements. For precise quantitation, measurement of the labeling efficiency, α for each perfusion measurement is recommended. Ideally, α should be measured in an artery just before its entry into the tissue of interest. This is not always possible because of the lack of an artery large enough to be imaged deep in tissue. In the rat brain, the labeling efficiency may be measured by imaging the carotid arteries distal to the labeling plane *(22)*. Typically, a flow-compensated gradient-echo sequence with sufficient spatial resolution is used to image the arteries about 0.5 cm distal to the imaging plane. Signal intensities of the carotid blood for labeled and unlabeled images are used to calculate the labeling efficiency *(22)*. Because images are obtained in magnitude mode, image intensity measurements do not provide information about the sign of the blood magnetization. Thus, it is necessary to first establish whether the AFP parameters used in the experiment do in fact result in inversion of spins. This can be easily confirmed by verifying that the intensity of blood passes through a minimum for a series of images obtained with varying B_1 values, starting from very low B_1 *(22)*. Labeling efficiency, α, is calculated as:

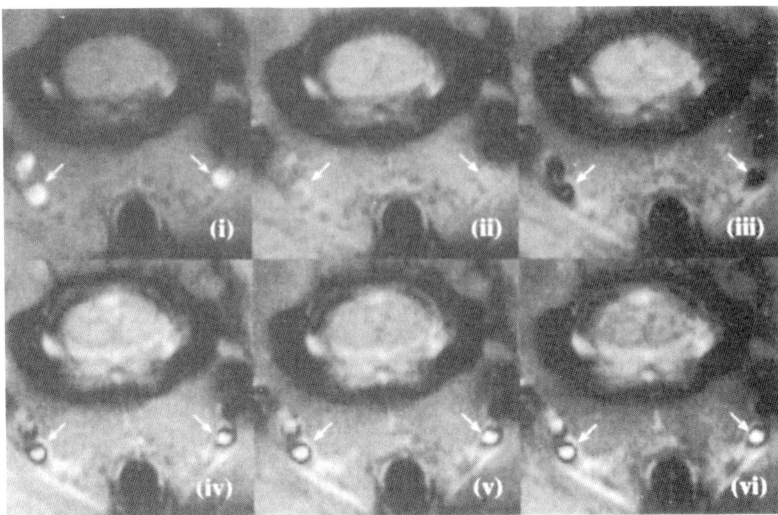

Fig. 5. Magnitude-calculated transverse magnetic resonance (MR) images of a rat neck with adiabatic fast passage arterial spin labeling using different B_1 strengths. The B_1 values used were 0 (i), 30 (ii), 60 (iii), 90 (iv), 120 (v), and 150 (vi) mG. Images were acquired using a gradient-echo sequence with echo time (TE) = 10 ms and repetition time (TR) = 530 ms. Radio frequency (RF) irradiation for spin labeling was applied for 500 ms during the TR period immediately before imaging. The original images had field of view (FOV) = 4.5 cm × 4.5 cm. Images presented were produced by zooming to FOV = 1.6 × 1.6 cm. Signal intensities in the carotid arteries (arrows) decrease and then increase as the B_1 power increases. The increase after minimum is caused by a change in phase (i.e., inversion) which shows up as increased signal intensity in the magnitude-calculated images. α is estimated using image intensies of carotid arteries (arrows) in **Eq. [21]**. (From **ref. *22***, courtesy of John Wiley and Sons.)

$$\alpha = \frac{S_c \pm S_L}{2S_c},$$
[21]

where S_C and S_L are signal intensities of blood in arteries in unlabeled and labeled images, respectively, with + or − being used depending on whether the spins are inverted or not. **Figure 5** shows typical images from a rat obtained for measurement of α.

2.1.2. Measurement of Transit Time

The spin label will, of course, relax because of T_1 relaxation during its transit from the labeling location to tissue of interest, and this loss of label can be accounted for if the T_1 for blood and the transit time are known. The transit

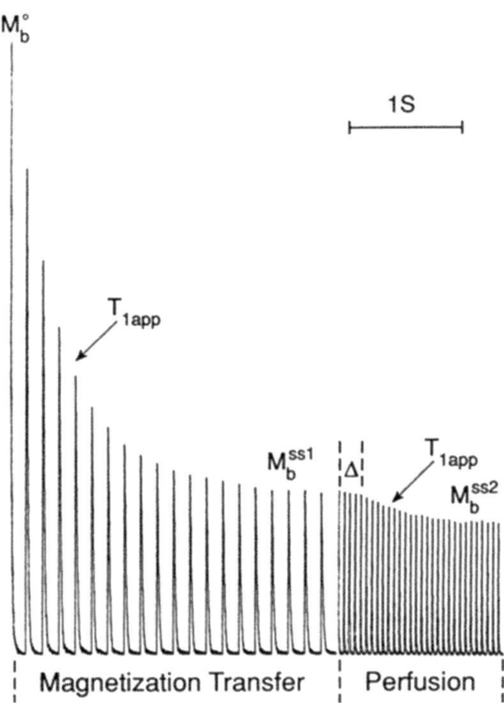

Fig. 6. Volume-localized brain tissue water Z-magnetization in a rat acquired with stimulated echo mode sequence for varying durations of radio frequency (RF) for saturation of macromolecules (magnetization transfer), and inversion of arterial water spins (perfusion). For the magnetization transfer period, RF irradiation was placed distal to the observed volume, and data show the behavior of magnetization, as described by **Eq. [12]**. Switching RF frequency to irradiate spins proximal to the observed volume results in inversion of spins, leading to a further, albeit small, decrease in Z-magnetization. Notice that after switching to inversion mode, magnetization remains constant for a time before it begins to decay; this delay, Δ, defines the transit time, the time taken for spins to travel from labeling location to tissue location. (From **ref.** *24*, courtesy of John Wiley and Sons.)

time has been measured by monitoring the signal intensity in brain after varying periods of delays after labeling. The arrival of labeled spins in the brain is signified by the beginning of a brain signal decrease, and the postlabeling delay at which this occurs is assumed to be a measure of transit time *(24,34,35)*. Measurement of transit time and several features of the CASL experiment are well illustrated in **Fig. 6**, reproduced from Zhang, et al. *(24)*. In this study, the first half of the experiment demonstrates how brain magnetization decreases due to magnetization transfer. For this part, the frequency of RF was placed on the control plane and Z-magnetization of brain tissue sampled with a stimulated echo mode sequence, for varying durations of RF. With increasing magnetization transfer times, brain Z-magnetization decreases exponentially with a time constant T_{1app} to a steady-state value, M_t^{ss1}. In the second half of the experiment, the frequency of RF is switched to the labeling plane and the brain water Z-magnetization sampled after varying delays after labeling. The magnetization stays constant until the labeled spins arrive at the tissue (transit time, Δ), and the signal then decays according to T_{1app} to a new steady state value, M_t^{ss2}, resulting from exchange of labeled spins with tissue water. If the transit time, Δ, is known, loss of label due to relaxation may be accounted for in the labeling efficiency as:

$$\alpha' = \alpha e^{\left(-\Delta/T_{1a}\right)}, \tag{22}$$

where T_{1a} is the T_1 relaxation time of arterial blood. Because the measurement of transit time is time consuming, it is not often carried out for each perfusion determination. Rather, a previously determined value is used. Alternatively, the sensitivity of the perfusion measurement to transit time may be minimized through the introduction of a postlabeling delay, a waiting period between the end of labeling period and the start of image acquisition *(33)*. It has been shown that transit time can be accounted for by carrying out the experiment with a postlabeling delay greater than the suspected transit time, and correcting the labeling efficiency for relaxation during the postlabeling delay, according to *(33)*:

$$\alpha' = \alpha e^{\left(-w/T_{1a}\right)}. \tag{23}$$

2.1.3. Measurement of Tissue T_1

T_{1obs}, as defined by **Eq. [16]** is the longitudinal relaxation time of tissue due to the natural T_1 of tissue water plus a component due to unperturbed water spins flowing into the tissue. It can be conveniently measured using a saturation recovery or inversion recovery (with slice-selective inversion pulse) sequence in the detection slice. The fact that a slice-selective T_1 sequence measures a T_1 as defined by **Eq. [16]** has been verified by measuring the slice-selective T_1 in an isolated perfused heart model; T_1 was measured for varying perfusate flow rates and the relaxation rate was shown to be linearly dependent on flow *(27)*. Generating perfusion maps require a T_{1obs} map, which can be calculated from a series of images constituting a saturation recovery sequence. Typically, a series of images in the detection slice are obtained, either at vary-

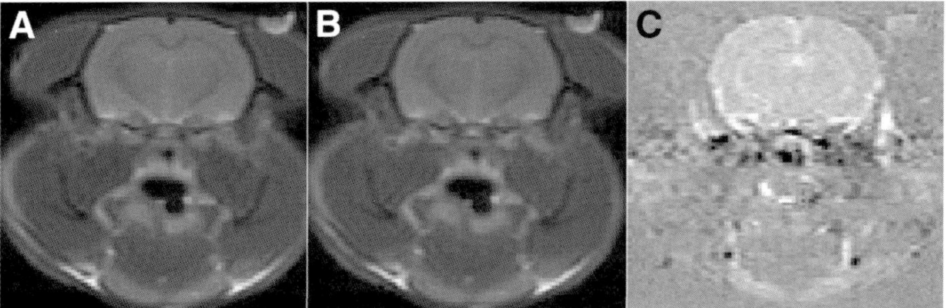

Fig. 7. Typical images obtained in a continuous arterial spin labeling experiment with adiabatic fast passage inversion of arterial spins for coronal slice in rat brain. (**A**) Control image, (**B**) labeled image, and (**C**) difference image. Note that in the difference image, that, with the exception of signals from blood vessels, image intensity outside the brain approaches zero because of very low blood flow to muscle compared with brain tissue.

ing TR values, or at varying recovery times after saturation pulses, and a pixel-by-pixel fit is carried out to the equation:

$$M_t(\tau) = A + Be^{-\left(\tau/T_{1obs}\right)} \tag{24}$$

where $M_t(\tau)$ is the pixel intensity of the image for a particular TR or recovery time τ, and A and B are constants.

The only other unknown quantity in **Eq. [15]** is the tissue:blood partition coefficient for water, λ, for which literature values are typically used; for the brain, a value of 0.9 mL/g is often used (*36*). A perfusion map may now be calculated using the labeled image, control image, and the T_{1obs} image, and carrying out a pixel-by-pixel calculation of f according to **Eq. [15]**. Alternatively, an average value for perfusion within a region of interest (ROI) may be calculated using the average values for M_t^{ss1}, M_t^{ss2}, and T_{1obs}, respectively, within the specified ROI in **Eq. [15]**. **Figure 7** shows typical images obtained in measurement of perfusion by CASL with flow-induced AFP inversion in the rat.

2.2. Three-Dimensional Perfusion Imaging

When a single coil is used for labeling and detection, the spatial dependence of MTC caused by the labeling RF limits perfusion image acquisition to planes parallel to the labeling plane. Also, the necessity of placing the control imaging plane symmetrically opposite and equidistant from the labeling plane means that each detection plane needs to have its control image acquired separately,

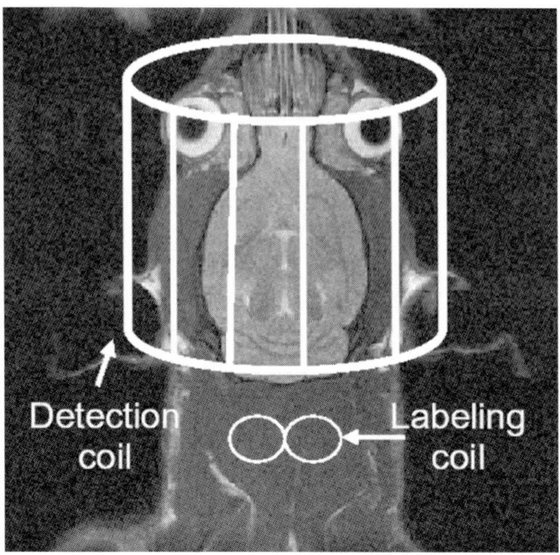

Fig. 8. Three-dimensional perfusion imaging in rat using two coils. Magnetization transfer effects are avoided using a separate labeling coil designed with a confined RF profile that does not reach brain tissue. Additional circuitry is often necessary to minimize cross talk between the labeling coil and the detection coil.

ruling out the option of acquiring control images for a slice group in multislice mode. One way to overcome this restriction is to use two RF coils, one for detection and a separate coil for labeling (**Fig. 8**). In this scheme, MTC from the labeling RF are eliminated if the labeling coil has sufficient RF coverage to label the arteries of interest but is small enough that its RF profile does not reach the tissue of interest *(37)*. Often, a small coil size itself is not sufficient to prevent the labeling RF field from reaching the tissue of interest because the labeling and detection coils can interact and alter each other's excitation profile. Additional circuitry actively decoupling the coils from each other during the time each coil is excited has provided excellent isolation of the coils for brain perfusion imaging in the rat *(37)* and human *(25,38)*. The details of coil geometry and decoupling circuits have been published elsewhere and needs to be adapted for the specific situation and scanner characteristics. For labeling blood in the carotid arteries, a butterfly or figure-8 coil of appropriate size can be constructed to give sufficient depth to label blood without exciting brain tissue *(37)*. The two-coil scheme places additional requirements on the capabilities of the scanner. It requires the scanner to possess two independent RF excitation channels for detection and labeling, respectively. In addition, control transistor-transistor logic (TTL) pulse outputs are required to actively decouple coils during transmission and need to be programmed into the pulse sequence. A two-coil arrangement can be used to carry out perfusion imaging in any slice direction and also in multislice mode, and the experiment and the quantitation are performed identical to the single-slice acquisition described in **Subheading 2.1.**

Several approaches have been proposed for multislice perfusion imaging by controlling for MTC without the use of additional hardware. In the modulated labeling RF procedure, a control image is acquired with application of cosine-modulated labeling RF in the neck region; the modulated RF produces two RF excitation sidebands separated by a frequency difference that can be controlled with the modulation frequency. The scheme is based on producing unperturbed blood by inversion at two closely spaced planes placed on either side of the labeling plane *(39)*. In this scheme, it is assumed that MTC on the brain can be made equal for the labeling and control images if the value of B_1 used for the modulated RF is half of that used for inversion, such that the total RF irradiation and frequency offset seen by brain tissue remains approximately the same. The technique has provided 3D coverage of perfusion images of the human brain but suffers from limitations. A true control image with unperturbed Z-magnetization is possible only if each AFP perturbation of the modulated RF pair produces complete inversion. In practice, inversion is rarely perfect ($\alpha > 1$) and will result in a control image with a Z-magnetization that is different from its equilibrium value. Although this can be accounted for in the perfusion quantitation by measuring the labeling efficiency for control and labeled images, sensitivity of the technique will drop rapidly as inversion efficiency deviates from 1. In brain perfusion of animals, brain tissue is much closer to the labeling plane and maintaining the same MTC in brain regions close to the labeling plane for the single and double inversion images may be difficult. A second technique attempts to minimize the spatial dependence of MTC by applying a cosine-modulated labeling RF excitation applied proximal and distal to the brain *(40)*. This excitation creates a region in the brain that exhibits constant MTC; repeating the sequence with no labeling gradient provides the control image. For 3D perfusion imaging of the human as well as animal brain, data in the literature suggest a two-coil arrangement as the most appropriate method to provide reliable perfusion quantitation.

2.3. Application of CASL to Other Organs

Although most applications using ASL have been on the brain, ASL has also been successfully applied to the kidneys in rats and humans *(18,40,41)*. Kidneys have a well-defined arterial input that can be labeled very effectively at either the descending aorta or the renal arteries. Transverse (short axis) perfusion images of the kidneys have been obtained in the rat by labeling blood in the supra-renal aorta in normal *(18)* and transplanted *(42)* kidneys, and in conscious rats *(43)* with cortical perfusion rates in excellent agreement with those obtained by traditional techniques. Because ASL is a difference technique, it is essential that motion artifacts are well controlled; a fast FLASH sequence has been found to provide artifact-free images of the kidneys in the rat *(18)*. Using a single coil for labeling and detection, arterial labeling may be carried out in the supra-renal aorta using a transverse labeling gradient and an optimized value for labeling B_1 strength. Labeling efficiency may be measured in the aorta distal to the labeling plane, as described in **Subheading 2.1.1.** Renal perfusion images have been obtained using a single labeling period (labeling time $>> T_{1app}$) for steady state to be reached, followed by a fast (imaging time $<< T_{1obs}$) acquisition of the image *(18,42,43)*. Centric phase encoding has been used to ensure that the image intensity represents a value as close as possible to steady state. Renal perfusion imaging using ASL is limited to the cortex; perfusion quantitation in the medulla or the papilla is not possible. This is because of the microcirculation path in the kidney; blood entering the medulla first passes through glomeruli, where the dense capillary network allows labeled water to freely exchange with cortical tissue water, thereby losing most of its spin label. Application of ASL techniques to measuring perfusion in other organs has been attempted with limited success; further development is required before routine measurements are possible.

3. Conclusions

Perfusion imaging using ASL has been successfully applied to the brain and kidneys in animal models and in humans. Most studies have used CASL because it offers the maximum possible sensitivity, but in cases in which hardware limitations or other restrictions rule out application of CASL, appropriate PASL techniques should be pursued. The totally noninvasive nature of ASL techniques allows repeated measurements to be made at a temporal resolution, in principle, limited only by tissue T_1. Absolute quantitation using ASL can be time consuming because of the need to measure ancillary parameters for each perfusion determination; relative changes in perfusion with a faster time resolution are often monitored by only measuring the tissue water signal change due to labeling.

Acknowledgments

The author thanks Lalith Talagala and Afonso Silva for helpful discussions.

References

1. Kety, S. S. and Schmidt, C. F. (1945) The determination of cerebral blood flow in man by the use of nitrous oxide in low concentrations. *Am. J. Physiol.* **143,** 53–66.
2. Bell, B. A. (1984) A history of the study of the cerebral circulation and the measurement of cerebral blood flow. *Neurosurgery* **14,** 238–246.

3. Kety, S. S. (1951) The theory and applications of the exchange of inert gas at the lungs and tissues. *Pharmacol. Rev.* **3,** 1–41.

4. Calamante, F., Thomas, D. L., Pell, G. S., Wiersma, J., and Turner, R. (1999) Measuring cerebral blood flow using magnetic resonance imaging techniques. *J. Cereb. Blood Flow Metab.* **19,** 701–735.

5. Koretsky, A. P., Silva, A. C., Williams, D. S., Zhang, W., and Detre, J. A. (1995) Magnetic resonance imaging of cerebral blood flow, in *Cerebrovascular Diseases Nineteenth Princeton Stroke Conference* (Moskowitz, M.A. and Caplan, L.R., eds.), Butterworth-Heinemann, Boston, MA, pp. 463–473.

6. Barbier, E., Lamalle, L., and Décorps, M. (2001) Methodology of brain perfusion imaging. *J. Magn. Reson. Imaging* **13,** 496–520.

7. Ackerman, J. J. H., Ewy, C. S., Becker, N. N., and Shalowitz, R. A. (1987) Deuterium nuclear magnetic resonance measurements of blood flow and tissue perfusion employing ^2H_2O as a freely diffusible tracer. *Proc. Natl. Acad. Sci. USA* **84,** 4099–4102.

8. Detre, J. A., Subramaniam, V. H., Mitchell, M. D., et al. (1990) Measurement of regional cerebral blood flow in cat brain using intracarotid injection of ^2H_2O and ^2H imaging. *Magn. Reson. Med.* **14,** 389–395.

9. Detre, J. A., Eskey, C. J., and Koretsky, A. P. (1990) Measurement of cerebral blood flow in rat brain by 19F-NMR detection of trifluoromethane washout. *Magn. Reson. Med.* **15,** 45–57.

10. Pekar, J., Ligeti, L., Ruttner, Z., et al. (1991) In vivo measurement of cerebral oxygen consumption and blood flow using ^{17}O magnetic resonance imaging. *Magn. Reson. Med.* **21,** 313–319.

11. Ostergaard, L., Sorensen, A. G., Kwong, K. K., Weisskoff, R. M., Gyldensted, C., and Rosen, B. R. (1996) High resolution measurement of cerebral blood flow using intravascular tracer bolus passages. II. Experimental comparison and preliminary results. *Magn. Reson. Med.* **36,** 726–736.

12. Ostergaard, L., Weisskoff, R. M., Chesler, D. A., Gyldensted, C., and Rosen, B. R. (1996) High resolution measurement of cerebral blood flow using intravascular tracer bolus passages. I Mathematical approach and statistical analysis. *Magn. Reson. Med.* **36,** 715–725.

13. Le Bihan, D., Breton, E., Lallemand, D., Grenier, P., Cabanis, E., and Laval-Jeantet, M. (1986) MR imaging of intravoxel incoherent motions: application to diffusion and perfusion in neurologic disorders. *Radiology* **161,** 401–407.

14. Ogawa, S., Lee, T. M., Nayak, A. S., and Glynn, P. (1990) Oxygenation-sensitive contrast in magnetic resonance image of rodent brain at high magnetic fields. *Magn. Reson. Med.* **14,** 68–78.

15. Ogawa, S., Tank, D. W., Menon, R., et al. (1992) Intrinsic signal changes accompanies sensory stimulation: functional brain mapping using magnetic resonance imaging. *Proc. Natl. Acad. Sci. USA* **89,** 5951–5955.

16. Detre, J. A., Leigh, J. S., Williams, D. S., and Koretsky, A. P. (1992) Perfusion imaging. *Magn. Reson. Med.* **23,** 37–45.

17. Williams, D. S., Detre, J. A., Leigh, J. S., and Koretsky, A. P. (1992) Magnetic resonance imaging of perfusion using spin inversion of arterial water. *Proc. Natl. Acad. Sci. USA* **89,** 212–216.

18. Williams, D. S., Zhang, W., Koretsky, A. P., and Adler, S. (1992) Perfusion imaging of the rat kidney with MR. *Radiology* **190,** 813–818.

19. Williams, D. S., Detre, J. A., Zhang, W., and Koretsky, A. P. (1993) Fast serial MRI of perfusion in the rat brain using spin inversion of arterial water. *Bulletin Magn. Reson.* **15,** 60–63.

20. Dixon, W. T., Du, L. N., Faul, D. D., Gado, M., and Rossnick, S. (1986) Projection angiograms of blood labeled by adiabatic fast passage. *Magn. Reson. Med.* **3,** 454–462.

21. Abragam A. (1961) *Principles of Nuclear Magnetism*, Clarendon, Oxford, UK.

22. Zhang, W., Williams, D. S., and Koretsky, A. P. (1993) Measurement of rat brain perfusion by NMR using spin labeling of arterial water: in vivo determination of the degree of spin labeling. *Magn. Reson. Med.* **29,** 416–421.

23. Uttig, J. F., Thomas, D. L., Gadian, D. G., and Ordidge, R. J. (2003) Velocity-driven adiabatic fast passage for arterial spin labeling: results from a computer model. *Magn. Reson. Med.* **49,** 398–401.

24. Zhang, W., Williams, D. S., Detre, J. A., and Koretsky, A. P. (1992) Measurement of brain perfusion by volume-localized NMR spectroscopy using inversion of arterial spins: Accounting for transit time and cross relaxation. *Magn. Reson. Med.* **25,** 362–371.

25. Talagala, S. L., Ye, F. Q., Ledden, P. J., and Chesnick, S. (2004) Whole brain 3D perfusion MRI at 3.0 T using CASL with a separate labeling coil. *Magn. Reson. Med.* **52,** 131–140.

26. Edelman, R. R., Siewert, B., Darby, D. G., et al. (1994) Qualitative mapping of cerebral blood flow and functional localization with echo planar MR imaging and signal targeting with alternating radiofrequency. *Radiology* **192,** 513–520.

27. Williams, D. S., Grandis, D. J., Zhang, W., and Koretsky, A. P. (1993) Magnetic resonance imaging of perfusion in the isolated rat heart using spin inversion of arterial water. *Magn. Reson. Med.* **30,** 361–365.

28. Kwong, K. K., Chesler, D. A., Weisskoff, R. M., et al. (1995). MR perfusion studies with T_1-weighted echo planar imaging. *Magn. Reson. Med.* **34,** 878–887.

29. Kim S-G. (1995) Quantification of relative cerebral blood flow change by flow-sensitive alternating inversion recovery (FAIR) technique: application to functional mapping. *Magn. Reson. Med.* **34,** 293–301.

30. Wong, E. C., Luh, W. M., and Liu, T. T. Turbo ASL: arterial spin labeling with higher SNR and temporal resolution. *Magn. Reson. Med.* 2000 **44,** 511–515.

31. Wolff, S. and Balaban, R. (1989) Magnetization transfer contrast (MTC) and tissue water proton relaxation in vivo. *Magn. Reson. Med.* **10,** 135–144.

32. Silva, A. C., Zhang, W., Williams, D. S., and Koretsky, A. P. (1997) Estimation of extraction fractions in rat brain using magnetic resonance measurement of perfusion with arterial spin labeling. *Magn. Reson. Med.* **35,** 58–68.

33. Alsop, D. C. and Detre, J. A. (1996) Reduced transit-time sensitivity in noninvasive magnetic resonance imaging of human cerebral blood flow. *J. Cereb. Blood Flow Metab.* **16,** 1236–1249.

34. Ye, F. Q., Mattay, V. S., Jezzard, P., Frank, F. A., Weinberger, D. R., and McLaughlin, A. C. (1997) Correction for vascular artifacts in cerebral blood flow values measured by using arterial spin tagging techniques. *Magn. Reson. Med.* **37,** 226–235.

35. Barbier, E. L., Silva, A. C., Kim, H. J., Williams, D. S., and Koretsky, A. P. (1999) Perfusion analysis using dynamic arterial spin labeling (DASL). *Magn. Reson. Med.* **41,** 299–308.

36. Herscovitch, P. and Raichle, M.E. (1985) What is the correct value for the brain–blood partition coefficient for water? *J. Cereb. Blood Flow Metab.* **5,** 65–69.

37. Silva, A. S., Zhang, W., Williams, D. S., and Koretsky, A. P. (1995) Multi-slice MRI of rat brain perfusion during amphetamine stimulation using arterial spin labeling. *Magn. Reson. Med.* **33,** 209–214.

38. Zaharchuck, G., Ledden, P. J., Kwong, K. K., Reese, T. G., Rosen, B. R., and Wald, L. L. (1999) Multislice perfusion and perfusion territory imaging in humans with separate label and image coils. *Magn. Reson. Med.* **41,** 1093–1098.

39. Alsop, D.C. and Detre, J.A. (1998) Multisection cerebral blood flow MR imaging with continuous arterial spin labeling. *Radiology* **202,** 410–416.

40. Talagala, S. L. and Kam, A. W. (2000) Multi-slice perfusion MRI of the kidney using SPDI-CASL. *Proc. Intl. Soc. Magn. Reson. Med.*, p. 705.

41. Roberts, D. A., Detre, J. A., Bolinger, L., et al. (1995) Renal perfusion in humans: MR imaging with spin tagging of arterial water. *Radiology* **196,** 281–286.

42. Wang, J.-J., Hendrich, K. S., Jackson, E. K., Ildstad, S. T., Williams, D. S., and Ho. C. (1998) Perfusion quantitation in transplanted rat kidney by MRI with arterial spin labeling. *Kidney Intl.* **53,** 1783–1791.

43. Kost, C. K., Jr, Li, P., Williams, D. S., and Jackson, E. K. (1998) Renal vascular responses to angiotensin II in conscious spontaneously hypertensive and normotensive rats. *J. Cardiovasc. Pharmacol.* **31,** 854–861.

Physiology of Functional Magnetic Resonance Imaging

Energetics and Function

Ikuhiro Kida and Fahmeed Hyder

Summary

Quantitative magnetic resonance spectroscopy (MRS) and imaging (MRI) measurements of energy metabolism (i.e., cerebral metabolic rate of oxygen consumption, $CMRo_2$), blood circulation (i.e., cerebral blood flow, CBF; and cerebral blood volume, CBV), and functional MRI (fMRI) were used to interpret the physiological basis of blood oxygenation level-dependent (BOLD) image contrast at 7 T in rat brain. Multimodal signals over a wide range of activity, for primarily glutamatergic neurons, were measured. Because each parameter that can influence the BOLD image contrast was measured quantitatively and separately, multimodal measurements of changes in $CMRo_2$, CBF, CBV, and BOLD signal allowed calibration as well as validation of fMRI. Good agreement between changes in $CMRo_2$ calculated from BOLD theory and measured by ^{13}C MRS reveal that BOLD signal changes at 7 T are closely linked with alterations in neuronal glucose oxidation of glutamatergic neurons, both for activation and de-activation paradigms. Additional neurochemical and neurophysiological studies with fMRI suggest that the BOLD response from the cerebral cortex is closely linked to neurotransmitter release and energetic demand of glutamatergic neurons. Thus, calibrated fMRI may be used to reflect energetic changes of ensembles of glutamatergic neurons in the cerebral cortex.

Key Words: Astrocyte; glucose; glutamate; glutamine; glycogen; lactate; neuronal activity; oxygen.

1. Introduction
1.1. BOLD fMRI: Window to Brain Function

The relationship between brain and mind remains poorly understood despite efforts by numerous scientists armed with an abundance of methodologies. Previous methods for measuring human brain function were limited to examining behavioral perturbations following selective brain injury or direct implantation of electrodes for measuring changes in electrical activity. Although development of positron emission topography (PET), which noninvasively

From: *Methods in Molecular Medicine, Vol. 124*
Magnetic Resonance Imaging: Methods and Biologic Applications
Edited by: P. V. Prasad © Humana Press Inc., Totowa, NJ

interprets changes in brain activity from alterations of cerebral metabolism and blood flow, began in the 1970s, its progress into mainstream studies of neuroscience was hindered by the need for special equipment and dependence on radioactive materials. However, the revolutionary idea of being able to visualize changes in brain function appealed to scientists in a wide range of disciplines, and magnetic resonance imaging (MRI) was a technology poised for being an integral part of the brain mapping revolution. Because MRI has long been a modality primarily used in a clinical capacity to visualize structural aspects of a patient's brain (and body), its evolution into the contemporary neuroimaging technique of choice among both scientists and clinicians makes an interesting narrative *(1)*. This technique, appropriately termed functional MRI (fMRI), can noninvasively, albeit indirectly, map changes in neuronal activity from a normal brain in healthy subjects in a repeated manner, and for these reasons, fMRI has become the preferred method for human neuroimaging in the last few years.

The basic principle of fMRI is captured by the blood oxygenation level-dependent (BOLD) effect discovered by Ogawa and coworkers *(2)*. They reported that the MRI contrast of a rat brain image was changed when the rodent inhaled high vs low fractions of oxygen. The magnetic properties of blood changing with oxygenation had been known for several decades *(3)*, because deoxyhemoglobin is paramagnetic, whereas oxyhemoglobin is diamagnetic. Ogawa and coworkers suggested that the MRI contrast was generated by the modified MRI signal (from protons of water molecules) in and around blood vessels and was caused by the presence (or absence) of deoxyhemoglobin in the vasculature *(2)*. Behaving as an endogenous contrast agent, presence of paramagnetic deoxyhemoglobin inside capillaries creates local magnetic field gradients that extend into the surrounding tissue, thus causing the (gradient or spin-echo) MRI signal within a voxel to dephase more than otherwise (e.g., in the presence of diamagnetic oxyhemoglobin). These local gradients are a consequence of the volume magnetic susceptibility difference between tissue and the compartmentalized paramagnetic material inside the vasculature. Following this surprising observation with BOLD contrast in rat brains, four groups independently, but almost simultaneously, reported that stimulation-induced fMRI signal changes based on this contrast mechanism could be mapped noninvasively in normal human volunteers *(4–7)*. This was the beginning of the fMRI revolution that has since swept through disciplines of psychology, radiology, neurology, and neuroscience.

1.2. What Do BOLD MRI Changes Reflect?

Although there has been great progress in the biophysical understanding of susceptibility-based contrast enhancement with BOLD *(8–10)*, the neurophysiological interpretation of fMRI has been lacking *(11–13)*. In this chapter, we will discuss both the biophysical and neurophysiological basis of BOLD contrast. However, we will specifically focus on some experimental data that shed light on the energetic basis of fMRI—an often ignored aspect of neuroimaging with fMRI—and the bright future of fMRI being made possible by higher magnetic field strengths.

2. Biophysics of BOLD Contrast Mechanism

More than half a century ago, Pauling and Coryell reported the relevance of hemoglobin for magnetic resonance: deoxyhemoglobin is paramagnetic and oxyhemoglobin is diamagnetic *(3)*. Because the hemoglobin molecule is contained within the erythrocyte (i.e., red blood cell), the presence of deoxygenated vs oxygenated blood in the microvasculature manifests an MRI contrast, and the variation of the magnetic susceptibility can be captured by the transverse relaxation times measured by MRI *(14)*.

The presence of paramagnetic deoxyhemoglobin in blood vessels, behaving as an endogenous MRI contrast agent, causes changes in the local magnetic field gradients between blood vessels and tissue (**Fig. 1A**) *(2)*. These microscopic local gradients are a consequence of the volume magnetic susceptibility difference between tissue and the compartmentalized paramagnetic material inside the capillary. The local gradients outside the capillaries enhance the rate of dephasing of water protons (i.e., spins) in the tissue which can be detected by decreased MRI signals in spin-echo (SE) and gradient-echo (GE) images or shorter transverse relaxation times of tissue water (i.e., T_2^{SE} and T_2^{GE}) (**Fig. 1B**). Although the physical factors that affect T_2^{SE} and T_2^{GE} of a given MRI voxel at steady-state conditions have been explored using mathematical modeling *(9–11)*, it is important to appreciate that intravascular and extravascular weightings in the BOLD data depend on actual values of transverse relaxation times of water in blood (T_2^{intra}) and tissue (T_2^{extra}) (**Fig. 1C**) *(15,16)*. A relaxation term (T_2^0) that is not linked to susceptibility-based effects (i.e., dipole–dipole) is also included in both image contrasts:

$$\frac{1}{T_2^{GE}} = \frac{1}{T_2^0} + \frac{1}{T_2'} + \frac{1}{T_2} + \frac{1}{T_2^{\Delta B_0}} \qquad [1a]$$

$$\frac{1}{T_2^{SE}} = \frac{1}{T_2^0} + \frac{1}{T_2'}, \qquad [1b]$$

where $T_2^{\Delta B_0}$ is the relaxation component that is assigned to local magnetic field inhomogeneity (ΔB_0), and T_2 and T_2' are the relaxation components attributed to the reversible and nonreversible terms caused by blood oxygenation effects, respectively. Because the SE sequence has a 180° refocusing pulse, the revers-

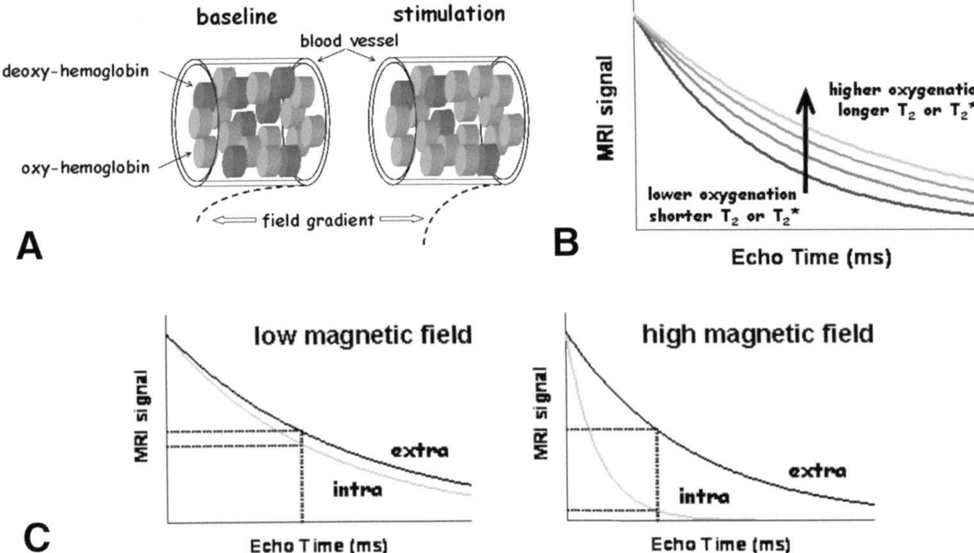

Fig. 1. The biophysical basis of fMRI. (**A**) Because deoxyhemoglobin is paramagnetic, the presence of this endogenous MRI contrast agent inside cerebral capillaries generates local magnetic field gradients that extend into cerebral tissue. The local gradients enhance dephasing of water protons in the tissue, which can be detected by decreased signals in T_2^{SE}- and T_2^{GE}-weighted images. (**B**) During activation, the amount of deoxyhemoglobin is decreased in comparison with the resting condition; this difference between the stimulation-induced susceptibility difference of blood can be observed as changes in T_2 by spin-echo (SE) sequence or in T_2^* by GE sequence. (**C**) At any given static magnetic field strength, the intravascular and extravascular weightings in BOLD data depend on the transverse relaxation times of water in blood (T_2^{intra}; gray) and tissue (T_2^{extra}; black). Prior studies have shown that T_2^{intra} T_2^{extra} at low fields, which suggests that both intravascular and extravascular compartments are equally contributing, whereas measured values show that $T_2^{intra} < T_2^{extra}$ at high fields, which indicates that the extravascular compartment is far more dominant.

ible (or susceptibility-based) blood oxygenation components (T_2) from GE are refocused. The combined SE and GE maps, after removal of the $T_2^{\Delta B_0}$ component using specific magnetic field tagging sequences (*17*), can provide a term that is closely related to the reversible term (T_2) and is mostly dependent on blood oxygenation effects from capillaries (*18*).

At low magnetic fields, because T_2^{intra} is usually slightly different from T_2^{extra}, the BOLD signal is often equally weighted by both compartments (**Fig. 1C**). However, at higher magnetic field strengths the BOLD signal is more heavily weighted by the extravascular compartment because T_2^{intra} is significantly shorter than T_2^{extra} (**Fig. 1C**). Therefore, at static magnetic field strengths of 4 T and higher, the BOLD effects with SE and GE signals are predominantly associated with the extravascular compartment *(19,20)*. Because the effect of the extravascular component may provide localization of neuronal activation *(21)*, the extravascular effects of BOLD are desired for neuroimaging.

Despite these advantages when working at high static magnetic fields, there are two types of vascular effects that should be avoided. Because the blood volume fraction tends to be small for a typical MRI voxel, there is an inherent partial volume bias toward signal from tissue water with either contrast. However, very large vessels (e.g., draining veins) can have larger partial volumes and these "false positives" in GE data can be removed by comparison with SE data *(22,23)*. Another type of vascular effect can be compressed by diffusion gradients in SE data *(21,22)* to reduce signals of slow and intermediate diffusion regimes.

Careful implementation of these precautions at high magnetic fields of modern scanners increase the signal-to-noise ratio (SNR) of the stimulation-induced positive BOLD signal change at steady-state *(19,20)*, depicting mainly increased blood oxygenation. Because the SNR of the so-called initial dip of the BOLD signal immediately after the stimulation onset is extremely low *(20)* and, therefore, its detection has been rather elusive *(24)*, we will not discuss this type of stimulation-induced BOLD signal change. Instead, we will focus on the delayed positive BOLD signal change, primarily reflecting increase in blood oxygenation from a steady-state baseline condition to a steady-state activated condition. It should be emphasized that the steady-state positive (or negative) BOLD signal change has been the focus of theoretical studies *(8–13)*. Furthermore, this type of BOLD imaging has also been successfully used for mapping columnar structures in the cerebral cortex *(25,26)*, similar to expectations from neuroimaging results by 2-deoxyglucose autoradiography *(27,28)*.

3. Physiological Basis of BOLD Signal Changes

The brain is a highly energy-demanding organ *(29)*, and neurons and astrocytes consume energy at all times to maintain the ionic gradients across the cell membranes *(30)*. However, unlike other organs in the body, the brain does not have very large energy reserves and, therefore, the brain is extremely vulnerable to transient lapses in energy supply. This necessitates that the local energy delivery system be appropriately coupled to local energy demands *(31)*. When sensory stimulation leads to local increases in cerebral metabolism (i.e., cerebral metabolic rates of oxygen and glucose use, $CMRo_2$ and CMR_{glc}), the delivery system responds by commensurate alterations of cerebral perfusion (i.e., cerebral blood flow and volume, CBF and CBV). The exact mechanisms that mediate the coupling between cerebral metabolism and perfusion, first noted by Roy and Sherrington *(32)*, are still under investigation. However, this metabolism–perfusion coupling is the basis of modern-day neuroimaging methods *(1)*.

The relationship between changes in oxidative metabolism in cells and blood perfusion in capillaries clarifies the physiological basis of BOLD. The classic observation that arterial blood is nearly always oxygenated *(33)* stipulates that a change in blood oxygenation for a bulk of tissue can primarily be manifested at the venous end of the capillary bed *(11)*. The process of oxygen extraction by cerebral tissue from capillaries can be modeled almost the same way as an exogenous indicator's diffusion curves *(34)* because the only source of oxygen is the blood (i.e., hemoglobin) and the major sink for oxygen is in the tissue (i.e., mitochondria). Thus at steady state, $CMRo_2$ and CBF can be theoretically related to the arterio-venous difference of oxygen (C_a–C_v) by Fick's principle *(18)*. The steady-state BOLD signal, which is dependent on the T_2 term of **Eq. [1]**, is related to blood oxygenation (*Y*) and CBV.

$$\frac{1}{T_2} \propto (1 - Y)b \, , \tag{2}$$

where the (1–*Y*) term is the blood deoxygenation, which is given by the ratio of $CMRo_2/(C_a\,CBF)$, and *b* is the CBV in terms of the volume fraction of blood for a typical MRI voxel *(11)*. Because, under steady-state conditions, (1–*Y*) is proportional to the amount of deoxyhemoglobin in the blood *(18,19)*, the biophysical models simulating the stimulation-induced changes in T_2 can indirectly infer alterations in metabolism and perfusion from changes in the intravascular paramagnetic contrast agent *(9,10)*. Thus stimulation-induced changes in $CMRo_2$, CBF, and CBV provide the physiological basis for the BOLD signal change ($\Delta S/S$),

$$\frac{\Delta S}{S} = M\left(\frac{\Delta CBF}{CBF} - \frac{\Delta CMRo_2}{CMRo_2}\right) - N\left(\frac{\Delta CBV}{CBV}\right) , \tag{3}$$

where M and N are measurable constants (related to $T_2{}^{SE}$ and $T_2{}^{GE}$), and $\Delta CMRo_2/CMRo_2$, $\Delta CBF/CBF$, and $\Delta CBV/CBV$ are respective changes in oxidative metabolism, blood flow, and blood volume *(18)*. Note that M is equal to N divided by (1+$\Delta CBF/CBF$). In **Eq. [3]**, on the right-hand side, the first term (metabolism–perfusion) should dominate the second term (blood volume) for a positive $\Delta S/S$. Thus, voxels with positive $\Delta S/S$ reflect regions that have undergone increased blood oxygenation caused by functional hyperemia. The $\Delta CMRo_2/CMRo_2$ term is the most relevant of these physiological parameters in

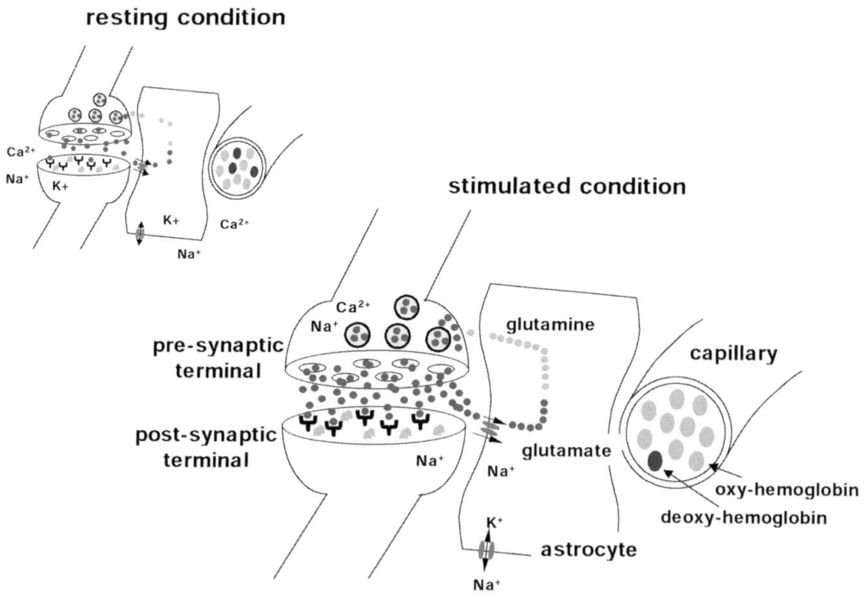

Fig. 2. The fMRI signal changes indirectly reflect alterations in energetics of glutamatergic synapses. Action potentials or spikes reach the presynaptic terminal to initiate the vesicular release of neurotransmitter molecules (glutamate) into the synaptic cleft. This activates the neurotransmitter receptors in the postsynaptic neuron, which is a step required in the propagation of electrical activity to the adjacent neuron in an all-or-none manner (in contrast, the subthreshold local or synaptic potentials do not function in an all-or-none manner). The extracellular glutamate (purple) is removed rapidly by Na^+-coupled transport into astrocytes, where it is converted into glutamine (gray). The glutamine is released and is transported into the neuron after reconversion to the neurotransmitter molecule, is repackaged into vesicles. A wide range of energy-consuming processes (which include action potential propagation, maintenance of membrane potentials, vesicular recycling, neurotransmitter release and uptake, and so on) are involved in signaling, in which the majority of the ATP used to support the cellular work is obtained from glucose oxidation in both neurons and astrocytes. Because the only source of oxygen is hemoglobin in the blood, and because the major sink for oxygen is the mitochondria, a tight relationship between CBF and CMo_2 is mandated.

Eq. [3] for studying brain activity *(35)*, because it is proportional to changes in energy use associated with alterations in neuronal activity *(36)*. To calibrate the BOLD effect, each term in **Eq. [3]** has to be measured *(18)*, not assumed or modeled.

When neurons are activated in a certain area of the brain (e.g., by stimulation of peripheral neurons), local blood flow and volume increase to supplement the substrate delivery (i.e., glucose and oxygen) by the amount needed to satisfy the increased energetic demands of the ensemble of neurons (**Fig. 2**).

Although the metabolic–perfusion changes underlying functional hyperemia provide a broad view for the physiology of BOLD, there are other features of neurotransmission that are important (**Fig. 2**). Cytological association between capillaries, astrocytes, and neurons in the brain provide the framework for the century-old hypothesis of activity–metabolic–perfusion coupling *(32)*. Astrocytes are preferentially located to provide a metabolic link between electrical activity and energy use *(37)*. Several energy-requiring processes are associated with neurotransmission. As a consequence of neurotransmission and passive ion leaks across the cell membrane, the active Na^+-K^+ pump uses ATP to restore Na^+ and K^+ concentrations across the membrane. An excited neuron generates short-lived (1–2 ms) presynaptic potentials (also known as action potentials or spikes) that propagate (micrometer scale) down axons to initiate Ca^{2+}-triggered neurotransmitter (e.g., glutamate) release via exocytocis of vesicles at the synaptic cleft, which in turn produce potentials in the postsynaptic neuron that can integrate over time (10–20 ms) and space (millimeter scale) to subsequently generate new trains of spikes once a threshold potential has been reached at a trigger zone near the cell body *(30)*. The astrocytic uptake of glutamate is a critical step in neurotransmission because high concentrations of neurotransmitters in the extracellular space impede cellular signaling. After synthesis of glutamine in the astrocyte and subsequent release, glutamine is taken up by the presynaptic neuron to form glutamate to replenish the neurotransmitter pool in the vesicles. Energy production, mainly via glucose oxidation, supports neurotransmission by reestablishing ionic gradients that prepare the cells to fire repetitively *(1)*. To establish the neurochemical basis of BOLD, some of these pathway(s) of neurotransmission must be impeded *(38)*.

4. Calibrated fMRI

To quantitatively understand the BOLD signal change caused by functional hyperemia, it is necessary to calibrate fMRI from direct measurements of BOLD signal, CBF, CBV, and $CMRo_2$, as shown in **Eq. [3]**. However, it is difficult to measure all of the parameters with the same spatial and temporal resolutions. An approach used by some groups (**Table 1**) is to perform the measurements of BOLD and CBF under hypercapnia perturbation to obtain values for the constants in **Eq. [3]** and then to measure CBF and BOLD signal during a functional challenge (e.g., a visual/motor stimulation in human subjects and sensory stimulation in animals). This hypercapnia method for calibration of fMRI must be treated with caution because it makes two critical assumptions.

First, it assumes that change in $CMRo_2$ during hypercapnia perturbation is negligible *(39,40)*, but statistically significant increases in $CMRo_2$ during hypercapnia have been reported *(41–43)*. The constants (M and N) in **Eq. [3]** are

Table 1
Summary of Calibrated fMRI Studies

	ΔCBF%	ΔCMRo$_2$%	ΔCBV%	$\dfrac{\Delta\text{CMRo}_2\%}{\Delta\text{CBF}\%}$	Subject; Area
Kim and Ugurbil *(81)*	43 ± 16	5.4 ± 7.3^a	15 ± 4^b	0.13	Human; visual
Kim et al. *(82)*	45 ± 12	7.5 ± 5.5^a	15 ± 4^b	0.17	Human; motor
Davis et al. *(83)*	45 ± 4	16 ± 1	15 ± 4^b	0.36	Human; visual
Hoge et al. *(84)*	32 (5–50)	16	11 ± 8^b	0.50	Human; visual
Kim et al. *(44)*	44 ± 9	15.6 ± 8.1	15 ± 3^b	0.35	Human; visual
Kastrup et al. *(85)*	61 ± 7	2.4 ± 4.9	20 ± 4^b	0.04	Human; visual
Mandeville et al. *(46)*	62 ± 16^c	19 ± 17	17 ± 2	0.31	Rat; sensory
Hyder et al. *(18)^d*	117 ± 41	93 ± 33	7 ± 4	0.79	Rat; sensory
Kastrup et al. *(86)*	71 ± 9	16 ± 9	23 ± 3^b	0.23	Human; motor
Smith et al. *(36)^d*	55 ± 15	40 ± 13	4 ± 2	0.73	Rat; sensory
Smith et al. *(36)^d*	156 ± 34	102 ± 22	9 ± 3	0.65	Rat; sensory
Feng et al. *(87)*	17.4 ± 1.4	10.4 ± 0.9	8 ± 1^e	0.60	Human; visual

[a]Assumed M and N in **Eq. [3]**.
[b]Estimated ΔCBV% with an assumed γ value of 0.38 in **Eq. [4]**.
[c]Measured ΔCBF% by laser Doppler flowmetry.
[d]Multimodal method (BOLD, CBF, and CBV).
[e]Estimated ΔCBV% with an assumed γ value of 0.50 in **Eq. [4]**.
CBF indicates cerebral blood flow; CMRo$_2$, cerebral metabolic rate of oxygen consumption; and CBV, cerebral blood volume.

determined from the ΔS/S and ΔCBF/CBF data during a hypercapnia challenge, and then these constants are used with the ΔS/S and ΔCBF/CBF data (and by assuming ΔCBV/CBV; *see* **Subheading 4.1.**) during a functional challenge to calculate the value of ΔCMRo$_2$/CMRo$_2$. However, if one assumes that CMRo$_2$ increases by 10% during mild hypercapnia, the stimulation-induced change in CMRo$_2$ during visual stimulation *(44)* may be underestimated by approximately a factor of two. Furthermore, there is the primary concern of hypercapnia altering the oxygen binding efficiency of hemoglobin in erythrocytes *(29)*, a confounding factor that cannot be corrected for because the hemoglobin saturation curve is not directly measured in vivo by MRI.

4.1. Relationship Between CBF and CBV

The second assumption in this hypercapnia method for calibration of fMRI is based on the perception of the perceived relationship between CBF and CBV—an assumption necessary because of the difficulty of measuring changes in CBV in human subjects because most currently approved MRI contrast agents have short lifetimes in circulation. As such, they assume that:

$$\left(\frac{\Delta CBV}{CBV}\right) = \left(\frac{\Delta CBF}{CBF}+1\right)^{\gamma} - 1 , \tag{5}$$

where γ is the power law factor for the relationship between changes in *CBV* and *CBF*. Most fMRI calibration studies in humans (**Table 1**) have used the γ value of 0.38, which was obtained in monkey brain with hypercapnia using PET *(45)*.

The γ value is still controversial, because several groups have observed different values of γ when measured by both MRI and other methods during functional challenge as opposed to hypercapnia *(18,46–48)*. However, these studies suggest that the γ value for functional and hypercapnia challenges are not identical, and, in fact, the γ value during a functional challenge is significantly smaller than the prior PET results *(45)*. Thus, all of the human results of $\Delta CMRo_2/CMRo_2$ listed in **Table 1** suffer from a slight underestimation, because γ values of 0.38 (or higher) were used. In the animal studies listed in **Table 1**, the same forepaw stimulation model *(28)* was used. During somatosensory stimulation in α-chloralose-anesthetized rats, Mandeville et al. *(46)* reported γ values that ranged from 0.18 and 0.36 using CBV changes measured by superparamagnetic MRI contrast agents and CBF changes measured by laser Doppler flowmetry. It is well known that the CBF changes measured by laser Doppler flowmetry are not quantitative and it may underestimate the actual fractional change in CBF by at least a factor of two *(49)*. Thus, the γ value from the Mandeville et al. study *(46)* during functional challenges may potentially be smaller. Similarly, during somatosensory stimulation in α-chloralose-anesthetized rats, Hyder et al. *(18)* reported γ values that ranged from 0.05 to 0.16 using CBV changes measured by superparamagnetic MRI contrast agents and CBF changes measured by arterial spin-tagging MRI. Because quantitative changes in CBF and CBV were measured sequentially in the same rodents in the same session, these γ values may be more reliable. Nevertheless, it should be noted that the variable reports of γ values from different studies may, in part, be caused by varied spatial resolutions for the different methods (i.e., MRI, PET, and optical imaging) and the actual source for the measurement of CBV (i.e., hemoglobin vs plasma content).

4.2. Multimodal Approach to Calibrated fMRI

To avoid these potential pitfalls affecting the calibration of fMRI, Hyder and colleagues *(17,18,36)* used a multimodal approach (at 7 T) in anesthetized rats by directly measuring changes in CBV, CBF, $CMRo_2$, and BOLD signal. Although the idea of this approach is quite simple (i.e., measure changes in all parameters in **Eq. [3]** induced by physiological perturbations, so that the constants M and N are used without complications), the realization of the experi-

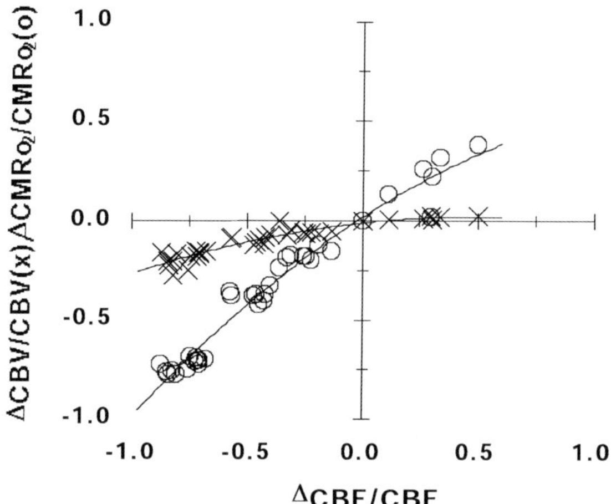

Fig. 3. Summary of quantitative magnetic resonance imaging (MRI) and magnetic resonance spectroscopy (MRS) measurements for blood oxygenation level-dependent (BOLD) in the anesthetized rat brain. Comparisons of $\Delta CBV/CBV$ (×) and $\Delta CMRo_2/CMRo_2$ (○) vs $\Delta CBF/CBF$ for the different conditions. The ratios of $(\Delta CMRo_2/CMRo_2)/(\Delta CBF/CBF)$ and $(\Delta CBV/CBV)/(\Delta CBF/CBF)$ are significantly different; the slopes through the origin are approx 0.7 and approx 0.1, respectively. The origin represents the resting awake state for rat cerebral cortex. CBV, cerebral blood volume; $CMRo_2$, cerebral metabolic rate of oxygen consumption; and CBF, cerebral blood flow.

ment is quite difficult because of methodological concerns. The multimodal measurement includes the arterial spin-tagging method for measuring CBF *(50)*, the use of long lifetime superparamagnetic MRI contrast agent for measuring CBV *(51)*, the ^{13}C glucose infusion in conjunction with heteronuclear magnetic resonance spectroscopy (MRS) for measuring $CMRo_2$ of glutamatergic neurons *(52)*, and the BOLD contrast as reflected by absolute measures of T_2^{SE} and T_2^{GE} *(17)*. For a region of interest in the somatosensory cortex, **Fig. 3** shows that for a specific magnitude of change in CBF from baseline, the change in $CMRo_2$ far exceeds the change in CBV. This indicates that the BOLD signal is influenced strongly by the neuroenergetics. An additional advantage with this multimodal approach is that the calibration of fMRI may also be validated. **Figure 4** shows a comparison between the predicted (from calibrated BOLD) and measured (from heteronuclear MRS) values of $\Delta CMRo_2/CMRo_2$. The $\Delta CMRo_2/CMRo_2$ values were predicted from changes in CBF, CBV, and T_2 based on **Eqs. [2]** and **[3]**. The prediction of $\Delta CMRo_2/CMRo_2$ is in good agreement with the measured values obtained from same region of interest by MRS over a wide range of neuronal activity *(17,18)*. This validation of the calibration makes it possible to map $\Delta CMRo_2/CMRo_2$ for

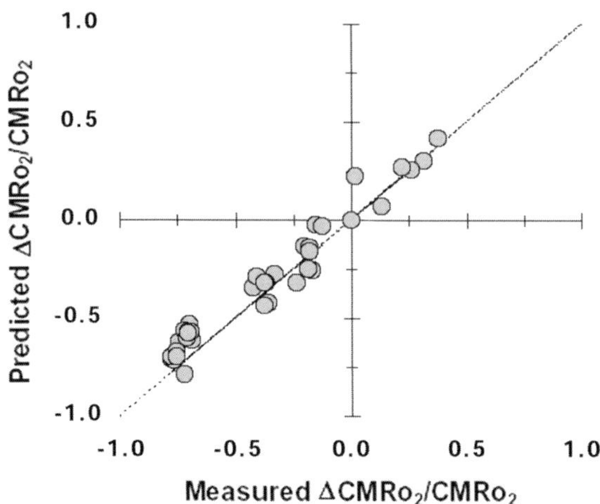

Fig. 4. Validation of calibrated fMRI. Comparison of predicted (by calibrated fMRI) and measured (by ^{13}C magnetic resonance spectroscopy) values of $\Delta CMR_{O_2}/CMR_{O_2}$ (cerebral metabolic rate of oxygen consumption) provide validation of the BOLD calibration at 7 T. The dotted line represents the line of identity. These results indicate that, at high fields, the microscopic susceptibility effects of deoxygenated hemoglobin dominates the relaxation effects in tissue, which can be accentuated by combining the GE and SE data (**Eqs. [1]** and **[2]**). Because the validation of BOLD calibration relies on standard errors of independent measures (for relaxation rate, blood flow, and volume), by comparing calculated and measured values of $\Delta CMR_{O_2}/CMR_{O_2}$, it can be estimated that the validation accuracy for high-resolution CMR_{O_2} mapping by multimodal MRI at 7 T in rat cortex is at least 80%.

functional activation studies in the rat brain (at 7 T) with a high spatial resolution (in the microliter range), whereas of [15]O PET, ^{13}C MRS, and ^{17}O MRS methods *(52–54)*, all provide measures of $\Delta CMR_{O_2}/CMR_{O_2}$ with slightly lower spatial resolutions.

Much of calibrated fMRI research pertains to measurements of activation-dependent changes in the physiological parameters mentioned (**Table 1**). However, it is important to characterize the molecular mechanisms linking the observed BOLD signal change to neurophysiology at the cellular level. Under physiological conditions, Ca^{2+}-dependent vesicular release of neurotransmitters (e.g., glutamate) occurs in response to depolarization, which results from influx of Na^+ ions through presynaptic voltage-dependent Na^+ channels *(55)*. Both neuronal excitability and neurotransmitter release can be suppressed by inhibitors of these channels and the Na^+ currents that these channels mediate. Thus, Na^+ and Ca^{2+} channel blockers, e.g., lamotrigine, can be applied in treatments in which excessive release of neurotransmitters is believed to contribute to neuronal injury (e.g., epilepsy). The hypothesis that activation of voltage-dependent Na^+ and Ca^{2+} channels is a necessary step in the neurochemical pathway leading to the BOLD and CBF responses during somatosensory activation in rat was tested *(38)*. Significant depression of localized hemodynamic responses was observed after lamotrigine treatment, which implies that voltage-dependent Na^+ and Ca^{2+} channels are involved in the BOLD response. However, more studies are required to determine the extent to which glutamate release or other neurotransmitters and modulators are involved in the generation of the BOLD neuroimaging signal.

5. The Future: Opportunities and Challenges

Much effort has recently been directed toward elucidating the relationship between neuronal activity measured by electrophysiological methods and fMRI signals *(36,56–59)*. Logothetis and coworkers *(59)* have successfully measured electrical activity of neurons (action and field potentials) and BOLD signal changes in the anesthetized monkey with temporal and spatial resolutions sufficient to correlate the different signals. They found that the dynamics of both the high SNR field potential signals and the low SNR action potential signals are qualitatively correlated with the dynamics of the BOLD response. However, because of a better temporal correlation between the field potential signals and the BOLD response, they concluded that the fMRI signal reflects signal input because local field potentials are believed to reflect the membrane potential changes in the dendritic branches *(30)*. In contrast, Hyder and coworkers separately measured quantitative changes in the spiking rate of a neuronal ensemble (measured by electrophysiology) and changes in energy consumption (measured by calibrated fMRI) for a rat forepaw model in a variety of conditions *(36)*. The preliminary results from a small ensemble of neurons presumably contained within an MRI voxel (in the microliter range) demonstrate a proportional relationship between changes in activity and energy. Unfortunately, even the smallest MRI voxel contains thousands of neurons—resulting in a large disparity in the spatial quality of electrophysiological vs fMRI measurements. Nevertheless, these are important initial steps toward revealing the connection between neuronal activity and fMRI, and toward being able to measure noninvasively the energy consumption from neuronal populations *(1)*.

Hardware developments for MRI have improved markedly in the recent years and continue to advance. Higher magnetic fields improve the SNR and, in addition, favorably alter the transverse relaxation rate (**Fig. 2**). These improvements make it possible to surpass submillimeter spatial resolutions and, thus, allow the examination of the correlation between BOLD signals and neuronal activity at the level of functional neuronal units. Numerous reports now exist that reveal successful measurements of such functional domains in animal models, and more recently in humans—all making use of the superior sensitivity of the delayed positive BOLD response *(25,26,60,61)*. In contrast to these studies using the positive fMRI signal change for mapping functional activation, studies using the decrease in fMRI signal immediately after stimulus onset, the so-called early negative dip, have imaged columnar-like structures in the visual system *(62,63)*, despite the unknown origin of the signal and the lower SNR *(20)*.

Although increasing the spatial resolution of fMRI enables multimodal measurements of $\Delta CMR_{O_2}/CMR_{O_2}$ at the level of functional units, it raises new problems as well. In particular, it becomes necessary to make careful fMRI calibrations because fMRI signal at high spatial resolution is subject to more physiological noise artifacts and very subtle motion artifacts. Therefore, it is very important to confirm the reliability of the fMRI signal as a measure of task-related changes. The reproducibility of fMRI in test-retest studies has been evaluated by very few investigators in visual *(64–68)*, motor *(69–72)*, and association cortices *(66,71,73–75)*. Recently, the activities of functional units, such as columnar-like structures in the cerebral cortex of humans *(26)* and glomeruli in the olfactory bulb *(60,61,76)* of rodents, have been reproducibly mapped at higher magnetic fields. Reproducibility is critical to maintain confidence in the data from the multimodal experiments for the prediction of $\Delta CMR_{O_2}/CMR_{O_2}$ with high spatial resolution. In our laboratory, the functional arrangement of glomerular activity in the olfactory bulb is preserved between animals and within animals when the same odorant (e.g., iso-amyl acetate) is used as a stimulant (**Fig. 5**). After ensuring the reproducibility of functional maps with the same odorant, we have shown that glomerular activity in olfactory bulbs of mice varies as a result of odorant structure *(77)*.

The dynamic changes in the fMRI signal can be characterized as delayed positive and negative responses (peaks at 4–6 s) and an early negative response (peaks at 1–2 s) after stimulus onset, and a delayed negative response (peaks at several seconds) after stimulus offset *(78,79)*, whereas the electrical signals respond on a millisecond time-scale after stimulus onset. Each of these fMRI responses can be explained on the basis of the mechanical manifestations of the microvasculature using the steady-state model of BOLD *(80)*. To understand the neurophysiological basis of the dynamic BOLD signal, dynamic multimodal fMRI calibration is necessary. Dynamic fMRI calibration can be used to derive values of $\Delta CMR_{O_2}/CMR_{O_2}$, which, in turn, would provide a "new" quantitative biophysical relationship between neuroimaging and neuronal activity. The steady-state calibration of fMRI described here cannot be easily applied for dynamic calibration.

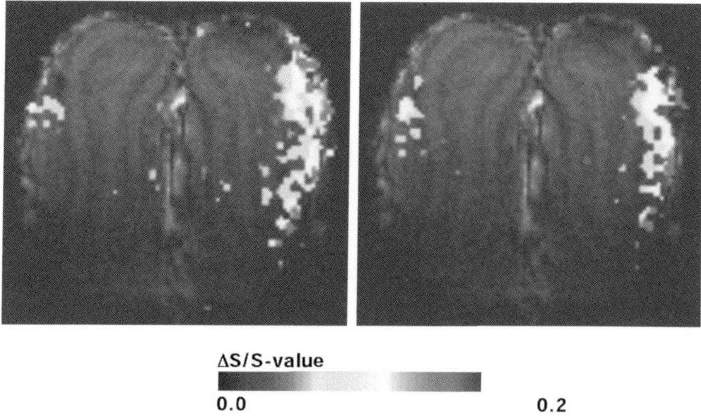

Fig. 5. Reproducibility of the high spatial resolution fMRI ($110 \times 110 \times 250$ μm³) in the rat olfactory bulb at 7 T. The coronal images, illustrated as BOLD signal change (ΔS/S) maps with the same threshold, were obtained from the same rat with repeated 2-min iso-amyl acetate exposures.

In the decade since the inception of fMRI, it has become commonplace to use BOLD contrast to identify areas of local brain activity in response to functional challenge. However, quantitative comparisons of signal changes of different magnitudes in either the same or different areas still cannot be made from conventional fMRI data. The multimodal fMRI approach outlined here makes it possible to evaluate how much energy is consumed by a given task and may be used in future physiological and pathological studies with high spatiotemporal resolution.

Acknowledgments

This work was supported by grants from the National Institutes of Health (NS-037203, DC-003710), MH-067528), National Science Foundation (DBI-9730892, DBI-0095173), and James S. McDonnell Foundation (21002033). FH thanks Arman Hyder for inspiration.

References

1. Shulman, R. G., Hyder, F., and Rothman, D. L. (2002) Biophysical basis of brain activity: implications for neuroimaging. *Q. Rev. Biophys.* **35,** 287–325.
2. Ogawa, S., Lee, T. M., Nayak, A. S., and Glynn, P. (1990) Oxygenation-sensitive contrast in magnetic resonance image on rodent brain at high magnetic fields. *Magn. Reson. Med.* **14,** 68–78.
3. Pauling, L. and Coryell, C. (1936) The magnetic properties of and structure of hemoglobin, oxyhemoglobin and carbon-monoxyhemoglobin. *Proc. Natl. Acad. Sci. USA* **22,** 210–216.

4. Bandettini, P. A., Wong, E. C., Hinks, R. S., Tikofsky, R. S., and Hyde, J. S. (1992) Time course EPI of human brain function during task activation. *Magn. Reson. Med.* **25,** 390–397.

5. Blamire, A. M., Ogawa, S., Ugurbil, K., et al. (1992) Dynamic mapping of the human visual cortex by high-speed magnetic resonance imaging. *Proc. Natl. Acad. Sci. USA* **89,** 11,069–11,073.

6. Kwong, K. K., Belliveau, J. W., Chesler, D. A., et al. (1992) Dynamic magnetic resonance imaging of human brain activity during primary sensory stimulation. *Proc. Natl. Acad. Sci. USA* **89,** 5675–5679.

7. Ogawa, S., Tank, D. W., Menon, R., et al. (1992) Intrinsic signal changes accompanying sensory stimulation: functional brain mapping with magnetic resonance imaging. *Proc. Natl. Acad. Sci. USA* **89,** 5951–5955.

8. Albert, M. S., Huang, W., Lee, J. H., Patlak, C. S., and Springer, C. S. Jr. (1993) Susceptibility changes following bolus injections. *Magn. Reson. Med.* **29,** 700–708.

9. Kennan, R. P., Zhong, J., and Gore, J. C. (1994) Intravascular susceptibility contrast mechanisms in tissues. *Magn. Reson. Med.* **31,** 9–21.

10. Weisskoff, R. M., Zuo, C. S., Boxerman, J. L., and Rosen, B. R. (1994) Microscopic susceptibility variation and transverse relaxation: theory and experiment. *Magn. Reson. Med.* **31,** 601–610.

11. Ogawa, S., Menon, R. S., Tank, D. W., et al. (1993) Functional brain mapping by blood oxygenation level-dependent contrast magnetic resonance imaging. *Biophys. J.* **64,** 803–812.

12. Buxton, R. B. and Frank, L. R. (1997) A model of the coupling between cerebral blood flow and oxygen metabolism during neural stimulation. *J. Cereb. Blood Flow Metab.* **17,** 64–72.

13. Hyder, F., Shulman, R. G., and Rothman, D. L. (1998) A model for the regulation of cerebral oxygen delivery. *J. Appl. Physiol.* **85,** 554–564.

14. Thulborn, K. R., Waterton, J. C., Matthews, P. M., and Radda, G. K. (1982) Oxygenation dependence of the transverse relaxation time of water protons in whole blood at high field. *Biochim. Biophys. Acta* **714,** 265–270.

15. Bauer, W. R. and Schulten, K. (1992) Theory of contrast agents in magnetic resonance imaging: coupling of spin relaxation and transport. *Magn. Reson. Med.* **26,** 16–39.

16. Yablonskiy, D. A. and Haacke, E. M. (1994) Theory of NMR signal behavior in magnetically inhomogeneous tissues: the static dephasing regime. *Magn. Reson. Med.* **32,** 749–763.

17. Kida, I., Kennan, R. P., Rothman, D. L., Behar, K. L., and Hyder, F. (2000) High-resolution CMR_{O2} mapping in rat cortex: a multi-parametric approach to calibration of BOLD image contrast at 7 Tesla. *J. Cereb. Blood Flow Metab.* **20,** 847–860.

18. Hyder, F., Kida, I., Behar, K. L., Kennan, R. P., Maciejewski, P. K., and Rothman, D. L. (2001) Quantitative functional imaging of the brain: towards mapping neuronal activity by BOLD fMRI. *NMR Biomed.* **14,** 413–431.

19. Ogawa, S., Menon, R. S., Kim, S. G., and Ugurbil, K. (1998) On the characteristics of functional magnetic resonance imaging of the brain. *Annu. Rev. Biophys. Biomol. Struct.* **27,** 447–474.
20. Ugurbil, K., Adriany, G., Andersen, P., et al. (2000) Magnetic resonance studies of brain function and neurochemistry. *Annu. Rev. Biomed. Eng.* **2,** 633–660.
21. Zhong, J., Kennan, R. P., Fulbright, R. K., and Gore, J. C. (1998) Quantification of intravascular and extravascular contributions to BOLD effects induced by alteration in oxygenation or intravascular contrast agents. *Magn. Reson. Med.* **40,** 526–536.
22. Lee, S. P., Silva, A. C., Ugurbil, K., and Kim, S. G. (1999) Diffusion-weighted spin-echo fMRI at 9.4T: microvascular/tissue contribution to BOLD signal changes. *Magn. Reson. Med.* **42,** 919–928.
23. Hyder, F., Renken, R., Kennan, R. P., and Rothman, D. L. (2000a) Quantitative multi-modal functional MRI with blood oxygenation level dependent exponential decays adjusted for flow attenuated inversion recoveries (BOLDED AFFAIR). *Magn. Reson. Imag.* **18,** 227–235.
24. Buxton, R. B. (2001) The elusive dip. *Neuroimage* **13,** 953–958.
25. Yang, X., Hyder, F., and Shulman, R. G. (1996) Single-whisker activation observed in rat cortex by functional magnetic resonance imaging. *Proc. Natl. Acad. Sci. USA* **93,** 475–478.
26. Cheng, K., Waggoner, R. A., and Tanaka, K. (2001) Human ocular dominance columns as revealed by high-field functional magnetic resonance imaging. *Neuron* **32,** 359–374.
27. Sokoloff, L., Reivich, M., Kennedy, C., et al. (1977) The [^{14}C]deoxyglucose method for the measurement of local cerebral glucose utilization: theory, procedure, and normal values in the conscious and anesthetized albino rat. *J. Neurochem.* **28,** 897–916.
28. Ueki, M., Linn, F., and Hossman, K. A. (1988) Functional activation of cerebral blood flow and metabolism and after global ischemia of rat brain. *J. Cereb. Blood Flow Metab.* **8,** 486–494.
29. Siesjo, B. K. (1978) *Brain Energy Metabolism.* Wiley, New York, NY.
30. Kandel, E. R., Schwartz, J. H., and Jessell, T. M. (1991) *Principles of Neural Science.* Appleton & Lange, Norwalk, CT.
31. Kuschinsky, W., Suda, S., and Sokoloff, L. (1981) Local cerebral glucose utilization and blood flow during metabolic acidosis. *Am. J. Physiol.* **241,** H772–H777.
32. Roy, C. S. and Sherrington, C. S. (1890) On the regulation of the blood supply of the rat brain. *J. Physiol. (Lond.)* **11,** 85–108.
33. Penfield, W. (1933) The evidence for a cerebral vascular mechanism in epilepsy. *Ann. Int. Med.* **7,** 303–310.
34. Crone, C. (1963) The permeability of capillaries in various organs as determined by the "indicator diffusion" method. *Acta Physiol. Scand.* **58,** 292–305.
35. Hyder, F., Rothman, D. L., and Shulman, R. G. (2002) Total neuroenergetics support localized brain activity: implications for the interpretation of fMRI. *Proc. Natl. Acad. Sci. USA* **99,** 10,771–10,776.

36. Smith, A. J., Blumenfeld, H., Behar, K. L., Rothman, D. L., Shulman, R. G., and Hyder, F. (2002) Cerebral energetics and spiking frequency: the neurophysiological basis of fMRI. *Proc. Natl. Acad. Sci. USA* **99,** 10,765–10,770.

37. Pellerin, L. and Magistretti, P. J. (1994) Glutamate uptake into astrocytes stimulates aerobic glycolysis: a mechanism coupling neuronal activity to glucose utilization. *Proc. Natl. Acad. Sci. USA* **91,** 10,625–10,629.

38. Kida, I., Hyder, F., and Behar, K. L. (2001) Inhibition of voltage-dependent sodium channels suppresses the functional MRI response to forepaw somatosensory activation in the rodent. *J. Cereb. Blood Flow Metab.* **21,** 585–591.

39. Kety, S. S. and Schmidt, C. F. (1948) The effects of altered arterial tensions of carbon dioxide and oxygen on cerebral blood flow and cerebral oxygen consumption of normal young men. *J. Clin. Invest.* **27,** 484–491.

40. Yang, S. P. and Krasney, J. A. (1995) Cerebral blood flow and metabolic responses to sustained hypercapnia in awake sheep. *J. Cereb. Blood Flow Metab.* **15,** 115–123.

41. Hemmingsen, R., Barry, D. I., and Hertz, M. M. (1979) Cerebrovascular effects of central depressants: a study of nitrous oxide, halothane, pentobarbital and ethanol during normocapnia and hypercapnia in the rat. *Acta Pharmacol. Toxicol. (Copenh.)* **45,** 287–295.

42. Berntman, L., Dahlgren, N., and Siesjo, B. K. (1979) Cerebral blood flow and oxygen consumption in the rat brain during extreme hypercarbia. *Anesthesiology* **50,** 299–305.

43. Horvath, I., Sandor, N. T., Ruttner, Z., and McLaughlin, A. C. (1994) Role of nitric oxide in regulating cerebrocortical oxygen consumption and blood flow during hypercapnia. *J. Cereb. Blood Flow Metab.* **14,** 503–509.

44. Kim, S. G., Rostrup, E., Larsson, H. B., Ogawa, S., and Paulson, O. B. (1999) Determination of relative CMR_{O_2} from CBF and BOLD changes: significant increase of oxygen consumption rate during visual stimulation. *Magn. Reson. Med.* **41,** 1152–1161.

45. Grubb, R. L., Raichle, M. E., Eichling, J. O., and Ter Pogosian, M. M. (1974) The effects of changes in pCO_2 on cerebral blood volume, blood flow, and vascular mean transit time. *Stroke* **5,** 630–639.

46. Mandeville, J. B., Marota, J. J., Ayata, C., Moskowitz, M. A., Weisskoff, R. M., and Rosen, B. R. (1999) MRI measurement of the temporal evolution of relative CMR_{O_2} during rat forepaw stimulation. *Magn. Reson. Med.* **42,** 944–951.

47. Ito, H., Takahashi, K., Hatazawa, J., Kim, S. G., and Kanno, I. (2001) Changes in human regional cerebral blood flow and cerebral blood volume during visual stimulation measured by positron emission tomography. *J. Cereb. Blood Flow Metab.* **21,** 608–612.

48. Jones, M., Berwick, J., and Mayhew, J. (2002) Changes in blood flow, oxygenation, and volume following extended stimulation of rodent barrel cortex. *Neuroimage* **15,** 474–487.

49. Silva, A. C., Lee, S. P., Yang, G., Iadecola, C., and Kim, S. G. (1999) Simultaneous blood oxygenation level-dependent and cerebral blood flow functional magnetic resonance imaging during forepaw stimulation in the rat. *J. Cereb. Blood Flow Metab.* **19,** 871–879.

50. Schwarzbauer, C., Morrissey, S. P., and Hasse, A. (1996) Quantitative magnetic resonance imaging of perfusion using magnetic labeling of water proton spins within the detection slice. *Magn. Reson. Med.* **35,** 540–546.

51. Kennan, R. P., Scanley, B. E., Innis, R. B., and Gore, J. C. (1998) Physiological basis for BOLD MR signal changes due to neuronal stimulation: separation of blood volume and magnetic susceptibility effects. *Magn. Reson. Med.* **40,** 840–846.

52. Hyder, F., Renken, R., and Rothman, D. L. (1999) In vivo carbon-edited detection with proton echo-planar spectroscopic imaging (ICED PEPSI): [3,4-^{13}CH$_2$]glutamate/glutamine tomography in rat brain. *Magn. Reson. Med.* **42,** 997–1003.

53. Mintun, M. A., Raichle, M. E., Martin, W. R., and Herscovitch, P. (1984) Brain oxygen utilization measured with O-15 radiotracers and positron emission tomography. *J. Nucl. Med.* **25,** 177–187.

54. Zhu, X. H., Zhang, Y., Tian, R. X., et al. (2002) Development of ^{17}O NMR approach for fast imaging of cerebral metabolic rate of oxygen in rat brain at high field. *Proc. Natl. Acad. Sci. USA* **99,** 13,194–13,199.

55. Leach, M. J., Marden, C. M., and Miller, A. A. (1986) Pharmacological studies on lamotrigine, a novel potential antiepileptic drug: II. neurochemical studies on the mechanism of action. *Epilepsia* **27,** 490–497.

56. Brinker, G., Bock, C., Busch, E., Krep, H., Hossmann, K. A., and Hoehn-Berlage, M. (1999) Simultaneous recording of evoked potentials and T$_2$*-weighted MR images during somatosensory stimulation of rat. *Magn. Reson. Med.* **41,** 469–473.

57. Rees, G., Friston, K., and Koch, C. (2000) A direct quantitative relationship between the functional properties of human and macaque V5. *Nat. Neurosci.* **3,** 716–723.

58. Ogawa, S., Lee, T. M., Stepnoski, R., Chen, W., Zhu, X. H., and Ugurbil, K. (2000) An approach to probe some neural systems interaction by functional MRI at neural time scale down to milliseconds. *Proc. Natl. Acad. Sci. USA* **97,** 11,026–11,031.

59. Logothetis, N. K., Pauls, J., Augath, M., Trinath, T., and Oeltermann, A. (2001) Neurophysiological investigation of the basis of the fMRI signal. *Nature* **412,** 150–157.

60. Kida, I., Xu, F., Shulman, R. G., and Hyder, F. (2002) Mapping at glomerular resolution: fMRI of rat olfactory bulb. *Magn. Reson. Med.* **48,** 570–576.

61. Xu, F., Kida, I., Hyder, F., and Shulman, R. G. (2000) Assessment and discrimination of odor stimuli in rat olfactory bulb by dynamic fMRI. *Proc. Natl. Acad. Sci. USA* **97,** 10,601–10,606.

62. Kim, D. S., Duong, T. Q., and Kim, S. G. (2000) High-resolution mapping of iso-orientation columns by fMRI. *Nat. Neurosci.* **3,** 164–169.

63. Duong, T. Q., Kim, D. S., Ugurbil, K., and Kim, S. G. (2000) Spatiotemporal dynamics of the BOLD fMRI signals: toward mapping submillimeter cortical columns using the early negative response. *Magn. Reson. Med.* **44,** 231–242.

64. Miki, A., Raz, J., Englander, S. A., et al. (2001) Reproducibility of visual activation in functional magnetic resonance imaging at very high field strength (4 Tesla). *Jpn. J. Ophthalmol.* **45,** 1–4.

65. Rombouts, S. A., Barkhof, F., Hoogenraad, F. G., Sprenger, M., and Scheltens, P. (1998) Within-subject reproducibility of visual activation patterns with functional magnetic resonance imaging using multislice echo planar imaging. *Magn. Reson. Imag.* **16,** 105–113.
66. Machielsen, W. C., Rombouts, S. A., Barkhof, F., Scheltens, P., and Witter, M. P. (2000) fMRI of visual encoding: reproducibility of activation. *Hum. Brain Mapp.* **9,** 156–164.
67. Moser, E., Teichtmeister, C., and Diemling, M. (1996) Reproducibility and postprocessing of gradient-echo functional MRI to improve localization of brain activity in the human visual cortex. *Magn. Reson. Imag.* **14,** 567–579.
68. Baumgartner, R., Scarth, G., Teichtmeister, C., Somorjai, R., and Moser, E. (1997) Fuzzy clustering of gradient-echo functional MRI in the human visual cortex. Part I: reproducibility. *J. Magn. Reson. Imaging* **7,** 1094–1101.
69. Tegeler, C., Strother, S. C., Anderson, J. R., and Kim, S. G. (1999) Reproducibility of BOLD-based functional MRI obtained at 4T. *Hum. Brain Mapp.* **7,** 267–283.
70. Yetkin, F. Z., McAuliffe, T. L., Cox, R., and Haughton, V. M. (1996) Test-retest precision of functional MR in sensory and motor task activation. *AJNR Am. J. Neuroradiol.* **17,** 95–98.
71. Noll, D. C., Genovese, C. R., Nystrom, L. E., et al. (1997) Estimating test-retest reliability in functional MR imaging. II: application to motor and cognitive activation studies. *Magn. Reson. Med.* **38,** 508–517.
72. Wexler, B. E., Fulbright, R. K., Lacadie, C. M., et al. (1997) An fMRI study of the human cortical motor system response to increasing functional demands. *Magn. Reson. Imag.* **15,** 385–396.
73. Casey, B. J., Cohen, J. D., O'Craven, K., et al. (1998) Reproducibility of fMRI results across four institutions using a spatial working memory task. *Neuroimage* **8,** 249–261.
74. Rutten, G. J., Ramsey, N. F., van Rijen, P. C., and van Veelen, C. W. (2002) Reproducibility of fMRI-determined language lateralization in individual subjects. *Brain Lang.* **80,** 421–437.
75. Chee, M. W., Lee, H. L., Soon, C. S., Westphal, C., and Venkatraman, V. (2003) Reproducibility of the word frequency effect: comparison of signal change and voxel counting. *Neuroimage* **18,** 468–482.
76. Yang, X., Renken, R., Hyder, F., et al. (1998) Dynamic mapping at the laminar level of odor-elicited responses in rat olfactory bulb by functional MRI. *Proc. Natl. Acad. Sci. USA* **95,** 7715–7720.
77. Xu, F., Liu, N., Kida, I., Rothman, D. L., Hyder, F., and Shepherd, G. M. (2003) Odor maps of aldehydes and esters revealed by fMRI in the glomerular layer of the mouse olfactory bulb. *Proc. Natl. Acad. Sci. USA* **100,** 11,029–11,034.
78. Ernst, T. and Hennig, J. (1994) Observation of a fast response in functional MR. *Magn. Reson. Med.* **32,** 146–149.
79. Harel, N., Lee, S. P., Nagaoka, T., Kim, D. S., and Kim, S. G. (2002) Origin of negative blood oxygenation level-dependent fMRI signals. *J. Cereb. Blood Flow Metab.* **22,** 908–917.

80. Buxton, R. B., Wong, E. C., and Frank, L. R. (1998) Dynamics of blood flow and oxygenation changes during brain activation: the balloon model. *Magn. Reson. Med.* **39,** 855–864.
81. Kim, S. G. and Ugurbil, K. (1997) Comparison of blood oxygenation and cerebral blood flow effects in fMRI: estimation of relative oxygen consumption change. *Magn. Reson. Med.* **38,** 59–65.
82. Kim, S. G., Tsekos, N. V., and Ashe, J. (1997) Multi-slice perfusion-based functional MRI using the FAIR technique: comparison of CBF and BOLD effects. *NMR Biomed.* **10,** 191–196.
83. Davis, T. L., Kwong, K. K., Weisskoff, R. M., and Rosen, B. R. (1998) Calibrated functional MRI: mapping the dynamics of oxidative metabolism. *Proc. Natl. Acad. Sci. USA* **95,** 1834–1839.
84. Hoge, R. D., Atkinson, J., Gill, B., Crelier, G. R., Marrett, S., and Pike, G. B. (1999) Linear coupling between cerebral blood flow and oxygen consumption in activated human cortex. *Proc. Natl. Acad. Sci. USA* **96,** 9403–9408.
85. Kastrup, A., Kruger, G., Glover, G. H., and Moseley, M. E. (1999) Assessment of cerebral oxidative metabolism with breath holding and fMRI. *Magn. Reson. Med.* **42,** 608–611.
86. Kastrup, A., Kruger, G., Neumann-Haefelin, T., Glover, G. H., and Moseley, M. E. (2002) Changes of cerebral blood flow, oxygenation, and oxidative metabolism during graded motor activation. *Neuroimage* **15,** 74–82.
87. Feng, C. M., Liu, H. L., Fox, P. T., and Gao, J. H. (2003) Dynamic changes in the cerebral metabolic rate of O_2 and oxygen extraction ratio in event-related functional MRI. *Neuroimage* **18,** 257–262.

8

Functional Magnetic Resonance Imaging of the Kidney

Pottumarthi V. Prasad

Summary

In addition to exquisite anatomical detail, magnetic resonance imaging (MRI) provides a variety of avenues to study functional status of tissue. These functional parameters could either provide additional information, in terms of pathophysiology, or may improve the specificity of the diagnosis. This chapter reviews some current state-of-the-art functional MRI (fMRI) methods as applied to the kidney. Three parameters, renal perfusion, filtration or excretory function, and oxygenation are reviewed in depth. Illustrative examples are provided and advantages discussed.

Key Words: Kidney; blood flow; glomerular filtration rate (GFR); oxygenation; BOLD; MRI.

1. Introduction

Magnetic resonance imaging (MRI) is already well established as a diagnostic imaging modality providing exquisite soft tissue contrast and anatomic detail. Over the last two decades, tremendous advances have been made in terms of improved image quality and spatial coverage. Also, unlike other diagnostic imaging modalities, contrast on MRI can be modified in many different ways. This has led to efficient tissue characterization paradigms. In addition to the inherent contrast properties of the magnetic resonance (MR), exogenous contrast can allow for further refinements in tissue characterization. Many believe that the next revolution in MRI will be one of exogenous contrast agents (e.g., tissue specific or targeted agents, smart contrast agents that are turned "on" only under specific conditions, such as the presence of a specific enzyme).

MRI offers additional avenues for functional evaluation of tissue, and this chapter elucidates such applications, specifically in the kidney. MRI has the advantage in that the methodology is equally applicable to small-animal models and, hence, allows for translation of results from preclinical to human applications.

In the spirit of a methods-based book, this review presents an overview of the different methodologies that MRI offers in terms of ability to characterize the functional status of renal tissue.

From: *Methods in Molecular Medicine, Vol. 124*
Magnetic Resonance Imaging: Methods and Biologic Applications
Edited by: P. V. Prasad © Humana Press Inc., Totowa, NJ

1.1. Small-Animal MRI on Human Whole-Body Scanners

Before starting the discussion on functional imaging of the kidneys, the possibility of small-animal MRI on whole-body scanners designed for routine human use is discussed. Compared with most of the other discussions within this book, in which data acquisitions were primarily made on dedicated small-animal MRI scanners (at least for small-animal work), the examples in this chapter were mostly obtained on whole-body scanners primarily designed for clinical use. These scanners afford some unique advantages and, of course, are associated with some disadvantages. We highlight them because of their practical significance to the potential end user.

Advantages of whole-body human scanners:

1. More widespread availability, especially within healthcare systems and academic medical centers.
2. When available, they are equipped with a greater variety of pulse sequences that can be easily adapted to small field of view imaging. Although it may be necessary to design custom radio frequency coils for signal reception, especially if high spatial resolution is of prime interest, many of the standard coils could be adequate for in vivo imaging. The examples in this chapter illustrate what may be possible.
3. The relatively open design of the whole-body scanners allow for better visual and physical monitoring of the animals during the scanning and can also easily accommodate ancillary equipment, if needed.
4. Translation of the studies to larger animal models, such as rabbits, pigs, dogs, and, ultimately, humans, is more straightforward. **Subheading 2.3.3.** provides an example with data from a 24-g mouse and all the way to a 70-kg human—all obtained from the same scanner platform.

Disadvantages of whole-body human scanners:

1. Although more widespread in availability, they may not be accessible for animal work because of priorities for human and mostly clinical use. Even when available, they may be relatively more expensive because of increased users' fees. However, at premier academic sites that have dedicated research scanners, this option is quite viable and, in many cases, preferable than using dedicated small-bore, high-field animal MRI scanners for certain applications, e.g., when susceptibility artifacts are of concern at higher field strengths.
2. Because of the larger physical size of the scanners and the associated rooms, monitoring equipment may need to accommodate certain changes, e.g., additional lengths of cables for instrumentation, such as blood pressure monitors, or longer infusion lines.

1.1.1. Examples of Microscopic MRI Obtained on a Whole-Body Scanner

Figure 1A illustrates MRI of an ex vivo rat kidney. These images were obtained with a custom microimaging coil (surface coil of 2-cm diameter, i.e., comparable to the length of the rat kidney). Shown is one representative image

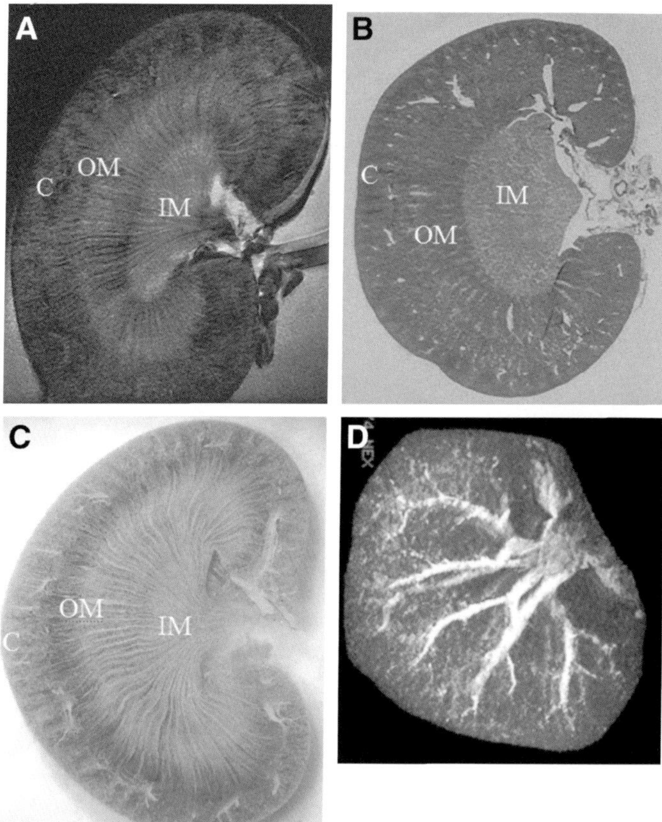

Fig. 1. **(A)** High-resolution (40-µm in-plane) anatomical magnetic resonance imaging (MRI) of ex vivo rat kidney acquired using a custom 2-cm radio frequency surface coil at 3.0 T. Shown is one representative slice from a 3D stack obtained with a fast spoiled gradient echo (SPGR) sequence (echo time, TE, 14.8 ms; repetition time, TR, 46; flip angle, 10°) with inversion recovery (IR) preparation time of 200 ms, which was used to acquire the magnetic resonance (MR) images in approx 20 min. Other relevant acquisition parameters were: field of view, 2 × 2 cm; matrix, 512 × 512; acquisition bandwidth of 6.94 kHz; slice thickness 0.5 mm; # of averages 2. The kidney was prepared by gadolinium (Gd) infusion with a concentration of 3.13 mg/mL before excision. For comparison, **(B)** is a textbook picture of a cross-section of a rat kidney, and **(C)** is an optical image of a rat kidney after perfusing with Microfil to fill the entire vascular space. **(D)** Shows a maximum intensity projection obtained from a 3D data set of MR images obtained with a Microfil-filled ex vivo rat kidney. The vascular contrast was obtained based only on inherent T_1 differences of renal tissue and the Microfil, using an IR preparation time of 500 ms. These images are provided to illustrate the level of anatomical detail in ex vivo tissue that can be achieved using a clinical scanner, which is more widely available than dedicated high-field small-animal MR scanners. C, IM, and OM stand of cortex, inner and outer medulla respectively.

from a 3D acquisition of 16 slices of 0.5 mm slice thickness with in-plane resolution of 40 μm. The total acquisition time was about 20 min. Note the exquisite contrast details and the ability to distinguish the different layers of the kidney (i.e., cortex, outer, and inner medulla). To put things in perspective, we have also included a standard textbook-type image (**Fig. 1B**), and an optical image (**Fig. 1C**) obtained after filling the vasculature with a colored resin (Microfil®, Flow Tech Inc., Carver, MA). The original picture was yellow in color, but for illustrative purposes we show a grayscale picture. The contrast is predominantly determined by the relative blood volume within the tissue and one can appreciate the structural differences in each of the layers of the kidney. **Figure 1D** shows an MRI of an ex vivo rat kidney that was perfused with Microfil before the removal of the kidney. The sequence (*viz.*, inversion recovery) and parameters were chosen to highlight the contrast from vascular structures (based on the significantly different T_1 values of the resin compared with tissue). Previous studies used similar preparations to obtain high-resolution images using micro-computed tomography (CT) *(1)*.

2. Methods: Functional Body MRI

In addition to the anatomical and structural information as illustrated above, MRI provides unique opportunities to probe tissue "function" or "physiological status." "Function" may mean different things to different types of tissues or organs. In neurological functional MRI (neuro fMRI), one may use the term "function" in the sense of cognitive brain function. Although the actual brain function takes place in terms of neuronal activity, MRI is very adept in characterizing the associated hemodynamic responses, as discussed in Chapter 7. Other organs and tissues within the body also are associated with specific functions and they may have significant implications in terms of our understanding of physiology and pathophysiology of human disease.

Functional MRI of tissue is motivated by the following:

1. to better understand physiology and pathophysiology,
2. to provide more comprehensive characterization of pathological lesions (e.g., functional or hemodynamic significance of ischemic/stenotic lesions), and
3. to provide either a more sensitive index, or an earlier index of disease progression.

There are several MRI-derived indices that can provide useful correlates to tissue function that may be useful for satisfying one or more of the above-mentioned motivating factors. The most commonly used functional parameter is perfusion. Although the intended meaning is to measure blood flow to a region of interest in absolute quantifiable terms (e.g., mL/s/100 g of tissue), MRI is capable of providing semiquantitative or qualitative indices that can be used to monitor changes in perfusion. There are many specific means to achieving the end results. In this chapter, we provide a review of these indices and provide illustrative specific examples and related discussion.

2.1. Perfusion MRI

Blood perfusion is a crucial and fundamental physiological process that controls delivery of nutrients to tissue *(2)*, and, thus, is a very important parameter in the assessment of tissue viability and function. Perfusion is usually expressed as milliliters of blood per minute per 100 g of tissue. Conventional in vivo perfusion measurements are based on the administration of exogenous tracers *(3)* detected by several different imaging techniques, such as X-ray CT *(4)* and positron emission tomography (PET) *(5)*. All of these techniques are based on the indicator-dilution method originally introduced a century ago by Stewart *(6)* and further developed by Zierler *(7)*. In practice, the indicator-dilution method involves introduction of a known quantity of indicator into the system under study and measurement of the concentration of the indicator as a function of time at one or more points downstream from the location of the injection.

There are number of applications of nuclear magnetic resonance (NMR) techniques proposed to image and measure tissue perfusion. Some are based on the indicator-dilution principle and others depend on inherent MR mechanisms. Although PET is still considered the gold standard for in vivo blood flow measurements, MR perfusion imaging is attractive because MR scanners are more readily available. Additionally, there is no ionizing radiation involved, and spatial resolution with MR is much superior to that obtained with PET. Furthermore, MRI offers the unique advantage of obtaining both anatomical and functional information with a single modality.

Like most applications in MRI, preliminary application of perfusion imaging was primarily targeted to the brain. Perfusion MRI in the brain is relatively well established and is part of routine clinical protocols. Although the fundamental principles are similar to the brain application, there are differences in implementation to different organs, such as the heart, kidney, lungs, liver, and so on. Although perfusion MRI of the heart is increasingly becoming part of clinical protocols, nonneurological applications still remain in the academic domain.

Before starting a discussion of the different types of techniques that have been proposed to perform perfusion MRI, it is worthwhile to make it clear that many of these techniques do not measure perfusion in classical terms (i.e., in units of mL/s/100 g of tissue). MR is sensitive to several physiological parameters that may be related to perfusion and could be used as indicators of local blood flow. A brief description of some of the parameters that could directly or indirectly influence the MRI signal and, thus, potentially be deduced from the MR measurements follows:

1. Perfusion (f): If a volume of tissue (V) is supplied with arterial blood at a rate of F (mL/min), then perfusion $f = F/V$, the milliliters of arterial blood delivered per minute per milliliter of tissue. Although this is slightly different from the classical description of perfusion, it is more applicable for imaging studies. Perfusion

f is the fundamental rate constant determining delivery of metabolic substrates to the local tissue and clearance of products of metabolism.

2. Blood Volume (V_b): V_b is the fraction of the total tissue volume within a voxel occupied by blood (including arteries, capillaries, and veins). Although V_b and f are principally distinct quantities, experimentally they are strongly correlated in normal brain *(8)*.

3. Blood velocity (u): Because MR is very sensitive to motion, u is used to describe the perfusion state of tissue, because changes in u could be correlated with changes in f. However, in general f, V_b, and u are distinct and independent parameters. Although they may be well correlated in normal states, the correlation may break down in pathological states.

4. Oxygen extraction fraction (E): As noted in **item 1**, f determines the rate of delivery of metabolic substrates, such as oxygen, to the tissue, but only a fraction of the supply is actually used for metabolism; thus, the extraction fraction, E, is a parameter of interest when considering perfusion imaging, especially because it is known that E could vary with f. By definition, E equals $(C_a–C_v)/C_a$, where C refers to arterial (a) and venous (v) oxygen concentrations.

5. Tissue–blood partition coefficient (p): When considering the kinetics of an agent as it passes through a tissue via blood, it is important to know the distribution of the agent between the blood and tissue compartments. The partition coefficient, p, usually refers to the ratio of tissue to blood concentration of the agent at equilibrium. For an agent that remains within the blood (intravascular agent), p equals the blood volume, V_b, and for a freely diffusible agent, such as labeled water, p is approx 1.0.

6. Mean transit time through the tissue (τ): Each molecule of an administered agent may trace a different path through a tissue element, so that there will be a range of transit times. Again, for agents that remain within the blood, the mean transit time, t, is usually only a few seconds, although for agents that diffuse out of the blood, t is much longer.

The central volume principle *(6)* relates the terms perfusion (f), blood tissue partition coefficient (p), and mean transit time (τ), by the equation: $f = p/\tau$. This principle applies to any agent, whether or not it is extracted from the blood.

2.1.1. MR Perfusion Imaging Techniques

In this section, we will describe a few of the established MR perfusion techniques, including a description of the basic mechanisms involved and how perfusion information can possibly be derived. For this discussion, it is useful to subdivide the techniques under two major categories:

1. techniques based on administration of exogenous contrast agent, and
2. techniques that obviate the need for exogenous contrast administration.

Each of these approaches has its own advantages and disadvantages.

2.1.1.1. Techniques Based on Exogenous Contrast Agent Administration

In nuclear medicine, the tissue concentration of a radioactive tracer is measured over time and, using suitable tracer kinetic models, several physiological parameters related to blood flow are estimated *(7,9)*. In principle, a similar approach is possible with MRI if a suitable tracer is available and measurements could be made with sufficient temporal resolution. With the evolution of ultrafast MRI techniques *(10,11)*, the possibility of monitoring exogenous tracer kinetics in vivo using MRI has become a reality, not only in the brain but in almost any organ in the body.

Currently approved and most widely available MR contrast agents are paramagnetic chelates, notably gadopentetate dimeglumine (Magnevist, Berlex, Wayne, NJ), sometimes referred to as Gd-DTPA. Gd-DTPA is a relaxivity agent, in that it decreases both T_1 and T_2 relaxation times. However, because T_1 rates $(1/T_1)$ are inherently smaller than T_2 rates in most tissues, relaxation time changes on a percentage basis are much greater for T_1 compared with T_2. For this reason, these agents are often characterized as T_1 agents. In organs such as the heart, the Gd-DTPA leaves the blood and accumulates in the interstitial space before being washed away by the venous supply. Thus, it is possible to follow the accumulation of the agent over time using appropriate MR techniques and to derive perfusion indices. In the brain, as a result of the blood–brain barrier, diffusion of the agent is prevented; thus, it behaves as an intravascular agent. This results in T_1 effects being small because only a small fraction of the tissue water can sample the agent, which is restricted within a small vascular volume. For this reason, neurological perfusion MRI is being performed based on T_2^* contrast. When Gd-DTPA is delivered as a compact bolus, it creates a transient drop in signal intensity as it passes through the brain because of magnetic susceptibility effects *(12)*. In humans, a typical iv injection rate of 5 mL/s is used to achieve optimum results. The high magnetic moment of gadolinium (Gd) alters the susceptibility of the blood compared with the surrounding water in the tissue, and the resulting magnetic field gradients produce signal loss. Variations in tissue magnetic susceptibility can affect MR images more profoundly than relaxivity changes when the agent remains in the vascular space. Thus, even though the agent is compartmentalized within 5% of the volume, the signal drop could be as high as 50% *(13)*.

Assuming that signal changes can be quantitatively related to changes in local concentration of Gd, one could apply tracer kinetic principles to relate the measured concentration time–curves to the different physiological parameters described above. From the measurements of the tissue and arterial concentration curves, $C_{tissue}(t)$ and $C_{arterial}(t)$, the volume of distribution of the agent can be calculated directly, as:

$$V = \frac{\int_0^\infty C_{tissue}(t)\,dt}{\int_0^\infty C_{arterial}(t)\,dt}$$

Because Gd-DTPA behaves as an intravascular agent in the intact brain, the volume of distribution of the contrast agent reflects the blood volume, V_b, within the tissue. The arterial concentration–time curve can be measured using additional images that include the feeding artery, acquired simultaneously *(14)*. However, in the absence of arterial sampling, one can still infer relative blood volumes, assuming all of the voxels within the image are fed by a single arterial source. It has been shown that with intravascular agents, robust blood volume measurements can be made, but measurement of perfusion is more difficult *(15)*. The estimate of blood flow based on the central volume principle involves estimates of blood volume and the mean transit time, τ.

Mean transit time is usually estimated by calculating the first moment of the measured concentration–time curve. However, as pointed out by Weisskoff et al. *(16)*, this calculation is not quite correct because the indicator-dilution principles call for concentration at the outlet, whereas MR (or any other imaging) measurements estimate the tissue concentration. In the same work, however, the authors point out that flow measurements made using the above calculation can yield a semiquantitative index that could be clinically useful. The measurement of τ using purely intravascular agents necessitates either ideal δ-function bolus injection of the contrast agent or an accurate measure of the arterial input function, which can then be deconvolved from the measured concentration–time curve. In the case of freely diffusible tracers, this is somewhat simplified by the slower transit times through the tissue; thus, the measurement of τ is less dependent on the arterial input curve.

2.1.1.1.1. Application of Perfusion MRI in Organs Other Than the Brain: Extracellular vs Intravascular Contrast Agents

In all other tissue except for the brain, Gd-DTPA leaves the vascular space and distributes within the interstitial space. Hence, one cannot equate V to the blood volume, and, for the same reason, the signal intensity vs time curve does not fully return to the equilibrium level over the measurement time. One can still estimate some useful perfusion indices that can be correlated with blood flow. This was shown in the heart by Wilke et al. *(17)*. They estimated $C_{tissue}(t)$ by fitting an empirically chosen portion of the *signal-intensity*$_{tissue}(t)$ curve to a γ-variate function *(18)*. Such a fitting method is also used to avoid contributions caused by recirculation. It is then possible to derive parameters such as apparent transit time, τ_{app}, for the tracer through the myocardium ("apparent" because it is different from the definition of mean transit time). It was shown that $1/\tau_{app}$ and slope of the signal intensity vs time during contrast agent wash-in exhibit good correlation with myocardial blood flow, as determined by radioactive microsphere technique. Thus, even if absolute flow measurements may not be available, the flow indices that can be estimated using this technique can provide relative flow distributions, which are usually more relevant in practice for most applications other than the ones in which the primary objective is to measure tissue blood flow.

Alternative pharmacokinetic models have been proposed to take into account the diffusion of contrast agent into the interstitium *(3)*. These models are being widely applied for functional evaluation of tumors because in tumor biology it is not only the blood flow but also the changes in the permeability of vessels that are of interest. With neoangiogenesis, there is an increase in vessel density. However, it turns out that the new vasculature is relatively more leaky. Dynamic contrast-enhanced MRI is widely being accepted as a mainstream clinical tool in clinical oncology *(19)*. Similar methods are also being used in the evaluation of renal function because most of the currently approved Gd chelates approved for human use are freely filtered and excreted through the kidneys *(20)*. These methods are discussed in **Subheading 2.2.**

Recent advances in MRI contrast agents have introduced the so-called intravascular agents. By virtue of their physical size or by attaching Gd to macromolecules, these agents remain within the vasculature for long periods of time. Although many have been proposed and shown to be efficacious in preclinical evaluation, not many have progressed toward approval for clinical use. One such agent is MS-325, which has completed testing in phase III clinical trials; the Food and Drug Administration is expected to approve MS-325 in the next year or so *(21)*. Ultrasmall superparamagnetic iron oxides (USPIO) are currently undergoing phase II clinical trials as potential intravascular contrast agents *(22)*.

2.1.1.2. TECHNIQUES BASED ON ENDOGENOUS CONTRAST MECHANISMS

Techniques relying on exogenous contrast administration have certain limitations. Repeat studies are limited by the total amount of contrast that can be administered in one sitting. Thus, it is desirable to use perfusion MRI techniques that do not require the use of exogenous contrast agents.

One approach that makes use of an endogenous contrast mechanism uses magnetically labeled water as a tracer. A number of approaches based on this basic idea have been proposed. All of these approaches are based on manipulating the magnetization of inflowing arterial blood and involve acquiring a flow-insensitive image and a flow-sensitive image then subtracting the former from the later to remove the background tissue signals. Because this technique was covered in detail in Chapter 6, we will not discuss this any further.

2.2. Renal Function

Kidneys maintain homeostasis by filtering and excreting metabolic waste products, regulating acid–base balance, and moderating blood pressure and fluid volume. Because decreasing renal function accompanies renal disease, monitoring renal function permits assessment of disease progression and is used to guide therapy. Many noninvasive tests of renal function are in use but all have their drawbacks. Serum creatinine levels and creatinine clearance are insensitive measures of global function and cannot provide information about individual renal function. CT and intravenous urography can provide functional and anatomic information, but both use nephrotoxic contrast agents and expose the patient to radiation. MRI is capable of providing functional information, which, when combined with the exquisite anatomical detail of MRI, allow for comprehensive examination of the kidneys with minimal risk or discomfort to the patient.

Like inulin and iodine contrast agents, Gd chelates, such as Gd-DTPA, have a predominant renal elimination (approx 98%) by glomerular filtration without tubular secretion or reabsorption. Therefore, calculation of the glomerular filtration rate (GFR) is feasible using Gd-DTPA by the formula:

$$GFR = U \cdot V/P,$$

where V is the urine flow rate (mL/min), U is the substance concentration in urine, and P is the substance concentration in plasma.

With MR, calculation of *GFR* requires measurement of the concentration of the agent via measurement of relaxivity changes in urine, blood, or kidney, or via measurement of signal intensity within the kidneys. Ideally, relaxation rate measurements allow for estimation of Gd concentrations. This approach necessitates fast T_1 mapping, such as with the Look-Locker method *(23)* or FARM *(24)*. These methods may not provide sufficient organ coverage. Under certain conditions (e.g., low concentration and heavily T_1-weighted sequences could eliminate T_2 dependence), signal intensity can be related to Gd concentration either empirically by measuring the signal intensity of phantoms with different concentrations or by converting MR signal intensity to Gd-DTPA concentration, using the following two relationships *(25)*:

$$\frac{1}{T_1} = \frac{1}{T_1'} + [Gd] \cdot R,$$

where T_1 and T_1' are the observed and precontrast relaxation times of the tissue being studied, respectively, $[Gd]$ is the concentration of Gd, and R is the relaxivity of Gd.

The second relationship is an empirical one,

$$SI = k \cdot f(T_1),$$

where *SI* is the observed signal intensity, *k* is a constant multiplicative factor, and *f* is a monotonic relationship between signal intensity and the tissue relaxation time, T_1.

Because Gd chelates get concentrated in the renal medulla and collecting system, it is important to use low doses of Gd. It was shown that 0.025 mmol/kg doses yield signal intensity vs time curves that were similar to the scintigraphic time activity curves *(25)*.

With imaging capability, one could extend the global GFR measurement to estimating single kidney GFR.

$$EF_{tracer} = \frac{[tracer]_{artery} - [tracer]_{vein}}{[tracer]_{artery}},$$

where *EF* refers to extraction fraction. Using the T_1 to [*Gd*] relationship, this can be rewritten as:

$$EF_{Gd} = \left(\frac{T_1^{precontrast}}{T_1^{vein}}\right)\left(\frac{T_1^{vein} - T_1^{artery}}{T_1^{precontrast} - T_1^{artery}}\right).$$

Once *EF* is determined, *GFR* can be calculated according to the following equation:

$$GFR = EF \cdot RBF \cdot (1 - Hct),$$

where RBF is the renal blood flow and *Hct* is the hematocrit.

Several groups have published results based on this approach to measure single kidney GFR *(26–28)*. However, it is not a technique viable for routine clinical use because of the need for quantitative estimation of concentrations in different compartments and determining RBF in small blood vessels.

Alternatively, single kidney GFR can be estimated based on monitoring intrarenal kinetics. Bauman and Rudin *(29)* proposed a first-order kinetic model of the kidney that consists of two compartments, the cortex and medulla, and a rate constant between the two representing the rate of clearance of tracer from the cortex:

$$\frac{d[Gd]_m}{dt} = k \cdot [Gd]_c,$$

where $[Gd]_{m,c}$ are the time varying concentrations of Gd in the medulla and cortex, respectively, and *k* is the flow rate between the two compartments.

Preliminary validation in a small-animal model has been reported *(30)*. An alternative two-compartment model *(31)* and a more expansive multicompartmental model have also been proposed *(32)*.

2.3. Oxygenation

Because oxygen is one of the key nutrients necessary for the viability of cells in any tissue, evaluation of tissue oxygenation is very important. There are number of direct and indirect methods of evaluating regional oxygenation using MRI. These, again, either depend on endogenous contrast mechanisms or on exogenous contrast administrations.

2.3.1. BOLD Technique, an Endogenous Contrast Mechanism

Blood oxygenation level-dependent (BOLD) MRI depends on the fact that deoxygenated hemoglobin is slightly paramagnetic and, hence, behaves as an intravascular endogenous contrast agent *(33,34)*. This mechanism is described in more detail in Chapter 7. In principle, one can monitor changes in tissue oxygenation using this technique by assuming that the regional blood oxygenation levels are in dynamic equilibrium with the surrounding tissue. The BOLD signal changes are influenced by both changes in regional blood flow (perfusion) and regional oxygenation consumption (or extraction). Hence, in principle, BOLD MRI measurements are not very specific, i.e., one cannot differentiate changes in perfusion from changes in oxygen extraction. However, by use of specific paradigms (physiological or pharmacological) it is possible to interpret changes observed on BOLD MRI as predominantly perfusion-related or oxygenation-related changes. With perfusion, BOLD is sensitive to either blood volume or blood flow change. The BOLD MRI signals are affected in opposite ways, i.e., an increase in blood volume results in increased signal decay, whereas an increase in blood flow results in an increase in signal, and *vice versa*. Because, in most tissue, changes in blood volume parallel those in blood flow, the opposing effects could potentially compromise the net observed changes in signal intensity. In neuro fMRI, the interpretation is based on the premise that observed signal changes are caused by changes in local perfusion with very little change in oxygen extraction. Blood volume only explains the poststimulus undershoot *(35)*. Although BOLD MRI is many times used synonymously with neuro fMRI, several applications in the rest of body are being actively pursued. We will provide a few representative examples in the kidney here.

2.3.2. Oxygen-Enhanced MRI, an Exogenous Contrast Mechanism

Molecular oxygen is weakly paramagnetic because of the presence of two unpaired electrons. Each electron has a magnetic moment that is 1000 times that of a nucleus, and the resulting fluctuating magnetic field can produce a greater dipole–dipole interaction than that of the neighboring nuclei, thus causing a faster rate of spin-lattice relaxation (R_1). Chiarotti et al. *(36)* first reported that an increase in dissolved oxygen in water shortens its T_1 ($1/R_1$). Young et al. *(37)* extended Chiarotti's study and reported the shortening of T_1 and an increase in signal intensity of blood in the left ventricle after volunteers inhaled 100% oxygen in their investigation of the potential use of oxygen as a paramagnetic contrast agent. Expanding on these results, Edelman et al. *(38)* proposed the use of oxygen for ventilation imaging of the lung. Though oxygen is only weakly paramagnetic, its overall effect on the lung is considerable given the large surface area of the lung and the large difference in partial pressures between room air and 100% oxygen. These two factors facilitate an environment that allows more oxygen to diffuse across the parenchyma and dissolve in blood. This topic is dealt in further detail in Chapter 13. Oxygen-enhanced MRI has been used in other organs, including the kidneys *(39–41)*, however, it has remained primarily of academic interest.

3. Examples and Applications
3.1. Renal Perfusion MRI

Renal blood flow (RBF) is approximately one-fourth of the cardiac output, the majority being devoted to the cortex for glomerular filtration. The cortical perfusion is about 500 mL/min/100 g and the medullary flow is only 20 mL/min/100 g *(42)*. In clinical practice, measurement of RBF or perfusion could have a significant effect in the evaluation of renal artery stenoses (RAS) or nephropathies with microvascular involvement because flow compromise is a source of hypertension and chronic renal failure. The technique may also allow for monitoring interventions.

Figure 2 is an example of first-pass perfusion MRI using a novel iron oxide-based contrast agent, ferumoxytol (Advanced Magnetics Inc., Cambridge, MA). Ferumoxytol consists of nanoparticles of iron oxide with a dextran coating for biocompatibility. Ferumoxytol is currently undergoing Phase II clinical trials *(22)*. Shown are gradient-echo (T_2*-weighted) images of the kidney obtained after a bolus administration of ferumoxytol (1 mg/kg) in an anesthetized rabbit. Using a similar agent, quantitative regional blood flow estimations were reported recently *(43,44)* using central volume principles.

3.2. Renal Function
3.2.1. Qualitative and Semiquantitative Approaches
to Evaluate Renal Function

Although the methods discussed in **Subheading 2.** are feasible and have been demonstrated in humans to provide quantitative measure of GFR *(26–28)*, they are not particularly amenable for routine clinical use. This is mainly

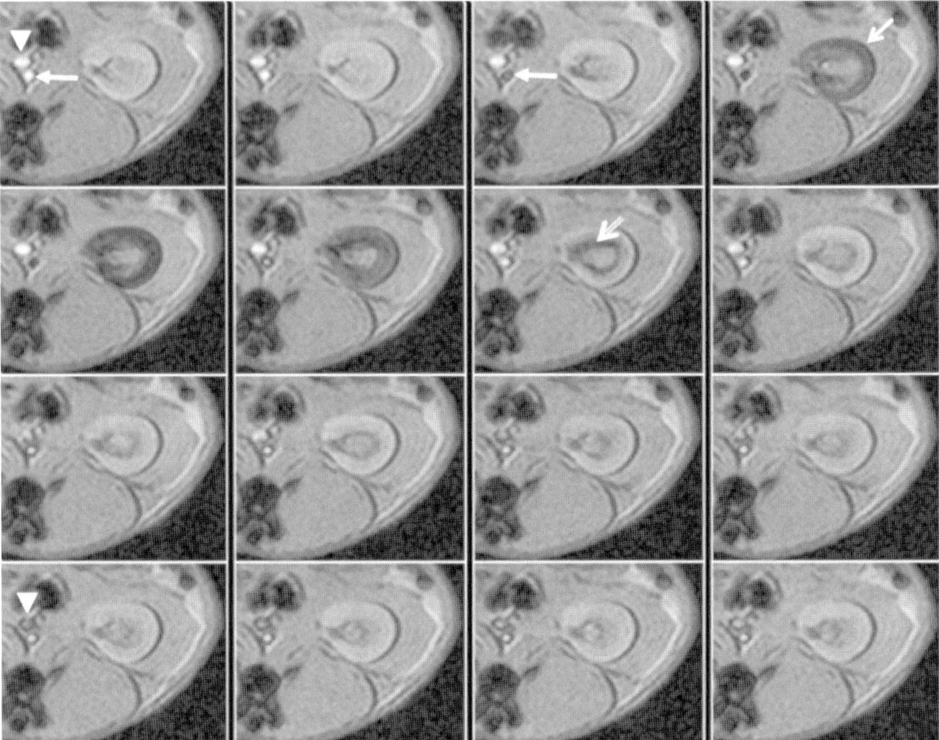

Fig. 2. Time series (left to right, top to bottom) of magnetic resonance (MR) images obtained before and during first pass of ferumoxytol, a negative contrast agent (i.e., with increasing concentration the signal becomes darker). Marked on the first time frame (precontrast) are the abdominal aorta (solid arrow) and vena cava (solid arrow head), respectively. Note that on the 3rd time point the aorta goes completely dark. In the next time frame, the cortex gets dark (arrow); by the 7th time frame, the medulla goes completely dark, whereas the cortex recovers; and by the 13th time frame, the vena cava becomes dark. Based on this type of dynamic scanning, one can obtain concentration vs time profiles and fit them to appropriate mathematical models to extract various perfusion indices *(44)*.

because of measurements necessitating quantitative measures of T_1 and blood flow in blood vessels. A more facile technique is based on dynamic imaging of the contrast passage through the renal parenchyma that is closely related to the nuclear medicine technique currently used in the clinic.

The signal intensity time curves obtained with predominantly T_1-weighted sequences can be used in concert with angiotensin-converting enzyme (ACE) inhibition to differentiate kidneys supplied by stenotic renal arteries *(45,46)*. This approach parallels ACE-I renal scintigraphy. The advantage with the MRI approach is that it can be readily combined with anatomical information, such as MR angiography. Preliminary feasibility has been reported both in animal models *(46)* and in human subjects *(45)*.

Hypertension is a common occurrence with almost 60 million diagnosed in the United States. Of these, an estimated 1 to 5% have renovascular disease (RVD) as the underlying cause *(47)*. As one of the few potentially curable causes of hypertension, RVD remains an important, yet challenging, diagnosis. Not all subjects with RAS have RVD; in fact, those with essential hypertension tend to develop accelerated atherosclerosis, which can lead to RAS. These diagnostic limitations have generated controversies surrounding treatment. Most anatomic tests, such as conventional angiography, MR angiography, and CT angiography, are limited in their ability to diagnose RVD because they rely on RAS as the sole criterion. ACE-inhibitor renal scintigraphy is the best predictor of response to therapy because it is a functional test of renal ischemia. However, it does not supply the anatomical information needed for therapeutic planning. Decreased renal perfusion pressure in subjects with RAS activates the renin–angiotensin system and increases production of angiotensin II. Angiotensin II causes vasoconstriction of the efferent glomerular arteriole and restores renal perfusion pressure and glomerular filtration to normal or near-normal levels. This compensated RAS may not manifest as any perfusion or filtration abnormalities on renal scintigraphy or MR renography. Administering ACE-I lowers GFR in the setting of RVD because it blocks the production of angiotensin II, and, hence, decreases efferent glomerular arteriolar vasoconstriction and reduces perfusion pressure. **Figure 3** is an example of captopril MR renography in a pig with unilateral RAS *(46)*. Although this example illustrates the efficacy of the method, for practical routine clinical use, other factors need to be considered. Because the objective is to combine such functional information with anatomical depiction of the RAS, the protocol should include MR angiography. Because contrast-enhanced MR angiography is the current standard clinical practice, the total dose administered is a key issue. Lee et al. *(48)* have implemented a protocol that uses a small dose of contrast for MR renography (2 mL or 0.013 mmol/kg of Gd-DTPA). The authors also take advantage of the higher spatial resolution available with MRI (compared with scintigraphy) to differentiate the signal intensity vs time curves independently for the cortex and medulla. Among patients with normal serum creatinine levels, ACE-I unmasked decreased GFR by depressing medullary enhancement in patients with RAS.

There are a number of other applications in which dynamic contrast enhancement kinetics could provide valuable information for comprehensive evaluation, such as ureteral obstruction *(49–51)*, and evaluation of renal transplants *(52,53)*.

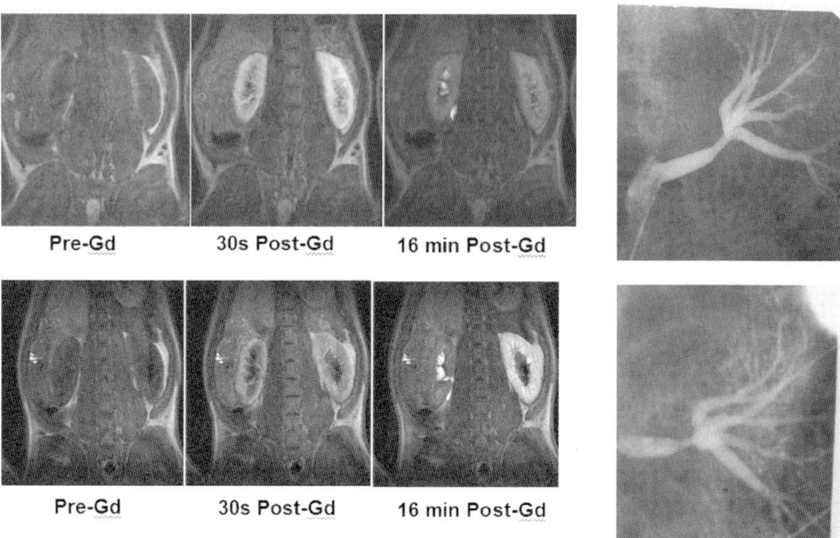

Fig. 3. Illustration of renal function as evaluated by dynamic magnetic resonance imaging (MRI) after administration of gadolinium diethylenetriamine pentaacetic acid (Gd-DTPA), a positive contrast agent (i.e., with higher concentrations the signal is increased). Shown are T_1-weighted magnetic resonance (MR) images obtained at representative time points after 0.05 mmol/kg Gd-DTPA administration and after administration of captopril *(46)*. The top row was obtained 1 wk after surgical placement of an MRI-compatible ameroid constrictor around the renal artery (seen on the X-ray angiograms on the right). The bottom row was obtained in the same animal 5 wk later. Note the severity of the renal artery stenosis, especially the poststenotic vessel dilatation, a classic sign of hemodynamically significant stenosis. At wk-1, the contrast wash-out is almost complete and symmetrical, whereas at wk-6, with the progression of the stenosis to being hemodynamically significant, the wash-out in the affected kidney is rather limited. In an independent series of animals (data not shown), it was shown that at wk-6 without captopril the wash-out appears symmetrical, confirming that only in the presence of a significant stenosis and after administration of captopril is the contrast accumulation observed. This is the basis of currently used captopril renography using radionuclide techniques. However, with MRI, the anatomical depiction is much more remarkable, and angiographic data can be obtained in the same setting to confirm the presence of the renal artery stenosis. (Reproduced with permission from **ref. *46*.**)

3.3. Intrarenal Oxygenation

It is now well recognized that the renal medulla operates at a low oxygenation level (renal medullary hypoxia) *(54,55)*. This makes it highly susceptible to even mild reductions in blood flow. Renal ischemia accounts for almost

50% of the observed cases of acute renal failure *(56)*. Over the years, based on several in vitro and in vivo animal studies, it has been shown that this type of acute renal failure usually involves hypoxic injury to renal medullary tubules *(57–63)*. Renal dysfunction may also play a role in the development of all forms of hypertension in humans and laboratory animals *(64)*. Many experiments have shown that medullary blood flow (and presumably medullary oxygenation status) is reduced in hypertension, and more importantly, that reduced medullary blood flow is sufficient to produce hypertension *(65–67)*. All these studies were performed using invasive microelectrodes and/or Doppler flow probes in rat kidneys. The availability of a noninvasive technique to monitor renal medullary blood flow in humans under normal conditions and during physiological and pharmacological stresses may allow for an extension of the observations to humans.

BOLD MRI has been used extensively in organs such as the brain *(68–70)*. The BOLD MRI technique exploits the fact that the magnetic properties of hemoglobin vary, depending on whether it is in the oxygenated or deoxygenated form. This affects the T_2^* relaxation time of the neighboring water molecules and, in turn, influences the MRI signal on T_2^*-weighted images. The rate of spin dephasing, R_2^* $(=1/T_2^*)$, is closely related to the tissue content of deoxyhemoglobin. Because the oxygen tension, pO_2, of capillary blood is thought to be in equilibrium with the surrounding tissue, changes estimated by BOLD MRI can be interpreted as changes in tissue pO_2 *(71,72)*. A strong correspondence has been demonstrated between renal BOLD MRI measurements in humans and earlier animal data obtained using invasive microelectrodes. **Figure 4** illustrates BOLD MRI application to intrarenal oxygenation in rat kidneys. Shown is the ability to follow dynamic changes in medullary oxygenation after administration of different vasoactive drugs. Also included are human and mouse examples, clearly demonstrating the advantage of the technique in terms of translation from preclinical to clinical setting.

Our own work is motivated by the hypothesis that medullary hypoxia is not necessarily the culprit in the pathophysiology of ischemic renal disease, but it is rather the compromise of endogenous protective molecular mechanisms that fail to maintain *status quo* and, hence, lead to manifestation of disease and disease progression. We have previously demonstrated, using the BOLD MRI technique, that age and diabetes (both recognized as predisposing factors for acute renal failure) are associated with reduced prostaglandin production, a hypothesized protective mechanism *(73,74)*. Similarly, using BOLD MRI, we have duplicated *(75)* prior observations using microelectrodes in which the authors had demonstrated that development of radiocontrast nephropathy necessitates elimination of prostaglandin and nitric oxide systems *(76)*. We are currently pursuing work in models of hypertension in which we have demon-

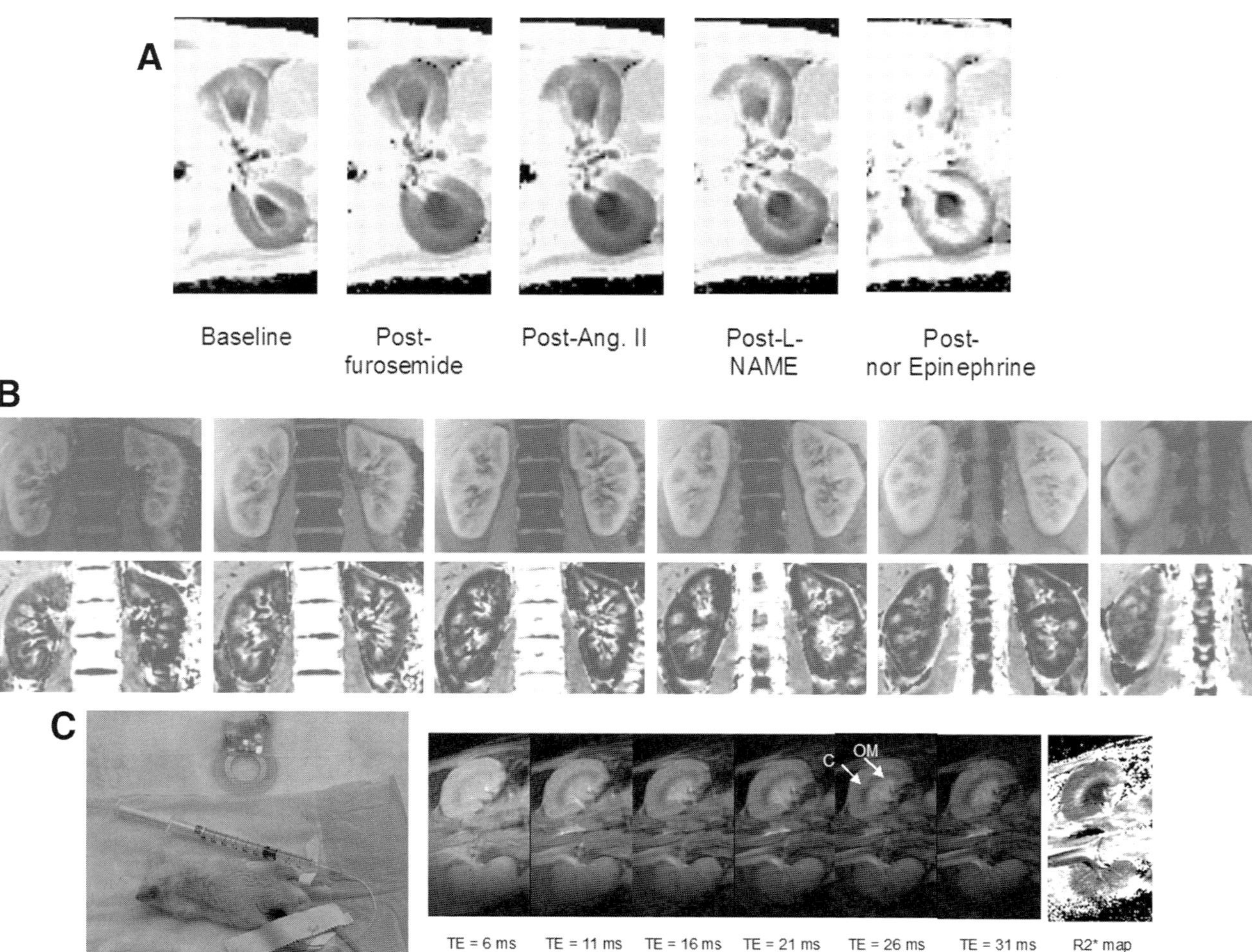
A
Baseline
Post-furosemide
Post-Ang. II
Post-L-NAME
Post-nor Epinephrine
B
C
C
OM
TE = 6 ms
TE = 11 ms
TE = 16 ms
TE = 21 ms
TE = 26 ms
TE = 31 ms
R2* map

strated lack of (or reduced) nitric oxide bioavailability *(77)*, and how that may be reversed by suitable pharmacological interventions *(78)*. With a better understanding of these and other such protective mechanisms (and, probably, the complicated interplay) one would be able to implement suitable interventions that could prevent certain disease progression. This thought process is very much in agreement with a theory that is now reaching wider acceptance; that several systemic disease processes actually start with a subclinical renal dysfunction *(64)*.

Other groups have adapted the BOLD MRI measurements to other applications, such as RAS *(79)* and diabetes *(80)*. In carefully performed, large-animal studies, Juillard et al. *(79)* found oxygenation in both cortex and medulla significantly reduced during acute reduction in blood flow. The authors also comment that:

Fig. 4. *(opposite page)* Blood oxygenation level-dependent (BOLD) magnetic resonance imaging (MRI) data obtained at 3.0 T in both rat and human kidneys. **(A)** Before and after pharmaceutical R_2^* maps in rat kidneys in the axial plane. Although this was not performed to address any specific scientific question, it is a very nice demonstration of the advantage and efficacy of the technique. These images were all acquired within 1 h, with approx 10 min between administrations of different agents. There is no other known technique that allows acquisition of such dynamic information. This is possible mainly because the technique does not rely on administration of exogenous agents. Of course, the observed effects would still depend on the pharmacokinetics of the agents used, however, that is not necessarily a limitation of the technique itself. Furosemide stops the reabsorptive function along the medullary thick ascending limbs and thereby reduces the oxygen consumption in the medullary segments. One can observe reduction in the brightness of R_2^* maps in the medulla (lower R_2^* implied better oxygenation). Angiotensin II (Ang. II) is a commonly used vasoconstrictor; we observed little effect on the R_2^* maps. However, after subsequent administration of N^G-nitro-L-arginine methylester (L-NAME) and norepinephrine (potent vasoconstrictors), there was a significant increase in R_2^*, predominantly in the renal medulla. **(B)** BOLD MRI data in a human kidney. Shown are data acquired with a 3D sequence in which the entire kidney in the coronal plane can be covered within a single breath-hold interval. Included are the first image of eight echo images acquired (top row) and the corresponding calculated R_2^* maps (bottom row). The cortico medullary differentiation both on the anatomical and R_2^* maps are remarkable. **(C)** BOLD MRI data in a mouse kidney. Shown are data acquired in a 24-g mouse using a dedicated 2-cm surface coil on a standard 3.0-T whole-body scanner, the same as in **(A)** and **(B)**. This figure provides a clear indication of the power of the technology in terms of its scaling, and how observations could easily be translated from a mouse model to humans. Included are the six individual echo images obtained in the coronal plane and the calculated R_2^* map. C, cortex; OM, outer medulla, IM, inner medulla

"BOLD MRI is the only technique currently available that allows noninvasive measurement of oxygen content in the kidney."

As concluding remarks, they also point out that:

"new functional tools, such as BOLD, capable of detecting ischemia and characterize patterns of intra-renal oxygen levels, may assist in identifying patients that would more likely to benefit from therapeutic benefits."

Using BOLD MRI, Ries et al. *(80)* showed that the oxygenation in all compartments of the kidney is significantly reduced in a rat streptozotocine-induced model of type I diabetes. They further interpreted this as being related to hyperfiltration-associated increase in oxygen consumption. By comparing the observed changes on BOLD MRI with histological changes, the authors further concluded that:

"the observed MR changes are not influenced by 'anatomical or pathological' changes, but by functional changes only."

3.4. Other Functional MRI Techniques as Applied to the Kidney

Although we tried to cover three major functional MRI methods in detail, there are other techniques that have been used as potential functional MRI methods. These include diffusion measurements in the kidney *(81–84)*; pH measurements *(85)*; and, more recently, sodium (Na) MRI *(86)*. Although diffusion measurements certainly provide opportunities for tissue characterization, it is not quite clear what the measured values represent in terms of the functional status of the kidney. pH measurements are discussed in detail in Chapter 14. A more recent development is the feasibility of performing Na MRI *(86)*, which allows one to follow the urinary concentrating process directly. MRI has the ability to directly measure the tissue sodium concentration noninvasively. However, Na MRI necessitates custom coils that either are tuned to the Na frequency or doubly tuned coils, so that one can perform both proton and Na MRI. The inherent sensitivity of Na MRI is at least an order of magnitude lower than proton MRI, and when combined with the fact that the availability of Na is couple of orders magnitude lower in the body, the signal-to-noise ratios are significantly lower on Na MRI compared with proton MRI images. Dynamic imaging after administration of a novel dendrimer-based contrast agent was recently reported in a mouse model of acute renal failure *(87)*. This particular example was also performed on a whole-body scanner.

4. Note

1. When planning BOLD MRI measurements in the kidneys, it is important to be aware of potential artifacts from bulk susceptibility effects from the surrounding bowels, which could be filled with gas. In our experience, this is more limiting in

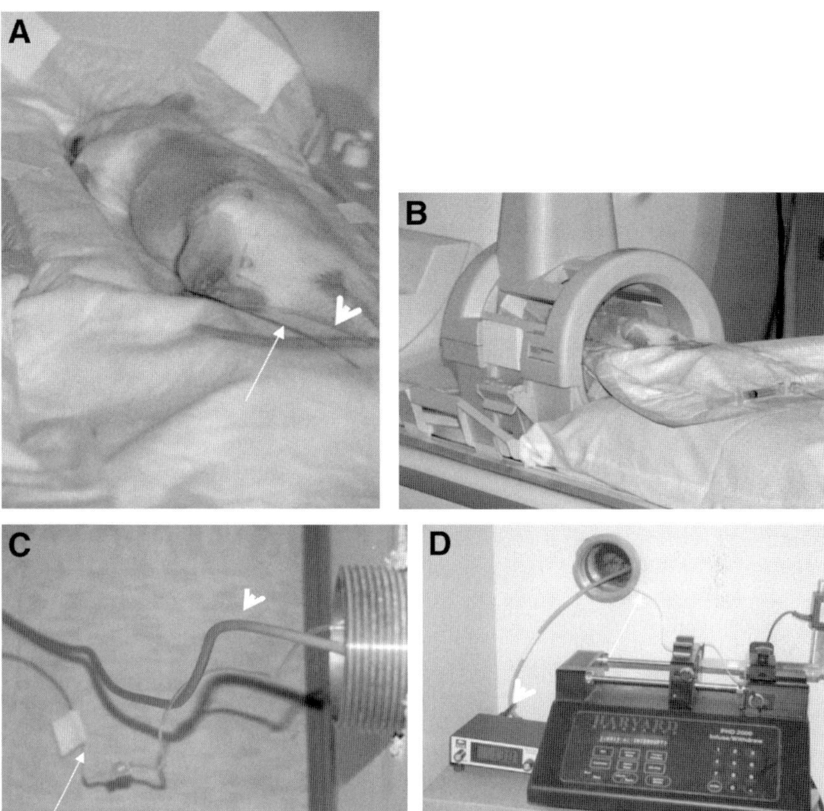

Fig. 5. Typical positioning of the rat for Blood oxygenation level-dependent (BOLD) magnetic resonance imaging (MRI) studies, lying on its side. The long arrow points to the iv line in the femoral vein, and the arrow head points to the arterial line placed in the femoral artery for monitoring blood pressure. The arterial line is then connected to a transducer at least 1 m away from the center of the magnet, and the cable is taken out of the scanner room via a wave guide (**C**). This will ensure minimization of any radio frequency interference with the scanner. (**D**) Shows the blood pressure gage, which can be connected either to a chart recorder or to a computer with charting software. The iv line is connected to an infusion pump. The typical length of the iv tubing and the cable is on the order of 5 m.

small animals, probably because of the relative proximity of the bowel loops to the kidney. We have primarily addressed this issue by positioning the animals on their side instead of supine (**Fig. 5**). With this arrangement, we can routinely image at least one kidney free of artifacts. However, Ries et al. *(80)* have used a home-built positioner (there is a figure in the cited article) that allows the isolation of one of the kidneys in the supine position away from the abdomen.

5. Summary Points

- Although primarily designed and optimized for human use, there are certain practical and logistical advantages in using whole-body scanners for small-animal MRI. The ultimate choice may be limited by availability to a particular user.
- "Functional" in the context of the kidney may mean several things. However, for our purposes we include all information other than anatomical as functional. In this chapter, we mainly focused on perfusion index, renal excretory functional index, and intrarenal oxygenation as functional parameters. This in no way exhausts all possible indices.
- Motivation to evaluate function arises from the hypothesis that it either adds value to anatomical characterization of disease and, hence, leads to comprehensive evaluation (e.g., captopril MR renography in combination with MR angiography) or it can provide early markers of change to study evolution of pathophysiology and/or to monitor therapeutic interventions.
- Dynamic imaging after administration of a suitable MR contrast agent (tracer) combined with an appropriate mathematical model allows for evaluation of useful functional indices, such as regional blood flow or GFR. Contrast agents can be either positive or negative with respect to the signal changes, based on concentration.
- Combining the ability to measure functional indices with suitable pharmacological and/or physiological paradigms, it is possible to study the dependence of pathophysiology on molecular mechanisms. By the same token, one can also follow the effects of novel interventions based on molecular medicine.
- An advantage of MRI methods for functional evaluation is that the techniques are easy to translate from small-animal models to humans.

Acknowledgments

The author was supported in part by a grant from the NIH (DK-53221). Images in **Figs. 1**, **3**, and **4C** were obtained with the help of Drs. Luping Li, Lin Ji, and Elizabete Santos.

References

1. Bentley, M. D., Ortiz, M. C., Ritman, E. L., and Romero, J. C. (2002) The use of microcomputed tomography to study microvasculature in small rodents. *Am. J. Physiol. Regul. Integr. Comp. Physiol.* **282,** R1267–R1279.
2. Edvinsson, L., MacKenzie, E. T., and McCulloch, J. (1993) *Cerebral Blood Flow and Metabolism.* Raven, New York, NY.
3. Kety, S. and Schmidt, C. F. (1948) Nitrous oxide method for the quantitative determination of cerebral blood flow in man: theory, procedure, and normal values. *J. Clin. Invest.* **27,** 475–483.
4. Gur, D., Good, W. F., Wolfson, S. K., Jr., Yonas, H., and Shabason, L. (1982) In vivo mapping of local cerebral blood flow by xenon-enhanced computed tomography. *Science* **215,** 1267–1268.
5. Fox, P. T., Raichle, M. E., Mintun, M. A., and Dence, C. (1988) Nonoxidative glucose consumption during focal physiologic neural activity. *Science* **241,** 462–464.

6. Stewart, G. N. (1894) Researches on the circulation time in organs, and on the influences which affect it: Parts I-III. *J. Physiol. (London)* **15,** 1–89.

7. Zeirler, K. L. (1962) Theoretical basis of indicator-dilution methods for measuring flow and volume. *Circ. Res.* **10,** 393–407.

8. Grubb, R. L., Jr., Raichle, M. E., Eichling, J. O., and Ter-Pogossian, M. M. (1974) The effects of changes in PaCO2 on cerebral blood volume, blood flow, and vascular mean transit time. *Stroke* **5,** 630–639.

9. Lassen, N. A. and Perl, W. (1979) *Tracer Kinetic Methods In Medical Physiology.* Raven, New York, NY.

10. Davis, C. P., McKinnon, G. C., Debatin, J. F., and von Schulthess, G. K. (1996) Ultra-high-speed MR imaging. *Eur. Radiol.* **6,** 297–311.

11. Nitz, W. R. (2002) Fast and ultrafast non-echo-planar MR imaging techniques. *Eur. Radiol.* **12,** 2866–82.

12. Villringer, A., Rosen, B. R., Belliveau, J. W., et al. (1988) Dynamic imaging with lanthanide chelates in normal brain: contrast due to magnetic susceptibility effects. *Magn. Reson. Med.* **6,** 164–174.

13. Rosen, B. R., Belliveau, J. W., Vevea, J. M., and Brady, T. J. (1990) Perfusion imaging with NMR contrast agents. *Magn. Reson. Med.* **14,** 249–265.

14. Perman, W. H., Gado, M. H., Larson, K. B., and Perlmutter, J. S. (1992) Simultaneous MR acquisition of arterial and brain signal-time curves. *Magn. Reson. Med.* **28,** 74–83.

15. Lassen, N. A. (1984) Cerebral transit of an intravascular tracer may allow measurement of regional blood volume but not regional blood flow. *J. Cereb. Blood Flow Metab.* **4,** 633–634.

16. Weisskoff, R. M., Chesler, D., Boxerman, J. L., and Rosen, B. R. (1993) Pitfalls in MR measurement of tissue blood flow with intravascular tracers: which mean transit time? *Magn. Reson. Med.* **29,** 553–558.

17. Wilke, N., Simm, C., Zhang, J., et al. (1993) Contrast-enhanced first pass myocardial perfusion imaging: correlation between myocardial blood flow in dogs at rest and during hyperemia. *Magn. Reson. Med.* **29,** 485–497.

18. Thompson, H. K., Stramer, C. F., Whalen, R. E., and McIntosh, H. D. (1964) Indicator transit time considered as a gamma variate. *Circ. Res.* 502–515.

19. Padhani, A. R. (2002) Dynamic contrast-enhanced MRI in clinical oncology: current status and future directions. *J. Magn. Reson. Imaging* **16,** 407–422.

20. Huang, A. J., Lee, V. S., and Rusinek, H. (2003) MR imaging of renal function. *Radiol. Clin. North Am.* **41,** 1001–1017.

21. Lauffer, R. B., Parmelee, D. J., Dunham, S. U., et al. (1998) MS-325: albumin-targeted contrast agent for MR angiography. *Radiology* **207,** 529–538.

22. Ersoy, H., Jacobs, P., Kent, C. K., and Prince, M. R. (2004) Blood pool MR angiography of aortic stent-graft endoleak. *AJR Am. J. Roentgenol.* **182,** 1181–1186.

23. Niendorf, E. R., Santyr, G. E., Brazy, P. C., and Grist, T. M. (1996) Measurement of Gd-DTPA dialysis clearance rates by using a look-locker imaging technique. *Magn. Reson. Med.* **36,** 571–578.

24. Chen, Z., Prato, F. S., and McKenzie, C. (1998) T1 fast acquisition relaxation mapping (T1-FARM): an optimized reconstruction. *I. E. E. E. Trans. Med. Imaging* **17,** 155–160.
25. Rusinek, H., Lee, V. S., and Johnson, G. (2001) Optimal dose of Gd-DTPA in dynamic MR studies. *Magn. Reson. Med.* **46,** 312–316.
26. Dumoulin, C. L., Buonocore, M. H., Opsahl, L. R., et al. (1994) Noninvasive measurement of renal hemodynamic functions using gadolinium enhanced magnetic resonance imaging. *Magn. Reson. Med.* **32,** 370–378.
27. Niendorf, E. R., Grist, T. M., Lee, F. T., Jr., Brazy, P. C., and Santyr, G. E. (1998) Rapid in vivo measurement of single-kidney extraction fraction and glomerular filtration rate with MR imaging. *Radiology* **206,** 791–798.
28. Coulam, C. H., Lee, J. H., Wedding, K. L., et al. (2002) Noninvasive measurement of extraction fraction and single-kidney glomerular filtration rate with MR imaging in swine with surgically created renal arterial stenoses. *Radiology* **223,** 76–82.
29. Baumann, D. and Rudin, M. (2000) Quantitative assessment of rat kidney function by measuring the clearance of the contrast agent Gd(DOTA) using dynamic MRI. *Magn. Reson. Imaging* **18,** 587–595.
30. Laurent, D., Poirier, K., Wasvary, J., and Rudin, M. (2002) Effect of essential hypertension on kidney function as measured in rat by dynamic MRI. *Magn. Reson. Med.* **47,** 127–134.
31. Smith, A. M., Materne, R., and Van Beers, B. E. (2001) Quantitative measurement of blood perfusion, GFR and arterial vascular fraction in the kidney cortex. *Proceedings of IX annual meeting of the International Society of Magnetic Resonance in Medicine*, Glasgow, Scotland, UK, April 21–27.
32. Lee, V. S., Rusinek, H., Kim, S., Leonard, E., Lee, P., and Johnson, G. (2001) Analysis of dynamic three-dimensional (3D) MR renography: regional characterization by multicompartmental modeling. *Proceedings of IX annual meeting of the International Society of Magnetic Resonance in Medicine* Glasgow, Scotland, UK, April 21–27.
33. Thulborn, K. R., Waterton, J. C., Matthews, P. M., and Radda, G. K. (1982) Oxygenation dependence of the transverse relaxation time of water protons in whole blood at high field. *Biochim. Biophys. Acta.* **714,** 265–270.
34. Ogawa, S., Lee, T. M., and Barrere, B. (1993) The sensitivity of magnetic resonance image signals of a rat brain to changes in the cerebral venous blood oxygenation. *Magn. Reson. Med.* **29,** 205–210.
35. Buxton, R. B., Wong, E. C., and Frank, L. R. (1998) Dynamics of blood flow and oxygenation changes during brain activation: the balloon model. *Magn. Reson. Med.* **39,** 855–864.
36. Chiarotti, G., Cristiani, G., and Bliulotto, L. (1955) Proton relaxation in pure liquids and in liquids containing paramagnetic gases in solution. *Nuovo Cimento* **1,** 863–873.
37. Young, I. R., Clarke, G. J., Bailes, D. R., Pennock, J. M., Doyle, F. H., and Bydder, G. M. (1981) Enhancement of relaxation rate with paramagnetic contrast agents in NMR imaging. *J. Comput. Tomogr.* **5,** 543–547.

38. Edelman, R. R., Hatabu, H., Tadamura, E., Li, W., and Prasad, P. V. (1996) Noninvasive assessment of regional ventilation in the human lung using oxygen-enhanced magnetic resonance imaging. *Nat. Med.* **2,** 1236–1239.

39. Berkowitz, B. A. and Wilson, C. A. (1995) Quantitative mapping of ocular oxygenation using magnetic resonance imaging. *Magn. Reson. Med.* **33,** 579–581.

40. Tadamura, E., Hatabu, H., Li, W., Prasad, P. V., and Edelman, R. R. (1997) Effect of oxygen inhalation on relaxation times in various tissues. *J. Magn. Reson. Imaging* **7,** 220–225.

41. Jones, R. A., Ries, M., Moonen, C. T., and Grenier, N. (2002) Imaging the changes in renal T1 induced by the inhalation of pure oxygen: a feasibility study. *Magn. Reson. Med.* **47,** 728–735.

42. Grenier, N., Basseau, F., Ries, M., Tyndal, B., Jones, R., and Moonen, C. (2003) Functional MRI of the kidney. *Abdom. Imaging* **28,** 164–175.

43. Aumann, S., Schoenberg, S. O., Just, A., et al. (2003) Quantification of renal perfusion using an intravascular contrast agent (part 1): results in a canine model. *Magn. Reson. Med.* **49,** 276–287.

44. Schoenberg, S. O., Aumann, S., Just, A., et al. (2003) Quantification of renal perfusion abnormalities using an intravascular contrast agent (part 2): results in animals and humans with renal artery stenosis. *Magn. Reson. Med.* **49,** 288–298.

45. Grenier, N., Trillaud, H., Combe, C., et al. (1996) Diagnosis of renovascular hypertension: feasibility of captopril-sensitized dynamic MR imaging and comparison with captopril scintigraphy. *AJR Am. J. Roentgenol.* **166,** 835–843.

46. Prasad, P. V., Goldfarb, J., Sundaram, C., Priatna, A., Li, W., and Edelman, R. R. (2000) Captopril MR renography in a swine model: toward a comprehensive evaluation of renal arterial stenosis. *Radiology* **217,** 813–818.

47. Pickering, T. G., Blumenfeld, J. D., and Laragh, J. H. (1996) Renovascular hypertension and ischemic nephropathy, in: *The Kidney* (Brenner, B. M., ed.), W.B. Saunders, Phildadelphia, PA, pp. 2106–2125.

48. Lee, V. S., Rusinek, H., Johnson, G., Rofsky, N. M., Krinsky, G. A., and Weinreb, J. C. (2001) MR renography with low-dose gadopentetate dimeglumine: feasibility. *Radiology* **221,** 371–379.

49. Mostafavi, M. R., Saltzman, B., and Prasad, P. V. (1997) Magnetic resonance imaging in the evaluation of ureteropelvic junction obstructed kidney. *Urology* **50,** 601–602; discussion 602–603.

50. Rohrschneider, W. K., Becker, K., Hoffend, J., et al. (2000) Combined static-dynamic MR urography for the simultaneous evaluation of morphology and function in urinary tract obstruction. II. Findings in experimentally induced ureteric stenosis. *Pediatr. Radiol.* **30,** 523–532.

51. Rohrschneider, W. K., Hoffend, J., Becker, K., et al. (2000) Combined static-dynamic MR urography for the simultaneous evaluation of morphology and function in urinary tract obstruction. I. Evaluation of the normal status in an animal model. *Pediatr. Radiol.* **30,** 511–522.

52. Agildere, A. M., Tarhan, N. C., Bozdagi, G., Demirag, A., Niron, E. A., and Haberal, M. (1999) Correlation of quantitative dynamic magnetic resonance imaging findings with pathology results in renal transplants: a preliminary report. *Transplant Proc.* **31,** 3312–3316.
53. Dorsam, J., Knopp, M. V., Carl, S., et al. (1997) Ureteral complications after kidney transplantation—evaluation with functional magnetic resonance urography. *Transplant Proc.* **29,** 132–135.
54. Brezis, M. and Rosen, S. (1995) Hypoxia of the renal medulla—its implications for disease. *N. Engl. J. Med.* **332,** 647–655.
55. Epstein, F. H., Agmon, Y., and Brezis, M. (1994) Physiology of renal hypoxia. *Ann. N. Y. Acad. Sci.* **718,** 72–81; discussion 81–82.
56. Thadhani, R., Pascual, M., and Bonventre, J. V. (1996) Acute renal failure. *N. Engl. J. Med.* **334,** 1448–1460.
57. Heyman, S. N., Fuchs, S., and Brezis, M. (1995) The role of medullary ischemia in acute renal failure. *New. Horiz.* **3,** 597–607.
58. Brezis, M. and Epstein, F. H. (1993) Cellular mechanisms of acute ischemic injury in the kidney. *Annu. Rev. Med.* **44,** 27–37.
59. Rosen, S., Epstein, F. H., and Brezis, M. (1992) Determinants of intrarenal oxygenation: factors in acute renal failure. *Ren. Fail.* **14,** 321–325.
60. Brezis, M., Dinour, D., Greenfeld, Z., and Rosen, S. (1991) Susceptibility of Henle's loop to hypoxic and toxic insults. *Adv. Nephrol. Necker Hosp.* **20,** 41–56.
61. Brezis, M., Rosen, S. N., and Epstein, F. H. (1989) The pathophysiological implications of medullary hypoxia. *Am. J. Kidney Dis.* **13,** 253–258.
62. Brezis, M., Rosen, S., Silva, P., and Epstein, F. H. (1984) Renal ischemia: a new perspective. *Kidney Int.* **26,** 375–383.
63. Brezis, M., Rosen, S., Silva, P., and Epstein, F. H. (1984) Selective anoxic injury to thick ascending limb: an anginal syndrome of the renal medulla? *Adv. Exp. Med. Biol.* **180,** 239–249.
64. Johnson, R. J., Herrera-Acosta, J., Schreiner, G. F., and Rodriguez-Iturbe, B. (2002) Subtle acquired renal injury as a mechanism of salt-sensitive hypertension. *N. Engl. J. Med.* **346,** 913–923.
65. Cowley, A. W., Jr., Mattson, D. L., Lu, S., and Roman, R. J. (1995) The renal medulla and hypertension. *Hypertension* **25,** 663–673.
66. Cowley, A. W., Roman, R. J., Fenoy, F. J., and Mattson, D. L. (1992) Effect of renal medullary circulation on arterial pressure. *J. Hypertens. Suppl.* **10,** S187–S193.
67. Cowley, A. W., Jr. (1997) Role of the renal medulla in volume and arterial pressure regulation. *Am. J. Physiol.* **273,** R1–R15.
68. Matthews, P. M. and Jezzard, P. (2004) Functional magnetic resonance imaging. *J. Neurol. Neurosurg. Psychiatry* **75,** 6–12.
69. Ugurbil, K., Hu, X., Chen, W., Zhu, X. H., Kim, S. G., and Georgopoulos, A. (1999) Functional mapping in the human brain using high magnetic fields. *Philos. Trans. R. Soc. Lond. B Biol. Sci.* **354,** 1195–1213.

70. Rajagopalan, P., Krishnan, K. R., Passe, T. J., and Macfall, J. R. (1995) Magnetic resonance imaging using deoxyhemoglobin contrast versus positron emission tomography in the assessment of brain function. *Prog. Neuropsychopharmacol. Biol. Psychiatry* **19,** 351–366.

71. Prasad, P. V., Edelman, R. R., and Epstein, F. H. (1996) Noninvasive evaluation of intrarenal oxygenation with BOLD MRI. *Circulation* **94,** 3271–3275.

72. Prasad, P. V., Chen, Q., Goldfarb, J. W., Epstein, F. H., and Edelman, R. R. (1997) Breath-hold R2* mapping with a multiple gradient-recalled echo sequence: application to the evaluation of intrarenal oxygenation. *J. Magn. Reson. Imaging* **7,** 1163–1165.

73. Prasad, P. V. and Epstein, F. H. (1999) Changes in renal medullary pO2 during water diuresis as evaluated by blood oxygenation level-dependent magnetic resonance imaging: effects of aging and cyclooxygenase inhibition. *Kidney Int.* **55,** 294–298.

74. Epstein, F. H., Veves, A., and Prasad, P. V. (2002) Effect of diabetes on renal medullary oxygenation during water diuresis. *Diabetes Care* **25,** 575–578.

75. Prasad, P. V., Priatna, A., Spokes, K., and Epstein, F. H. (2001) Changes in intrarenal oxygenation as evaluated by BOLD MRI in a rat kidney model for radiocontrast nephropathy. *J. Magn. Reson. Imaging* **13,** 744–747.

76. Agmon, Y., Peleg, H., Greenfeld, Z., Rosen, S., and Brezis, M. (1994) Nitric oxide and prostanoids protect the renal outer medulla from radiocontrast toxicity in the rat. *J. Clin. Invest.* **94,** 1069–1075.

77. Li, L., Storey, P., Kim, D., Li, W., and Prasad, P. (2003) Kidneys in hypertensive rats show reduced response to nitric oxide synthase inhibition as evaluated by BOLD MRI. *J. Magn. Reson. Imaging* **17,** 671–675.

78. Li, L., Fogelson, L., Li, B., Li, W., Storey, P., and Prasad, P. (2003) Effect of oxygen free radical scavenger on renal medullary oxygenation in hypertensive rats as evaluated by BOLD MRI. *Proceedings of the XI annual meeting of the* 79. Juillard, L., Lerman, L. O., Kruger, D. G., et al. (2004) Blood oxygen level-dependent measurement of acute intra-renal ischemia. *Kidney Int.* **65,** 944–950.

80. Ries, M., Basseau, F., Tyndal, B., et al. (2003) Renal diffusion and BOLD MRI in experimental diabetic nephropathy. Blood oxygen level-dependent. *J. Magn. Reson. Imaging* **17,** 104–113.

81. Muller, M. F., Prasad, P. V., Bimmler, D., Kaiser, A., and Edelman, R. R. (1994) Functional imaging of the kidney by means of measurement of the apparent diffusion coefficient. *Radiology* **193,** 711–715.

82. Siegel, C. L., Aisen, A. M., Ellis, J. H., Londy, F., and Chenevert, T. L. (1995) Feasibility of MR diffusion studies in the kidney. *J. Magn. Reson. Imaging* **5,** 617–620.

83. Ries, M., Jones, R. A., Basseau, F., Moonen, C. T., and Grenier, N. (2001) Diffusion tensor MRI of the human kidney. *J. Magn. Reson. Imaging* **14,** 42–49.

84. Liu, A. S. and Xie, J. X. (2003) Functional evaluation of normothermic ischemia and reperfusion injury in dog kidney by combining MR diffusion-weighted imaging and Gd-DTPA enhanced first-pass perfusion. *J. Magn. Reson. Imaging* **17,** 683–963.

85. Raghunand, N., Howison, C., Sherry, A. D., Zhang, S., and Gillies, R. J. (2003) Renal and systemic pH imaging by contrast-enhanced MRI. *Magn. Reson. Med.* **49,** 249–257.

86. Maril, N., Margalit, R., Mispelter, J., and Degani, H. (2004) Functional sodium magnetic resonance imaging of the intact rat kidney. *Kidney Int.* **65,** 927–935.

87. Kobayashi, H., Kawamoto, S., Jo, S. K., et al. (2002) Renal tubular damage detected by dynamic micro-MRI with a dendrimer-based magnetic resonance contrast agent. *Kidney Int.* **61,** 1980–1985.

9

Cardiac Magnetic Resonance Spectroscopy

A Window for Studying Physiology

Michael Horn

Summary

Cardiac magnetic resonance spectroscopy (MRS) opens a window to the metabolism of the heart. Various intermediates of metabolic pathways can be observed and followed over time. Most applications of cardiac MRS have been performed with the ^{31}P nuclei, which reflect the metabolites from the high-energy phosphate metabolism. Other nuclei, such as ^{1}H or ^{13}C, have also been investigated but less intensively, most likely because of either large background signals (e.g., water) or inherent low sensitivity of the method. MRS can be used for the examination of tissue extracts, isolated organs, whole animals in vivo, as well as healthy human subjects and patients. Although the primary motivation is to gain an understanding of metabolism using animal models, a potential for diagnostic applications in humans certainly exists.

Key Words: Heart; myocardium; metabolism; magnetic resonance; spectroscopy; imaging; metabolite map; acidity; ATP; phosphocreatine; TCA cycle; creatine kinase; human; rodent; animal; mouse; rat; fat; water suppression; creatine.

1. Introduction

Magnetic resonance imaging (MRI) has evolved into an important diagnostic tool in clinical application as well as in biomedical research. The number of clinical MR scanners is growing continuously. The use of MRI for evaluating cardiac function has been shown to be more accurate than other modalities (*1*), with a potential to reduce the number of patients in clinical trials.

Although MR spectroscopy (MRS) is the older technique compared with MRI and MRS is widely used in chemistry and biochemistry for the evaluation of chemical structures and conformations, its use in humans and laboratory animals is not as widespread as MRI. Using the biochemical information of in vivo processes, one can potentially measure steady-state concentrations, changes of concentrations over time, and kinetics of various complex meta-

From: *Methods in Molecular Medicine, Vol. 124*
Magnetic Resonance Imaging: Methods and Biologic Applications
Edited by: P. V. Prasad © Humana Press Inc., Totowa, NJ

bolic patterns. In other words, MRS allows direct investigation of tissue metabolites. The acquisition of data can be performed repetitively, in contrast to other methods, which, for instance, involve the injection of radioactive tracers. Thus, MRS provides a unique opportunity to observe biological systems with minimal interference to their function or metabolism.

The nuclei ^{31}P, ^{13}C, and ^{1}H reflect the metabolites of the high-energy phosphate metabolism, the tricarboxylic acid cycle (TCA) cycle, and the creatine kinase system as well as fat metabolism, respectively. In experimental applications with isolated organs, even ion homeostasis, i.e., the flux of ^{23}Na and ^{39}K, can be investigated. Although data acquisition and interpretation of in vivo MRS of the myocardium is challenging, the unique opportunity to monitor in vivo biochemical changes in a noninvasive fashion remains attractive.

2. Technical Requirements

Cardiac MRS is demanding in terms of technique because of several reasons. Nuclei other than protons are low in relative and absolute sensitivity (^{31}P: 6.6% of ^{1}H; and ^{13}C: 0.018% of ^{1}H) *(2)*. The heart is hidden behind the chest wall, i.e., there is quite a distance between the sensor (coil) and the object of interest. Furthermore, the heart and the chest are in constant motion. Although these problems also affect MRI, the implications in terms of quantitation of metabolite is rather severe with MRS.

2.1. Radio Frequency Coils

Low inherent sensitivity leads to low signal-to-noise ratios (SNR), which necessitate the use of coils producing high signal, e.g., surface coils. SNR is best with the smallest surface coils; however, the penetration into the tissue is approximately half the diameter of the surface coil. Because most of the heart needs to be within the reach of the surface coil, an appropriate diameter has to be used. Furthermore, one has to overcome the thickness of the chest wall, which differs by almost an order of magnitude between mice and men.

Linearly polarized surface coils with a diameter of 2 to 15 cm have been used in the past. **Figure 1** illustrates a rat instrumented with electrocardiogram (ECG), breathing control, and a surface coil. Bottomley et al. investigated the use of coil arrays *(3)*, which combine the benefits of small single surface coils (high SNR) and the larger spatial coverage of volume coils. During the last few years, coils with quadrature detection became available, which yield up to 41% (square root of 2) more signal than linearly polarized coil.

2.2. Trigger to Motion

The effects of heart movement can be compensated for by triggering the MR sequence to the ECG. A recording of the electrical signals from the heart is

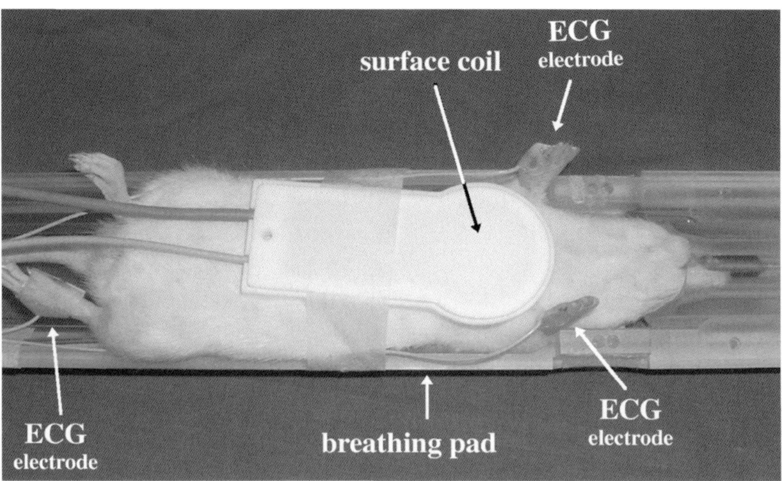

Fig. 1. Anesthetized rat in supine position on a warming bed. The animal is equipped with electrocardiogram (ECG) electrodes on both front paws and the left hind paw. A pressure-sensitive pad is placed next to the thorax for breathing control. Both ECG and breathing are used for triggered measurements. A 3-cm, receive-only ^{31}P surface coil is placed on the thorax for acquisition of the resonance signal. For the measurement, the animal is placed in an outer volume resonator for radio frequency transmission, which is located in the center of the magnet.

amplified and used for timing of the MR system. In contrast to MRI examinations, in which small variations of repetition time (TR) in the sequence are not considered to be a major issue, timing problems can have serious implications in MRS. Because MRS examinations are performed with a distinct saturation of the signal (TR < 5 T_1), changes in the timing schedule caused by waiting for a trigger signal before starting the data acquisition might cause severe alterations in the TR of the sequence. Variations in TR cause changes in saturation and cause major problems for corrections and interpretation. Data acquired after a prolonged waiting period are less saturated and might have stronger contributions to the result than other, correctly timed, data points in measurements. The severity of the problem depends on heart rate, i.e., is more prominent in humans (with low heart rates) than in small animals (with higher heart rates).

Breathing artifacts can be lowered by triggering on the movement of the thorax, which is done by a thorax belt, pressure sensitive cushions, or optical systems. Practically, this causes an increase in the total time in the magnet, a factor that might be critical for ill patients. Placing the patients in a prone position on the surface coil shifts most of the movement from breathing to the back of the patient and, thus, outside the sensitive volume of the surface coil. Additionally, the heart moves slightly to the front toward the thoracic wall and, thus, is closer to the sensitive region of the surface coil. Of course, the prone position is the least comfortable for cardiac patients, which might limit the time of examination. In animals, timing is not such a sensitive issue, and spectroscopy is triggered to ECG and breathing simultaneously. However, the risk of variation in TR, as explained for the ECG trigger, is even greater when combining both triggers.

2.3. Water Suppression (^{1}H MRS Only)

Protons have a concentration of 110 M in water and approx 80 M in tissue, whereas the concentrations of the metabolites of interest are in the millimolar range *(2)*. Hence, effective suppression of water signal is imperative for MRS. Suppression of the water signal can be achieved by saturation methods or by a narrow, frequency-selective 90° pulse on the water resonance followed by spoiler gradients. One should be aware of the shift of the resonance frequency of water with temperature, which is on the order of 0.01 ppm/°C *(4)*. Water suppression optimized in phantoms at room temperature may not be sufficient in living objects at 37°C.

2.4. Pulse Sequences

In MRS, the signal has to be acquired from a defined and well-localized volume. The spectral information of the target organ has to be clearly separated from the signal of surrounding tissue, which might contain different concentrations of the same metabolites as the localized volume. A thorough discussion of the different localization techniques is beyond the scope of this chapter (for reviews, *see* **refs. 2**, and **5–7**).

Because the position of the heart is not aligned to a direct line from nose to tail (**Fig. 2**), and it does not follow the Cartesian coordinates of the magnet, the orientation of the localized voxels is mainly in a double-oblique fashion. The long and the short heart axes are determined in pilot images, and a series of images in the short heart axis view is used to define the exact spot of the localized volume element.

Basic information about commonly used localization techniques is given below (*see* **Subheadings 2.4.1.** and **2.4.3.**).

2.4.1. Single-Voxel Techniques

One single volume element is placed in the anterior heart wall close to the septum. **Figure 3** shows an example of a single voxel in the rat heart. To reach sufficient signal in small voxels, a magnet with a high field strength has to be used. Typical small-animal MRS/MRI scanners are 4.7 T or higher. Some field strengths currently in use are 7.0, 9.4, and 11.0 T. Clinical scanners typically are 3.0 T and lower, the most common being 1.5 T.

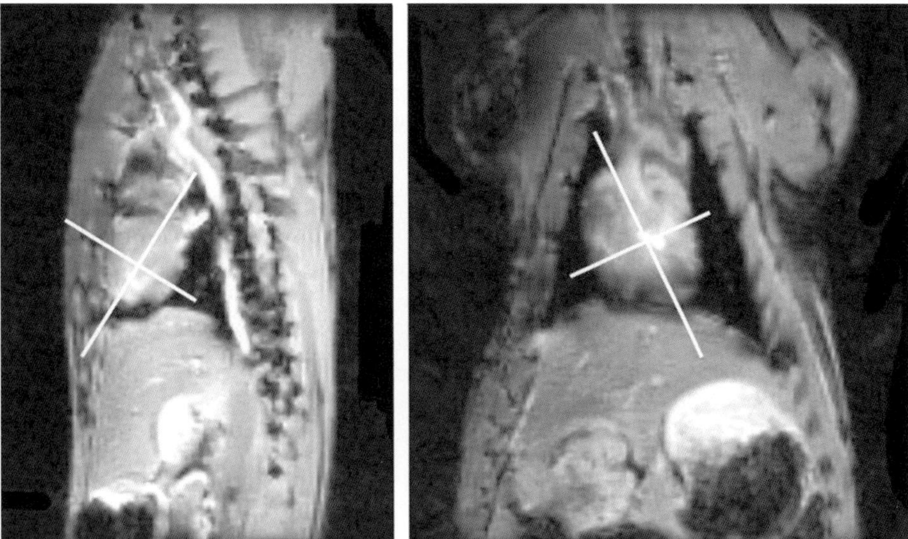

Fig. 2. Gradient-echo images of the thorax region of a rat. Sagittal (left) and coronal slices (right) show the oblique position of the heart in the thorax. White lines are added to show the direction of the long and short heart axes.

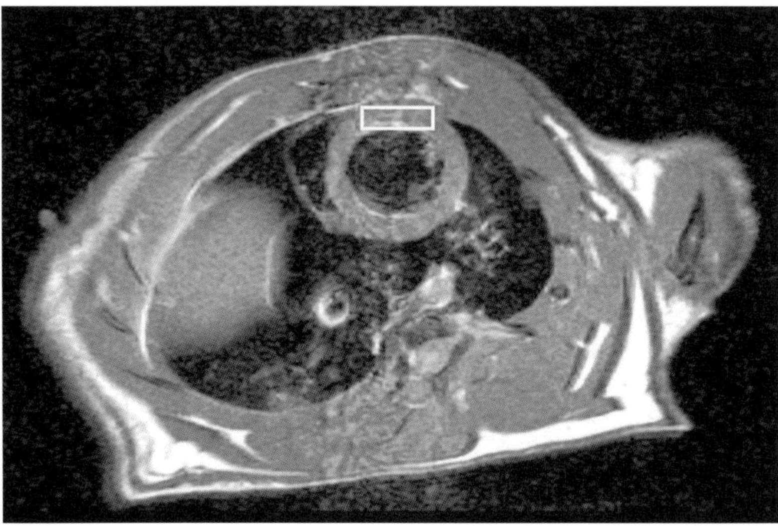

Fig. 3. Axial slice of a rat thorax from a spin-echo sequence. The left ventricular wall chamber appears as a circular structure because of the double-oblique orientation of the slice. A single voxel is placed in the anterior wall close to the septum. The placement of the voxel is critical. Neither thorax wall (same metabolites as the heart) nor left ventricular chamber (blood contributing to ATP signal) should be part of the localized volume.

2.4.1.1. POINT-RESOLVED SPECTROSCOPY (PRESS)

PRESS (point-resolved spectroscopy) uses the sequence *(8,9)*:

$$90°: TE1; 180°: TE1 + TE2; 180°: TE2; \text{acquire},$$

where TE is the echo time. Each of the three radio frequency (RF) pulses is slice selective in three orthogonal planes. An echo is generated after the first $90°$, $180°$ pulse combination in the region intersected by the two pulses. The last $180°$ pulse causes an echo after TE2 from those spins that were excited by all three RF pulses. Additional spoiler gradients are implemented in the sequence to avoid signal observation from spins that experience not all of the RF pulses. Because TE is quite large in this sequence to accommodate the three RF pulses, a problem arises for metabolites with short T_2 values or complex coupling patterns, which are lost at long TE times. Thus, PRESS is used only in ^{1}H MRS and is not suitable for ^{31}P MRS. Use of three pulses affords spatial selection in all three directions and, hence, localization of an arbitrary volume within the object.

2.4.1.2. STIMULATED ECHO ACQUISITION MODE (STEAM)

Stimulated echo acquisition mode (STEAM) *(10)* is used for compounds with a short T_2, i.e., STEAM is suitable for ^{31}P MRS. The spatial selection is performed by three RF pulses, similar to PRESS, however, using $90°$ pulses. The sequence can be written as: $90°$: TE/2; $90°$: TM; $90°$: TE/2; acquire. TM is the delay during which the magnetization is in the longitudinal rather than in the transversal plane and, thus, relaxation is by T_1 rather than T_2 (please refer to Chapter 1 for more description).

Spoiler gradients are incorporated to eliminate unwanted signals. With the STEAM sequence, only half of the available signal is recaptured, and, hence, the sensitivity is lower than in the PRESS sequence. However, the STEAM sequence can achieve shorter TE times compared with PRESS and, thus, can be used for metabolites with short T_2 or with complex coupling patterns.

2.4.1.3. IMAGE-SELECTED IN VIVO SPECTROSCOPY (ISIS)

Image-selected in vivo spectroscopy (ISIS) *(11)* is a technique that involves accumulation of multiple acquisitions with different combination of inversion pulses before the signal-generating $90°$ RF pulse. A multiple of eight measurements has to be added for a complete cycle. The sequence involves no echo formation, which, in turn, allows the accumulation of signal from metabolites with very short T_2.

In its original form, ISIS could be used only if TR $> 3T_1$, because of the influence of remaining longitudinal magnetization on the result of the $180°$ inversion pulse in the next preparation step of the sequence. The main disadvantage of the method is the subtraction of a large signal from outside the volume of interest from a very small signal in the volume of interest. The combination of eight measurements does not allow suppression of the water signal, which is possible only in single-shot methods. Furthermore, any movement by the subject within the eightfold TR time will not only place the voxel in wrong spatial location but even destroy the results from the other acquisitions of the ISIS cycle.

2.4.2. Validation of Single-Voxel Techniques

All of the localization techniques mentioned above suffer from the disadvantage that metabolic information can be acquired only from one region. A technique capable of acquiring data from two regions of interest simultaneously is feasible and allows inclusion of another volume of interest as a control or to verify the correct placement of the volume of interest. Furthermore, in the single-voxel methods mentioned, the origin of frequency differences cannot be distinguished between chemical shift and spatial location. Resonances of metabolites are shifted with the spatial location of their origin, i.e., they do not appear exactly at the location of their origin, which might lead to acquisition of data from the neighboring tissue. Thus, one has to evaluate the spatial origin of the metabolite resonance signal in phantoms before in vivo applications.

2.4.3. Multivoxel Techniques

The chemical shift imaging (CSI) *(12,13)* technique uses an excitation pulse followed by phase encoding and acquisition of the free induction decay (FID). Spatial resolution in one, two, or three directions can be achieved depending upon the number of gradients involved (**Fig. 4**). Please note that there is some confusion in literature about the number of dimensions. For this chapter, the numbers given are for spatial resolution, not taking into account the additional spectroscopic dimension. Users might be tempted to measure a large number of volume elements, e.g., $16 \times 16 \times 16$ in 3D CSI, to get high spatial resolution. However, the acquisition time could be prohibitively long (4096 TRs) for in vivo human application. An effective compromise is to use 1D CSI. A stack of several CSI voxels is placed orthogonal to the chest wall. The signal of the chest wall can even be saturated by a slice-selective presaturation pulse, which eliminates the risk of signal contamination in the CSI voxels accumulating data from the heart *(14)*. By reduction of the numbers of voxels, total measurement time for one experiment is reduced and allows averaging of data.

Independent of the technique used, the voxel size needed to yield a sufficient SNR is still a limiting factor for spatial resolution. Currently, voxel size for ^{31}P in humans is approx 16 mL in clinical standard systems (1.5 T), whereas ^{1}H MRS makes it feasible to have voxel size on the order of a few microliters.

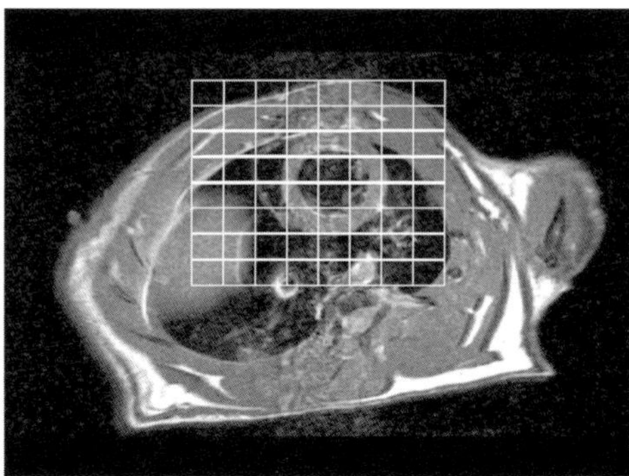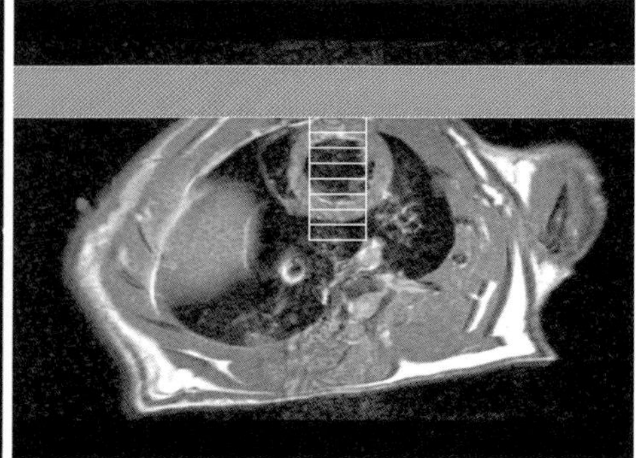

Fig. 4. Axial slice of a rat thorax from a spin-echo sequence. The left ventricular wall chamber appears as circular structure because of the double-oblique orientation of the slice. A 3D chemical shift imaging (CSI) grid (left) is placed over the entire heart. Because of a large number of phase encoding steps (e.g., $8 \times 8 \times 8 = 512$), data acquisition is time consuming. Using a 1D CSI cuboid (right) reduces the number of phase encoding steps, which allows an increased number of averages. An additional saturation slab on the thorax wall eliminates signal contribution from skeletal muscle. Both CSI methods allow collection of a spectrum of blood, which can be used for correction of signal contamination originating from blood. In both CSI setups, the voxels reach beyond the sensitive area of the surface coil. Voxels outside the sensitive area will contain only noise information.

2.4.4. Validation of Multivoxel Techniques

Comparing single-voxel techniques with CSI measurements, examination with a single-voxel technique is always faster, which allows additional averaging of the data. However, the content from CSI experiments is much greater compared with single-voxel techniques. One problem with CSI is that the signal attributed to each volume element contains significant contributions from neighboring volume elements. Further development of CSI with correct filtering and acquisition weighting may overcome this problem to a certain extent *(15)*.

3. Resonances in MRS and Values to Calculate From Spectra

3.1. ^{31}P MRS

The spectra of the isolated heart (**Fig. 5**) from a rat shows five clear resonance signals. The most prominent peak is the resonance signal from phosphocreatine (PCr; in older literature, creatine phosphate), which is used as internal standard for the chemical shift and set to 0 ppm. This is in not in accordance with the standard in ^{31}P NMR in chemistry, which uses 85% H_3PO_4 in D_2O. The reader should be aware of a shift difference in biological and chemical

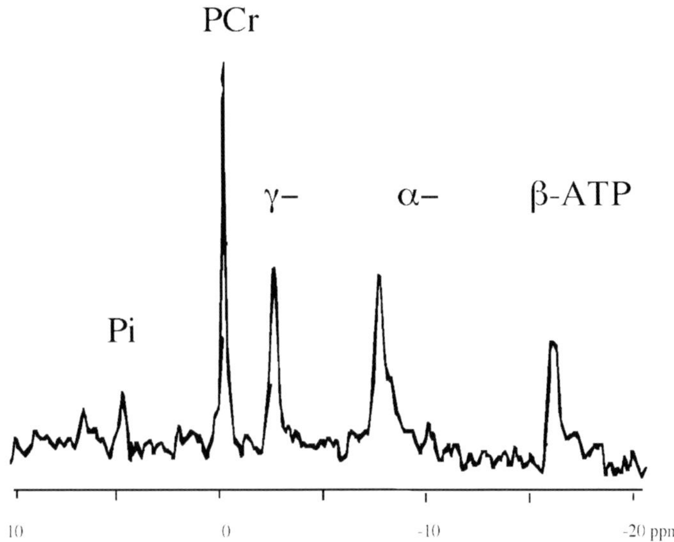

Fig. 5. ^{31}P magnetic resonance spectroscopy (MRS)of an isolated rat heart at 7.05 T. Resonance frequency is 121.5 MHz. The resonance signals represent inorganic phosphate (Pi), phosphocreatine (PCr), and the three resonances from adenosine triphosphate (γ-, α-, and β-ATP). The spectra is recorded as an average of 152 single acquisitions over a 5-min time period, with a TR of 1.93 s. Saturation correction for PCr is 1.12, and for Pi is 1.08.

measurements of approx 4 ppm. This information might be helpful when looking up chemical shifts for concentration measurements, which should be outside the range of the resonance signals from the biological system. To the left of PCr, at a chemical shift range of 4 to 5 ppm, the signal from inorganic phosphate (Pi) is seen.

This resonance moves dependant upon the proton concentration, i.e., of the pH value *(16)*. Chemical shift difference can be converted into pH values by the formula:

$$\text{pH} = 6.9 - \log_{10}[(\Delta\partial - 5.805) / (3.29 - \Delta\partial)],$$

where $\Delta\partial$ is the difference in the chemical shift between PCr and Pi in parts per million (ppm).

In other species, e.g., guinea pig, an additional resonance frequency at 8 ppm arises that originates from phosphorylated sugars. On the right of the PCr signal, there are three signals from the three phosphorous atoms of ATP. These resonances belong to the γ-P-atom at –2.5 ppm; the α-P-atom at –8 ppm; and the β-P-atom at –15 ppm. The different chemical surrounding of the phosphorous atoms cause resonance at slightly different frequencies. At high field, the signals appear as a single resonance signal; however, at lower field, e.g., 1.5 T, the spin coupling between the phosphorous atoms can be seen at approx 16 Hz. The γ-signal as well as the α-signal split into doublets, whereas the β-signal is coupled to a triplet. The shift difference between the α and β resonance mirrors the concentration of free Mg^{2+} *(17)*.

Because the α- and β-phosphorous atoms in adenosine diphosphate (ADP) and the phosphorous atom in adenosine phosphate (AMP) are in a chemically similar positions to those in adenosine triphosphate (ATP), they contribute to the respective signal of ATP. Taking into account that ADP has a very low concentration in the heart, despite a high turnover, the contribution from ADP and AMP to the resonance signal is negligible. When calculating ratios of the metabolites in ^{31}P MR spectra, one has to decide whether to take the β- or γ-signal of ATP. There are two arguments for the use of the γ-signal:

1. Even when a surface coil is used for the RF excitation pulse, there is little off-resonance effect when the center frequency of the spectra is set between the PCr and the γ-signal.
2. The γ-signal is more narrow (because of coupling to a doublet, which collapses at high field) than the β signal and, thus, a higher SNR will be reached, which, in turn, allows for easier definition of the borders of the signal, even in noisy spectra.

The argument for the usage of the β-signal, that is, the falsification of the integration caused by contribution of ADP to the resonance signal, seems to be a minor one.

At the right shoulder of the α-signal, a contribution from nicotinamide adenine dinucleotide phosphate oxidized form/reduced form ($NADP^+/NADPH^+$) is seen. Because the signal cannot be resolved from the α-signal, direct quantification is not feasible. A calculation of the difference in the integral of the α- and the β-signal is performed in a limited number of publications.

In vivo spectra are distorted by the signal from the blood. Besides the signal from 2,3-bisphosphoglycerate (2,3-DPG) and phosphodiester, there are the three signals of ATP from the red blood cells *(18)*. 2,3-DPG covers the resonance frequency of Pi, which prevents the calculation of pH values. ^1H decoupling of ^{31}P MR spectra of the human heart reduces the width of the resonance signal and allows determination of the chemical shift of Pi at low field strength (1.5 T) *(19)*. Decoupling causes changes in signal strength by the nuclear Overhauser effect (NOE), which is discussed in **Subheading 3.3.** If a visible resonance signal from 2,3-DPG is present in in vivo ^{31}P MR spectra, a correction of the ATP values should be performed. The ratio of 2,3-DPG and ATP changes with species *(20)* and disease *(18)*, thus, determination of correction values for the research model used is recommended.

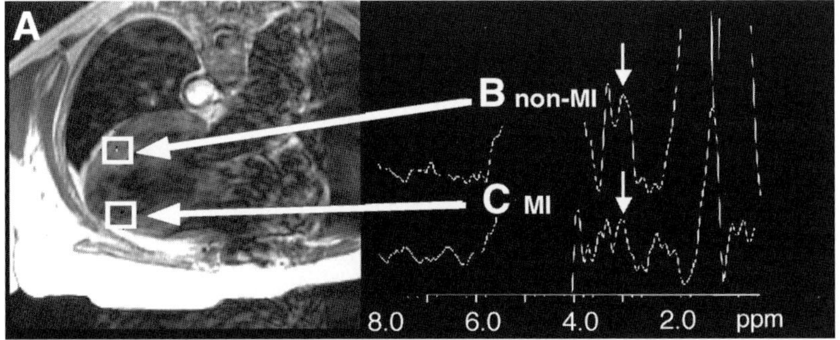

Fig. 6. ¹H magnetic resonance image (MRI) of a patient with anterior wall infarction (**A**). The spectra (right panel) represent ¹H MRS from the noninfarcted (remote) region, non-MI (**B**) and the infarcted region, MI (**C**). A clear reduction in the signal of total creatine at 3 ppm can be seen. (From **ref. *47***, with permission from Elsevier.)

3.2. ¹H MRS

A large number of resonance signals in ¹H MRS reflect a number of metabolites. Compared with ¹H MR spectra of the brain, only a small number of metabolites can be identified in cardiac spectra. The most prominent resonance signals in ¹H MR spectra of the heart reflect lipids in the range of 0.8 to 2 ppm, total creatine (sum of creatine and PCr) at 3 ppm and at 3.8 ppm, as well as overlapping signals from taurine and carnitine at 3.2 to 3.5 ppm. **Figure 6** shows spectra of human myocardium from normal (upper panel) and infarcted myocardium (lower panel).

A resonance at approx 72 ppm was reported *(21)* as the signal of deoxymyoglobin, whereas no deoxyhemoglobin was visible in the canine myocardium when using an appropriate Gaussian excitation pulse.

Besides major differences in the metabolism of brain and heart, broad and overlapping resonances result in limited spectral resolution in cardiac ¹H MRS. The broadening of the signal is caused by the challenge of optimized field homogeneity of a moving organ. Thus, compared with brain ¹H MRS, cardiac applications are not as extensive as applications in the brain.

3.3. ¹³C MRS

The chemical shift range of ¹³C MRS is very wide *(22)*, which avoids signal overlap and allows easier discrimination of the metabolites. Because ¹³C nuclei couple with ¹H nuclei over several bonds, causing complex coupling patterns, biological applications of ¹³C MRS are mostly performed in decoupled mode. Off-resonant irradiation of the ¹H frequency causes the collapse of the coupling patterns, and single lines per ¹³C atom are visible. In return, SNR

Table 1
Chemical Shifts of ^{13}C Atoms (in ppm)

	C1	C2	C3	C4	C5	C6
Glutamate	175.1	55.2	27.6	34.2	181.8	
α–Glucose	93.1	72.5	73.8	70.7	72.5	61.7
β–Glucose	97.0	75.2	77.0	70.7	76.8	61.8
Aspartate	175.0	55.2	37.4	178.3		
Alanine	176.3	51.9	17.3			
β–Hydroxybutyrate	181.1	47.6	66.6	22.7		

increases significantly. In vivo, the specific absorption rate limits might be limiting when using continuous decoupling. Gated decoupling with WALTZ pulses *(23)* overcomes this problem. Besides the suppression of the ^{13}C–^{1}H coupling, sensitivity of ^{13}C is enhanced by the NOE *(24,25)*. For the calculation of absolute values from the spectra, one has to consider that the strength of the NOE is different for each resonance and, thus, integral values might need to be corrected.

The natural abundance of ^{13}C is only 1.1% of all nuclei. Thus, sensitivity is very low. This can be overcome by enrichment of ^{13}C substrates. However, these isotope-enriched substrates are expensive and, often, physiological concentrations of a specific substrates might be low. Depending on the substrate given, several spots in the TCA cycle can be highlighted by ^{13}C MRS. The chemical shifts (in ppm) of ^{13}C atoms of some compounds are given in **Table 1**.

If several ^{13}C-enriched atoms are located in one molecule, ^{13}C–^{13}C coupling will split up the peaks into complex patterns. An estimation of the spectra and planning of these studies can be performed by a program that is provided by the University of Texas Southwestern Medical Center at Dallas, TX (http://www4.utsouthwestern.edu/rogersmr/software.htm, last accessed: June 14, 2005). Transfer of magnetization from ^{1}H to neighboring ^{13}C nuclei by heteronuclear coherent polarization transfer increases sensitivity without the need of ^{13}C-enriched substances and was shown to be effective in a canine model *(26)*.

4. Performing a MRS Examination

Because of the differences in performing an examination in humans vs animals and because of the differences in the MR systems from different vendors, there is no way to describe exactly how to perform a MRS examination. **Table 2** tries to list the thoughts and steps one has to go through when performing an examination. The left column describes the step of the measurement; the middle column, the animal-specific items; and the right column, the human-specific items.

5. Processing of Data

Data accumulated in MRS are stored in the FID, which is a sum of decaying waves over time. Processing of spectroscopy data is mostly performed by Fourier transformation, a mathematical operation that brings the data from the time domain into the frequency domain. Frequency domain is the encoding familiar to use, however, the content of information is the same in an FID as in a spectrum. Increase of SNR can be achieved by applying windows to the FID, e.g., multiplication with an exponential function, which accentuates the information in the early time-points of the FID and lessens the contribution from the late time-points. Because location and size is mainly encoded in the beginning of the FID, whereas fine structure and coupling is contained at the end of the FID, the signal will not be affected in strength; however, noise will be reduced. Because exponential multiplication increases linewidth, the decay of the exponential function is mostly expressed as line broadening, in Hertz. A commonly accepted rule for the degree of exponential multiplication is that linewidth at half-height of the signal should not be more than doubled.

The information about the number of molecules measured, equal to the concentration, is in the area of the resonance signal. An integration of the area under the resonance signal yields area values, which have to be compared with standards of known concentration. Sometimes, when SNR is low, integration is tricky and the definition of the borders of a resonance signal is an informed guess. Furthermore, nonmobile compounds, e.g., from cell membranes, contribute with a hump of the baseline. Any correction of the baseline might compromise the integration of the signal in frequency domain.

Another way to determine concentration is to use a mathematical fit in the time domain. As stated above, the FID is a combination of decaying waves. Because the frequency of each of the signals is known, these values can be provided to a mathematical model that suits the amplitude of each frequency. A variety of programs is available. A complete list and description is beyond the scope of this chapter. It is recommended that those interested in processing other than Fourier transformation try the programs MRUI (Magnetic Resonance User Interface) and LCModel. MRUI was developed with support from the European community and is available for free for academic users (after registration), at: http://www.mrui.uab.es (last accessed: June 14, 2005).

LCModel is a commercial program written by S. Provencher. This program deals with ^{1}H MRS only and has its origin in brain applications. After adaption for cardiac parameters, it is a useful tool for ^{1}H spectra (http://www.s-provencher.com/pages/lcmodel.shtml; last accessed: June 14, 2005).

The presentation of these two programs does not reflect the variety of other possibilities available.

Table 2
Important Steps Involved in Performing MRS Experiment

Step of measurement	Animal specific	Human specific
Decide for nucleus: ^{1}H, ^{31}P, ^{13}C		
Choose coil	Transmitter: volume coil	^{1}H:like animal
	Receiver: surface coil	^{31}P, ^{13}C: surface coil
	anesthesia	
Position object in magnet	Prone position	Preferably prone
	ECG trigger, breath trigger, warming	ECG trigger
	pad/heating	Ask about a blanket
Optimize coil to RF frequency: tune & match (if not fixed t&m coil or done automatically)		
Run localizer ^{1}H MRI, often 3 perpendicular slices*		
Homogenize magnetic field (shim)	Use X, Y, Z, Z^2. With large changes in animal size (e.g., species), use XY, XZ and YZ as well	Use X, Y, Z, and Z^2 or map shim
Check width of water signal at half height = quality measurement of shim, value depends on field strength		
Choose volume selection method	Single voxel: PRESS; STEAM, ISIS	Time constraints!
	Multi multivoxel: 1D CSI, 3D CSI	
Place voxel only inside myocardium (if possible), might be double oblique.	In mice, wall thickness forces to accept ventricular cavity as well	
Avoid chest wall!		
For ^{1}H: select water suppression (might need to optimize!)		Check for SAR limits
For ^{31}P and ^{13}C: decide for ^{1}H decoupling at of resonance position	Be aware of NOE effect	Be aware of NOE effect

238

For ^{31}P and CSI: decide whether to use saturation slab on chest wall		
Calculate time for MRS measurement, decide about number of averages	Keep time in anesthesia limited	Time is limited by patients disease
		Inform patient about start of spectroscopy to keep level of motivation
Start data accumulation		
If possible, sample ECG or heart rate during measurement		
If time allows: run basic images after spectroscopy to calculate some parameters of cardiac funtion parameters (wall thickness, EF, heart mass)		Check for patient movement compared to initial images
		Remove patient as soon as possible from magnet!
Always save FID data, not only spectra		
Processing: use Fourier transformation with low line broadening OR use time domain fitting. Be careful with low SNR and where to set the limits of your integration area		
Correct for saturation, NOE effect, blood contamination	Use species specific values for blood contamination	Correction factors are values from volunteers, disease might influence the correction fact

---

* During this step, automatic calculation of 90° or 180° pulses as well as RF power and receiver gain will be performed by the imaging software

6. Biological Information From MR Spectra

6.1. ^{31}P MRS in Animals and Humans

The most extensive work in cardiac MRS was performed using ^{31}P nuclei. Studies from the isolated heart to in vivo examination in humans give rich and detailed information of the effects of various disease states to the high-energy phosphate cycle.

PCr/ATP ratios given in the literature differ depending on the technique used *(27)* as well as the model. In the isolated heart, the dependence of the PCr/ATP ratio from the substrate can be easily seen, with a ratio of 1.3 in glucose-only perfused hearts *(28)*, and up to 2.0 in glucose plus fatty acid-perfused hearts *(29)*. In all states of disease, PCr/ATP ratios are lowered *(28,30–33)*. PCr/ATP drops with the severity of disease *(34,35)*. ATP content is found to be either stable *(28,32)* or slightly decreased *(31,33)*. Patients with congestive heart failure show low PCr/ATP ratios during hand grip exercise *(36)* in cases in which an irreversible defect was detected *(37)*. Athletes developing hypertrophy similar to patients did not show any changes in the high-energy phosphate content of the heart *(38)*. Treatment of heart failure was shown to be beneficial in patients *(34)* and animals *(32)*. In a small study involving 31 patients, the PCr/ATP ratio was a predictor of mortality *(39)* in dilative cardiomyopathy patients.

All of these studies suffer from the expression of relative concentrations (PCr/ATP ratio) instead of absolute concentrations of the metabolites. Studies of the isolated heart allow inclusion of a concentration standard to the sensitive volume of the coil. In contrast, in in vivo studies using surface coils, the sensitivity of the coil is not equally distributed, which makes calculations of absolute concentrations even more complex. Measurement of ^1H MR spectra and ^{31}P MRS with the same coil was used to calculate the ^{31}P metabolites by comparing signal intensity of the proton signal with a know concentration of protons in water *(40)*. The method of spatial localization with optimal pointspread function (SLOOP) allows acquisition of data from nonrectangular voxels *(41)* and can be used for the calculation of absolute metabolite concentrations *(42,43)*. Using SLOOP, the results of clinical examination of patients with hypertrophied or failing myocardium showed alterations of PCr and ATP *(44)*, even when the ratio of these metabolites was unchanged. Further research is necessary to calculate absolute values to increase our understanding of the alterations in the high-energy metabolism before or during heart failure.

6.2. ^1H MRS in Animals and Humans

Creatine is an important metabolite in the creatine kinase shuttle *(45)*. Creatine is phosphorylated on the outer membrane of the mitochondria *(46)* to PCr. These two molecules are small and diffuse easily between the mitochondria and the myofibrils, thus, transporting ATP between the place of origin and the place of usage. A resonance signal at 3.0 ppm in ^{1}H MR spectrum reflects the sum of PCr and creatine. Because PCr can be measured by ^{31}P MRS, the combination of both nuclei allows the calculation of creatine concentration. As shown in **Subheading 6.1.**, PCr is reduced in disease. This is true for creatine as well, because the concentration of both molecules is coupled by the law of mass action for the creatine kinase reaction. Work from Bottomley and Weiss show the reduction of creatine in the infarcted heart *(47)* in humans and a canine model. In this paper, a second voxel was chosen from the noninfarcted area and served as control. The same group also demonstrated an increase of PCr and creatine in GLUT 4-null mice *(48)*.

Myocardial triglycerides are suspected to damage the heart by deposition of triglycerides, a process known as myocardial steatosis. ^{1}H MRS can be used for the investigation of the triglycerides in the heart *(49)*. A resonance at approx 1.3 ppm reflects the CH_2-groups of triglycerides, whereas a second resonance at approx 0.8 ppm originates from the CH_3-groups. The method showed a good correlation of the MR-acquired data with biochemical assays in rats ex vivo. In humans, good reproducibility was shown for repetitive measurements. Another resonance signal appeared in humans, originating from epicardial fat. The shift of the resonance signals depending on the origin is well-known from investigation in skeletal muscle *(50)*. Recently, Schneider *et al.* have shown ^{1}H MR spectra of a mouse heart with a voxel size of 2 µL *(51)*.

6.3. ^{13}C MRS in Animals and Humans

Studies involving ^{13}C MRS of the heart are performed with enrichment of the ^{13}C isotope of carbon. Taking into account the price of the enriched isotopes and the size and volume of the human body, these studies are performed mainly in small rodents. Often, isolated organs are used, which show an even better ratio of enriched isotope to metabolic information. One has to be careful to keep the ^{13}C-enriched substances at physiological levels. Increase of the concentration of ^{13}C-enriched substrate will shorten the time for the measurement markedly; however, nonphysiologically high concentrations of substrate might lead to preference of metabolic pathways different from the baseline situation.

Because of a wide variety of substrates, the number of potential results is high. ^{13}C MRS has provided access to key metabolites in glycolysis, the TCA cycle *(52–54)*, and in glycogen and fat use *(55–57)*. In the human heart, resonances of CH_2-, CH_3- and C=O groups were detected at natural abundance *(58)*.

Figure 7 gives a schematic representation of glucose metabolism. 1-^{13}C marked glucose is metabolized in several steps to acetyl-coenzyme A and then fed into the TCA cycle. All intermediates marked with an asterisk are detectable by MRS starting from 1-^{13}C marked glucose. If fatty acids inhibit the

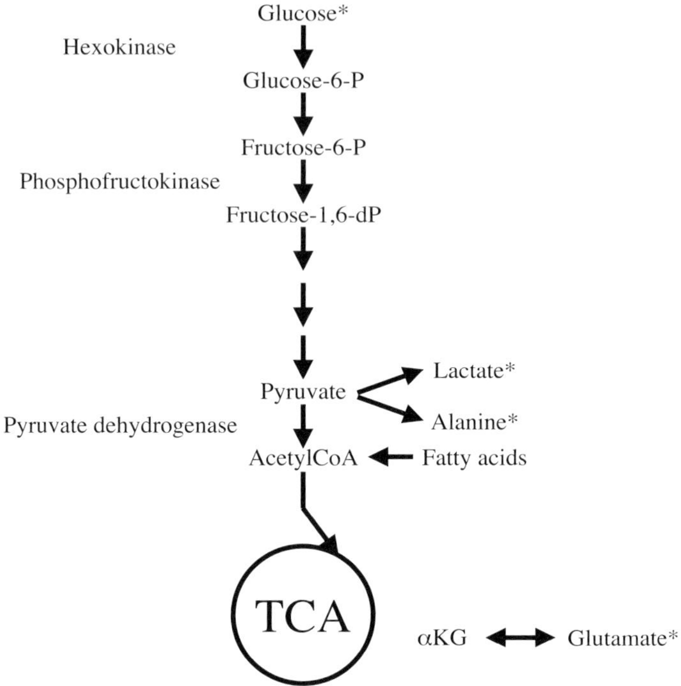

Fig. 7. Schematic representation of glucose metabolism. The reactions highlighted (hexokinase, phosphofructokinase, and pyruvate dehydrogenase) indicate steps that might be inhibited by fatty acids. The metabolites marked by * represent intermediates detectable by MRS.

reactions highlighted to the left (hexokinase, phosphofructokinase, and pyruvate dehydrogenase), changes in the ratio of the MR-visible metabolites will be seen *(59)*.

Fatty acids are an important source of energy in the heart. More than 60% of the energy requirements of the heart are met by fatty acid oxidation *(60,61)*. Perfusion of isolated hearts with labeled fatty acids $^{13}C_8$-palmitate vs $^{13}C_8$-palmitate plus unlabeled butyrate showed an increase in the ratio of (flux via TCA)/(palmitate uptake) *(62)*. The change in the ratio was induced by the increase of the flux through the TCA cycle by butyrate; however, the palmitate transport into the mitochondria was not significantly reduced. These selected examples demonstrate the opportunities of ^{13}C MRS. The labeling of the substrate decides which metabolites will be observed. As mentioned in **Subheading 3.3.**, web tools are available for more information on this topic.

7. Limitations

Cardiac MRS has inherent problems that limit the usage of the technique for in vivo examination. Three limitations are outlined in this section; however, these are not the only limitations, merely ones to be overcome in a first step.

7.1. Low Sensitivity

All MRS suffers from low inherent SNR. The metabolite content is low compared with the metabolites observed in MRI, and, with the exception of ^{1}H MRS, sensitivity of the nuclei observed is reduced. The low signal forces long measurement times and a limitation in the smallest volume element to be measured. An impressive example might be the use of ^{31}P MRS for the determination of viability, in which the smallest volumes measured in humans at 1.5 T are currently 16 mL. In contrast, using contrast-enhanced MRI with late-enhancement technique, a volume element of 16 µl could be realized *(63)*. Currently, only disease states that affect the entire heart (dilative cardiomyopathy, valve incompetence, or stenosis) or the surviving myocardium remote from local events (myocardial infarction) can be addressed by MRS. An exception is ^{1}H MRS, in which the volume of interest can be smaller *(47)*; however, the spatial resolution is still limited to a volume on the order of milliliters.

7.2. Number of Users

The number of centers capable to perform MRS of the heart is limited. A tight cooperation of different disciplines is required to perform and understand these examinations. Experimental MRS means to yield biochemical information by a physical technique in a biological model of a human disease. The manufacturers of clinical MR scanners put effort into making MRS work as a "push one button" technique, which would allow more users to acquire data. Interpretation and understanding of the data, however, is not delivered with the system. There is clearly a need for more education as well as for exchange of knowledge and expertise within the MR community.

7.3. Relative vs Absolute Values

The limitation to relative values, i.e., ratios of the metabolites, may be the largest problem in understanding the results. There are some developments toward absolute concentrations of metabolites *(44)*, which show that constant metabolite ratios can be caused by a comparable reduction in both metabolites. Absolute numbers will help to understand the origin of a disease or to optimize the model used for the understanding of the disease.

8. Conclusion

MRS is a technique that could potentially provide a wealth of information for better understanding of diseases in terms of the underlying biochemistry. MRS is able to document the alterations of metabolites that might lie behind the development of disease and disorder. MRS opens a window to the molecular level of the functional organization of cells and the organism. Coupled with the noninvasive character of MRS, which allows repetitive examinations, direct measurement of metabolites and their reactions makes MRS an important tool for molecular biology and medicine. However, further developments in the methodologies involved, as well as an expansion in the number of users are necessary to increase the awareness of MRS and to broaden its application for more routine use.

References

1. Bellenger, N. G., Burgess, M. I., Ray, S. G., et al. (2000) Comparison of left ventricular ejection fraction and volumes in heart failure by echocardiography, radionuclide ventriculography and cardiovascular magnetic resonance; are they interchangeable? *Eur. Heart J.* **21,** 1387–1396.
2. Gadian, D. (1982) *Nuclear Magnetic Resonance and its Application to Living Systems.* Oxford University Press, New York, NY.
3. Bottomley, P. A., Lugo Olivieri, C. H., and Giaquinto, R. (1997) What is the optimum phased array coil design for cardiac and torso magnetic resonance? *Magn. Reson. Med.* **37,** 591–599.
4. Ackerman, J. J. H., Gadian, D. G., Radda, G. K., and Wong, G. G. (1981) Observation of 1H NMR signal with receiver coils tuned for other nuclei. *J. Magn. Reson.* **42,** 498–500.
5. Ordidge, R. J., Helpern, J. A., Hugg, J. W., and Matson, G. B. (2000) Single voxel whole body phosphorus MRS, in *Methods in Biomedical Magnetic Resonance Imaging and Spectroscopy,* 1 ed., vol. 2 (Young, I. R., ed.), John Wiley & Sons, Chicester, UK, pp. 729–734.
6. Brown, T. (2000) Chemical shift imaging, in *Methods in Biomedical Magnetic Resonance Imaging and Spectroscopy,* 1 ed., vol. 2 (Young, I. R., ed.), John Wiley & Sons, Chicester, UK, pp. 751–762.
7. Frahm, J. and Hänicke, W. (2000) Single voxel localized proton nmr spectroscopy of human brain in vivo, in *Methods in Biomedical Magnetic Resonance Imaging and Spectroscopy,* 1 ed., vol. 2 (Young, I. R., ed.), John Wiley & Sons, Chicester, UK, pp. 735–750.
8. Bottomley, P. A. (1987) Spatial localization in NMR-spectroscopy in vivo. *Ann. N. Y. Acad. Sci.* **508,** 333–348.
9. Ordidge, R. J., Bendall, M. R., Gordon, R. E., and Conelly, A. (1985) Volume selection for in-vivo biological spectroscopy, in *Magnetic Resonance in Biology and Medicine* (Govil, G., Khetrapal, C. L., and Saran, A., eds.), Tata McGraw-Hill, New Dehli, India, pp. 387–397.

10. Frahm, J., Merboldt, K. D., and Hänicke, W. (1987) Localized proton spectroscopy using stimulated echoes. *J. Magn. Reson.* **72,** 501–508.

11. Ordidge, R. J., Conelly, A., and Lohman, J. A. B. (1986) Image selected in vivo spectroscopy (ISIS). A new technique for spatially selective NMR spectroscopy. *J. Magn. Reson.* **66,** 283–294.

12. Brown, T. R., Kincaid, B. M., and Ugurbil, K. (1982) NMR chemical shift imaging in three dimensions. *Proc. Natl. Acad. Sci. USA* **79,** 3523–3526.

13. Maudsley, A. A., Hilal, S. K., Perman, W. H., and Simon, H. E. (1983) Spatially resolved high-resolution spectroscopy by "four-dimensional" NMR. *J. Magn. Reson.* **51,** 147–152.

14. Bottomley, P. A., Atalar, E., and Weiss, R. G. (1996) Human cardiac high-energy phosphate metabolite concentrations by 1D-resolved NMR spectroscopy. *Magn. Reson. Med.* **35,** 664–670.

15. Pohmann, R. and von Kienlin, M. (2001) Accurate phosphorus metabolite images of the human heart by 3D acquisition-weighted CSI. *Magn. Reson. Med.* **45,** 817–826.

16. Moon, R. and Richards, J. (1973) Determination of intracellular pH by 31P magnetic resonance. *J. Biol. Chem.* **248,** 7276–7278.

17. Williams, G. D., Mosher, T. J., and Smith, M. B. (1993) Simultaneous determination of intracellular magnesium and pH from the three 31P NMR Chemical shifts of ATP. *Anal. Biochem.* **214,** 458–467.

18. Horn, M., Neubauer, S., Bomhard, M., Kadgien, M., Schnackerz, K., and Ertl, G. (1993) 31P-NMR spectroscopy of human blood and serum: first results from volunteers and patients with congestive heart failure, diabetes mellitus and hyperlipidemia. *MAGMA* **1,** 55–60.

19. Sieverding, L., Jung, W. I., Breuer, J., et al. (1997) Proton-decoupled myocardial 31P NMR spectroscopy reveals decreased PCr/Pi in patients with severe hypertrophic cardiomyopathy. *Am. J. Cardiol.* **80,** 34A–40A.

20. Horn, M., Kadgien, M., Schnackerz, K., and Neubauer, S. (2000) 31P-NMR spectroscopy of blood: a species comparison. *J. Cardiovasc. Magn. Reson.* **2,** 143–149.

21. Chen, W., Cho, Y., Merkle, H., et al. (1999) In vitro and in vivo studies of 1H NMR visibility to detect deoxyhemoglobin and deoxymyoglobin signals in myocardium. *Magn. Reson. Med.* **42,** 1–5.

22. Stothers, J. B. (1982) *Carbon 13-NMR Spectroscopy*, Academic, New York, NY.

23. Shaka, A. J., Keeler, J., and Freeman, R. (1983) An improved sequence for broadband decoupling: WALTZ-16. *J. Magn. Reson.* **53,** 313–340.

24. Overhauser, A. W. (1953) Polarization of nuclei in metals. *Phys. Rev.* **92,** 411–415.

25. Solomon, I. (1955) Relaxation processes in a system of two spins. *Phys. Rev.* **99,** 559–565.

26. Wei, H., Merkle, H., Xu, Y., Ellermann, J., Sipprell, K., and Ugurbil, K. (1997) Detection of 13C-labeled metabolites in the in vivo canine heart by B1 insensitive heteronuclear coherent polarization transfer and comparison of signal enhancement with NOE. *Magn. Reson. Med.* **37,** 327–330.

27. Bottomley, P. A. (1994) MR spectroscopy of the human heart: the status and the challenges. *Radiology* **191,** 593–612.

28. Neubauer, S., Horn, M., Naumann, A., et al. (1995) Impairment of energy metabolism in intact residual myocardium of rat hearts with chronic myocardial infarction. *J. Clin. Invest.* **95,** 1092–1100.
29. Schwartz, G. G., Greyson, C., Wisneski, J. A., and Garcia, J. (1994) Inhibition of fatty acid metabolism alters myocardial high-energy phosphates in vivo. *Am. J. Physiol.* **267,** H224–H231.
30. Hardy, C. J., Weiss, R. G., Bottomley, P. A., and Gerstenblith, G. (1991) Altered myocardial high-energy phosphate metabolites in patients with dilated cardiomyopathy. *Am. Heart J.* **122,** 795–801.
31. Zhang, J., Wilke, N., Wang, Y., et al. (1996) Functional and bioenergetic consequences of postinfarction left ventricular remodeling in a new porcine model. MRI and 31 P-MRS study. *Circulation* **94,** 1089–1100.
32. Horn, M., Neubauer, S., Frantz, S., et al. (1996) Preservation of left ventricular mechanical function and energy metabolism in rats after myocardial infarction by the angiotensin-converting enzyme inhibitor quinapril. *J. Cardiovasc. Pharmacol.* **27,** 201–210.
33. Liao, R., Nascimben, L., Friedrich, J., Gwathmey, J. K., and Ingwall, J. S. (1996) Decreased energy reserve in an animal model of dilated cardiomyopathy. Relationship to contractile performance. *Circ. Res.* **78,** 893–902.
34. Neubauer, S., Krahe, T., Schindler, R., et al. (1992) 31P magnetic resonance spectroscopy in dilated cardiomyopathy and coronary artery disease. Altered cardiac high-energy phosphate metabolism in heart failure. *Circulation* **86,** 1810–1888.
35. Conway, M. A., Allis, J., Ouwerkerk, R., Niioka, T., Rajagopalan, B., and Radda, G. K. (1991) Detection of low phosphocreatine to ATP ratio in failing hypertrophicd human myocardium by 31P magnetic resonance spectroscopy. *Lancet* **338,** 973–976.
36. Weiss, R. G., Bottomley, P. A., Hardy, C. J., and Gerstenblith, G. (1990) Regional myocardial metabolism of high-energy phosphates during isometric exercise in patients with coronary artery disease. *N. Engl. J. Med.* **323,** 1593–1600.
37. Yabe, T., Mitsunami, K., Okada, M., Morikawa, S., Inubushi, T., and Kinoshita, M. (1994) Detection of myocardial ischemia by 31P magnetic resonance spectroscopy during handgrip exercise. *Circulation* **89,** 1709–1716.
38. Pluim, B. M., Lamb, H. J., Kayser, H. W., et al. (1998) Functional and metabolic evaluation of the athlete's heart by magnetic resonance imaging and dobutamine stress magnetic resonance spectroscopy. *Circulation* **97,** 666–672.
39. Neubauer, S., Horn, M., Cramer, M., et al. (1997) Myocardial phosphocreatine-to-ATP ratio is a predictor of mortality in patients with dilated cardiomyopathy. *Circulation* **96,** 2190–2196.
40. Bottomley, P. A., Hardy, C. J., and Roemer, P. B. (1990) Phosphate metabolite imaging and concentration measurements in human heart by nuclear magnetic resonance. *Magn. Reson. Med.* **14,** 425–434.
41. von Kienlin, M., Beer, M., Greiser, A., et al. (2001) Advances in human cardiac 31P-MR spectroscopy: SLOOP and clinical applications. *J. Magn. Reson. Imaging* **13,** 521–527.

42. Landschütz, W., Meininger, M., Beer, M., et al. (1998) Concentration of human cardiac 31P-metabolites determined by SLOOP 31P- MRS. *MAGMA* **6,** 155–156.

43. Meininger, M., Landschütz, W., Beer, M., et al. (1999) Concentrations of human cardiac phosphorus metabolites determined by SLOOP 31P NMR spectroscopy. *Magn. Reson. Med.* **41,** 657–663.

44. Beer, M., Seyfarth, T., Sandstede, J., et al. (2002) Absolute concentrations of high-energy phosphate metabolites in normal, hypertrophied, and failing human myocardium measured noninvasively with (31)P-SLOOP magnetic resonance spectroscopy. *J. Am. Coll. Cardiol.* **40,** 1267–1274.

45. Ingwall, J., Kramer, M., Fifer, M., et al. (1985) The creatine kinase system in normal and diseased human myocardium. *N. Engl. J. Med.* **313,** 1050–1054.

46. Wallimann, T. and Eppenberger, H. M. (1990) The subcellular compartmentation of creatine kinase isozymes as a precondition for a proposed phosphoryl-creatine circuit. *Prog. Clin. Biol. Res.* **344,** 877–889.

47. Bottomley, P. A. and Weiss, R. G. (1998) Non-invasive magnetic-resonance detection of creatine depletion in non-viable infarcted myocardium. *Lancet* **351,** 714–718.

48. Weiss, R. G., Chatham, J. C., Georgakopolous, D., et al. (2002) An increase in the myocardial PCr/ATP ratio in GLUT4 null mice. *FASEB J.* **16,** 613–615.

49. Szczepaniak, L. S., Dobbins, R. L., Metzger, G. J., et al. (2003) Myocardial triglycerides and systolic function in humans: in vivo evaluation by localized proton spectroscopy and cardiac imaging. *Magn. Reson. Med.* **49,** 417–423.

50. Szczepaniak, L. S., Dobbins, R. L., Stein, D. T., and McGarry, J. D. (2002) Bulk magnetic susceptibility effects on the assessment of intra- and extramyocellular lipids in vivo. *Magn. Reson. Med.* **47,** 607–610.

51. Schneider, J. E., Tyler, D. J., ten Hove, M., et al. (2004) In vivo cardiac ^{1}H-MRS in the mouse. *Magn. Reson. Med.* **52,** 1029–1035.

52. Neurohr, K. J., Barrett, E. J., and Shulman, R. G. (1983) In vivo carbon-13 nuclear magnetic resonance studies of heart metabolism. *Proc. Natl. Acad. Sci. USA* **80,** 1603–1607.

53. Chance, E. M., Seeholzer, S. H., Kobayashi, K., and Williamson, J. R. (1983) Mathematical analysis of isotope labeling in the citric acid cycle with applications to 13C NMR studies in perfused rat hearts. *J. Biol. Chem.* **258,** 13,785–13,794.

54. Weiss, R. G., Chacko, V. P., Glickson, J. D., and Gerstenblith, G. (1989) Comparative 13C and 31P NMR assessment of altered metabolism during graded reductions in coronary flow in intact rat hearts. *Proc. Natl. Acad. Sci. USA* **86,** 6426–6430.

55. Stevens, A. N., Iles, R. A., Morris, P. G., and Griffiths, J. R. (1982) Detection of glycogen in a glycogen storage disease by 13C nuclear magnetic resonance. *FEBS Lett.* **150,** 489–493.

56. Sillerud, L. O. and Shulman, R. G. (1983) Structure and metabolism of mammalian liver glycogen monitored by carbon-13 nuclear magnetic resonance. *Biochemistry* **22,** 1087–1094.

57. Canioni, P., Alger, J. R., and Shulman, R. G. (1983) Natural abundance carbon-13 nuclear magnetic resonance spectroscopy of liver and adipose tissue of the living rat. *Biochemistry* **22,** 4974–4980.
58. Bottomley, P. A., Hardy, C. J., Roemer, P. B., and Mueller, O. M. (1989) Proton-decoupled, Overhauser-enhanced, spatially localized carbon-13 spectroscopy in humans. *Magn. Reson. Med.* **12,** 348–363.
59. Weiss, R. G., Chacko, V. P., and Gerstenblith, G. (1989) Fatty acid regulation of glucose metabolism in the intact beating rat heart assessed by carbon-13 NMR spectroscopy: the critical role of pyruvate dehydrogenase. *J. Mol. Cell. Cardiol.* **21,** 469–478.
60. Belke, D. D., Larsen, T. S., Lopaschuk, G. D., and Sevenson, D. L. (1999) Glucose and fatty acid metabolism in the isolated working mouse heart. *Am. J. Phys. Regulatory Integrative Comp. Physiol.* **277,** R1210–R1217.
61. Goodwin, G. W. and Taegtmeyer, H. (1999) Regulation of fatty acid oxidation of the heart by MCD and ACC during contractile stimulation. *Am. J. Physiol. Endocrinol. Metab.* **277,** E772–E777.
62. O'Donnell, J. M., Alpert, N. A., White, L. T., and Lewandowski, E. D. (2002) Coupling of mitochondrial fatty acid uptake to oxidative flux in the intact heart. *Biophys. J.* **82,** 11–18.
63. Kim, R. J., Wu, E., Rafael, A., Chen, E. L., et al. (2000) The use of contrast-enhanced magnetic resonance imaging to identify reversible myocardial dysfunction. *N. Engl. J. Med.* **343,** 1445–1453.

IV

PATHOPHYSIOLOGY

10

Application of Magnetic Resonance Imaging to Study Pathophysiology in Brain Disease Models

Rick M. Dijkhuizen

Summary

Magnetic resonance imaging (MRI) provides a noninvasive and multimodal tool to study neurological disorders in experimental models. MRI experiments can be sensitized to various contrast parameters and, hence, enable comprehensive assessment of normal and abnormal brain physiology. Different conventional and novel MRI techniques have been developed that supply specific information on lesion location and size (e.g., T_2- and diffusion-weighted MRI), alterations in tissue structure (e.g., magnetization transfer imaging and diffusion tensor imaging), perfusion deficits (perfusion MRI), brain activation (functional MRI), cell migration (cellular MRI), gene expression (molecular MRI), and more. The advantages of in vivo, longitudinal, and multiparametric studies with MRI provide unique opportunities for characterizing and delineating experimental models of neurological diseases and pathophysiological mechanisms, as well as spontaneous and treatment-induced recovery mechanisms.

Key Words: Magnetic resonance imaging; brain diseases; physiopathology; animal models; diffusion; perfusion; fMRI; brain ischemia; neurodegenerative diseases; therapy.

1. Introduction

Much of our understanding of the pathophysiology of neurological disorders, as well as development of therapeutic strategies, is based on studies that use animal models of human brain diseases. In recent times, neurology and basic neuroscience has been significantly advanced by imaging tools that enable in vivo monitoring of the brain. In particular, magnetic resonance imaging (MRI) has proven to be a powerful and versatile brain imaging modality that allows noninvasive longitudinal and 3D assessment of tissue morphology, metabolism, physiology, and function. During the last two decades, numerous studies have demonstrated the potential of MRI techniques to obtain multiparametric information on the pathophysiology, recovery mechanisms, and treatment strategies in experimental models of stroke, brain tumors, mul-

From: *Methods in Molecular Medicine, Vol. 124*
Magnetic Resonance Imaging: Methods and Biologic Applications
Edited by: P. V. Prasad © Humana Press Inc., Totowa, NJ

tiple sclerosis, neurodegenerative diseases, traumatic brain injury, epilepsy, and other brain disorders. Importantly, because MRI is available in preclinical and clinical settings, optimal translational research can be achieved. The combination of diverse MRI methods creates an excellent opportunity for a comprehensive diagnosis of brain injury and a thorough analysis of therapeutic intervention strategies. This chapter describes applications of conventional and novel MRI methods in studies using experimental brain disease models.

2. Application of MRI Methods in Brain Disease Models

2.1. Proton Density, T_1-, T_2-, and T_2^*-Weighted MRI

Proton density, T_1-, and T_2-weighted MRI are sensitized to the concentration, the longitudinal magnetic resonance (MR) relaxation time (T_1) and the transverse MR relaxation time (T_2) of tissue water, respectively. T_2^*-weighted MRI is sensitized to transverse MR relaxation that is not corrected for phase shifts caused by local field inhomogeneities. These MR techniques have been widely applied to detect brain lesions, because many types of pathology, such as tumors, edema, and hemorrhage, are associated with changes in water content and relaxation rates.

2.1.1. Proton Density, T_1-, and T_2-Weighted MRI

Proton density, T_1-, and T_2-weighted MRI techniques demonstrated their potential to detect cerebral lesions in various animal studies during the 1980s *(1–5)*. Increases in proton density, as well as in T_1 and T_2 in pathological tissue are mostly caused by an increase in interstitial water associated with the development of vasogenic edema (*see* Van Bruggen et al., **ref. *6***, and references therein). T_1 and T_2 values correlate well with tissue water content *(7)*; however, the relative prolongation of T_2 in edematous tissue is usually larger than the T_1 (or proton density) increase *(7–9)*. For example, in acute stroke lesions *(9)* and intracerebral tumors in rats *(8)*, increases in T_2, T_1, and proton density were about 45 to 50%, 30 to 35%, and 5 to 10%, respectively. Because of its histologically validated superior sensitivity for detecting tissue damage *(10–12)*, T_2-weighted MRI has been the most favored MRI method for delineating lesions in clinical and experimental diagnostic studies. To illustrate, the bottom row of **Fig. 1** shows T_2 maps that clearly depict a stroke lesion in rat brain.

Although changes on proton density, T_1-, and T_2-weighted MRI are predominantly associated with late and irreversible neuropathological damage (vasogenic edema typically develops during subacute and chronic stages), early T_1 and T_2 changes of a few percent have been observed in the hyperacute stages of experimental cerebral ischemia *(13)*. Hyperacute prolongation of T_1 may be related to cessation of blood flow *(13,14)*, whereas T_2 reduction directly following cerebral ischemia is believed to be the result of tissue deoxygenation *(13,15,16)*.

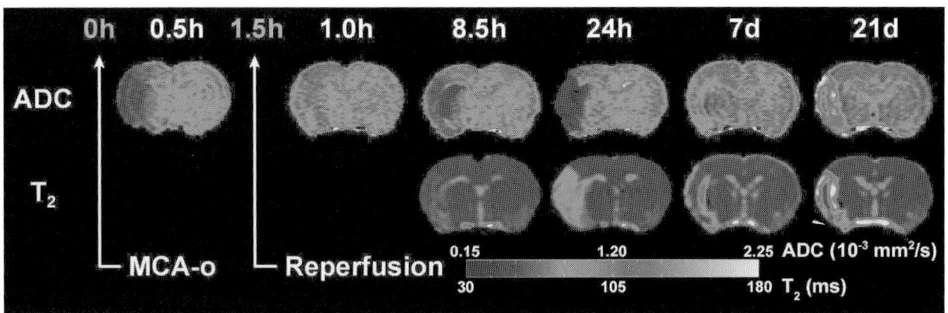

Fig. 1. Apparent diffusion coefficient (ADC; top row) and T_2 maps (bottom row) of a coronal rat brain slice at different time points after transient unilateral occlusion of the middle cerebral artery (MCA). The reduction of the brain tissue water ADC in the MCA-territory acutely after cerebral ischemia is reflective of cellular swelling. After reperfusion, the ADC initially recovers, followed by a secondary reduction. Subsequently, the ADC increases because of tissue lysis and cavitation. Prolongation of T_2 becomes evident several hours after cerebral ischemia and is indicative of formation of vasogenic edema. (Reproduced courtesy of Dr. W. B. Veldhuis.)

2.1.2. T_2^*-Weighted MRI

Tissue deoxygenation-induced MR signal loss, as described in **Subheading 2.1.1.**, is caused by an increase in the amount of deoxyhemoglobin and is most clearly observed on T_2^*-weighted MR images. The deoxygenated form of hemoglobin is paramagnetic, which causes increased local magnetic susceptibility differences between intravascular and extravascular compartments, thereby resulting in shortening of T_2 and, in particular, T_2^*. Gradient-echo T_2^*-weighted MRI is more sensitive to susceptibility effects than spin-echo T_2-weighted MRI because phase shifts caused by local field inhomogeneities are not compensated for. The sensitivity of MRI to the magnetic property of blood forms the basis of blood oxygenation level-dependent (BOLD) MRI *(17)*. BOLD MRI can be applied to assess hemodynamic factors in normal and diseased brain physiology. For example, deoxygenation of hemoglobin after hemorrhage allows detection of acute hematomas, which appear as clear hypointensities on spin-echo T_2-weighted and especially on gradient-echo T_2^*-weighted MR images *(18)*. Cerebrovascular reactivity, an important hemodynamic index in brain disease, can be examined by combining BOLD MRI with a specific challenge. A vasodilatory challenge, induced by injection of the vasodilator acetazolamide, or by CO_2 inhalation, leads to increases in BOLD MR signal intensity in normal but not in ischemic tissue, suggesting failure of autoregulatory response *(19,20)*. In a rat brain tumor study performed in a clinical 1.5 T MR scanner, hyperemia and hyperoxygenation induced by acetazolamide injection in combination with 100% O_2 inhalation, resulted in BOLD MR signal intensity increases of up to 25% in viable tumor tissue with functioning microvessels, whereas necrotic regions showed minimal BOLD changes *(21)*.

BOLD MRI also forms the basis for functional MRI (fMRI). During neuronal activation in the brain, the local rise in cerebral metabolic rate results in an elevation of both oxygen demand and local cerebral blood flow (CBF). However, the increase in oxygen supply exceeds the increase in oxygen consumption in the activated neuronal network. The consequent increase in local blood oxygenation leads to an increase of BOLD MR signal. fMRI allows noninvasive generation of indirect functional brain activation maps and will be further discussed in **Subheading 5.**

2.1.3. Contrast-Enhanced T_1-Weighted MRI

Tissue contrast on MR images can be enhanced by administration of a paramagnetic contrast agent. Paramagnetic agents, such as gadolinium-based dimeglumine gadopentetate (Gd-DTPA), interact with nearby proton spins via dipole–dipole connections, which affects relaxation times of the proton MR signal. The predominant effect is observed on T_1 (i.e., T_1 shortening). The use of exogenous contrast agents to achieve T_1-weighted contrast has gained widespread use for the study of blood–brain barrier (BBB) integrity. BBB disruption results in leakage of intravascularly injected contrast agent into brain tissue, thereby causing local signal enhancement on T_1-weighted images *(22)* (proton spins with relatively short T_1 give rise to relatively high MR signal). Contrast-enhanced T_1-weighted MRI has been applied to delineate the presence and extent of brain tumors *(23,24)*, ischemic injury *(25,26)*, and inflammatory lesions *(27–29)* (*see* **Fig. 2**). Besides detection of BBB breakdown, contrast-enhanced T_1-weighted MRI can provide additional pathophysiological details. For example, Van der Sanden et al. *(30)* demonstrated that the rate of Gd-DTPA accumulation in rat tumor tissue correlates with perfused microvessel density and vascular surface area. In experimental stroke studies, Gd-DTPA tissue enhancement has been shown to be predictive of subsequent vasogenic edema formation *(31)* and hemorrhagic transformation *(32,33)*.

2.2. Magnetization Transfer Imaging

Magnetization transfer (MT) effects are caused by chemical exchange or dipole–dipole interactions between protons from water and macromolecules and can be used as an MR contrast mechanism *(34)*. MT imaging can yield information on the ratio between free and bound proton pools (MT ratio; MTR), on the rate of magnetization exchange, and on the magnetic properties of the immobilized proton pool.

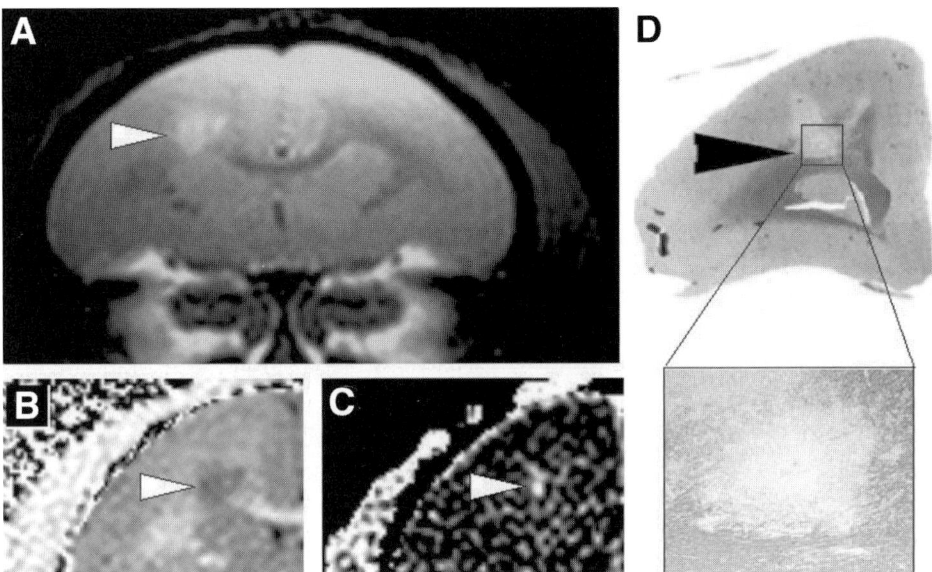

Fig. 2. In vivo T_2-weighted magnetic resonance (MR) image **(A)**; magnetization transfer ration (MTR) map **(B)**; and postcontrast T_1-weighted difference image (difference between T_1-weighted MR images acquired before and 13 min after intravenous injection of 0.3 mmol/kg of Gd-DTPA) **(C)**; of a coronal brain slice of a marmoset (a small nonhuman primate) with experimental allergic encephalomyelitis (EAE). **(D)** Klüver Barrera staining for myelin of postmortem brain section. The EAE lesion is characterized by prolongation of T_2 (i.e., vasogenic edema), decrease of MTR (i.e., tissue degradation), post Gd-DTPA contrast enhancement (i.e., blood–brain barrier disruption), and loss of Klüver Barrera staining (i.e., myelin destruction). (Reproduced courtesy of Dr. E. L. A. Blezer.)

MT imaging has been successfully applied in pathologies that alter the structural integrity of brain tissue, such as multiple sclerosis (**Fig. 2**) and other white matter disorders *(35)*. Reductions in MTR in demyelinating lesions correlate with myelin and axon destruction *(36)*, and recovery of MTR corresponds with remyelination *(37)*. Nevertheless, other pathological features may also be involved in the MTR decrease. Prevention or reversal of MTR without accompanying recovery of myelin water percentage has been found after modulation of inflammation after experimental allergic encephalomyelitis (EAE; a model for multiple sclerosis) in guinea pig brain *(35,38)*. In experimental cerebral ischemia, reductions in the magnetization change rate between the free and immobile proton pool in the brain have been reported, which may be related to an increase in tissue water content and to degradation of macromolecular structures *(39,40)*. A small increase in MT (<5%), in combination with an increase in the on-resonance T_1 in the rotating frame, $T_{1\rho}$, within the first hour after experimental stroke suggests that the interaction between water and macromolecules is altered acutely after cerebral ischemia *(41)*. Finally, MTR reductions have also been reported in studies on experimental brain tumors *(42,43)* and experimental traumatic brain injury *(44,45)*.

2.3. Diffusion-Weighted MRI

Diffusion-weighted MRI is sensitized to microscopic incoherent motion of water and allows quantification of the apparent diffusion coefficient (ADC) of tissue water *(46)*. This technique is sensitive to several cellular changes and tissue abnormalities and can detect diseased regions at acute stages. A cerebral ischemia-induced increase of diffusion-weighted MR signal intensity within approx 15 min was first described by Moseley et al. *(47)*. A signal intensity increase on diffusion-weighted MR images points toward a reduction in the ADC of brain tissue water, which most likely reflects cell swelling as a result of an osmotically obliged shift of extracellular water to intracellular compartments caused by ion homeostasis disruption (i.e., cytotoxic edema) *(47–50)*. The tissue water ADC decline can be explained by the enlarged fraction of intracellular water, which encounters a high density of barriers and restrictions, as compared with the more freely diffusing extracellular water. In addition, increases in extracellular and intracellular tortuosity are also likely to contribute to the tissue water ADC decrease (*see* reviews by Nicolay et al., **refs.** *51* and *52*, and Gass et al., **ref.** *53*).

The application of diffusion-weighted MRI has been extensively investigated in stroke models in which acute ADC decreases of 10 to 60% are found after ischemia *(54,55)* (*see* also **Fig. 1**). However, early ADC reductions have also been detected in other neurological disease models, such as neonatal hypoxia/ischemia *(56–58)*, traumatic brain injury *(44,59,60)*, and subarachnoid hemorrhage *(61–63)*. In cerebral ischemia, a reduction in the tissue water ADC develops when tissue perfusion has decreased below a certain threshold; e.g., below 15 to 20 mL/100 g/min in a gerbil model of global cerebral ischemia *(64)* , and below 35 mL/100 g/min after focal ischemia in rat brain *(65)*. The perfusion threshold for ADC changes increases as a function of time of ischemia *(66–68)*. On the other hand, ADC reductions may also occur without concomitant ischemia and/or energy depletion. For example, the ADC changes that are induced by certain excitotoxins *(69,70)* and seizures *(71–73)* could be the result of chronic perturbation of ion homeostasis and consequent intracellular water accumulation, and they could occur without severe changes in blood flow and tissue energy status.

Cell swelling as a result of impaired ion homeostasis in itself may not be injurious and, in theory, is reversible. Treatment studies in a neonatal rat excitotoxicity model have demonstrated that lowered ADC values in cortex and striatum as a result of injection of the excitotoxin *N*-methyl-D-aspartate (NMDA), can completely renormalize after treatment with an NMDA antagonist *(69,74)*. Importantly, these initially affected regions were free of signs of histological damage at later stages. Nevertheless, a prolonged disrupted ion homeostasis initiates a variety of injurious processes that can ultimately lead to cell death. Thus, tissue in which cytotoxic edema has existed for an extended period may have advanced into a state of irreversible damage. Under these conditions, normalization of the cellular volume, for example, by restoration of blood supply after stroke, does not necessarily represent actual tissue recovery. This has been demonstrated by different groups, who showed that brain regions with an acute water ADC reduction during cerebral ischemia could initially recover after reperfusion but eventually exhibited a secondary ADC decrease and irreversible tissue damage *(56,75–78)* (*see* **Fig. 1**). Thus, ADC normalization after spontaneous reperfusion or therapeutic intervention after an ischemic insult is not necessarily a good predictor of ultimate tissue recovery.

At subacute stages, the water ADC reduction becomes less pronounced. ADC levels return to preischemic levels at 2 to 3 d after onset of focal ischemia in rats *(79)* and subsequently increase above preischemic control values (up to 1.5×10^{-3} mm^2/s; *see* **Fig. 1**) *(80,81)*. The elevated ADC of tissue water is associated with cellular lysis *(82,83)*. The loss of cellular barriers combined with the excessive accumulation of (more freely diffusing) edematous water would explain the high water ADC values. This implies that diffusion-weighted MRI may also be informative about loss of tissue structure that occurs at more chronic stages. Indeed, diffusion-weighted MRI in chronic demyelinating disease models, such as EAE, demonstrated increased water diffusion in white matter areas *(84,85)*. Similarly, white matter edema in hydrocephalic rat brain also exhibits an increased ADC *(86)*. In addition, cystic, necrotic, and edematous tissue in and near brain tumors can be identified as areas with high ADC values *(8,42,87)*. Diffusion-weighted MRI has also been examined as a tool to monitor responses to tumor therapy (*see* Kauppinen, **ref.** *87* and Ross et al., **ref.** *88*, for reviews). Treatment-induced killing of tumor cells in a 9L brain glioma model, resulting in a decrease of cellular density in tumor tissue, is accompanied by an increase of the ADC *(89)*. The elevated ADC may be explained by destruction of tumor cells, widening of the extracellular space, and a consequent increase in extracellular, relatively mobile, water. At later timepoints, the ADC subsequently decreased, purportedly caused by cellular repopulation.

2.3.1. Diffusion Tensor Imaging

Because of the organized structure of tissues, diffusion is often not the same in all directions, i.e., the rate of diffusion is anisotropic, and the measured ADC depends on the direction of the diffusion sensitization. The 3D displacement of a molecule can be characterized by a tensor containing nine matrix elements, which can be measured using diffusion tensor imaging (DTI) *(90)*. The trace of the water diffusion tensor (i.e., the sum of the three diagonal elements of the tensor) divided by three can be used to create a direction-independent average diffusivity (ADC_{av}) map, which provides a more accurate delineation of actual ischemic lesions than an ADC map obtained with diffusion encoding in only one direction *(91,92)*.

DTI allows the calculation of indices of diffusion anisotropy, e.g., the fractional anisotropy *(93)*. In rat brain, increased anisotropy has been found during the first hours of permanent focal ischemia *(94)*, possibly caused by increased intracellular and/or extracellular tortuosity. At chronic stages, diffusion anisotropy declines, which is believed to reflect loss of structural integrity of brain tissue *(57,94)*. In shiverer mice with incomplete myelin formation, water diffusivity perpendicular to axonal fiber tract was significantly higher than in control mice, whereas diffusion along axonal tracts was unaffected *(95)*. Importantly, it has recently been demonstrated that modeling of neuronal tracts based on diffusion anisotropy measures is feasible in small animal brain *(96,97)*. Hence, DTI provides a unique means to study integrity of axons and myelin in particular neurological disorders.

2.4. Perfusion MRI

Several MR techniques are able to measure brain hemodynamics (*see* Hossmann and Hoehn-Berlage, **ref. 98** and Calamante et al., **ref. 99**, for reviews). The most popular MR approaches to assess cerebral microcirculation are dynamic susceptibility contrast-enhanced (DSC) and steady-state susceptibility contrast-enhanced MRI, which measure signal changes after intravascular bolus injection of an exogenous contrast agent; and arterial spin labeling (ASL) techniques, which are based on the detection of signal from endogenous arterial water.

2.4.1. Dynamic Susceptibility Contrast-Enhanced MRI

DSC (or "bolus tracking") MRI typically makes use of rapidly acquired T_2- or T_2^*-weighted MR images to assess the first passage of an intravenously injected bolus of paramagnetic contrast agent through the microvascular bed *(100)*. In addition to the earlier mentioned T_1-shortening effect (**Subheading 2.1.3.**), paramagnetic contrast agents also induce shortening of T_2 or T_2^* via magnetic susceptibility effects; the T_2 or T_2^* shortening extends over a larger distance than the local T_1-shortening effect caused by direct dipole–dipole interactions. Various hemodynamic parameters, e.g., bolus peak time, maximal change of the transverse relaxation rate, i.e., $\Delta R_2^*{}_{max}$ [$R_2^* = 1/T_2^*$], relative cerebral blood volume (CBV), relative mean transit time and relative CBF index (CBF_i), can be calculated from the time-course of the contrast agent-induced change of the effective transverse relaxation rate [$\Delta R_2^*(t)$]. The tissue response function can be calculated by deconvolution with a measured arterial input function *(99–101)*. Significant correlations have been demonstrated between relative CBF indices, as determined from DSC MRI, and CBF values quantified by autoradiography *(102)* or positron emission tomography *(103)* in normal and ischemic animal brain.

DSC MRI has been used to study the pattern of perfusion deficits in various animal models of ischemia *(98,99)*. Spatial assessment of multiple hemodynamic parameters can identify brain regions in which microcirculation is preserved but compromised *(66,104,105)*. For example, a mismatch between relative CBF_i and relative CBV could indicate compensatory vasodilatation, whereas a delayed bolus peak time in perifocal areas may reflect alternative routes of blood supply via collaterals. DSC MRI can also evaluate the hemodynamic consequences of induction of reperfusion (e.g., no reflow, hyperemia, or hypoperfusion) *(106–108)*. **Figure 3** shows the effect of thrombolysis on CBF_i maps as derived from repetitive DSC MRI experiments in a rat stroke model. Finally, DSC MRI-based CBV mapping of 9L gliosarcomas in rats has been evaluated as a potential means of measuring of tumor vascularity and angiogenesis *(109,110)*. It was shown that MRI-derived CBV correlated with histologically measured fractional volume of vessels.

2.4.2. Steady-State Susceptibility Contrast-Enhanced MRI

As described above, DSC MRI allows calculation of relative CBV and CBF_i from the first passage of intravascularly injected contrast agent. For repetitive measurements, however, the contrast agent needs to be cleared from the blood first, resulting in limitations to how often the experiment can be repeated in a single scan session. A MRI methodology in which relative CBV can be measured continuously is steady-state susceptibility contrast-enhanced MRI *(111)*. This method makes use of T_2- or T_2^*-weighted MRI in combination with a MR contrast agent that is not rapidly washed out from the blood but instead remains in the blood pool over a prolonged period (e.g., superparamagnetic iron oxide particles, SPIOs). In this way, dynamic relative CBV changes can be calculated by making use of the relationship between the change in ΔR_2^* and the local relative CBV change *(111,112)*. Accordingly, with the use of ultrasmall SPIOs (USPIOs), Hamberg et al. *(111)* measured rapid hyperemic responses in a feline global cerebral ischemia model. Zaharchuk et al. *(113)*

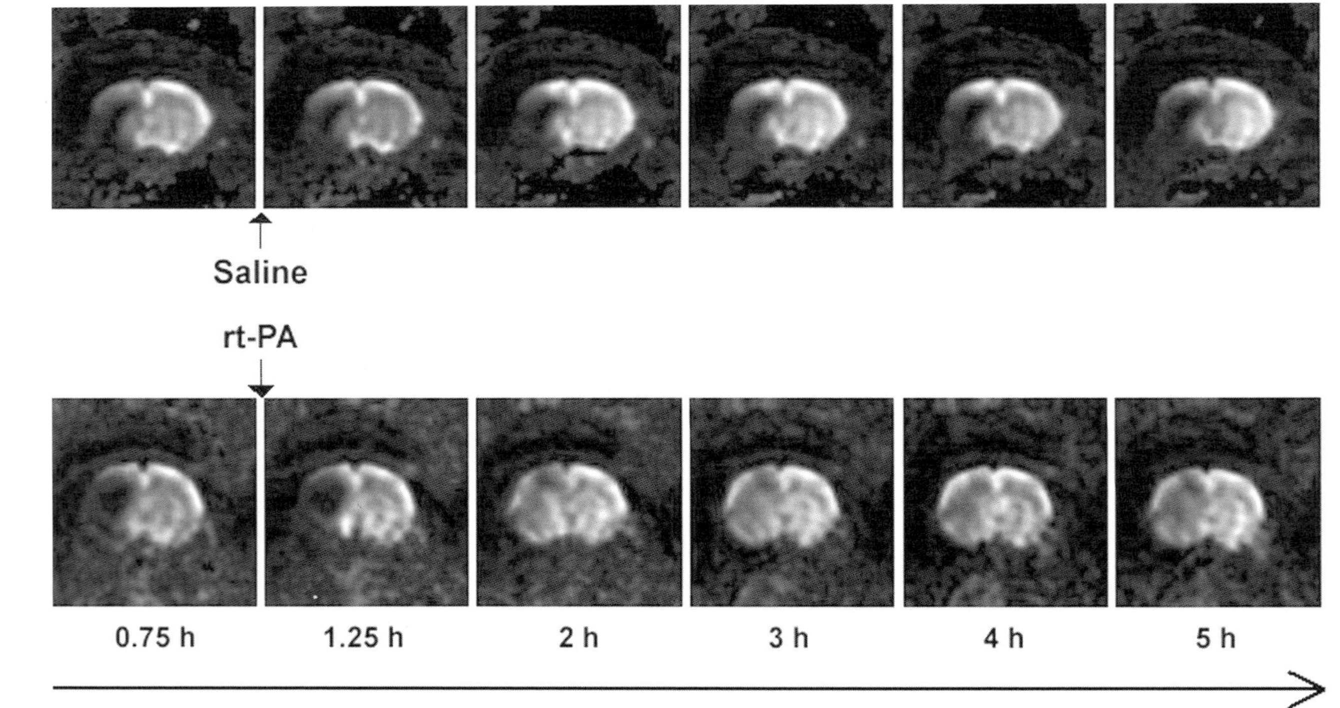

Fig. 3. Serial cerebral blood flow index (CBF_i) maps of a coronal rat brain slice before and after treatment with saline (top row) or thrombolytic recombinant tissue plasminogen activator (rt-PA) (1 mg/kg of pamiteplase; Yamanouchi Pharmaceutical Co., Tsukuba, Ibaraki, Japan) (bottom row). Onset of treatment was at approx 1 h after unilateral embolic middle cerebral artery occlusion. Data demonstrate thrombolysis-induced reperfusion after rt-PA treatment and absence of CBF recovery after saline treatment.

applied this technique with gradient-echo and spin-echo MR sequences to demonstrate differences in temporal changes in total CBV and microvascular CBV, respectively, after unilateral middle cerebral artery (MCA) occlusion in rats. This experimental approach is based on the concept that gradient-echo sequences are sensitive to changes in both microvessels and macrovessels, whereas spin-echo sequences predominantly measure changes in microvasculature *(114)*.

Steady-state susceptibility contrast-enhanced MRI has also been applied to measure brain tumor vascularization. Because gradient-echo and spin-echo steady-state susceptibility contrast-enhanced MRI are sensitive to varying sizes of blood vessels *(114)*, combining these approaches can provide information on growth and distribution of vessels in glioma models *(115–117)*. Two-dimensional maps of $\Delta R_2^*/\Delta R_2$ demonstrated increased vessel size in tumors as compared with surrounding tissue, thereby yielding information on local differences in vascular morphology and angiogenesis *(115)*.

2.4.3. Arterial Spin Labeling

ASL uses endogenous water as a tracer to quantify the regional CBF and is based on inversion or saturation of a plane through which arterial water spins flow before entering the region of interest where they exchange with tissue water *(118)*. The arterial spin tagging can be executed by a single pulse, such as in a flow-sensitive alternating inversion recovery (FAIR) sequence *(119,120)* or by continuous inversion or saturation of inflowing spins *(118,121)*.

ASL techniques are completely noninvasive (they do not require intravascular injection of exogenous MR contrast agent) and have been applied with increasing frequency in animal models of neurological disorders. Serial CBF measurements with continuous or pulsed ASL have been performed after acute cerebral ischemia in rats *(79,122,123)*, gerbils *(124)*, and mice *(125)*. In animal models of traumatic brain injury *(126)* and brain cancer *(127)*, ASL measurements revealed reduced CBF values in impaired regions. Schepers et al. *(128)* demonstrated that relative CBF measures derived from FAIR and DSC MRI after permanent or transient unilateral occlusion of the MCA in rats correlated well in regions of normal and elevated perfusion. However, in regions with moderate perfusion deficits, CBF values calculated from FAIR MRI were lower than those calculated from DSC MRI, which may be explained by the long mean transit time. In addition, ASL loses sensitivity in areas with very low CBF. Sensitivity to longer arrival times may be reduced by using a two-coil system, in which arterial spins are labeled by one radio frequency coil in the neck region, whereas the other coil detects exchange of arterial and tissue water in the brain *(129)*. This approach eliminates MT effects associated with single-coil ASL experiments and allows straightforward multislice imaging.

2.5. Functional MRI

The application of MRI for mapping cerebral activity, i.e., fMRI, has become a major research field over the past years. Standard fMRI techniques measure hemodynamic responses to neural activity in the functioning brain during cognitive, perceptual, sensory, or motor processes, or during a pharmacological challenge (i.e., pharmacological MRI, phMRI). fMRI studies in animal models have been performed using BOLD MRI *(130)*, ASL *(131,132)*, or steady-state susceptibility contrast-enhanced MRI *(112,133,134)*. In addition, Lin and Koretsky *(135)* have shown that intracellular accumulation of intravenously administered paramagnetic Mn^{2+} may enable direct detection of brain activation on T_1-weighted MR images. Mn^{2+} is a Ca^{2+} analog that can enter cells through Ca^{2+} channels during neuronal activation and that is relatively slowly cleared, thereby allowing detection of activated sites on a prolonged time scale. Manganese-enhanced MRI has also been applied as an in vivo tract tracing method; intracerebrally injected Mn^{2+} can be taken up by neurons and is subsequently transported along connective pathways *(136)*.

Animal fMRI studies allow the assessment of spatial and temporal dynamics of brain reorganization in relation to cerebral pathophysiology and functional recovery. With the use of BOLD and perfusion fMRI, Schmitz et al. *(137)* demonstrated loss of hemodynamic responses in the somatosensory cortex evoked by electrical forelimb stimulation in rats recovering from cardiac arrest. Changes in limb stimulation-induced brain activation patterns have also been reported after focal cerebral ischemic damage in rats *(138–142)*. Steady-state contrast-enhanced CBV-weighted fMRI studies by Dijkhuizen et al. *(140,142)* and Abo et al. *(139)* have described extensive contralesional activity and perilesional activation foci after cerebral ischemia, thereby providing evidence for brain reorganization after stroke (*see* **Fig. 4**). Altered brain activation patterns, i.e., bilateral overactivation in the sensorimotor cortex, have also been demonstrated in a rodent model of Parkinson's disease *(143)*. Furthermore, the potential of fMRI to analyze the origin and propagation of seizures has been illustrated in a sheep model of penicillin-induced partial epilepsy, in which BOLD signal changes were detected at the seizure focus and ipsilateral amygdala *(144)*.

2.5.1. Pharmacological MRI

phMRI is an fMRI variant that measures hemodynamic changes associated with cerebral activity in response to centrally acting pharmacological agents *(131,145,146)*. For example, injection of pharmacological agents that increase synaptic dopamine levels (e.g., D-amphetamine) results in an increase in BOLD MRI signal intensity in brain regions with high dopamine receptor density *(146)*. Pharmacological MRI can aid in the detection of compromised regions in pathological brain and has been applied in models of Parkinson's disease,

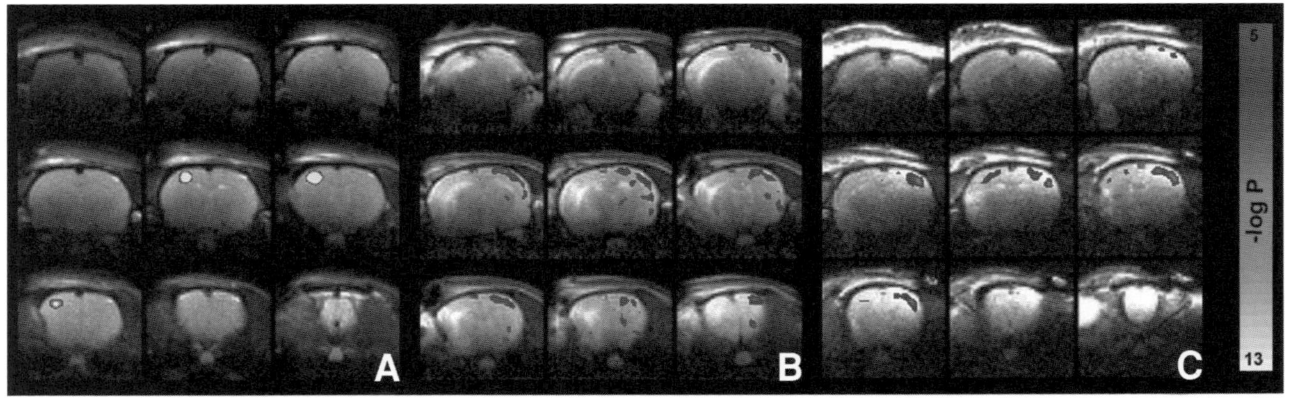

Fig. 4. Functional activation maps overlaid on T_2-weighted images of coronal rat brain slices. Functional magnetic resonance imaging (MRI) was performed by combining steady-state contrast-enhanced CBV-weighted MRI with an electrical forelimb stimulation paradigm as described by Dijkhuizen et al. *(140)*. Statistical activation maps were generated by a voxel-wise *t*-test of differences in CBV response between stimulation and rest conditions. The map of p values has been color-coded, corresponding to the degree of significance. Unilateral forelimb stimulation induced significant activation responses in the contralateral sensorimotor cortex in control rats (**A**). At 3 d after unilateral stroke, no significant activation was detected in the ipsilesional sensorimotor cortex in response to stimulation of the impaired forelimb (contralateral to the lesion side) (**B**). However, clear responses were found in the contralesional hemisphere. After 14 d, activation responses appeared both contralesional and ipsilesional (**C**). Infarction areas are characterized by increased T_2-weighted signal intensity.

stroke and Alzheimer's disease. In a rat model for Parkinson's disease, in which the dopaminergic neurotoxin 6-hydroxydopamine was unilaterally injected in the striatum, phMRI responses to dopamine transporter ligands (e.g., amphetamine) was shown to be ablated in the ipsilateral hemisphere, and could be restored by transplantation of fetal dopamine neurons in the striatum *(147)*. In hemiparkinsonian rhesus monkeys, treatment with the dopamine precursor, levodopa, resulted in increased BOLD phMRI responses in the striatum, which temporally correlated with increases in dopamine levels *(148)*. In an experimental stroke study, systemic administration of bicuculline, a γ-aminobutyric acid receptor type A antagonist, gave rise to a strong steady-state contrast-enhanced phMRI response in normal brain (up to a 50% rise in CBV), which was diminished after unilateral MCA occlusion in rats *(149)*. Similar findings were observed in amyloid precursor protein transgenic mice *(150)*, a model of Alzheimer's disease.

2.6. Cellular and Molecular MRI
2.6.1. Cellular MRI

Labeling of cells with MR contrast agent provides a tool to detect and track cells with MRI *(151,152)*. Intravascularly administered SPIOs have been shown to accumulate in rat brain tumor as a result of phagocytosis by glioma cells *(153)*. Similarly, uptake of SPIOs by macrophages accumulating in inflammatory sites has been demonstrated in rats with clinical EAE (**Fig. 5**) *(154,155)*. In recent years, stem cell therapy has proven to be a promising means to improve neurological function in various brain pathologies. Hoehn et al. *(156)* and Modo et al. *(157)* performed longitudinal, in vivo MRI-based tracking of stem cells labeled with USPIOs or with a gadolinium complex that were implanted in the contralateral hemisphere after unilateral stroke in rats. Both studies demonstrated directed transhemispheric movement of the transplanted cells along the corpus callosum toward the peri-infarct region, which illustrates the potential of MRI to map the distribution, migration, and destination of transplanted cells for therapeutic purposes.

2.6.2. Molecular MRI

Molecular imaging involves the detection of biological processes at the cellular and molecular level (*see* reviews by Weissleder and Mahmood, **ref. *158*** and Blasberg, **ref. *159***). Molecular MRI makes use of dedicated MRI reporter probes that consist of a specific targeting element (e.g., monoclonal antibodies) and a MR-detectable label (e.g., paramagnetic atoms). Examples of molecular MRI in models of brain disorders are starting to emanate. Tumor-specific imaging can be achieved with tumor-targeted monoclonal antibodies conjugated to monocrystalline iron oxide nanoparticles, which has been shown to result in contrast enhancement of rat gliomas with the strongest

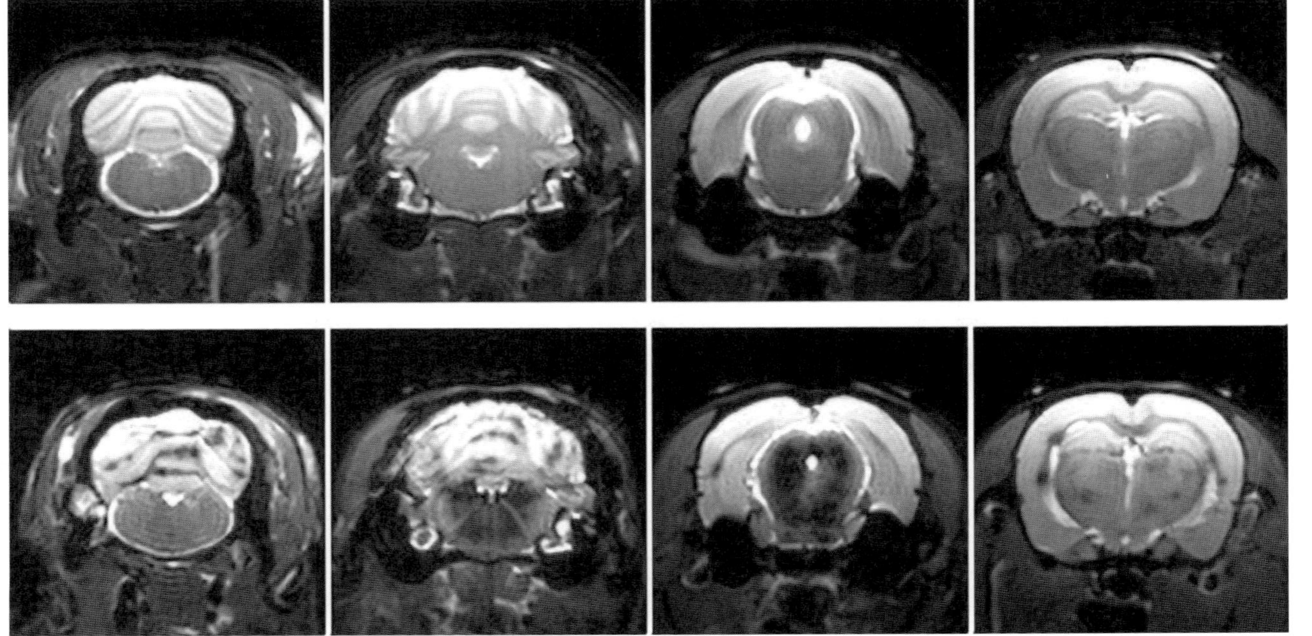

Fig. 5. T_2-weighted images of coronal brain slices at 24 h after intravenous injection of ultrasmall superparamagnetic iron oxide particles (USPIOs) (600 µmol Fe/kg; Sinerem, Guerbet, Aulnay sous Bois, France) at 9 d (top row) and 14 d (bottom row) after induction of experimental allergic encephalomyelitis (EAE) in rats. Monocyte-derived macrophages incorporate USPIOs and accumulate in inflammatory sites. These regions can be detected as hypointensities on T_2-weighted images because of the paramagnetic properties of the USPIOs. Massive accumulation of USPIO-containing macrophages was observed at the peak of the disease (i.e., 14 d after immunization; bottom row), but not at d-9, when neurological deficits were still absent (top row). (Modified from Floris et al., ref. *155*. Reprinted with permission from Oxford University Press. Courtesy of Drs. S. Floris and E. L. A. Blezer.)

effect in areas with highest tumor cell density *(160)*. Endothelial antigens that are expressed under pathophysiological conditions, such as leukocyte adhesion molecules, also provide significant targets for molecular MRI. Antibody-conjugated gadolinium-containing liposomes targeted to intracellular adhesion molecule-1 have been used to highlight areas with strong intracellular adhesion molecule-1 expression with ex vivo high-resolution T_1-weighted MRI after in vivo administration in mice with EAE *(161)*. With use of a specific Gd-DTPA complex that binds the adhesion molecule, E-selectin, Sibson et al. *(162)* recently detected acute in vivo neuroinflammation in rats after intracerebral injection of proinflammatory cytokines. In a transgenic mouse model for Alzheimer's disease, intravenously injected putrescine–gadolinium–amyloid-β peptide was shown to bind to β-amyloid plaques, resulting in selective plaque enhancement on postmortem T_1-weighted MR microscopic images *(163)*. Molecular MRI is still in its infancy in terms of in vivo application in brain injury models. Nevertheless, it has a promising future for the characterization of cellular and molecular processes in neurological disorders and in the assessment of gene-based therapy.

This review has given an overview of the potential of MRI to provide wide-ranging in vivo insight on brain pathophysiology in models of neurological disorders. Importantly, advances in MR technology (e.g., magnets with higher field strength, more powerful gradient systems, refined radio frequency coil design and increasing availability of targeted MR contrast agents) will allow MRI with even higher sensitivity, faster acquisition, and improved specificity. These progressions are expected to lead to unique insights into in vivo molecular and functional aspects of brain diseases and novel treatment strategies (e.g., cell-based therapies).

Acknowledgments

Drs. E. L. A. Blezer, W. B. Veldhuis, and O. Wu are gratefully acknowledged for critically reading the manuscript.

References

1. Buonanno, F. S., Pykett, I. L., Kistler, J. P., et al. (1982) Cranial anatomy and detection of ischemic stroke in the cat by nuclear magnetic resonance imaging. *Radiology* **143,** 187–193.
2. Levy, R. M., Mano, I., Brito, A., and Hosobuchi, Y. (1983) NMR imaging of acute experimental cerebral ischemia: time course and pharmacologic manipulations. *Am. J. Neuroradiol.* **4,** 238–241.
3. Stewart, W. A., Alvord, E. C., Hruby, S., Hall, L. D., and Paty, D. W. (1985) Early detection of experimental allergic encephalomyelitis by magnetic resonance imaging. *Lancet* **2,** 898.

4. Bederson, J. B., Bartkowski, H. M., Moon, K., et al. (1986) Nuclear magnetic resonance imaging and spectroscopy in experimental brain edema in a rat model. *J. Neurosurg.* **64,** 795–802.
5. O'Brien, J. T., Noseworthy, J. H., Gilbert, J. J., and Karlik, S. J. (1987) NMR changes in experimental allergic encephalomyelitis: NMR changes precede clinical and pathological events. *Magn. Reson. Med.* **5,** 109–117.
6. van Bruggen, N., Roberts, T. P., and Cremer, J. E. (1994) The application of magnetic resonance imaging to the study of experimental cerebral ischaemia. *Cerebrovasc. Brain Metab. Rev.* **6,** 180–210.
7. Kato, H., Kogure, K., Ohtomo, H., et al. (1986) Characterization of experimental ischemic brain edema utilizing proton nuclear magnetic resonance imaging. *J. Cereb. Blood Flow Metab.* **6,** 212–221.
8. Eis, M., Els, T., and Hoehn-Berlage, M. (1995) High resolution quantitative relaxation and diffusion MRI of three different experimental brain tumors in rat. *Magn. Reson. Med.* **34,** 835–844.
9. Hoehn-Berlage, M., Eis, M., Back, T., Kohno, K., and Yamashita, K. (1995) Changes of relaxation times (T1, T2) and apparent diffusion coefficient after permanent middle cerebral artery occlusion in the rat: temporal evolution, regional extent, and comparison with histology. *Magn. Reson. Med.* **34,** 824–834.
10. Bose, B., Jones, S. C., Lorig, R., Friel, H. T., Weinstein, M., and Little, J. R. (1988) Evolving focal cerebral ischemia in cats: spatial correlation of nuclear magnetic resonance imaging, cerebral blood flow, tetrazolium staining, and histopathology. *Stroke* **19,** 28–37.
11. Allegrini, P. R. and Sauer, D. (1992) Application of magnetic resonance imaging to the measurement of neurodegeneration in rat brain: MRI data correlate strongly with histology and enzymatic analysis. *Magn. Reson. Imaging* **10,** 773–778.
12. Palmer, G. C., Peeling, J., Corbett, D., Del Bigio, M. R., and Hudzik, T. J. (2001) T2-weighted MRI correlates with long-term histopathology, neurology scores, and skilled motor behavior in a rat stroke model. *Ann. N. Y. Acad. Sci.* **939,** 283–296.
13. Calamante, F., Lythgoe, M. F., Pell, G. S., et al. (1999) Early changes in water diffusion, perfusion, T1, and T2 during focal cerebral ischemia in the rat studied at 8.5 T. *Magn. Reson. Med.* **41,** 479–485.
14. Kettunen, M. I., Grohn, O. H., Lukkarinen, J. A., Vainio, P., Silvennoinen, M. J., and Kauppinen, R. A. (2000) Interrelations of T(1) and diffusion of water in acute cerebral ischemia of the rat. *Magn. Reson. Med.* **44,** 833–839.
15. Quast, M. J., Huang, N. C., Hillman, G. R., and Kent, T. A. (1993) The evolution of acute stroke recorded by multimodal magnetic resonance imaging. *Magn. Reson. Imaging* **11,** 465–471.
16. van der Toorn, A., Verheul, H. B., Berkelbach van der Sprenkel, J. W., Tulleken, C. A., and Nicolay, K. (1994) Changes in metabolites and tissue water status after focal ischemia in cat brain assessed with localized proton MR spectroscopy. *Magn. Reson. Med.* **32,** 685–691.
17. Ogawa, S., Lee, T. M., Kay, A. R., and Tank, D. W. (1990) Brain magnetic resonance imaging with contrast dependent on blood oxygenation. *Proc. Natl. Acad. Sci. USA* **87,** 9868–9872.

18. Gustafsson, O., Rossitti, S., Ericsson, A., and Raininko, R. (1999) MR imaging of experimentally induced intracranial hemorrhage in rabbits during the first 6 hours. *Acta Radiol.* **40,** 360–368.

19. Moseley, M. E., de Crespigny, A. J., Roberts, T. P., Kozniewska, E., and Kucharczyk, J. (1993) Early detection of regional cerebral ischemia using high-speed MRI. *Stroke* **24,** 160–165.

20. Ono, Y., Morikawa, S., Inubushi, T., Shimizu, H., and Yoshimoto, T. (1997) T2*-weighted magnetic resonance imaging of cerebrovascular reactivity in rat reversible focal cerebral ischemia. *Brain Res.* **744,** 207–215.

21. Mazurchuk, R., Zhou, R., Straubinger, R. M., Chau, R. I., and Grossman, Z. (1999) Functional magnetic resonance (fMR) imaging of a rat brain tumor model: implications for evaluation of tumor microvasculature and therapeutic response. *Magn. Reson. Imaging* **17,** 537–548.

22. Runge, V. M., Price, A. C., Wehr, C. J., Atkinson, J. B., and Tweedle, M. F. (1985) Contrast enhanced MRI. Evaluation of a canine model of osmotic blood-brain barrier disruption. *Invest. Radiol.* **20,** 830–844.

23. Whelan, H. T., Clanton, J. A., Moore, P. M., Tolner, D. J., Kessler, R. M., and Whetsell, W. O., Jr. (1987) Magnetic resonance brain tumor imaging in canine glioma. *Neurology* **37,** 1235–1239.

24. Wilkins, D. E., Raaphorst, G. P., Saunders, J. K., Sutherland, G. R., and Smith, I. C. (1995) Correlation between Gd-enhanced MR imaging and histopathology in treated and untreated 9L rat brain tumors. *Magn. Reson. Imaging* **13,** 89–96.

25. McNamara, M. T., Brant-Zawadzki, M., Berry, I., et al. (1986) Acute experimental cerebral ischemia: MR enhancement using Gd-DTPA. *Radiology* **158,** 701–705.

26. Van de Vyver, F. L. and Peersman, G. V. (1990) Experimental cerebral infarction in the rat: utility of Gd-DOTA for MR imaging. *Magn. Reson. Imaging* **8,** 333–340.

27. Hawkins, C. P., Munro, P. M., MacKenzie, F., et al. (1990) Duration and selectivity of blood-brain barrier breakdown in chronic relapsing experimental allergic encephalomyelitis studied by gadolinium-DTPA and protein markers. *Brain* **113 (Pt 2),** 365–378.

28. Namer, I. J., Steibel, J., Poulet, P., Armspach, J. P., Mauss, Y., and Chambron, J. (1992) In vivo dynamic MR imaging of MBP-induced acute experimental allergic encephalomyelitis in Lewis rat. *Magn. Reson. Med.* **24,** 325–334.

29. Karlik, S. J., Grant, E. A., Lee, D., and Noseworthy, J. H. (1993) Gadolinium enhancement in acute and chronic-progressive experimental allergic encephalomyelitis in the guinea pig. *Magn. Reson. Med.* **30,** 326–331.

30. van der Sanden, B. P., Rozijn, T. H., Rijken, P. F., et al. (2000) Noninvasive assessment of the functional neovasculature in 9L-glioma growing in rat brain by dynamic 1H magnetic resonance imaging of gadolinium uptake. *J. Cereb. Blood Flow Metab.* **20,** 861–870.

31. Neumann-Haefelin, T., Kastrup, A., de Crespigny, A., et al. (2000) Serial MRI after transient focal cerebral ischemia in rats: dynamics of tissue injury, blood-brain barrier damage, and edema formation. *Stroke* **31,** 1965–1972; discussion 1972–1963.

32. Knight, R. A., Barker, P. B., Fagan, S. C., Li, Y., Jacobs, M. A., and Welch, K. M. (1998) Prediction of impending hemorrhagic transformation in ischemic stroke using magnetic resonance imaging in rats. *Stroke* **29,** 144–151.

33. Dijkhuizen, R. M., Asahi, M., Wu, O., Rosen, B. R., and Lo, E. H. (2001) Delayed rt-PA treatment in a rat embolic stroke model: diagnosis and prognosis of ischemic injury and hemorrhagic transformation with magnetic resonance imaging. *J. Cereb. Blood Flow Metab.* **21,** 964–971.

34. Balaban, R. S. and Ceckler, T. L. (1992) Magnetization transfer contrast in magnetic resonance imaging. *Magn. Reson. Q* **8,** 116–137.

35. Brochet, B. and Dousset, V. (1999) Pathological correlates of magnetization transfer imaging abnormalities in animal models and humans with multiple sclerosis. *Neurology* **53,** S12–S17.

36. Dousset, V., Brochet, B., Vital, A., et al. (1995) Lysolecithin-induced demyelination in primates: preliminary in vivo study with MR and magnetization transfer. *Am. J. Neuroradiol.* **16,** 225–231.

37. Deloire-Grassin, M. S., Brochet, B., Quesson, B., et al. (2000) In vivo evaluation of remyelination in rat brain by magnetization transfer imaging. *J. Neurol. Sci.* **178,** 10–16.

38. Gareau, P. J., Rutt, B. K., Karlik, S. J., and Mitchell, J. R. (2000) Magnetization transfer and multicomponent T2 relaxation measurements with histopathologic correlation in an experimental model of MS. *J. Magn. Reson. Imaging* **11,** 586–595.

39. Ordidge, R. J., Helpern, J. A., Knight, R. A., Qing, Z. X., and Welch, K. M. (1991) Investigation of cerebral ischemia using magnetization transfer contrast (MTC) MR imaging. *Magn. Reson. Imaging* **9,** 895–902.

40. Ewing, J. R., Jiang, Q., Boska, M., et al. (1999) T1 and magnetization transfer at 7 Tesla in acute ischemic infarct in the rat. *Magn. Reson. Med.* **41,** 696–705.

41. Makela, H. I., Kettunen, M. I., Grohn, O. H., and Kauppinen, R. A. (2002) Quantitative T(1rho) and magnetization transfer magnetic resonance imaging of acute cerebral ischemia in the rat. *J. Cereb. Blood Flow Metab.* **22,** 547–558.

42. Ikezaki, K., Takahashi, M., Koga, H., et al. (1997) Apparent diffusion coefficient (ADC) and magnetization transfer contrast (MTC) mapping of experimental brain tumor. *Acta Neurochir. Suppl. (Wien)* **70,** 170–172.

43. Quesson, B., Bouzier, A. K., Thiaudiere, E., Delalande, C., Merle, M., and Canioni, P. (1997) Magnetization transfer fast imaging of implanted glioma in the rat brain at 4.7 T: interpretation using a binary spin-bath model. *J. Magn. Reson. Imaging* **7,** 1076–1083.

44. Smith, D. H., Meaney, D. F., Lenkinski, R. E., et al. (1995) New magnetic resonance imaging techniques for the evaluation of traumatic brain injury. *J. Neurotrauma* **12,** 573–577.

45. Kimura, H., Meaney, D. F., McGowan, J. C., et al. (1996) Magnetization transfer imaging of diffuse axonal injury following experimental brain injury in the pig: characterization by magnetization transfer ratio with histopathologic correlation. *J. Comput. Assist. Tomogr.* **20,** 540–546.

46. Le Bihan, D. (1988) Intravoxel incoherent motion imaging using steady-state free precession. *Magn. Reson. Med.* **7,** 346–351.
47. Moseley, M. E., Cohen, Y., Mintorovitch, J., et al. (1990) Early detection of regional cerebral ischemia in cats: comparison of diffusion- and T2-weighted MRI and spectroscopy. *Magn. Reson. Med.* **14,** 330–346.
48. Benveniste, H., Hedlund, L. W., and Johnson, G. A. (1992) Mechanism of detection of acute cerebral ischemia in rats by diffusion-weighted magnetic resonance microscopy. *Stroke* **23,** 746–754.
49. Verheul, H. B., Balazs, R., Berkelbach van der Sprenkel, et al. (1994) Comparison of diffusion-weighted MRI with changes in cell volume in a rat model of brain injury. *NMR Biomed.* **7,** 96–100.
50. van der Toorn, A., Sykova, E., Dijkhuizen, R. M., et al. (1996) Dynamic changes in water ADC, energy metabolism, extracellular space volume, and tortuosity in neonatal rat brain during global ischemia. *Magn. Reson. Med.* **36,** 52–60.
51. Nicolay, K., van der Toorn, A., and Dijkhuizen, R. M. (1995) In vivo diffusion spectroscopy. An overview. *NMR Biomed.* **8,** 365–374.
52. Nicolay, K., Braun, K. P., Graaf, R. A., Dijkhuizen, R. M., and Kruiskamp, M. J. (2001) Diffusion NMR spectroscopy. *N. M. R. Biomed.* **14,** 94–111.
53. Gass, A., Niendorf, T., and Hirsch, J. G. (2001) Acute and chronic changes of the apparent diffusion coefficient in neurological disorders—biophysical mechanisms and possible underlying histopathology. *J. Neurol. Sci.* **186 (Suppl. 1),** S15–S23.
54. Hoehn-Berlage, M. (1995) Diffusion-weighted NMR imaging: application to experimental focal cerebral ischemia. *NMR Biomed.* **8,** 345–358.
55. Hoehn, M., Nicolay, K., Franke, C., and van der Sanden, B. (2001) Application of magnetic resonance to animal models of cerebral ischemia. *J. Magn. Reson. Imaging* **14,** 491–509.
56. Rumpel, H., Nedelcu, J., Aguzzi, A., and Martin, E. (1997) Late glial swelling after acute cerebral hypoxia-ischemia in the neonatal rat: a combined magnetic resonance and histochemical study. *Pediatr. Res.* **42,** 54–59.
57. Thornton, J. S., Ordidge, R. J., Penrice, J., et al. (1997) Anisotropic water diffusion in white and gray matter of the neonatal piglet brain before and after transient hypoxia-ischaemia. *Magn. Reson. Imaging* **15,** 433–440.
58. D'Arceuil, H. E., de Crespigny, A. J., Rother, J., et al. (1998) Diffusion and perfusion magnetic resonance imaging of the evolution of hypoxic ischemic encephalopathy in the neonatal rabbit. *J. Magn. Reson. Imaging* **8,** 820–828.
59. Hanstock, C. C., Faden, A. I., Bendall, M. R., and Vink, R. (1994) Diffusion-weighted imaging differentiates ischemic tissue from traumatized tissue. *Stroke* **25,** 843–848.
60. Ito, J., Marmarou, A., Barzo, P., Fatouros, P., and Corwin, F. (1996) Characterization of edema by diffusion-weighted imaging in experimental traumatic brain injury. *J. Neurosurg.* **84,** 97–103.
61. Busch, E., Beaulieu, C., de Crespigny, A., and Moseley, M. E. (1998) Diffusion MR imaging during acute subarachnoid hemorrhage in rats. *Stroke* **29,** 2155–2161.

62. Piepgras, A., Elste, V., Frietsch, T., Schmiedek, P., Reith, W., and Schilling, L. (2001) Effect of moderate hypothermia on experimental severe subarachnoid hemorrhage, as evaluated by apparent diffusion coefficient changes. *Neurosurgery* **48,** 1128–1134; discussion 1134–1125.

63. van den Bergh, W. M., Zuur, J. K., Kamerling, N. A., et al. (2002) Role of magnesium in the reduction of ischemic depolarization and lesion volume after experimental subarachnoid hemorrhage. *J. Neurosurg.* **97,** 416–422.

64. Busza, A. L., Allen, K. L., King, M. D., van Bruggen, N., Williams, S. R., and Gadian, D. G. (1992) Diffusion-weighted imaging studies of cerebral ischemia in gerbils. Potential relevance to energy failure. *Stroke* **23,** 1602–1612.

65. Perez-Trepichio, A. D., Xue, M., Ng, T. C., et al. (1995) Sensitivity of magnetic resonance diffusion-weighted imaging and regional relationship between the apparent diffusion coefficient and cerebral blood flow in rat focal cerebral ischemia. *Stroke* **26,** 667–674; discussion 674–665.

66. Verheul, H. B., Tamminga, K. S., Dijkhuizen, R. M., et al. (1994) Focal ischemia in cat brain as studied by diffusion-weighted and dynamic susceptibility-contrast magnetic resonance imaging. *MAGMA* **2,** 367–370.

67. Kohno, K., Hoehn-Berlage, M., Mies, G., Back, T., and Hossmann, K. A. (1995) Relationship between diffusion-weighted MR images, cerebral blood flow, and energy state in experimental brain infarction. *Magn. Reson. Imaging* **13,** 73–80.

68. Mancuso, A., Karibe, H., Rooney, W. D., et al. (1995) Correlation of early reduction in the apparent diffusion coefficient of water with blood flow reduction during middle cerebral artery occlusion in rats. *Magn. Reson. Med.* **34,** 368–377.

69. Verheul, H. B., Balazs, R., Berkelbach van der Sprenkel, J. W., Tulleken, C. A., Nicolay, K., and van Lookeren Campagne, M. (1993) Temporal evolution of NMDA-induced excitotoxicity in the neonatal rat brain measured with 1H nuclear magnetic resonance imaging. *Brain Res.* **618,** 203–212.

70. Dijkhuizen, R. M., van Lookeren Campagne, M., Niendorf, T., et al. (1996) Status of the neonatal rat brain after NMDA-induced excitotoxic injury as measured by MRI, MRS and metabolic imaging. *NMR Biomed.* **9,** 84–92.

71. Zhong, J., Petroff, O. A., Prichard, J. W., and Gore, J. C. (1993) Changes in water diffusion and relaxation properties of rat cerebrum during status epilepticus. *Magn. Reson. Med.* **30,** 241–246.

72. Righini, A., Pierpaoli, C., Alger, J. R., and Di Chiro, G. (1994) Brain parenchyma apparent diffusion coefficient alterations associated with experimental complex partial status epilepticus. *Magn. Reson. Imaging* **12,** 865–871.

73. Wall, C. J., Kendall, E. J., and Obenaus, A. (2000) Rapid alterations in diffusion-weighted images with anatomic correlates in a rodent model of status epilepticus *Am. J. Neuroradiol.* **21,** 1841–1852.

74. van Lookeren Campagne, M., Verheul, J. B., Nicolay, K., and Balazs, R. (1994) Early evolution and recovery from excitotoxic injury in the neonatal rat brain: a study combining magnetic resonance imaging, electrical impedance, and histology. *J. Cereb. Blood Flow Metab.* **14,** 1011–1023.

75. Zarow, G. J., Graham, S. H., Mintorovitch, J., Chen, J., Yang, G., and Weinstein, P. R. (1995) Diffusion-weighted magnetic resonance imaging during brief focal cerebral ischemia and early reperfusion: evolution of delayed infarction in rats. *Neurol. Res.* **17**, 449–454.

76. Dijkhuizen, R. M., Knollema, S., van der Worp, H. B., et al. (1998) Dynamics of cerebral tissue injury and perfusion after temporary hypoxia-ischemia in the rat: evidence for region-specific sensitivity and delayed damage. *Stroke* **29**, 695–704.

77. Li, F., Han, S. S., Tatlisumak, T., et al. (1999) Reversal of acute apparent diffusion coefficient abnormalities and delayed neuronal death following transient focal cerebral ischemia in rats. *Ann. Neurol.* **46**, 333–342.

78. van Lookeren Campagne, M., Thomas, G. R., Thibodeaux, H., et al. (1999) Secondary reduction in the apparent diffusion coefficient of water, increase in cerebral blood volume, and delayed neuronal death after middle cerebral artery occlusion and early reperfusion in the rat. *J. Cereb. Blood Flow Metab.* **19**, 1354–1364.

79. Jiang, Q., Zhang, Z. G., Chopp, M., et al. (1993) Temporal evolution and spatial distribution of the diffusion constant of water in rat brain after transient middle cerebral artery occlusion. *J. Neurol. Sci.* **120**, 123–130.

80. Verheul, H. B., Berkelbach van der Sprenkel, J. W., Tulleken, C. A., Tamminga, K. S., and Nicolay, K. (1992) Temporal evolution of focal cerebral ischemia in the rat assessed by T2-weighted and diffusion-weighted magnetic resonance imaging. *Brain Topogr.* **5**, 171–176.

81. Knight, R. A., Dereski, M. O., Helpern, J. A., Ordidge, R. J., and Chopp, M. (1994) Magnetic resonance imaging assessment of evolving focal cerebral ischemia. Comparison with histopathology in rats. *Stroke* **25**, 1252–1261; discussion 1261–1252.

82. Pierpaoli, C., Righini, A., Linfante, I., Tao-Cheng, J. H., Alger, J. R., and Di Chiro, G. (1993) Histopathologic correlates of abnormal water diffusion in cerebral ischemia: diffusion-weighted MR imaging and light and electron microscopic study. *Radiology* **189**, 439–448.

83. Matsumoto, K., Lo, E. H., Pierce, A. R., Wei, H., Garrido, L., and Kowall, N. W. (1995) Role of vasogenic edema and tissue cavitation in ischemic evolution on diffusion-weighted imaging: comparison with multiparameter MR and immunohistochemistry. *Am. J. Neuroradiol.* **16**, 1107–1115.

84. Heide, A. C., Richards, T. L., Alvord, E. C., Jr., Peterson, J., and Rose, L. M. (1993) Diffusion imaging of experimental allergic encephalomyelitis. *Magn. Reson. Med.* **29**, 478–484.

85. Richards, T. L., Alvord, E. C., Jr., He, Y., et al. (1995) Experimental allergic encephalomyelitis in non-human primates: diffusion imaging of acute and chronic brain lesions. *Mult. Scler.* **1**, 109–117.

86. Braun, K. P., Dijkhuizen, R. M., de Graaf, R. A., et al. (1997) Cerebral ischemia and white matter edema in experimental hydrocephalus: a combined in vivo MRI and MRS study. *Brain Res.* **757**, 295–298.

87. Kauppinen, R. A. (2002) Monitoring cytotoxic tumour treatment response by diffusion magnetic resonance imaging and proton spectroscopy. *NMR Biomed.* **15**, 6–17.

88. Ross, B. D., Chenevert, T. L., and Rehemtulla, A. (2002) Magnetic resonance imaging in cancer research. *Eur. J. Cancer* **38**, 2147–2156.

89. Chenevert, T. L., McKeever, P. E., and Ross, B. D. (1997) Monitoring early response of experimental brain tumors to therapy using diffusion magnetic resonance imaging. *Clin. Cancer Res.* **3**, 1457–1466.

90. Basser, P. J., Mattiello, J., and LeBihan, D. (1994) Estimation of the effective self-diffusion tensor from the NMR spin echo. *J. Magn. Reson. B* **103**, 247–254.

91. van Gelderen, P., de Vleeschouwer, M. H., DesPres, D., Pekar, J., van Zijl, P. C., and Moonen, C. T. (1994) Water diffusion and acute stroke. *Magn. Reson. Med.* **31**, 154–163.

92. Lythgoe, M. F., Busza, A. L., Calamante, F., et al. (1997) Effects of diffusion anisotropy on lesion delineation in a rat model of cerebral ischemia. *Magn. Reson. Med.* **38**, 662–668.

93. Basser, P. J. and Pierpaoli, C. (1996) Microstructural and physiological features of tissues elucidated by quantitative-diffusion-tensor MRI. *J. Magn. Reson. B* **111**, 209–219.

94. Sotak, C. H. (2002) The role of diffusion tensor imaging in the evaluation of ischemic brain injury—a review. *NMR Biomed.* **15**, 561–569.

95. Song, S. K., Sun, S. W., Ramsbottom, M. J., Chang, C., Russell, J., and Cross, A. H. (2002) Dysmyelination revealed through MRI as increased radial (but unchanged axial) diffusion of water. *Neuroimage* **17**, 1429–1436.

96. Xue, R., van Zijl, P. C., Crain, B. J., Solaiyappan, M., and Mori, S. (1999) In vivo three-dimensional reconstruction of rat brain axonal projections by diffusion tensor imaging. *Magn. Reson. Med.* **42**, 1123–1127.

97. Zhang, J., van Zijl, P. C., and Mori, S. (2002) Three-dimensional diffusion tensor magnetic resonance microimaging of adult mouse brain and hippocampus. *Neuroimage* **15**, 892–901.

98. Hossmann, K. A. and Hoehn-Berlage, M. (1995) Diffusion and perfusion MR imaging of cerebral ischemia. *Cerebrovasc. Brain Metab. Rev.* **7**, 187–217.

99. Calamante, F., Thomas, D. L., Pell, G. S., Wiersma, J., and Turner, R. (1999) Measuring cerebral blood flow using magnetic resonance imaging techniques. *J. Cereb. Blood Flow Metab.* **19**, 701–735.

100. Rosen, B. R., Belliveau, J. W., Vevea, J. M., and Brady, T. J. (1990) Perfusion imaging with NMR contrast agents. *Magn. Reson. Med.* **14**, 249–265.

101. Ostergaard, L., Weisskoff, R. M., Chesler, D. A., Gyldensted, C., and Rosen, B. R. (1996) High resolution measurement of cerebral blood flow using intravascular tracer bolus passages. Part I: Mathematical approach and statistical analysis. *Magn. Reson. Med.* **36**, 715–725.

102. Wittlich, F., Kohno, K., Mies, G., Norris, D. G., and Hoehn-Berlage, M. (1995) Quantitative measurement of regional blood flow with gadolinium diethylenetriaminepentaacetate bolus track NMR imaging in cerebral infarcts in rats: validation with the iodo[14C]antipyrine technique. *Proc. Natl. Acad. Sci. USA* **92**, 1846–1850.

103. Sakoh, M., Rohl, L., Gyldensted, C., Gjedde, A., and Ostergaard, L. (2000) Cerebral blood flow and blood volume measured by magnetic resonance imaging bolus tracking after acute stroke in pigs: comparison with [(15)O]H(2)O positron emission tomography. *Stroke* **31,** 1958–1964.

104. Maeda, M., Itoh, S., Ide, H., et al. (1993) Acute stroke in cats: comparison of dynamic susceptibility-contrast MR imaging with T2- and diffusion-weighted MR imaging. *Radiology* **189,** 227–232.

105. Roberts, T. P., Vexler, Z., Derugin, N., Moseley, M. E., and Kucharczyk, J. (1993) High-speed MR imaging of ischemic brain injury following stenosis of the middle cerebral artery. *J. Cereb. Blood Flow Metab.* **13,** 940–946.

106. Hamberg, L. M., Macfarlane, R., Tasdemiroglu, E., et al. (1993) Measurement of cerebrovascular changes in cats after transient ischemia using dynamic magnetic resonance imaging. *Stroke* **24,** 444–450; discussion 450–441.

107. Kucharczyk, J., Vexler, Z. S., Roberts, T. P., et al. (1993) Echo-planar perfusion-sensitive MR imaging of acute cerebral ischemia. *Radiology* **188,** 711–717.

108. Minematsu, K., Fisher, M., Li, L., and Sotak, C. H. (1993) Diffusion and perfusion magnetic resonance imaging studies to evaluate a noncompetitive N-methyl-D-aspartate antagonist and reperfusion in experimental stroke in rats. *Stroke* **24,** 2074–2081.

109. Pathak, A. P., Schmainda, K. M., Ward, B. D., Linderman, J. R., Rebro, K. J., and Greene, A. S. (2001) MR-derived cerebral blood volume maps: issues regarding histological validation and assessment of tumor angiogenesis. *Magn. Reson. Med.* **46,** 735–747.

110. Cha, S., Johnson, G., Wadghiri, Y. Z., et al. (2003) Dynamic, contrast-enhanced perfusion MRI in mouse gliomas: correlation with histopathology. *Magn. Reson. Med.* **49,** 848–855.

111. Hamberg, L. M., Boccalini, P., Stranjalis, G., et al. (1996) Continuous assessment of relative cerebral blood volume in transient ischemia using steady state susceptibility-contrast MRI. *Magn. Reson. Med.* **35,** 168–173.

112. Mandeville, J. B., Marota, J. J., Kosofsky, B. E., et al. (1998) Dynamic functional imaging of relative cerebral blood volume during rat forepaw stimulation. *Magn. Reson. Med.* **39,** 615–624.

113. Zaharchuk, G., Yamada, M., Sasamata, M., Jenkins, B. G., Moskowitz, M. A., and Rosen, B. R. (2000) Is all perfusion-weighted magnetic resonance imaging for stroke equal? The temporal evolution of multiple hemodynamic parameters after focal ischemia in rats correlated with evidence of infarction. *J. Cereb. Blood Flow Metab.* **20,** 1341–1351.

114. Boxerman, J. L., Bandettini, P. A., Kwong, K. K., et al. M. (1995) The intravascular contribution to fMRI signal change: Monte Carlo modeling and diffusion-weighted studies in vivo. *Magn. Reson. Med.* **34,** 4–10.

115. Dennie, J., Mandeville, J. B., Boxerman, J. L., Packard, S. D., Rosen, B. R., and Weisskoff, R. M. (1998) NMR imaging of changes in vascular morphology due to tumor angiogenesis. *Magn. Reson. Med.* **40,** 793–799.

116. Le Duc, G., Peoc'h, M., Remy, C., et al. (1999) Use of T(2)-weighted suscepti-bility contrast MRI for mapping the blood volume in the glioma-bearing rat brain. *Magn. Reson. Med.* **42,** 754–761.

117. Jensen, J. H. and Chandra, R. (2000) MR imaging of microvasculature. *Magn. Reson. Med.* **44,** 224–230.

118. Detre, J. A., Leigh, J. S., Williams, D. S., and Koretsky, A. P. (1992) Perfusion imaging. *Magn. Reson. Med.* **23,** 37–45.

119. Kwong, K. K., Belliveau, J. W., Chesler, D. A., et al. (1992) Dynamic magnetic resonance imaging of human brain activity during primary sensory stimulation. *Proc. Natl. Acad. Sci. USA* **89,** 5675–5679.

120. Kim, S. G. (1995) Quantification of relative cerebral blood flow change by flow-sensitive alternating inversion recovery (FAIR) technique: application to func-tional mapping. *Magn. Reson. Med.* **34,** 293–301.

121. Detre, J. A., Zhang, W., Roberts, D. A., et al. (1994) Tissue specific perfusion imaging using arterial spin labeling. *NMR Biomed.* **7,** 75–82.

122. Tsekos, N. V., Zhang, F., Merkle, H., Nagayama, M., Iadecola, C., and Kim, S. G. (1998) Quantitative measurements of cerebral blood flow in rats using the FAIR technique: correlation with previous iodoantipyrine autoradiographic stud-ies. *Magn. Reson. Med.* **39,** 564–573.

123. Zaharchuk, G., Bogdanov, A. A., Jr., Marota, J. J., et al. (1998) Continuous as-sessment of perfusion by tagging including volume and water extraction (CAP-TIVE): a steady-state contrast agent technique for measuring blood flow, relative blood volume fraction, and the water extraction fraction. *Magn. Reson. Med.* **40,** 666–678.

124. Pell, G. S., Lythgoe, M. F., Thomas, D. L., et al. (1999) Reperfusion in a gerbil model of forebrain ischemia using serial magnetic resonance FAIR perfusion imaging. *Stroke* **30,** 1263–1270.

125. van Dorsten, F. A., Hata, R., Maeda, K., et al. (1999) Diffusion- and perfusion-weighted MR imaging of transient focal cerebral ischaemia in mice. *NMR Biomed.* **12,** 525–534.

126. Forbes, M. L., Hendrich, K. S., Kochanek, P. M., et al. (1997) Assessment of cerebral blood flow and CO2 reactivity after controlled cortical impact by perfu-sion magnetic resonance imaging using arterial spin-labeling in rats. *J. Cereb. Blood Flow Metab.* **17,** 865–874.

127. Silva, A. C., Kim, S. G., and Garwood, M. (2000) Imaging blood flow in brain tumors using arterial spin labeling. *Magn. Reson. Med.* **44,** 169–173.

128. Schepers, J., Veldhuis, W. B., Pauw, R. J., et al. (2004) Comparison of FAIR perfusion kinetics with DSC-MRI and functional histology in a model of tran-sient ischemia. *Magn. Reson. Med.* **51,** 312–320.

129. Zhang, W., Silva, A. C., Williams, D. S., and Koretsky, A. P. (1995) NMR mea-surement of perfusion using arterial spin labeling without saturation of macro-molecular spins. *Magn. Reson. Med.* **33,** 370–376.

130. Hyder, F., Behar, K. L., Martin, M. A., Blamire, A. M., and Shulman, R. G. (1994) Dynamic magnetic resonance imaging of the rat brain during forepaw stimulation. *J. Cereb. Blood Flow Metab.* **14,** 649–655.

131. Silva, A. C., Zhang, W., Williams, D. S., and Koretsky, A. P. (1995) Multi-slice MRI of rat brain perfusion during amphetamine stimulation using arterial spin labeling. *Magn. Reson. Med.* **33,** 209–214.

132. Kerskens, C. M., Hoehn-Berlage, M., Schmitz, B., et al. (1996) Ultrafast perfusion-weighted MRI of functional brain activation in rats during forepaw stimulation: comparison with T2 -weighted MRI. *N. M. R. Biomed.* **9,** 20–23.

133. Kennan, R. P., Scanley, B. E., Innis, R. B., and Gore, J. C. (1998) Physiological basis for BOLD MR signal changes due to neuronal stimulation: separation of blood volume and magnetic susceptibility effects. *Magn. Reson. Med.* **40,** 840–846.

134. van Bruggen, N., Busch, E., Palmer, J. T., Williams, S. P., and de Crespigny, A. J. (1998) High-resolution functional magnetic resonance imaging of the rat brain: mapping changes in cerebral blood volume using iron oxide contrast media. *J. Cereb. Blood Flow Metab.* **18,** 1178–1183.

135. Lin, Y. J. and Koretsky, A. P. (1997) Manganese ion enhances T1-weighted MRI during brain activation: an approach to direct imaging of brain function. *Magn. Reson. Med.* **38,** 378–388.

136. Pautler, R. G., Silva, A. C., and Koretsky, A. P. (1998) In vivo neuronal tract tracing using manganese-enhanced magnetic resonance imaging. *Magn. Reson. Med.* **40,** 740–748.

137. Schmitz, B., Bock, C., Hoehn-Berlage, M., Kerskens, C. M., Bottiger, B. W., and Hossmann, K. A. (1998) Recovery of the rodent brain after cardiac arrest: a functional MRI study. *Magn. Reson. Med.* **39,** 783–788.

138. Reese, T., Porszasz, R., Baumann, D., et al. (2000) Cytoprotection does not preserve brain functionality in rats during the acute post-stroke phase despite evidence of non-infarction provided by MRI. *NMR Biomed.* **13,** 361–370.

139. Abo, M., Chen, Z., Lai, L. J., Reese, T., and Bjelke, B. (2001) Functional recovery after brain lesion–contralateral neuromodulation: an fMRI study. *Neuroreport* **12,** 1543–1547.

140. Dijkhuizen, R. M., Ren, J., Mandeville, J. B., Wu, O., et al. (2001) Functional magnetic resonance imaging of reorganization in rat brain after stroke. *Proc. Natl. Acad. Sci. U. S. A.* **98,** 12,766–12,771.

141. Tuor, U. I., Hudzik, T. J., Malisza, K., Sydserff, S., Kozlowski, P., and Del Bigio, M. R. (2001) Long-term deficits following cerebral hypoxia-ischemia in four-week-old rats: correspondence between behavioral, histological, and magnetic resonance imaging assessments. *Exp. Neurol.* **167,** 272–281.

142. Dijkhuizen, R. M., Singhal, A. B., Mandeville, J. B., et al. (2003) Correlation between brain reorganization, ischemic damage, and neurologic status after transient focal cerebral ischemia in rats: a functional magnetic resonance imaging study. *J. Neurosci.* **23,** 510–517.

143. Pelled, G., Bergman, H., and Goelman, G. (2002) Bilateral overactivation of the sensorimotor cortex in the unilateral rodent model of Parkinson's disease—a functional magnetic resonance imaging study. *Eur. J. Neurosci.* **15,** 389–394.

144. Opdam, H. I., Federico, P., Jackson, G. D., et al. (2002) A sheep model for the study of focal epilepsy with concurrent intracranial EEG and functional MRI. *Epilepsia* **43,** 779–787.

145. Chen, Q., Andersen, A. H., Zhang, Z., Ovadia, A., Gash, D. M., and Avison, M. J. (1996) Mapping drug-induced changes in cerebral R2* by multiple gradient recalled echo functional MRI. *Magn. Reson. Imaging* **14,** 469–476.

146. Chen, Y. C., Galpern, W. R., Brownell, A. L., et al. (1997) Detection of dopaminergic neurotransmitter activity using pharmacologic MRI: correlation with PET, microdialysis, and behavioral data. *Magn. Reson. Med.* **38,** 389–398.

147. Chen, Y. I., Brownell, A. L., Galpern, W., et al. (1999) Detection of dopaminergic cell loss and neural transplantation using pharmacological MRI, PET and behavioral assessment. *Neuroreport* **10,** 2881–2886.

148. Chen, Q., Andersen, A. H., Zhang, Z., et al. (1999) Functional MRI of basal ganglia responsiveness to levodopa in parkinsonian rhesus monkeys. *Exp. Neurol.* **158,** 63–75.

149. Reese, T., Bochelen, D., Baumann, D., Rausch, M., Sauter, A., and Rudin, M. (2002) Impaired functionality of reperfused brain tissue following short transient focal ischemia in rats. *Magn. Reson. Imaging* **20,** 447–454.

150. Mueggler, T., Sturchler-Pierrat, C., Baumann, D., Rausch, M., Staufenbiel, M., and Rudin, M. (2002) Compromised hemodynamic response in amyloid precursor protein transgenic mice. *J. Neurosci.* **22,** 7218–7224.

151. Norman, A. B., Thomas, S. R., Pratt, R. G., Lu, S. Y., and Norgren, R. B. (1992) Magnetic resonance imaging of neural transplants in rat brain using a superparamagnetic contrast agent. *Brain Res.* **594,** 279–283.

152. Bulte, J. W., Duncan, I. D., and Frank, J. A. (2002) In vivo magnetic resonance tracking of magnetically labeled cells after transplantation. *J. Cereb. Blood Flow Metab.* **22,** 899–907.

153. Zimmer, C., Weissleder, R., Poss, K., Bogdanova, A., Wright, S. C., Jr., and Enochs, W. S. (1995) MR imaging of phagocytosis in experimental gliomas. *Radiology* **197,** 533–538.

154. Dousset, V., Delalande, C., Ballarino, L., et al. (1999) In vivo macrophage activity imaging in the central nervous system detected by magnetic resonance. *Magn. Reson. Med.* **41,** 329–333.

155. Floris, S., Blezer, E. L., Schreibelt, G., et al. (2004) Blood-brain barrier permeability and monocyte infiltration in experimental allergic encephalomyelitis: a quantitative MRI study. *Brain* **127,** 616–627.

156. Hoehn, M., Kustermann, E., Blunk, J., et al. (2002) Monitoring of implanted stem cell migration in vivo: a highly resolved in vivo magnetic resonance imaging investigation of experimental stroke in rat. *Proc. Natl. Acad. Sci. USA* **99,** 16,267–16,272.

157. Modo, M., Mellodew, K., Cash, D., et al. (2004) Mapping transplanted stem cell migration after a stroke: a serial, in vivo magnetic resonance imaging study. *Neuroimage* **21,** 311–317.
158. Weissleder, R. and Mahmood, U. (2001) Molecular imaging. *Radiology* **219,** 316–333.
159. Blasberg, R. (2002) Imaging gene expression and endogenous molecular processes: molecular imaging. *J. Cereb. Blood Flow Metab.* **22,** 1157–1164.
160. Remsen, L. G., McCormick, C. I., Roman-Goldstein, S., et al. (1996) MR of carcinoma-specific monoclonal antibody conjugated to monocrystalline iron oxide nanoparticles: the potential for noninvasive diagnosis. *Am. J. Neuroradiol.* **17,** 411–418.
161. Sipkins, D. A., Gijbels, K., Tropper, F. D., Bednarski, M., Li, K. C., and Steinman, L. (2000) ICAM-1 expression in autoimmune encephalitis visualized using magnetic resonance imaging. *J. Neuroimmunol.* **104,** 1–9.
162. Sibson, N. R., Blamire, A. M., Bernades-Silva, M., et al. (2004) MRI detection of early endothelial activation in brain inflammation. *Magn. Reson. Med.* **51,** 248–252.
163. Poduslo, J. F., Wengenack, T. M., Curran, G. L., et al. (2002) Molecular targeting of Alzheimer's amyloid plaques for contrast-enhanced magnetic resonance imaging. *Neurobiol. Dis.* **11,** 315–329.

11

Magnetic Resonance Imaging of Tumor Physiology

Arvind P. Pathak

Summary

Cancer is one of the most mutable diseases known, exhibiting a superfluity and heterogeneity of molecular pathways that impart an almost chimerical nature to it. Exploiting these pathways for patient therapy demands an understanding of the physiology of tumors from the molecular to the systemic level. To this end, multiparametric functional and molecular imaging play a vital role in not only tracking delivery and efficacy of therapy, but also in discovering novel therapeutic targets. The plethora of available magnetic resonance (MR) contrast mechanisms, in conjunction with its superior dynamic functional range, bestow on magnetic resonance imaging (MRI) the potential to be a formidable tool in the noninvasive, in vivo, multilevel assessment of tumor physiology.

This chapter begins with a description of the aberrant pathophysiology of tumors, including a description of tumor angiogenesis and how MRI affords us a window into such processes. Following a discussion of endogenous and exogenous contrast, a specific example of measuring a tumor's vascular parameters with a macromolecular contrast agent is considered. This is followed by a description of revolutionary developments in the molecular imaging of tumors with MRI and complementary modalities.

Key Words: Cancer; tumor; angiogenesis; MRI; contrast agent; blood volume; permeability.

1. Introduction

The cells in our body replicate millions of times, with each cell knowing where, when, and what it is supposed to do. Any breakdown of this tightly regulated cell cycle, i.e., uncontrolled proliferation, often accompanied by cells spreading to distant sites (i.e., metastases) is the process we have broadly come to label cancer. In the past century, several diseases have fallen before the scythe of human ingenuity in the form of biomedical advances in our understanding of various disease processes; however, cancer, by virtue of its mercurial and adaptive nature, remains a scourge of humankind. Over the past several decades, we have slowly but surely been chipping away at the edifice of cancer. Whether these advances include the unmasking of critical molecular pathways, antiangiogenic therapy, or the identification of novel therapeutic targets,

From: *Methods in Molecular Medicine, Vol. 124*
Magnetic Resonance Imaging: Methods and Biologic Applications
Edited by: P. V. Prasad © Humana Press Inc., Totowa, NJ

there remains an exigent need for a safe method of monitoring and assessing the efficacy of such approaches. Moreover, any assessment method preferably needs to be noninvasive, enabling us to conduct such evaluations in vivo. As you will learn from this chapter, magnetic resonance imaging (MRI) with its plethora of contrast mechanisms is well up to this challenge.

2. Why Monitor Tumor Physiology?

Advances in cancer treatments have occurred at several levels, including, but not limited to, the molecular, cellular, tissue, and systemic levels. The degree of success of most of these therapies crucially depends on the underlying tumor physiology. This physiology, in turn, depends on the interaction between the tumor cells and their micro-milieu. Some of the aberrant microenvironmental factors in solid tumors are described briefly in **Subheading 3.** These include the abnormal architecture of tumor blood vessels, the resulting spatio–temporal heterogeneities in blood flow, which, in turn, results in variations in tumor oxygenation, pH, and energy status. Thus, an understanding of tumor structure, physiology, and metabolism has the potential to provide important insights into any treatment modality.

3. The Anomalous Pathophysiology of Tumors
3.1. Morphological Aspects of Tumor Angiogenesis

Tumor angiogenesis is the process via which avascular aggregates of tumor cells establish a blood supply derived from the host stroma, and angiogenesis is necessary for the establishment, proliferation, and metastasis of the tumor *(1)*. In addition to the process of *de novo* angiogenesis, certain tumors do not originate avascularly but initially grow by co-opting, i.e., incorporating preexisting host vessels into the tumor *(2)*. Several exquisite ultrastructural studies of the tumor vasculature have identified a variety of structural and functional discrepancies between tumor and normal vasculature *(3–5)*. Briefly, tumor microvessels are sinusoidal, fragile, and hyperpermeable, with discontinuous basement membranes. The additional hallmarks of such vessels are poor differentiation, leakiness, lack of smooth muscle cell lining, spatial heterogeneity, chaotic branching hierarchies, arterio–venous shunts, acute and transient collapse, and an inability to match the rapid proliferation of cancer cells, often producing areas of hypoxia and necrosis within the tumor.

3.2. Tumor Blood Flow

Because, as described in **Subheading 3.1.**, tumor microvessels exhibit such a superfluity of structural and functional anomalies, it is no surprise that the blood circulation or perfusion within such vessels is seldom correlated to the metabolic demands of the solid tumor. In fact, the high permeability of the tumor vessels often results in extravasation of erythrocytes and plasma, producing an elevated interstitial fluid pressure *(6)*. This elevated interstitial fluid pressure, in conjunction with the resulting hemoconcentration, leads to a rise in the viscous resistance to blood flow. The drastically altered vessel architecture and density also results in an increase in the geometric resistance to flow. Thus, overall, there exists a huge heterogeneity in tumor blood flow, with no correlation between either the blood flow rate or the perfusion efficiency within tumor vessels and the size or functional state of the tumor *(7)*.

3.3. Tumor Oxygenation

The irregularities in tumor perfusion, described in **Subheading 3.2.**, result in variations in supply of oxygen to the proliferating tumor cells. Thus, cancer cells in solid tumors and many human tumors often exist under hypoxic conditions. However, hypoxia found in solid tumors is usually of two kinds, depending on its cause. The first kind of hypoxia is caused by the poor perfusion efficiency of tumor blood vessels and is called perfusion-limited hypoxia. The second kind of hypoxia mainly arises from the fact that oxygen has to diffuse across larger intervessel distances to reach tumor cells, and is called diffusion-limited hypoxia. Overall, like tumor perfusion, the oxygenation of tumors is heterogeneous, compromised, and mostly unrelated to factors such as metabolic demand, tumor stage, and so on.

3.4. Tumor Metabolism and pH

In addition to hypoxia, the compromised tumor vasculature also results in the inadequate clearance of metabolic byproducts. Tumors rely mainly on the glycolytic pathway for satisfying their energy requirements *(8)*, resulting in the production of lactate and hydrogen ions. Not only does the poor clearance of hydrogen ions result in acidosis, but also, the pH gradient across the cell membranes in tumors has been found to be the reverse of that found in normal tissues, i.e., the extracellular pH is less than the intracellular pH *(9)*. This reversal in the pH gradient is thought to be mainly attributable to the rapid removal of hydrogen ions from the tumor cells *(10)*.Thus, an understanding of the anomalous pathophysiology of tumors is extremely important from both a diagnostic and treatment perspective.

4. MRI Affords a Window Into Tumor Physiology

Unlike other noninvasive imaging modalities, such as computed tomography, ultrasound, positron emission tomography (PET), and single-photon emission computerized tomography (SPECT), MRI is unique in that it offers a profuse array of contrast mechanisms that enable radiologists to probe several aspects of a tumor's physiology. This superior dynamic functional range of MRI in conjunction with its superior spatio–temporal resolution bestows on it the potential to be a formidable tool for probing the physiology of tumors noninvasively and in vivo. Magnetic resonance (MR) contrast mechanisms can be broadly classified into intrinsic or extrinsic contrast mechanisms.

4.1. Intrinsic or Endogenous Contrast

Intrinsic contrast is that which arises from a substance that occurs naturally within the body and in sufficiently high concentrations to influence the MR signal via some kind of magnetic property, such as susceptibility or magnetization transfer. An example of such a substance is deoxyhemoglobin.

4.1.1. The BOLD Contrast Mechanism

Probing the tumor vasculature using the endogenous contrast produced by deoxyhemoglobin in tumor vessels is based on the blood oxygenation level-dependent (BOLD) contrast mechanism first revealed by Ogawa et al. *(11)*. In this case, the concentration of paramagnetic deoxyhemoglobin (the endogenous contrast agent) is the primary determinant of the contrast observed in the final MR image. When deoxyhemoglobin (dHb) is present within a blood vessel, it not only produces a difference between the susceptibility of the vessel and the surrounding tissue (i.e., the extravascular component), but also between the red blood cells carrying dHb and the plasma (i.e., the intravascular component). During a typical MR measurement time, water rapidly exchanges between red blood cells and the plasma, and the diffusion of proton spins through the many microscopic dHb-induced magnetic fields results in motional averaging (i.e., time-irreversible averaging), which produces dephasing of the MR signal, that, in turn, leads to a reduction in the value of the blood water, T_2. On the other hand, additional phase dispersion arising from extravascular susceptibility-induced magnetic field gradients leads to a reduction in the value of T_2^*. Thus, the presence of deoxyhemoglobin in blood vessels causes image voxels containing vessels to appear darker in a T_2- or T_2^*-weighted imaging experiment. Because oxyhemoglobin is diamagnetic and does not induce an analogous dephasing of proton spins, blood oxygenation changes can be monitored as MR signal changes on T_2^*-weighted images. Some applications of the BOLD MR contrast mechanism include generation of maps of the functional tumor vasculature in genetically modified animal models *(12)*, as well as assessment of the risk of radiation resistance in cancer patients *(13)*. It is worth mentioning that BOLD MRI contrast is not solely determined by the deoxygenation status of the blood vessels and the MR pulse sequence used but is also affected by other factors, such as local hematocrit, oxygen saturation, blood flow, vessel orientation, and geometry *(14)*.

4.1.2. The ASL Contrast Mechanism

Native blood flow of tumors can be imaged using another endogenous MR contrast mechanism, arterial spin labeling (ASL) *(15)*. In this approach, the water protons within the arterial blood pool serve as the perfusion marker. More recently, this approach has been used for determining relative changes in the cerebral blood flow of patients with brain metastases, wherein it was demonstrated that after stereotaxic radiosurgery, ASL in conjunction with contrast agent-enhanced MRI had potential to predict treatment outcome *(16)*.

MRI using endogenous contrast has the additional advantages of being completely noninvasive, of not requiring the administration of any contrast agent or tracer pharmaceutical, and of allowing the radiologist to conduct the measurement of interest as many times as desired, yielding dynamic data with high temporal resolution. On the other hand, most endogenous MRI methods do not provide quantitative measures of the angiogenic tumor parameters, such as the vascular volume or vascular permeability; one has to resort to exogenous contrast MRI if such information is desired.

4.2. Extrinsic or Exogenous Contrast

Extrinsic contrast is that which arises from a pharmaceutical agent that is injected into the subject to alter the local magnetic field in a tissue of interest, thereby producing contrast in the MR image. Unlike the dyes or contrast agents developed for nuclear medicine or X-ray imaging, MR contrast agents are unique in that they are not visualized directly on the image, but indirectly, by virtue of the changes they induce in water relaxation behavior. The most commonly used contrast agents in MRI are paramagnetic gadolinium (Gd) chelates. These contrast agents are complexes of the rare earth element, Gd, and various chelating agents. The unpaired electrons of Gd produce a large magnetic moment that results in shortening of both the T_1 (spin–lattice relaxation time) and T_2 (spin–spin relaxation time) values of tissue water. Thus, on a T_1-weighted MR scan, tissues that take up the paramagnetic agent are brightened (i.e., positive enhancement), whereas on a T_2-weighted scan, the observed contrast is reversed (i.e., negative enhancement). Using tracer kinetic principles, the tissue concentration of Gd-based agents can be calculated from the MR image intensity. The Gd-based agents currently in use or under development can broadly be classified as either being low molecular weight (~0.57 kDa), e.g., the gadolinium diethylenetriamine pentaacetid acid (Gd-DTPA) compounds used in clinical studies of various pathologies including malignant tumors, or macromolecular agents (~65 kDa), such as albumin-(Gd-DTPA) compounds that remain in the intravascular space for up to several hours.

4.2.1. Low Molecular Weight Contrast Agents

The low molecular weight contrast agents class is the only class of paramagnetic agents approved for clinical use. As a result, there are several studies describing the use of such agents for imaging a variety of tumors, including those of the breast *(17)*, brain *(18)*, and uterus *(19)*. On the basis of one of

Table 1
Summary of Various Physiological Parameters of Tumors That Can Be Probed Using Different MRI Contrast Mechanisms and Techniques[a]

Contrast mechanism	Angiogenic parameter	Reference
Endogenous	Tumor oxygenation (BOLD)	*(11–13)*
	Tumor vascular volume	*(12)*
	Tumor blood flow (ASL)	*(15,16)*
Exogenous	Tumor vessel influx/outflux constants	*(20,21)*
	Tumor vascular volume	*(18,19,21–23,25–27)*
	Tumor permeability–surface area product	*(31,33,37)*
	Tumor blood flow	*(25)*
	Tumor vessel size	*(18,24)*
	Tumor vessel density	*(14,19,26)*
	Tumor leakiness	*(37)*
	Tumor grade	*(18,26)*
	Tumor receptor targeted	*(44,45)*

[a]BOLD, blood oxygenation level-dependent; ASL, arterial spin labeling.

several multicompartment models *(20)*, most T_1-based techniques involve the analyses of relaxivity changes induced by the contrast agent followed by the determination of influx/outflux transfer rates, as well as the extracellular extravascular volume fractions *(21)*. A large range of clinically relevant tumor parameters can be inferred from such approaches *(22)*. T_2 and T_2^* methods have also been used in the study of tumor angiogenesis. These methods rely on the susceptibility-induced effects of these contrast agents. In addition to the traditional tumor blood volume measurements by both T_1 *(22,23)* and T_2 *(18)* techniques, indices of tumor vessel size *(24)* and predictors of tumor grade *(25,26)* have been added to the clinician's repertoire (**Table 1**). With the advent of novel methods for the histological validation of low molecular weight MR approaches *(27)*, as well as techniques for correcting for the effects of agent extravasation that occurs by means of hyperpermeable tumor vessels *(18,28)*, the use of some of the parameters summarized in **Table 1** might soon become more widespread in the clinical assessment of the angiogenic status of tumors. Finally, it has also been demonstrated in a tumor xenograft study that the uptake kinetics of these low molecular weight MR contrast agents might be used to assess the efficacy of chemotherapeutic agent delivery to solid tumors *(29)*.

4.2.2. High Molecular Weight Contrast Agents

One drawback in the quantitation of tumor vascular parameters with low molecular weight contrast agents is their rapid leakage from the hyperpermeable tumor vasculature. The availability of high molecular weight or macromolecular contrast agents (MMCA) such as albumin-(Gd-DTPA) complexes or synthetic compounds, such as polylysine-Gd-DTPA and gadomer-17, provide a unique opportunity for the quantitative determination of tumor vascular volume and the permeability–surface area (PS) product for molecules of comparable sizes. The relatively slow leakage of these agents from the vasculature results in a long circulation half-life and rapid equilibration of plasma concentrations within the tumor. Assuming fast exchange of water protons between all of the tumor compartments, the concentration of the MMCA within any given voxel is proportional to the changes in relaxation rate ($\Delta R_1 = \Delta 1/T_1$) before ($1/T_{1pre}$) and after ($1/T_{1post}$) administration of the contrast agent, i.e., $\Delta R_1 = 1/T_{1post} - 1/T_{1pre}$. The changes in T_1 relaxation rates can be measured directly using either dynamic *(30)* or steady-state T_1 methods *(31)*. Voxel-wise maps constructed from the acquired relaxation data and fit to the appropriate compartmental model provide spatial maps of tumor vascular volume and PS. Briefly, assuming a simple two-compartment model and negligible reflux of the contrast agent, the contrast uptake can be modeled as a linear function of time. In this case, the slope of the concentration–time curve provides the parameter PS and the *y*-intercept provides the vascular volume *(32,33)*. Quantification of these parameters requires normalization to the changes in the relaxation rate of the blood, which can be obtained separately from blood samples taken before administration of the contrast agent and again at the end of the MR experiment. Details of this approach are given in the ensuing section. One should keep in mind that there exist several more complicated models of contrast uptake, and that the accuracy of the tissue vascular volume measurement depends on the rate of water exchange between the vascular and extracellular compartments *(34)*. Investigators have also used the MMCA approach for detecting the efficacy of different antiangiogenic therapies *(35,36)*. MRI was also used to explore whether there were any differences between the tumor vasculature of cancer xenografts of varying metastatic potential *(37)*. The study was not only able to noninvasively assess the role of the functional tumor vasculature in metastasis but also demonstrated that, although invasion was necessary, without adequate vascularization invasion was not sufficient for metastasis to occur.

5. Specific Example: Measurement of Tumor Vascular Volume and PS Product Using an MMCA

As mentioned in **Subheading 4.2.2.**, T_1-weighted MRI methods involve the analyses of relaxivity changes induced by the contrast agent based on one of several compartmental models *(21)*. Although these agents are not freely diffusible and remain in the extracellular compartment, three standard kinetic parameters can be derived from dynamic contrast-enhanced, T1-weighted MRI. These are:

1. K_{trans} (min^{-1})—the volume transfer constant between the intravascular and extravascular extracellular space (EES),
2. k_{ep} (min^{-1})—the rate constant describing transport between the EES and intravascular space, and
3. v_e (%)—the volume fraction of the EES *(20)*.

These three parameters are related by:

$$k_{ep} = \frac{K^{trans}}{v_e}. \tag{1}$$

K_{trans} has varying connotations, depending on the balance between blood flow and capillary permeability in the tissue of interest. For the purposes of this example, we will only consider a special case of the simple two-compartment (blood space and the EES) model, known as the PS-limited model. An excellent review of the different kinds of compartment models and their oncological applications may be found in *(20)* and *(38)*, respectively.

5.1. Modeling the Kinetics of the MMCA in the Blood

The differential equation for the simple model comprising of two compartments, i.e., the blood space and the EES, that relates the concentration in the EES (C_e) to that in the plasma (C_p) is given by:

$$\frac{dC_e}{dt} = K_{trans} C_p(t) - k_{ep} C_e(t), \tag{2}$$

where all concentrations are measured in mmol/mL. The solution to **Eq. [2]** in terms of the convolution integral is given by:

$$C_e(t) = K_{trans} \int_0^t C_p(t) e^{-k_{ep}(t-t')} dt', \tag{3}$$

where, initially, at $t = 0$, $C_e(t) = 0$. Because the concentration of the MMCA in the tumor at any time t, $C_t(t)$ consists of the concentrations in both the plasma space and the EES (i.e., the interstitial space of the tumor) we may express the total concentration in the tumor as:

$$C_t(t) = K_{trans} \int_0^t C_p(t) e^{-k_{ep}(t-t')} dt' + v_p C_p(t), \tag{4}$$

where v_p is the fractional plasma volume of the tumor (mmol/cc of tissue). Now, we introduce certain approximations that enable us to solve and implement **Eq. [4]** in a computationally efficient manner, which, in turn, allows us to generate spatial maps of the necessary tumor tissue parameters.

5.2. How Do We Get from MMCA Concentration to the Tumor Blood Volume and PS Product?

First, K_{trans} is related to the plasma flow rate (F, mL/min/cc of tissue) and the first-pass extraction fraction according to the Renkin-Crone model *(39)* by:

$$K^{trans} = EF\rho(1-Hct) = F\rho(1-Hct)\left[1-e^{-\frac{PS}{F(1-Hct)}}\right], \qquad [5]$$

where *Hct* is the hematocrit. However, as mentioned in **Subheading 5.**, we are considering a special case of the two-compartment model called the PS-limited model. For this model, if the blood flow (F) is high, the arterial and venous concentrations may be considered equal, and the rate of MMCA uptake within that tissue is then limited by the PS product of the vessel wall and the concentration gradient between the plasma and EES compartments. Thus, when *PS* << *F* and *E* << 1, we may simplify **Eq. [5]** to:

$$K^{trans} = F\rho(1 - Hct)\left[1-e^{-\frac{PS}{F(1-Hct)}}\right] \approx F\rho(1 - Hct)\frac{PS}{F(1 - Hct)} = PS\rho, \qquad [6]$$

i.e., $K_{trans}=PS\,\rho$ for the PS-limited model.

We can define an apparent PS product, PS' = PSρ. Also, $v_p = (1 - Hct)v_b$, where v_b is the fractional vascular volume. Using these approximations, the result from **Eq. [6]**, ignoring back-flux of the MMCA (i.e., setting $k_{ep} = 0$) and dividing both sides of **Eq. [4]** by $Cp(t)$, we can rewrite **Eq. [4]** as:

$$\frac{C_t(t)}{C_p(t)} = PS'\frac{\int_0^t C_p(t')dt'}{C_p(t)} + v_b. \qquad [7]$$

As described by Demsar et al., we may approximate the rate of clearance of the MMCA from the blood as a monoexponential, i.e., $C_p(t) \approx e^{-\beta t}$ *(33)*. For instances in which the rate of clearance (β) of the MMCA is small, we can simplify the plasma terms in **Eq. [7]** as follows:

$$\frac{\int_0^t C_p(t')dt'}{C_p(t)} = \frac{\int_0^t e^{-\beta t'}dt'}{e^{-\beta t'}} = \frac{1 - e^{-\beta t}}{\beta e^{-\beta t}} \approx t. \qquad [8]$$

Using **Eq. [8]** in **Eq. [7]**, we get:

$$\frac{C_t(t)}{C_p(t)} \cong v_b + PS't \, . \tag{9}$$

If we assume that $C_e(t) = 0$, at $t \approx 1$ min, **Eq. [9]** gives us:

$$\frac{C_t(t = 1\ min)}{C_p(t = 1\ min)} = v_b \, . \tag{10}$$

Thus, **Eq. [9]** is nothing but the equation of a straight line with y-intercept v_b and slope PS'. Thus, in our MRI experiment we can use any kind of T_1-weighted imaging sequence that allows us to measure the changes in relaxation rate ($\Delta R_1 = \Delta 1/T_1$) before ($1/T_{1pre}$) and after ($1/T_{1post}$) administration of the contrast agent, i.e., $\Delta R_1 = 1/T_{1post} - 1/T_{1pre}$ (**Fig. 1A**). We do this over time, such that we have $\Delta R_{1tissue}(t)$ for the tumor tissue, or equivalently $C_t(t)$ (**Fig. 1**). At the end of the experiment, we extract some blood from the animal and determine ΔR_1 for the blood, or, equivalently, $C_p(t)$ (**Fig. 1B**). Because we use an MMCA, blood concentrations of the contrast agent can be approximated to be constant for the duration of the MR experiment and, under these conditions, contrast uptake is a linear function of time *(32,33)* (**Fig. 2**):

$$\frac{C_t(t)}{C_p(t)} = \frac{\Delta R1_t(t)}{\Delta R1_{Blood}} = v_b + PS't \, . \tag{11}$$

On a plot of contrast agent concentration vs time, the slope of the line provides the parameter PS, and the intercept of the line with the vertical axis at time zero provides the vascular volume (**Fig. 2**). These can easily be obtained by performing straightforward linear regression analysis of the tumor on a voxel-by-voxel basis (**Fig. 2**). The algorithm for the entire experiment is summarized in **Fig. 3**. Changes in blood T_1 can not only be obtained separately from blood samples taken before administration of the contrast agent at the end of the experiment but can be measured noninvasively as well *(40)*.

5.3. What is MMCA Albumin-(Gd-DTPA)?

For macromolecular agents, such as albumin-(Gd-DTPA) (molecular weight ≈ 90 kDa) blood concentrations equilibrate within 2 to 3 min and do not change for at least 40 min after an iv injection. The tissue concentration of the MMCA increases linearly with time from 5 to 40 min after the iv injection. Therefore, the simple linear model is preferable for analysis of intrinsically noisy relaxation data because it is much more stable in comparison with nonlinear fitting

A

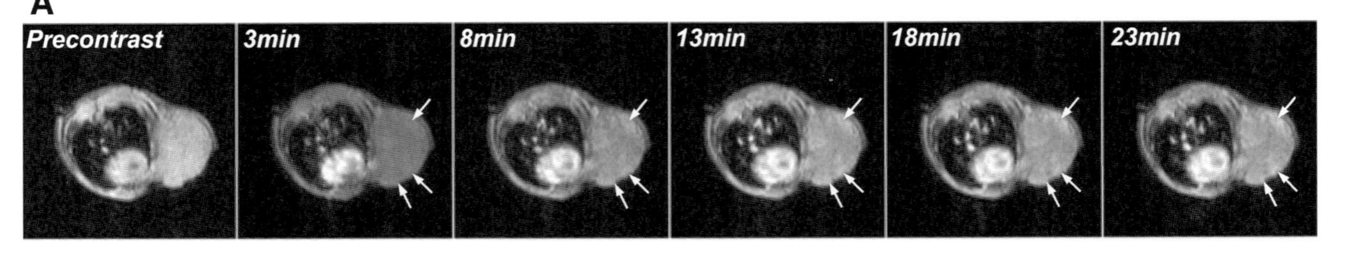

B

Experimental MRI Protocol

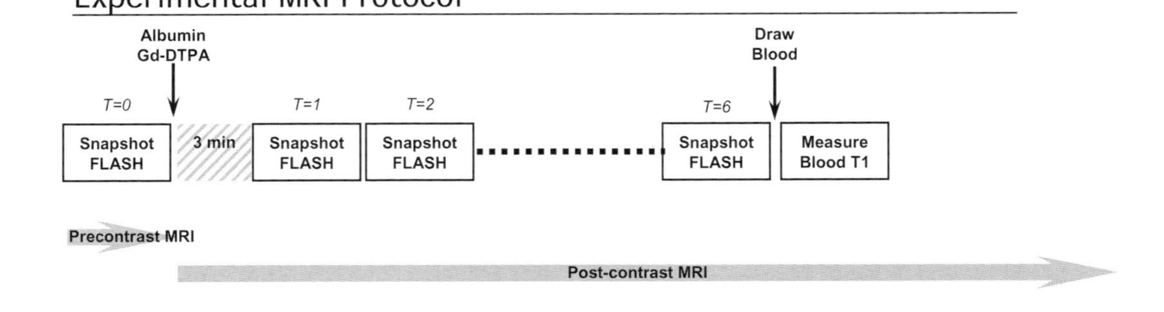

Fig. 1. (**A**) Magnetic resonance (MR) images obtained from a mouse bearing a breast cancer xenograft. A time series of cross-sectional images of one precontrast and five albumin-(Gd-DTPA) postcontrast MR images acquired with a saturation recovery time of 1 s, illustrating the enhancement of the tumor ($\rightarrow$) from 3 min to 23 min postcontrast. Note that for illustration purposes the window and level setting for all the postcontrast images are kept constant, whereas the precontrast image is displayed with a different window level. (**B**) Summary of a typical T_1-weighted experimental MR imaging protocol to obtain data shown in (**A**).

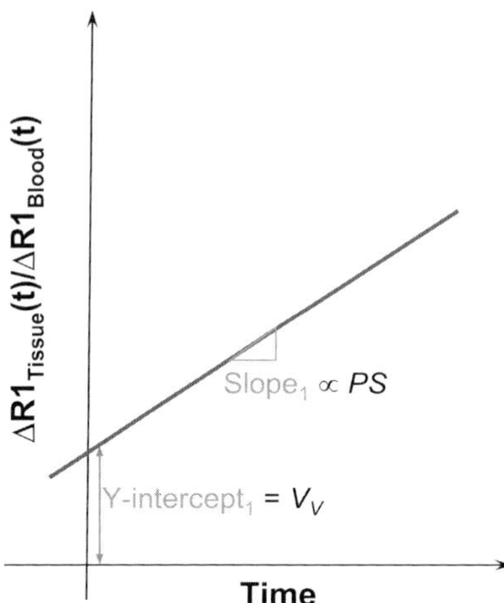

Fig. 2. Schematic illustrating how macromolecular contrast agent uptake is modeled as a linear function of time for the first 30 min of the magnetic resonance acquisition. The slope of the concentration-time curve provides the permeability–surface area product, PS (µL/g·min); and the y-intercept, the vascular volume, V_V (µL/g).

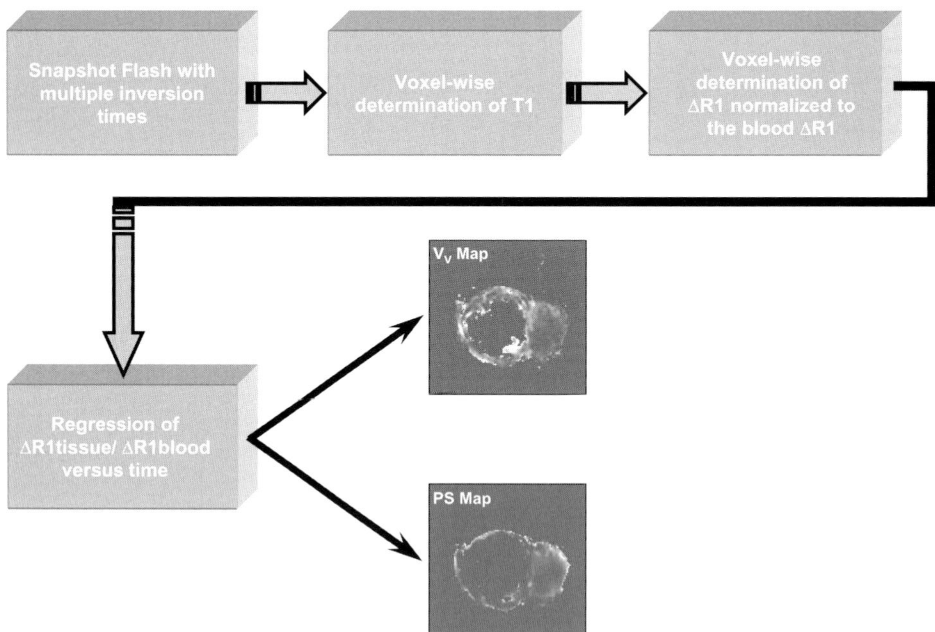

Fig. 3. Illustration of the algorithm for computing vascular volume (V_v) and permeability–surface area (PS) product maps based on T_1-weighted imaging measurements, such as described in **Fig. 1**.

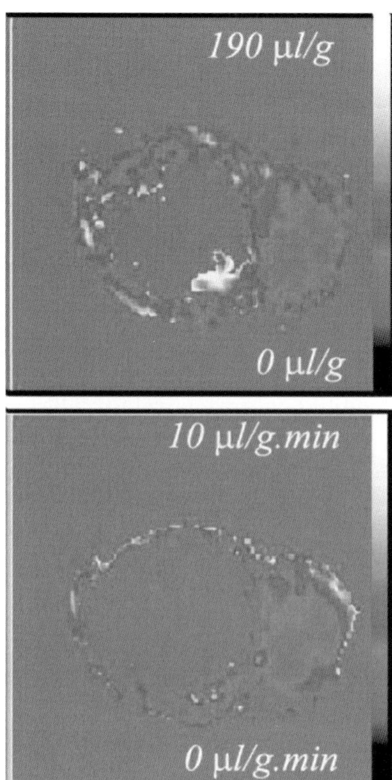

Fig. 4. Representative blood volume and permeability–surface area product (PS) maps obtained from the data set shown in **Fig. 1**. (Pathak, A. P., Artemov, D., and Bhujwalla, Z. M., unpublished data).

algorithms usually employed for two-compartment models. The entire algorithm is summarized in **Fig. 3**. Sample vascular volume and PS maps derived using this technique are shown in **Figs. 4** and **5**. However, the accuracy of the measurement of tissue vascular volume using this approach does depend on the water exchange rate between the vascular and extracellular compartments. Using a simplified model of fast exchange when there actually may exist intermediate to slow exchange can lead to significant underestimation of vascular volume *(41)*. Experimental approaches to minimize these errors are being developed *(42)*.

When administered intravenously, the MMCA albumin labeled with Gd-DTPA or albumin-(Gd-DTPA) is mostly confined to the intravascular compartment. It is an extremely efficient T_1 relaxation agent and its effects persist for up to 45 min after injection *(40)*. A detailed description of its biodistribution can be found in *(43)*.

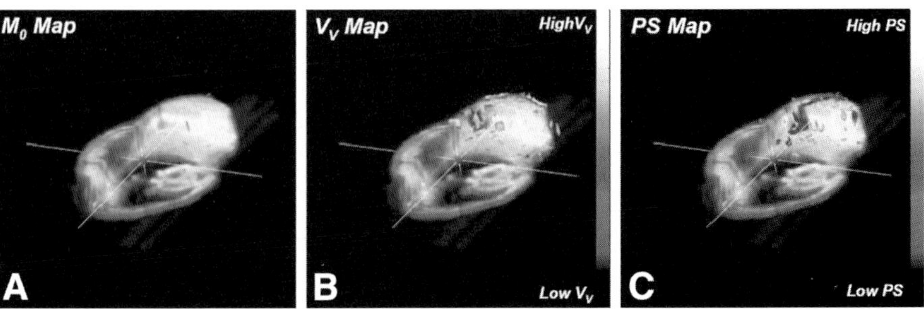

Fig. 5. Overlay of functional maps on anatomical template. Information, such as shown in **Fig. 4**, can be fused with underlying anatomy. Shown here is a representative 3D reconstruction of the longitudinal magnetization (M_0) map of a breast tumor xenograft-bearing mouse, cutaway to show the tumor interior. (**B**) Three-dimensional M_0 map overlaid with a vascular volume map. (**C**) Three-dimensional M_0 map overlaid with a PS map, enabling us to see the spatial distribution of these two parameters within the tumor mass.

6. Molecular Imaging of Tumors

As mentioned in **Subheading 4.2.**, by using exogenous contrast agents one can drastically improve the contrast-to-noise ratio when performing MRI of tumor physiology. However, the visualization of selected molecular targets or receptors and the molecular processes fundamental to tumor physiology, i.e., true "molecular imaging" using MRI was not possible until very recently. This was primarily attributable to the relative insensitivity of MRI compared with PET and optical imaging, and to target concentrations in the picomolar and nanomolar ranges in conjunction with problems of contrast agent delivery to the molecular target and dilution of the label within the blood pool. Recent improvements in the design of contrast agents with higher relaxivities, as well as novel strategies for MR signal and receptor target amplification have finally brought the functional assessment of tumors under the purview of molecular imaging. Studies involving the detection of tumor cell-surface receptors using novel receptor-specific contrast agents have added a new dimension to our ability to probe the tumor pathophyisology using MRI.One such study used an MR contrast agent composed of Gd-labeled polymerized liposomes conjugated with biotinylated antibodies targeted against the $\alpha_V\beta_3$ receptors commonly found on endothelial cell surfaces *(44)*. On a standard T_1-weighted image, the observed contrast was then proportional to the density of receptors and thus to the density of the neovasculature. In yet another recent study, Artemov et al. demonstrated the feasibility of using MRI to detect the Her-2/neu receptor, an important cell-surface receptor in breast cancer prognosis *(45)*. The use of targeted contrast agents in conjunction with the functional imaging techniques described in **Subheading 4.**, provide unique opportunities for understanding receptor-mediated pathways in cancer using MRI.

7. Imaging Tumors With Complementary Imaging Modalities

Although it may seem that MRI is unmatched in its ability to probe tumor angiogenesis and other important pathways in cancer, several pioneering studies using alternative imaging modalities have proved this untrue. Regarding the molecular imaging of tumor angiogenesis, an innovative study using SPECT recently demonstrated the viability of imaging an antibody fragment to fibronectin, an important cell-adhesion molecule and angiogenic marker *(46)*. With this technique, the authors were able to able to distinguish between inactive and actively growing lesions in patients with lung, colorectal, or brain cancer. Advances in ultrasound imaging instrumentation and ultrasound blood pool contrast agents have enabled the sonographic detection of tumor angiogenesis. An innovative study using microbubbles targeted to α_V-integrins, an endothelial cell surface receptor expressed in neovessels, enabled the noninvasive assessment of angiogenesis in vivo by ultrasound *(47)*. More recently, the quantification of tumor vascularity was achieved using a multimodal approach *(48)*. In this study, the authors used another microbubble contrast agent and contrast-enhanced sonography in mice to quantify tumor vascularization using fractal analysis. Their ultrasound measurements were compared with fractional vascular volume measurements using MRI and with fluorodeoxyglucose autoradiography measurements, to identify the viable regions within the tumor. They found an excellent correlation between the ultrasound and MRI, as well as between the ultrasound and fluorodeoxyglucose measurements, respectively. The high sensitivity of photon detection, widespread availability of a large range of novel fluorescent probes and targets, and the development of near-infrared techniques has made optical imaging a favored modality for imaging molecular targets. More recently, diffuse near-infrared optical spectroscopy was used to quantify the dynamics of optical contrast agents in a rat tumor model in vivo, in conjunction with MRI *(49)*. The kinetics of the optical contrast agents, indocyanine green and methylene blue, were found to be analogous to those of a macromolecular and low molecular weight MR contrast agent, respectively.

In addition to these novel imaging approaches, the development of multimodal contrast agents, i.e., contrast agents that are simultaneously observable or visible to two or more imaging modalities allow researchers to simultaneously enjoy the advantages of both imaging modalities. One such study developed a near-infrared fluorescent and magnetic nanoparticle as an MRI contrast agent and optical probe *(50)*. The long blood half-life superparamagnetic iron oxide nanoparticle served as the MR contrast agent, and a cyanine conjugate served as the near-infrared fluorescent probe. In a model surgical setting, using gliosarcoma-bearing rats, the authors were able to accurately delineate the extent of the brain tumors both presurgically, using MRI, and intraoperatively, using near-infrared optical imaging. This was possible because the contrast agent was naturally sequestered in the microglia because of iron oxide nanoparticle metabolism.

Finally, Dafni et al. describe the development of a contrast agent based on albumin that was triply labeled with biotin, a fluorescent tag, and Gd-DTPA, allowing optical, plasma mass spectrometry, and MRI detection of the same agent *(51)*. This was an elegant solution for mapping the clearance of interstitial MMCA after it had extravasated from hyperpermeable blood vessels, because the biotin tag allowed in vivo chasing of the contrast material from the blood by intravenous administration of avidin. The avidin caused the contrast agent to disappear from the blood vessels, whereas contrast agent that had extravasated before administration of avidin was not cleared and continued to be transported in the interstitium via convection.

Although nuclear medicine techniques, such as SPECT and PET, tend to be limited in their spatial resolution and require the administration of radioisotopes, and light scattering in soft tissues often limits the effective depth of optical techniques, the development of multimodal probes promises to circumvent these drawbacks by allowing us to exploit the sensitivity of these techniques, while combining them with the advantages of MRI, such as high spatial resolution.

Acknowledgments

Support from NIH-NCI-RO1-CA90471 is gratefully acknowledged.

References

1. Baillie, C. T., Winslet, M. C., and Bradley, N. J. (1995) Tumor vasculature—a potential therapeutic target. *Br. J. Cancer* **72,** 257–267.
2. Holash, P., Maisonpierre, P. C., Compton, D., et al. (1999) Vessel cooption, regression, and growth in tumors mediated by angiopoietins and VEGF. *Science* **284,** 1994–1998.
3. Deane, B. R. and Lantos, P. L. (1981) The vasculature of experimental brain tumors—part 1: a sequential light and electron microscope study of angiogenesis. *J. Neurol. Sci.* **49,** 55–66.
4. Deane, B. R. and Lantos, P. L. (1981) The vasculature of experimental brain tumors—part 2: a quantitative assessment of morphological abnormalities. *J. Neurol. Sci.* **49,** 67–77.
5. Konerding, M. A., van Ackern, C., Fait, E., Steinberg, F., and Streffer, C. (2000) Morphological aspects of tumor angiogenesis and microcirculation, in *Blood Perfusion and Microenvironment of Human Tumors: Implications for Clinical Radiooncology (Medical Radiology)* (Molls, M., Vaupel, P., Brady, L. W., and Heilmann, H. P., eds.), Springer Verlag, New York, NY, pp. 5–17.

6. Jain, R. K. (1988) Determinants of tumor blood flow: a review. *Cancer Res.* **48,** 2641–2658.

7. Vaupel, P. (2000) Tumor blood flow, in *Blood Perfusion and Microenvironment of Human Tumors: Implications for Clinical Radiooncology (Medical Radiology)* (Molls, M., Vaupel, P., Brady, L. W., and Heilmann, H. P., eds.), Springer Verlag, New York, NY, pp. 5–17.

8. Vaupel, P., Schaefer, C., and Okunieff, P. (1994) Intracellular acidosis in murine fibrosarcomas coincides with ATP depletion, hypoxia, and high levels of lactate and total Pi. *NMR Biomed.* **7,** 128–136.

9. Stubbs, M., Bhujwalla, Z. M., Tozer, G. M., et al. (1992) An assessment of 31P MRS as a method of measuring pH in rat tumours. *NMR Biomed.* **5,** 351–359.

10. Stubbs, M., Rodrigues, L., Howe, F. A., et al. (1994) Metabolic consequences of a reversed pH gradient in rat tumors. *Cancer Res.* **54,** 4011–4016.

11. Ogawa, S. (1990) Oxygenation-sensitive contrast in MR image of rodent brain at high magnetic fields. *Mag. Reson. Med.* **14,** 68–78.

12. Carmeliet, P., Dor, Y., Herbert, J-M, et al. (1998) Role of HIF-1 in hypoxia-mediated apoptosis, cell proliferation and tumor angiogenesis. *Nature* **394,** 485–490.

13. Taylor, N. J., Baddeley, H., Goodchild, K. A., et al. (2001) BOLD MRI of human tumor oxygenation during carbogen breathing. *J. Magn. Reson. Imaging* **14,** 156–163.

14. Pathak, A. P., Rand, S. D., and Schmainda, K. M. (2003) The effect of brain tumor angiogenesis on the in vivo relationship between the gradient-echo relaxation rate change (DeltaR2*) and contrast agent (MION) dose. *J. Magn. Reson. Imaging* **18,** 397–403.

15. Silva, A. C., Zhang, W., Williams, D.S., and Koretsky, A. P. (1995) Multi-slice MRI of rat brain perfusion during amphetamine stimulation using arterial spin labeling. *Mag. Reson. Med.* **33,** 209–214.

16. Weber, M. A., Thilmann, C., Lichy, M. P., et al. (2004) Assessment of irradiated brain metastases by means of arterial spin-labeling and dynamic susceptibility-weighted contrast-enhanced perfusion MRI: initial results. *Invest. Radiol.* **39,** 277–287.

17. Morris, E. A. (2003) Screening for breast cancer with MRI. *Semin. Ultrasound CT MR.* **24,** 45–54.

18. Donahue, K. M., Krouwer, H. G., Rand, S. D., et al. (2000) Utility of simultaneously acquired gradient-echo and spin-echo cerebral blood volume and morphology maps in brain tumor patients. *Magn. Reson. Med.* **43,** 845–853.

19. Hawighorst, H., Knapstein, P. G., Weikel, W. et al. (1997) Angiogenesis of uterine cervical carcinoma: characterization by pharmacokinetic magnetic resonance parameters and histological microvessel density with correlation to lymphatic involvement. *Cancer Res.* **57,** 4777–4786.

20. Tofts, P. S., Brix, G., Buckley, D. L., et al. (1999) Estimating kinetic parameters from dynamic contrast-enhanced T(1)-weighted MRI of a diffusible tracer: standardized quantities and symbols. *J. MRI.* **10,** 223–232.

21. Tofts, P. S. (1997) Modeling tracer kinetics in dynamic Gd-DTPA MR imaging. *J. MRI.* **7,** 91–101.

22. Hacklander, T. (1996) Cerebral blood volume maps with dynamic contrast-enhanced T1-weighted FLASH imaging: normal values and preliminary clinical results. *J. CAT.* **20,** 532–539.
23. Hacklander, T., Reichenbach, J. R., Hofer, M., and Modder, U. (1996) Measurement of cerebral blood volume via the relaxing effect low-dose gadopentetate dimeglumine during bolus transit. *A. J. N. R.* **17,** 821–830.
24. Dennie, J., Mandeville, J. B., Boxerman, J. L., Packard, S. D., Rosen, B. R., and Weisskoff, R. M. (1998) NMR imaging of changes in vascular morphology due to tumor angiogenesis. *Mag. Reson. Med.* **40,** 793–799.
25. Aronen, H. J., Gazit, I. E., Louis, D. N., et al. (1994) Cerebral blood volume maps of gliomas: comparison with tumor grade and histological findings. *Radiology* **191,** 41–51.
26. Maeda, M., Itoh, S., Kimura, H., et al. (1993) Tumor vascularity in the brain: evaluation with dynamic susceptibility-contrast MR imaging. *Radiology* **189,** 233–238.
27. Pathak, A. P., Schmainda, K. M., Ward, B. D., Linderman, J. R., Rebro, K. J., and Greene, A. S. (2001) MR-derived cerebral blood volume maps: issues regarding histological validation and assessment of tumor angiogenesis. *Magn. Reson. Med.* **46,** 735–747.
28. Weisskoff, R. M., Boxerman, J. L., Sorenson, A. G., Kulke, S. M., Campbell, T. A., and Rosen, B. R. (1994) *2nd Annual Meeting, Society of Magnetic Resonance in Medicine, San Francisco, CA.*
29. Artemov, D., Solaiyappan, M., and Bhujwalla, Z. M. (2001) Magnetic resonance pharmacoangiography to detect and predict chemotherapy delivery to solid tumors. *Cancer Res.* **61,** 3039–3044.
30. Schwarzbauer, C., Syha, J., and Haase, A. (1993) Quantification of regional cerebral blood volumes by rapid T1 mapping. *Mag. Reson. Med.* **29,** 709–712.
31. Brasch, R., Pham, C. Shames, D., et al. (1997) Assessing tumor angiogenesis using macromolecular MR imaging contrast media. *J. MRI.* **7,** 68–74.
32. Patlak, C. S., Blasberg, R. G., and Fenstermacher, J. D. (1983) Graphical evaluation of blood-to-brain transfer constants from multiple-time uptake data. *J. Cereb. Blood Flow Metab.* **3,** 1–7.
33. Demsar, F., Roberts, T. P., Schwickert, H. C. , et al. (1997) A MRI spatial mapping technique for microvascular permeability and tissue blood volume based on macromolecular contrast agent distribution. *Magn. Reson. Med.* **37,** 236–242.
34. Kim, Y. R., Rebro, K. J., and Schmainda, K. M. (2002) Water exchange and inflow affect the accuracy of T1-GRE blood volume measurements: implications for the evaluation of tumor angiogenesis. *Mag. Reson. Med.* **47,** 1110–1120.
35. Badruddoja, M. A., Krouwer, H. G., Rand, S. D., Rebro, K. J., Pathak, A. P., and Schmainda, K. M. (2003) Antiangiogenic effects of dexamethasone in 9L gliosarcoma assessed by MRI cerebral blood volume maps. *Neuro-oncol.* **5,** 235–243.
36. Turetschek, K., Preda, A., Novikov, V., et al. (2004) Tumor microvascular changes in antiangiogenic treatment: assessment by magnetic resonance contrast media of different molecular weights. *J. Magn. Reson. Imaging* **20,** 138–144.

37. Bhujwalla, Z. M., Artemov, D., Natarajan, K., Ackerstaff, E., and Solaiyappan, M. (2001) Vascular differences detected by MRI for metastatic versus nonmetastatic breast and prostate cancer xenografts. *Neoplasia* **3,** 143–153.
38. Evelhoch, J. L. (1999) Key factors in the acquisition of contrast kinetic data for oncology. *J. Magn. Reson. Imaging* **10,** 254–259.
39. Crone, C. (1963) The permeability of capillaries in various organs as determined by use of the 'indicator diffusion' method. *Acta Physiol. Scand.* **58,** 292–305.
40. Pathak, A. P., Artemov, D., and Bhujwalla, Z. M. (2004) Novel system for determining contrast agent concentration in mouse blood in vivo. *Magn. Reson. Med.* **51,** 612–615.
41. Kim, Y. R. and Donahue, K. M. (2000) *8th Annual Meeting, International Society of Magnetic Resonance Medicine, Denver, CO.*
42. Yankeelov, T. E., Rooney, W. D., Li, X., and Springer, C. S., Jr. (2003) Variation of the relaxographic "shutter-speed" for transcytolemmal water exchange affects the CR bolus-tracking curve shape. *Magn. Reson. Med.* **50,** 1151–1169.
43. Ogan, M. D., Schmiedl, U., Mosley, M.E., Grodd, W., Paajanen, H., and Brasch, R.C. (1987) Albumin labeled with Gd-DTPA; an intravascular contrast enhancing agent for magnetic resonance blood pool imaging: preparation and characterization. *Invest. Radiol.* **22,** 665–671.
44. Sipkins, D. A., Cheresh, D. A., Kazemi, M. R., Nevin, L. M., Bednarski, M. D., and Li, K. C. P. (1998) Detection of tumor angiogenesis in vivo by AB-targeted magnetic resonance imaging. *Nat. Med.* **4,** 623–626.
45. Artemov, D., Mori, N., Ravi, R., and Bhujwalla, Z. (2003) Magnetic resonance molecular imaging of the HER-2/neu receptor. *Cancer Res.* **63,** 2723–2727.
46. Santimaria, M., Moscatelli, G., Viale, G. L., et al. (2003) Immunoscintigraphic detection of the ED-B domain of fibronectin, a marker of angiogenesis, in patients with cancer. *Clin. Cancer Res.* **9,** 571–579.
47. Leong-Poi, H., Christiansen, J., Klibanov, A. L., Kaul, S., and Lindner, J. R. (2003) Noninvasive assessment of angiogenesis by ultrasound and microbubbles targeted to alpha(v)-integrins. *Circulation* **107,** 455–460.
48. Fleischer, A. C., Donnelly, E. F., Grippo, R. J., Black, A. S., and Hallahan, D. E. (2004) Quantification of tumor vascularity with contrast-enhanced sonography: correlation with magnetic resonance imaging and fluorodeoxyglucose autoradiography in an implanted tumor. *J. Ultrasound Med.* **23,** 37–41.
49. Cuccia, D. J., Bevilacqua, F., Durkin, A. J., et al. (2003) In vivo quantification of optical contrast agent dynamics in rat tumors by use of diffuse optical spectroscopy with magnetic resonance imaging coregistration. *Appl. Opt.* **42,** 2940–2950.
50. Kircher, M. F., Mahmood, U., King, R. S., Weissleder, R., and Josephson, L. (2003) A multimodal nanoparticle for preoperative magnetic resonance imaging and intraoperative optical brain tumor delineation. *Cancer Res.* **63,** 8122–8125.
51. Dafni, H., Gilead, A., Nevo, N., Eilam, R., Harmelin, A., and Neeman, M. (2003) Modulation of the pharmacokinetics of macromolecular contrast material by avidin chase: MRI, optical, and inductively coupled plasma mass spectrometry tracking of triply labeled albumin. *Magn. Reson. Med.* **50,** 904–914.

12

MRI in Preclinical Drug Development

Matthew D. Silva and Sudeep Chandra

Summary

This chapter outlines the challenges that the pharmaceutical industry faces during the course of drug development and discusses the role of magnetic resonance imaging in preclinical drug discovery.

Key Words: MRI; drug discovery; preclinical imaging,

1. Introduction

The application of imaging experiments in the pharmaceutical industry needs to be cleverly optimized to realize value in the development cycle of a drug. In that regard, it is often not the optimization of a novel imaging technique that is of interest, *per se*, but rather, the novel application of understood and validated techniques. Specific tertiary application development encompasses a variety of magnetic resonance imaging (MRI) techniques discussed in detail elsewhere in this book and, as such, a review of the techniques again will be redundant. The purpose of this chapter is to present an operational overview of how MRI has contributed to the drug-discovery process and provide guidance for application development in the context of drug-discovery research.

1.1. The Drug Development Process

Pharmaceutical drug development is an expensive and risk-intensive process that needs cross-functional expertise. It is marked by long development life cycles and substantial *a priori* fixed costs. In 2003, pharmaceutical companies spent $33 billion on research to develop new treatments of diseases *(1)*. As a percentage of revenue, it was the highest amount, an estimated 17.7% among all of the research and development (R&D)-intensive industries (such as aeronautics, electronics, and so on) *(1)*. In a recent, comprehensive review of the pharmaceutical industry, DiMasi and colleagues estimated that the capi-

From: *Methods in Molecular Medicine, Vol. 124*
Magnetic Resonance Imaging: Methods and Biologic Applications
Edited by: P. V. Prasad © Humana Press Inc., Totowa, NJ

talized total cost for the development of a new drug is approx $802 million, with $335 and $467 million in investments in preclinical and clinical research, respectively *(2)*. These estimates are based on R&D costs only of 68 randomly selected new drugs from 10 firms and are pre-FDA approval values not counting commercial expenses. In comparison to a similar analysis performed in 1991 *(3)*, the cost of drug development has increased by 152% (from $318 million in 1991); however, the success rate of candidates and the life cycle of product (which remains at ~12 yr) have not changed. Because the average patent cycle of new chemical entities is on the order of 17 to 20 yr, it is imperative that pharmaceutical companies bear a significant upfront burden of R&D costs before any return on investment is achievable.

Although a variety of new improvements have been introduced to the R&D process over the last decade or so (microfluidics, high-throughput chemistry, modern lead-optimization techniques, pharmacokinetic modeling, and so on), the attrition rates of lead agents is still extremely high *(4,5)*. More specifically, typically only 5% of all molecules identified in discovery research advance into human trials; even within that pool, typically only one in five makes it through the complete approval process for marketed use in humans. Clearly, improving the attrition rate would significantly impact the development (and ultimately the market cost) of drugs. In fact, estimates of the cost savings indicate that an increase in the success rate from one in five to one in three would reduce the capitalized total cost by approx 30% ($230 million) *(6)*.

As a first approximation, the drug development process can be thought of as a linear process, comprised of key "stage gates" and leading ultimately to regulatory approval for human testing and subsequent clinical trials of a test agent. During preclinical development, researchers usually first identify, prioritize, and validate cellular and genetic targets of relevance for an unmet clinical need. Subsequent to this, a variety of chemical designs and optimizations are usually undertaken to arrive at compounds that are considered "leads" or potential drug-like agents. Lead compounds are then subjected to extensive in vitro and in vivo investigation that may span more than 6 yr. Once properly characterized, and after initial regulatory approval, three successive phases of clinical testing are undertaken. During Phase I, healthy volunteers are tested to establish safety requirements and biophysical parameters (absorption, distribution, metabolism, excretion, and toxicity). After this phase, in Phase II, diseased patients are tested to establish an understanding of preliminary efficacy of the compound. Finally, in Phase III, large patient cohorts are tested, typically in multiple centers, for proof of efficacy. The duration of each phase is variable and, in many cases, can be dictated by the disease itself. Clearly, the cost burden is extremely high in the last two phases of the drug development cycle. Moreover, the failure rates are very high beyond Phase I *(2,3,6)*. A small change in the success rate of Phase II or Phase III, therefore, can lead to enormous cost savings. It is estimated that shifting a failure rate of 10% from Phase III to Phase II would lead to an approx 40% reduction in cost of the whole cycle *(6)*.

It is imperative, therefore, that compounds are interrogated carefully and that, at different drug-discovery stages, resources are applied to rate-limiting disconnects, such that more confidence can be gained regarding the potential clinical success of a drug-like candidate. A key area of focus in the drug-discovery area currently is on the transition period between proof-of-concept testing in animal models to Phase II proof-of-concept demonstration in humans. Improving success rates of candidates in this period requires dedicated efforts to understand animal models of disease and capabilities of developing readouts similar to those that would be used in humans for monitoring the outcome of clinical trials. It is in this domain that a variety of imaging modalities and tools will find greater use in the drug-discovery process. Specifically, the ever-increasing role of MRI in drug development has been reviewed previously *(7,8)*. It has been recognized that proper application of imaging in preclinical stages can lead to a better understanding of the disease process as well as the effects of treatment downstream. The preclinical setting offers several advantages to characterize markers of disease. Numerous constraints—cost, compliance, control of study design, access to instrumentation, multiplicity of protocols in multiple centers, lack of validated markers, and so on—make it harder to develop new markers during clinical trials *(2–6)*. Hence, despite some incongruity with the human disease phenotypes, disease modeling in animals is an important and critical area necessary for the development of new drugs. It is in this arena that imaging is being applied extensively to develop novel, validated, and translatable surrogate markers for efficacy of test agents. Efforts to make such imaging biomarkers translatable to human studies would facilitate and enhance clinical application development; and, in parallel, imaging may also find greater use in clinical trials.

2. Imaging Application Development in Pharmaceutical Research: Specific Role of MRI

The usefulness of MRI in in vivo research is ever expanding—from novel applications in pathophysiology to biochemistry, and, in turn, to molecular domains *(7–10)*. One of the most significant advantages of MRI is its versatility, which could lead to consolidation of cost via development of rapid/simultaneous functional and pathological readouts. In this context, MRI offers several key opportunities to interrogate in vivo physiology: MRI is noninvasive, is inherently 3D, and has high spatial resolution. Additionally, there are a variety of physiologically relevant contrasts *in situ* (e.g., diffusion rates of water, transfer rates of water between free and bound states, blood flow, and so on). Hence, numerous indices can be developed that correlate with therapeutic modulations of a test drug with high spatial accuracy and with novel information content. The noninvasive property of MRI is enormously valuable for serial interrogation of disease status, allowing development of clinically relevant, statistically robust readout tools and important information on disease profiles without the use of expanded cohorts of animals or resources. Moreover, as a platform tool, methods developed in the preclinical stages can be directly adapted to the clinic, minimizing the need for *de novo* method development. This ability of MRI—to connect preclinical and clinical applications—is an important capability to facilitate the practice of translational medicine, wherein the tools used to gage the preclinical efficacy of a therapy may also be used in clinical development and treatment plans.

MRI remains the premier anatomical imaging tool, and anatomical information obtained by MRI can be significantly enhanced by the higher sensitivity offered by nuclear tools—e.g., positron emission tomography and single-photon emission computed tomography—or novel readouts from optical (i.e., fluorescence and bioluminescence) imaging methods *(9–11)*. The emerging field of molecular imaging would explore this issue and attempt to integrate the benefits of most optimal modes simultaneously. Multimodal imaging couples sensitivity and resolution from different modes simultaneously during scanning. Such combined systems are rapidly becoming available for the small-animal domain and will offer unique opportunities for drug design in combination with MRI.

2.1. Representative Examples

Imaging technology has made numerous contributions to advancement of candidates to the clinic and for development of therapeutic profiles of putative drug candidates, some of which are listed in **Table 1**. As the industry learns more about the rapidly expanding field of medical imaging and reorients its focus on the disconnects from the bench to the bedside, important advances will occur in the areas of R&D process design and integration of imaging modalities.

The reader is urged to consult **Table 1** and to review articles for some perspective on the breadth of MRI work conducted in support of drug advancement. From the perspective of drug-discovery assay development, three such examples are briefly presented next.

2.1.1. Arterial Restenosis

Animal models of arterial restenosis have been used extensively to model the human condition that occurs after percutaneous transluminal coronary angioplasty. Application of MRI to characterize preclinical vessel diameter in

Table 1[a]
Pharmaceutical Drugs Studied by Magnetic Resonance Imaging

Stroke	Calcium antagonists	Isradipine *(57–60)*; Nimodipine *(61)*; Nicardipine *(62,63)*; SNX-111 *(64,65)*
	Serotonin antagonists	Levemopamil *(66)*
	Glycine receptor antagonists	GV150526 *(67)*; ACEA 1021 *(68)*; ZD9379 *(69,70)*
	AMPA antagonist	NBQX *(71)*
	Calcium channel entry blockers	RS-87476 *(72)*; LOE 908 MS *(73)*
	N-methyl-D-aspartate receptor antagonists	Dizocilpine (MK 801) *(74,75)*; CGP 40116 *(76,77)*; CNS 1102 *(78,79)*; CGS 19755 *(80)*
	Calcineurin inhibitors	FK506 and SDZ ASM 981 *(81)*
	Nitric oxide synthase inhibitors	NG-nitro-L-arginine methyl ester *(82,83)*; TRIM *(84)*
	Cellular phosphodiesterase III inhibitor	Cilostazol *(85)*
	Free-radical scavengers	Tirilazad; U74006F *(86)*; U74389G *(87)*
	Thromboxane A2 synthase inhibitor	Isbogrel (CV-4151) *(88)*
	Growth factors	Basic fibroblast growth factor *(89)*; VEGF antagonist, mFlt(1-3)-IgG *(90)*; nerve growth factor *(91)*
	Anti-inflammatory chemokine inhibitor	NR58-3.14.3 *(92)*
	Thrombolytic	Prourokinase *(38)*
Cancer	Chemotherapeutics	Dexamethasone *(93,94)*; Tamoxifen *(95)*; 5-Fluorouracil *(96,97)*
	Somatostatin analogs	Sandostatin *(98,99)*; RC-160 *(100)*
	VEGF signaling inhibitors	ZD6474 *(101)*; ZD4190 *(102)*; PTK787/ZK 222584 *(103)*
	5 α-reductase inhibitors	Finasteride *(104)*; azasteroids *(105)*
	PSMA-targeted chemotherapeutic	MLN2704 *(106)*
Cardiovascular	Restenosis	SB 217242 *(12,13)*
	Cardiac hypertrophy	Spirapril *(107)*; Captopril and Metoprolol *(108)*; Eprosartan *(109)*; Benazepril *(110)*; Valstartan *(110)*
	Cardiac ischemia	OPC-18790 *(111)*; Verapamil *(112)*; Nicorandil *(113)*; Cariporide *(114)*; Glibenclamid *(115)*; Pinacidil *(115)*; Bumetanide *(115)*

(continued)

Table 1[a] *(Continued)*
Pharmaceutical Drugs Studied by Magnetic Resonance Imaging

Additional studies	Traumatic brain injury	Diketopiperazine and Lubeluzole (*116,117*); MDL 74,180 (*118*)
	Antimigraine/ anticonvulsant	Sumatriptan and Tonabersat (*119*)
	Renal dysfunction	p38 MAPK inhibitors (*120*)
	Adipose tissue remodeling caused by obesity and insulin-resistance	Pioglitazone (*121*)
	Arthritis	SK&F 106615 (*122*); SB 242235 (*123*); SB 273005 (*124*); Indomethacin (*126*); Neoral (*126*)

[a]AMPA, α-amino-3-hydroxy-5-methyl-4-isoxazolepropionic acid; VEGF, vascular endothelial growth factor; PSMA, prostate-specific membrane antigen; MAPK, mitogen-activated protein kinase.

a restenosis model was deemed helpful because of its serial and noninvasive nature. **Figure 1** shows the results of a serial MRI study designed to test SB 217242, a dual endothelin antagonist in a rat restenosis model (*12,13*). The serial in vivo profile of the disease development shown in the study provides novel information—for example, the fact that the loss in vessel patency occurs between d-10 and d-14 of the experiment. Such information is important for

Fig. 1. *(opposite page)* (**A**) The three panels show the lumen caliber measured using high-resolution, cardiac-gated magnetic resonance imaging (MRI) under placebo, treatment, and sham balloon angioplasty conditions. All three groups must be monitored carefully to ensure calculable difference (data window) between sham and placebo, proper operation of the MRI scanner (stability of sham group), and the effects of therapeutic modulation (obtained by monitoring the drug treatment groups with respect to sham and placebo). Quantitative indices were developed and compared for titrating efficacy of test agents. (**B**) The volume obtained for the unballooned contralateral artery and the ballooned artery using magnetic resonance images like those shown in (**A**). The volume is calculated from seven contiguous slices over a predefined section on each carotid artery at each time point. On d-14, the mean lumen volume of the ballooned artery was significantly smaller than the corresponding mean baseline value (*$*p <$* 0.05). The mean volume of the drug-treated group ($n = 11$) at this time point was found to be significantly larger than the vehicle-treated control group ($n = 12$) (#$p < 0.05$). The data indicate that on d-14, approx 20% protection in terms of lumen patency is provided by chronic use of SB 217242. All numbers are expressed as mean ± SEM. The number of animals used in each group is indicated by *n*. In each case, the vehicle-treated (filled bar), the drug-treated (hatched bar), and the sham group (open bar) are shown. (Reproduced from **ref.** *12*.) http://lww.com

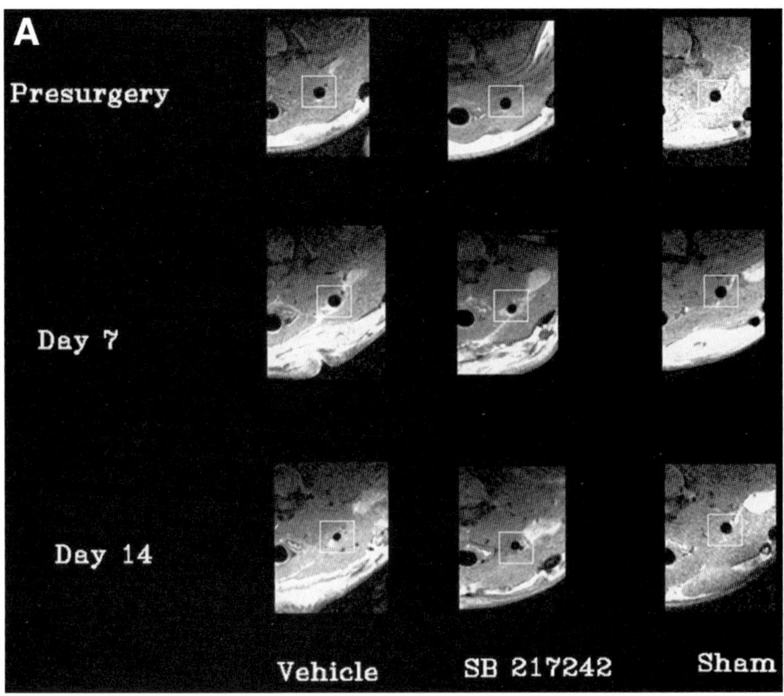
A
Presurgery
Day 7
Day 14
Vehicle
SB 217242
Sham

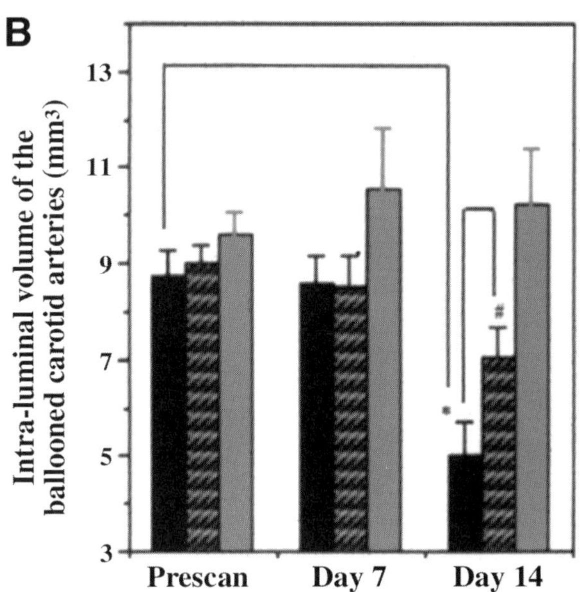
B
Intra-luminal volume of the
ballooned carotid arteries (mm3)
13
11
9
7
5
3
#
*
Prescan
Day 7
Day 14

discussions of late vascular effects and perhaps new ideas on dosing schedules. The disease group with treatment shows the effects of therapy with a dual endothelin antagonist and shows the ameliorating effects the antagonist can have on the lumen patency. Note that the study detailed the relationship of such measurements with histopathological cross-sectional measures and alluded to additional factors that can affect such internal measurements. Additionally, variability between animals also dictates the need to set up experiments with appropriate throughput, such that quantitative indices can be developed for meaningful measures of disease status and for robust analysis of test agents.

2.1.2. Pulmonary Inflammation

Another example of a serial study in a model of allergic pulmonary inflammation and the ability of MRI to pick up a marker of local inflammation after ovalbumin challenge has been carefully demonstrated in the literature *(14)* and shown in **Fig. 2**. The authors compared the MRI signal volumes with broncho-alveolar lavage measurements (of proteins, methoxyperoxidases, eosinophils, and lymphocytes) to better understand the MRI observations. The authors carefully established the assay in terms of validation with histological markers and used control drugs (a gluco-corticosteroid, budesonide) to demonstrate resolution of the MRI-signal volume after treatment with budesonide and NVP-ABE171 (a phosphodiesterase 4 inhibitor) *(15)*. Interestingly, the authors also demonstrated that such readouts can be obtained without the need for complicated setups, such as respiratory gating. This study and other studies of inflammatory pulmonary dysfunctions *(16)* that model diseases such as chronic obstructive pulmonary disease, emphysema, and asthma, provide guidance on adapting MRI in this domain. Another potential application of MRI readout is in using hyperpolarized ^{3}He-enhanced pulmonary imaging, in which anatomical contrast can be obtained either for the larger airways or for highlighting tissue parenchyma *(17)*, which may find more and more application in monitoring small-animal models of airways disease *(18)*.

2.1.3. Arthritis

MRI has also been extensively studied in degenerative disorders of the joints (rheumatoid arthritis and osteoarthritis) *(19,20)* and predictive markers of disease, such as bone spacing *(16)* and synovial hyperplasia *(16)*, have been investigated as a part of disease profiling in rheumatoid arthritis. For longitudinal studies, the usefulness of such markers has been demonstrated; especially in the context of late times after disease onset, when the paw-swelling data is less reliable. Of late, dynamic imaging of mobile cells (i.e., cell-trafficking studies) has become important and gained attention. **Figure 3** shows the ability to follow cell trafficking (in this case, labeled monocytes) in a rat arthritis model

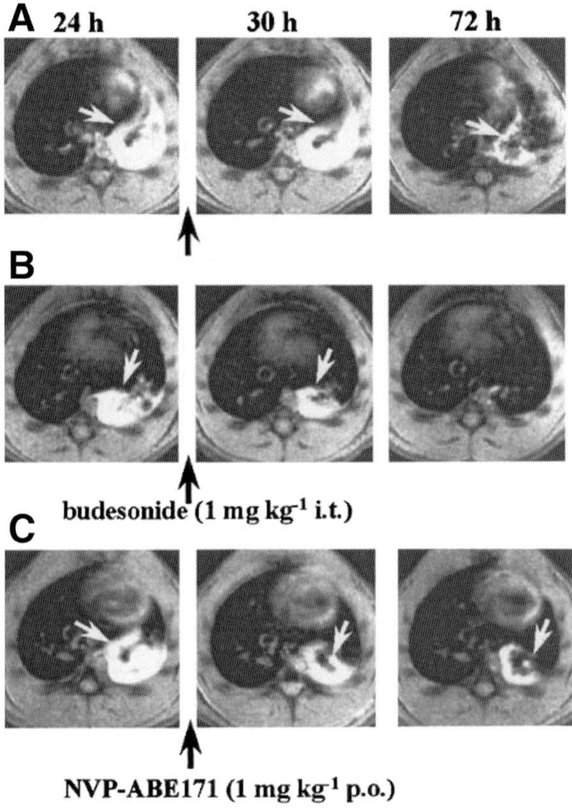

Fig. 2. Transverse section through the thorax of Brown Norway rats acquired at different time points after challenge with ovalbumin (OVA). Images correspond to approximately the same anatomical location in each animal. For each animal, the area corresponding to the edematous signal (indicated by the white arrows) was assessed on 25 transverse sections analogous to those shown here and covering the chest. (**A**) Oral NVP-ABE171 (2 mg/kg); (**B**) intrathecal budesonide (1 mg/kg); or (**C**) oral NVPABE171 (1 mg/kg) was administered immediately after the 24-h magnetic resonance imaging (MRI) acquisition (indicated by the black arrows). MRI images were acquired at 24, 30, and 72 h after intrathecal challenge with OVA (0.3 mg/kg; at time 0). Neither respiratory nor cardiac gating was used, and the animals respired spontaneously during image acquisition. (Reproduced from **ref. *15*.)

and the opportunity to study the efficacy of test agents against such an outcome *(16)*. Test agents affecting such trafficking outcomes are currently in clinical development and, hence, such noninvasive markers may serve as critical decision-making criteria for efficacy of compounds.

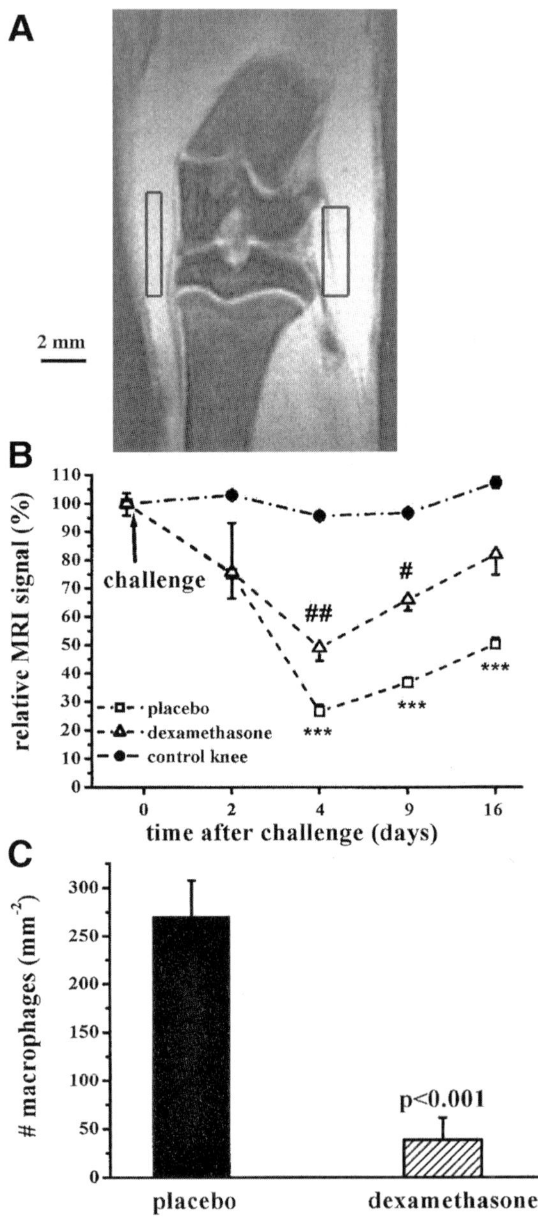

Fig. 3. (**A**) Anatomical location of region of interest on an arthritic knee joint of a female Lewis rat from which measurements are made in (**B**) and (**C**). (**B**) Time course of changes in magnetic resonance (MR) signal intensity; and (**C**) macrophage numbers measured from histology at the same sites shown in (**A**) on d-16 after challenge. (Reproduced from **ref. *23*.**)

2.2. Other Applications

In addition to titration studies of test agents and all associated requirements (identification and validation of a marker, time of measurement, quantitative robustness, and so on) several studies have been undertaken to profile an MRI capability in the context of a disease paradigm. For example, studies reported in the prostate cancer models *(24)*, in which diffusion-weighted MRI was used to detect a cancerous lesion on a mouse prostate or in high-resolution imaging of apolipoprotein E-deficient *(25)* and low-density lipoprotein-deficient *(26)* knockout mice. MRI has played an integral role in the evaluation of animal models of cerebral ischemia because it offers a full set of tools to capture the earliest events in this very traumatic disease *(7,8,27–29)*. Various agents (*see* **Table 1**) have been interrogated using combinations of T_1-, T_2-, diffusion-, and perfusion-weighted MRI. Despite such large-scale efforts, the clinical success in this area has not been exemplary. To that point, the only approved treatment for an acute cerebral ischemic attack is fibrinolysis (thrombolysis) with tissue plasminogen activator, and a huge unmet clinical need remains. Of late, careful considerations of diffusion/perfusion mismatch in animals *(30,31)* and humans *(32)* have attempted to better describe the ischemic progression. However, early hopes *(33)* that this method would revolutionize the treatment and prognosis of stroke patients have not yet been fully realized, and this continues to be an active area of research *(34)*. Further, advanced animals models of thrombolytic stroke have attempted to investigate imaging signatures in rat stroke models relevant to human disease *(35–39)*. It remains to be seen whether these studies can add beneficial information to decision making in the clinic.

MRI has also been used to screen compounds in xenograft-based testing methods on rodents (*see* **ref. *40***; additional information in **Table 1**). Although primary outcome measures have still focused on tumor burden and size reductions, in recent times, a variety of imaging readouts have added value *(41)*. MRI has also provided information on anatomical heterogeneity of tumors and, coupled with MRS, has generated observations of molecular markers *(42–44)*. There has been recent literature demonstrating the prognostic value of diffusion-weighted MRI for the early visualization of chemotherapeutic or radiotherapeutic response in solid tumors *(45)*. Advanced magnetic resonance angiography has demonstrated value in anatomical (morphometric) phenotyping in focal ischemia studies *(46)* and also in cardiovascular studies of vessel compliance *(47)*.

All of these studies ultimately contribute to annotate the efficacy of a drug-like lead along its evolution path to the clinic, presumably increasing the probabilities of future success.

2.3. Molecular Imaging With MRI

Molecular imaging is a broad, evolving field of research that includes a wide variety of imaging modalities and approaches *(9–11)*. Specific to the task of drug discovery, molecular imaging has the potential to provide dose–response relationships, to target modulation readouts, and to aid in the development of markers with prognostic value for disease evolution prediction.

MRI is likely to play a dual role in this evolving paradigm. First, the intricate pathological detail obtainable from MR can help guide the anatomical origin of molecular events measured by highly sensitive techniques (i.e., optical or nuclear techniques). Examples of such usefulness have already been described using fluorescence approaches *(10,11)*. Second, MRI will be useful in direct visualization of molecular events of interest to pharmacological disease processes. In this context, gene expression studies with MRI have been demonstrated, using controllable contrast agents *(48,49)* and engineered transferrin receptors *(41)*. Magnetic relaxation switches and high-throughput chemistry with superparamagnetic iron oxide particles have also been notably demonstrated *(50)*. Further method development and experimental optimization is ongoing to make these assays robust and viable for industrial grade scale-up.

3. Insights for Executing an MRI Experiment Within a Drug-Discovery Context

From the perspective of the need for MRI and the evidence of extensive use of MRI within the pharmaceutical industry, it is worthwhile to capture a practitioner's overview of how MRI experiments need to be developed and deployed within a drug-discovery environment. Clearly, there is no unique way of achieving this, and we only intend to provide the following as a framework for discussions; we fully recognize that many other novel applications will and need to occur outside of this framework.

Generation of an imaging assay for large-scale testing usually requires significant planning *a priori*. The most important requirement is to conceptually separate studies of analytical response characterization of test agents (e.g., dose–response, ED50, studies) from those of disease profiling. For studies with test agents, the capability to robustly quantify imaging markers is the key determinant of success. This implies that observations from images must have a high degree of fidelity and relevance to the disease process, and that the spatial features must have enough contrast to visualize and quantitate the features with confidence and reproducibility. It is equally important to establish a window of opportunity—i.e., to establish a quantifiable index with statistically significant difference between sham (naive animals) and controls (placebo-treated groups), within which, efficacy of test agents can be demonstrated. In investigational disease-profiling studies, appropriate focus needs to be targeted to build radio frequency (RF) coils, to optimize MRI pulse sequences, to capture the appropriate biomarker in conjunction with other available markers (e.g., from histopathology and histomorphometry), and, ultimately, to explore the feasibility of temporal staging of disease status by serial interrogation of such noninvasive markers. In each of these domains, there is much discussion and debate in the literature, and it is up to the imaging scientists to capture the full value from the opinions expressed.

With this general guidance, a specific path to implementing diffusion-weighted MRI (DWI) to study cerebral ischemia is presented below. Although DWI is used here as an example, the reader should recognize that a similar approach will be necessary for any imaging assay development. For example, developing a method for T_2-weighted and perfusion-weighted MRI for cerebral ischemic studies of test agents would require equal scrutiny and meticulous preparation.

3.1. Pilot Phase

Consider a pilot first, in which the following parameters can be optimized before undertaking a full-scale compound evaluation study:

3.1.1. The Model and the Appropriate Time Points

In general, DWI or calculated maps of the apparent diffusion coefficient would be able to map evolving ischemic lesions as early as minutes after an ischemic event. Such time precision is achievable and controllable with surgical models of ischemic stroke. If preocclusion and acute ischemic periods are critical, the use of an in-bore stroke model (e.g., via suture *(51,52)*, clot *(53)*, or macrosphere *(54)* occlusion) might be considered relevant, despite the complexity of this method. In other cases, a traditional bench-top occlusion method *(55,56)* might achieve the desired time points. In either case, the imaging scientist has to decide if an early readout will provide crucial information on the action of a test agent. Typically, this would also depend on the type of compound and its pharmacokinetics; for example, subcutaneous administration may be much slower to have an effect as opposed to intravenous administration. Hence, the time course of treatment relative to the modulation of water diffusion contrast with DWI may or may not always be the most optimal way of assessing efficacy-related outcomes, despite the attractive proposition of presenting the earliest in vivo signatures of tissue damage. In that case, it is imperative that negative imaging results attributable to compound pharmacokinetics and bioavailability not be (mis)interpreted as negative for treatment efficacy.

The most appropriate range of diffusion sensitivities to use (b values > 1000 s/mm^2, for example) needs to be addressed in the pilot stage as well. It is important to recognize the balance between the DWI contrast needed to see a drug-related modulation and the need to have appropriate image quality and signal-to-noise ratio to have confidence in those measurements. Additionally, given that the apparent diffusion coefficient can be influenced by a number of physiological parameters, it is important to ensure that normothermia, normocapnia, and normal heart rates are maintained during the MR examination.

3.1.2. Shimming/Tuning/RF Pulse Calibration Issues

Although this part is routine in most MRI experiments, it is important to remember that, in high-throughput studies of diseased animals, the imaging scientists may not always get the opportunity to tune and shim on every sample every time. Hence, shim files need to optimized, saved, and reloaded to save time; the tuning of the RF coil used must be robust enough to handle different animals without significant variability. One comforting point in this is the fact that most animals in focal ischemic studies (and many pharmacological studies, for that matter) are chosen to be similar (in weight, size, strain, and so on) for surgical and dosing needs. Hence, for MRI, usually shimming and tuning on one animal is sufficient.

3.1.3. Development of Quantitative Indices

Once the marker (for example, a DWI hyperintensity corresponding to an ischemic lesion in the brain) is identified and shown to be robustly registered as a surrogate for the disease in a small batch of animals, the issue of quantitation needs to be seriously reviewed. It is important to recognize that several indices can be devised to capture different features of a disease marker. For example, the complexity of the marker may range from lesion volume to modeling the temporal–spatial progression of ischemia in specific cerebral regions. Within each of these frames of thinking, three issues need to be clearly explored:

1. Sources of variability and relevance of the index to the disease process or its alleviation;
2. Sensitivity of the index to modulation by drug candidates; and
3. Feasibility and resources needed to calculate the index in a high-throughput mode.

Furthermore, in the cross-functional world of interdisciplinary results, acceptance of a new outcome measure is more widespread if it is appreciable not only to physicists but also to collaborating chemists and biologists.

3.1.4. Validation/Sensitivity With a Control Drug

Once an index is adapted, it is important to obtain histopathological signatures of events closest to the imaging readouts. This is not a trivial exercise because it is often challenging to localize histology to similar anatomical locations and measure appropriate processes that reflect the in vivo imaging readout. Therefore, it is not uncommon to find relatively low correlations between histological readouts and imaging readouts. Another aspect of interest at this level of testing is to check the sensitivity of the index with a control drug of known dramatic efficacy. This allows one to understand the window available in the index to capture the efficacy readout when an unknown test agent is used.

3.2. Scale-Up

Once the method of acquisition is settled via a pilot study, the biggest hindrance to robust application is throughput. Imaging studies, although sometimes only in perception, tend to be slower in their interrogation capabilities unless they are actively optimized to match the required industrial-grade throughput. This has to be done by careful optimization from the pilot stages of the assay development; otherwise, the full potential of MRI may not be fully realized.

Therefore, after the pilot, described in **Subheading 3.1.**, and the analysis of the results, and before scaling up, a detailed discussion about the need for such early signatures (predictive, serial value, and so on) should be undertaken. At this stage, careful planning of throughput is necessary, as is the ability to monitor different therapeutic groups. Typically, sham groups (i.e., groups with no surgical modifications or treatments) and placebo groups provide data on instrumental stability and model robustness, respectively. Such monitoring is critical to establish an imaging assay that can be used routinely for large-scale *ad hoc* testing of unknown test agents.

4. Summary

MRI has contributed significantly to the understanding of basic biological events in intact animal models of disease and also in trials of agents in both animals and man. As MRI evolves more in its throughput capabilities and in its capabilities to map molecular domain information in analytically robust ways, it is likely to have more and more influence on the drug-discovery processes (safety studies, pharmacokinetics, toxicological studies, target modulation and dose–response studies, and so on). In parallel, the appreciation of in vivo data and the value of noninvasive serial interrogation from intact animals will gain more importance, such that imaging may become an integral stage in the decision-making process of advancing lead compounds into the clinic. In combination with such capabilities, process-related mandates, and validated data, imaging is likely to play an increasingly significant role in drug discovery. Significant challenges exist along the path—the most important of which is the ability to produce robust data with *ad hoc* flexibility to participate in ongoing studies.

The indispensable value and, hence, the need of MRI is certainly beyond debate and MRI is currently well positioned to make dramatic contributions in pharmaceutical research and development.

References

1. http://www.phrma.org/issues/researchdev/.
2. DiMasi, J. A., Hansen, R. W., and Grabowski, H. G. (2003) The price of innovation: new estimates of drug development costs. *J. Health Econ.* **22,** 151–185.
3. DiMasi, J. A., Hansen, R. W., Grabowski, H. G., and Lasagna, L. (1991) Cost of innovation in the pharmaceutical industry. *J. Health Econ.* **10,** 107–142.
4. Roberts, S. A. (2003) Drug metabolism and pharmacokinetics in drug discovery. *Curr. Opin. Drug Discov. Devel.* **6,** 66–80.
5. Franks, R. and Hargeaves, R. (2003) Clinical biomarkers in drug discovery and development. *Nature Drug Discov.* **2,** 566–580.
6. DiMasi, J. A. (2002) The value of Imroving the productivity of the drug development process. *Pharmacoeconomics* **20 (Suppl. 3),** 1–10.
7. Beckmann, N., Mueggler, T., Allegrini, P. R., Laurent, D., and Rudin, M. (2001) From anatomy to the target: contributions of magnetic resonance imaging to pre-clinical pharmaceutical research. *Anat. Rec.* **265,** 85–100.
8. Rudin, M., Beckmann, N., Porszasz, R., Reese, T., Bochelen, D., and Sauter, A. (1999) In vivo magnetic resonance methods in pharmaceutical research: current status and perspectives. *NMR Biomed.* **12,** 69–97.
9. Rudin, M. and Weissleder, R. (2003) Molecular imaging in drug discovery and development. *Nat. Rev. Drug Discov.* **2,** 123–131.
10. Weissleder, R. and Mahmood, U. (2001) Molecular imaging. *Radiology* **219,** 316–333.
11. Weissleder, R. (2002) (Scaling down imaging: molecular mapping of cancer in mice. *Nat. Rev. Cancer* **2,** 11–18.
12. Chandra, S., Clark, L. V., Coatney, R. W., Phan, L., Sarkar, S. K., and Ohlstein, E. H. (1998) Application of serial in vivo magnetic resonance imaging to evaluate the efficacy of endothelin receptor antagonist SB 217242 in the rat carotid artery model of neointima formation. *Circulation* **97,** 2252–2258.
13. Chandra, S., Sarkar, S., Elliot, J. D., and Ohlstein, E. H. (1998) Application of magnetic resonance imaging for evaluation of the efficacy of SB 217242 in neointimal formation. *J. Cardiovasc. Pharmacol.* **31 (Suppl 1),** 317–319.
14. Beckmann, N., Tigani, B., Ekatodramis, D., Borer, R., Mazzoni, L., and Fozard, J. R. (2001) Pulmonary edema induced by allergen challenge in the rat: noninvasive assessment by magnetic resonance imaging. *Magn. Reson. Med.* **45,** 88–95.
15. Tigani, B., Cannet, C., Zurbrugg, S., et al. (2003) Resolution of the oedema associated with allergic pulmonary inflammation in rats assessed noninvasively by magnetic resonance imaging. *Br. J. Pharmacol.* **140,** 239–246.
16. Hellings, P. W., Hessel, E. M., Van Den Oord, J. J., Kasran, A., Van Hecke, P., and Ceuppens, J. L. (2001) Eosinophilic rhinitis accompanies the development of lower airway inflammation and hyper-reactivity in sensitized mice exposed to aerosolized allergen. *Clin. Exp. Allergy.* **31,** 782–790.

17. Middleton, H., Black, R. D., Saam, B., et al. (1995) Magnetic Resonance Imaging with hyperpolarized 3He gas. *Magn. Reson. Med.* **33,** 271–275.
18. Samee, S., Altes, T., Powers, P., et al. (2003). Imaging the lungs in asthmatic patients using hyperpolarized Helium-3 magnetic resonance assessment of response to methcholine exercise challenge. *J. Allergy Clin. Immun.* **111,** 1205–1211.
19. Waterton, J. C., Rajanayagam, V., Ross, B. D., Whittemore, A., and Johnstone, D. (1993). Magnetic Resonance methods for measurement of disease progression in rheumatoid arthritis. *Magn. Reson. Imaging* **11,** 1033–1038.
20. Dawson, J., Gustard, S., and Beckmann, N. (1999) High Resolution three dimensional magnetic resonance imaging for the investigation of knee joint damage during the time course of antigen induced arthiritis in rabbits. *Arthritis Rheum.* **42,** 119–128.
21. Beckmann, N., Bruttel, K., Mir, A., and Rudin, M. (1995) Non invasive 3D MR microscopy as a tool in pharmacological research: Applications to a model of arthritis. *Magn. Reson. Imaging* **13,** 1013–1017.
22. Beckmann, N., Bruttel, K., Schuurman, H., and Mir, A. (1998). Effects of sandimmune neural on collagen-induced arthritis in DA rats: Characterization by high resolution three dimensional magnetic resonance imaging and by histology. *J. Magn. Reson.* **131,** 8–16.
23. Beckmann, N., Falk, R., Zurbrugg, S., Dawson, J., and Engelhardt, P. (2003) Macrophage infiltration into the rat knee detected by MRI in a model of antigen-induced arthritis. *Magn. Reson. Med.* **49,** 1047–1055.
24. Song, S. K., Qu, Z., Garabedian, E. M., Gordon, J. I., Milbrandt, J., and Ackerman, J. J. (2002) Improved magnetic resonance imaging detection of prostate cancer in a transgenic mouse model. *Cancer Res.* **62,** 1555–1558.
25. Fayad, Z. A., Fallon, J. T., Shinnar, M., et al. (1998) Noninvasive In vivo high-resolution magnetic resonance imaging of atherosclerotic lesions in genetically engineered mice. *Circulation* **98,** 1541–1547.
26. Hockings, P. D., Roberts, T., Galloway, G. J., et al. (2002) Repeated three-dimensional magnetic resonance imaging of atherosclerosis development in innominate arteries of low-density lipoprotein receptor-knockout mice. *Circulation* **106,** 1716–1721.
27. Fisher, M. and Takano, K. (1995) The penumbra, therapeutic time window and acute ischaemic stroke. *Baillieres Clin. Neurol.* **4,** 279–295.
28. Hoehn, M., Nicolay, K., Franke, C., and van der Sanden, B. (2001) Application of magnetic resonance to animal models of cerebral ischemia. *J. Magn. Reson. Imaging* **14,** 491–509.
29. Tatlisumak, T. and Li, F. (2003) Use of diffusion- and perfusion-weighted magnetic resonance imaging in drug development for ischemic stroke. *Curr. Drug Targets CNS Neurol. Disord.* **2,** 131–141.
30. Quast, M. J., Huang, N. C., Hillman, G. R., and Kent, T. A. (1993) The evolution of acute stroke recorded by multimodal magnetic resonance imaging. *Magn. Reson. Imaging* **11,** 465–471.

31. Hata, R., Mies, G., Wiessner, C., et al. (1998) A reproducible model of middle cerebral artery occlusion in mice: hemodynamic, biochemical, and magnetic resonance imaging. *J. Cereb. Blood Flow Metab.* **18,** 367–375.

32. Baird, A. E., Benfield, A., Schlaug, G., et al. (1997) Enlargement of human cerebral ischemic lesion volumes measured by diffusion-weighted magnetic resonance imaging. *Ann. Neurol.* **41,** 581–589.

33. Albers, G. W. (1999) Expanding the window for thrombolytic therapy in acute stroke. The potential role of acute MRI for patient selection. *Stroke.* **30,** 2230–2237.

34. Guadagno, J. V., Donnan, G. A., Markus, R., Gillard, J. H., and Baron, J. C. (2004) Imaging the ischaemic penumbra. *Curr. Opin. Neurol.* **17,** 61–67.

35. de Crespigny, A. J., Tsuura, M., Moseley, M. E., and Kucharczyk, J. (1993) Perfusion and diffusion MR imaging of thromboembolic stroke. *J. Magn. Reson. Imaging* **3,** 746–754.

36. Zhang, Z., Zhang, R. L., Jiang, Q., Raman, S. B., Cantwell, L., and Chopp, M. (1997) A new rat model of thrombotic focal cerebral ischemia. *J. Cereb. Blood Flow Metab.* **17,** 123–135.

37. Busch, E., Kruger, K., Allegrini, P. R., et al. (1998) Reperfusion after thrombolytic therapy of embolic stroke in the rat: magnetic resonance and biochemical imaging. *J. Cereb. Blood Flow Metab.* **18,** 407–418.

38. Takano, K., Carano, R. A., Tatlisumak, T., et al. (1998) Efficacy of intra-arterial and intravenous prourokinase in an embolic stroke model evaluated by diffusion-perfusion magnetic resonance imaging. *Neurology* **50,** 870–875.

39. Jiang, Q., Zhang, R. L., Zhang, Z. G., Ewing, J. R., Divine, G. W., and Chopp, M. (1998) Diffusion-, T2-, and perfusion-weighted nuclear magnetic resonance imaging of middle cerebral artery embolic stroke and recombinant tissue plasminogen activator intervention in the rat. *J. Cereb. Blood Flow Metab.* **18,** 758–767.

40. Gillies, R. J., Bhujwalla, Z. M., Evelhoch, J., et al. (2000) Applications of Magnetic Resonance in Model Systems: Tumor Biology and Physiology. *Neoplasia* **2,** 139–151.

41. Weissleder, R., Moore, A., Mahmood, U., et al. (2000) In vivo Magnetic Resonance Imaging of Transgene Expression, *Nat. Med.* **63,** 351–354.

42. Stegman, L. D., Rehemetullah, A., Beattle, B., et al. (1999) Noninvasive quantitation of cytosine deaminase transgene expression in human tumor xenografts with in vivo magnetic resonance spectroscopy. *Proc. Natl. Acad. Sci. US A* **96,** 9821–9826

43. Nordsmark, M., Maxwell, R. J., Wood, P. J., et al. (1996) Effects of hydralazine in spontaneous tumors assessed by oxygen electrodes and 31P magnetic resonance spectroscopy. *Br. J.Cancer Suppl.* **27,** S232–235.

44. Shine, N., Palladino, M. A., Patton, J. S., et al. (1989) Early metabolic response to tumor necrosis factoring mouse sarcoma: a phophorus -31 nuclear magnetic resonance study. *Cancer Res.* **49,** 2123–2127.

45. Song, S.-K., Qu, Z., Garabedian, E. M., Milbrandt, J., and Ackerman, J. J. (2002) Improved magnetic resonance imaging detection of prostate cancer in a transgenic mouse model. *Cancer Res.* **62,** 1555–1558.

46. Beckmann, N. (2000) High resolution magnetic resonance angiography non-invasively reveals mouse strain differences in the cerebrovascular anatomy in vivo. *Magn. Reson. Med.* **44,** 252–258.
47. Chandra, S., Willette, R., Sauermelch, C., et al. (1999) Angiographic Determination of Vessel Distensibility in vivo. Effects of Eprosartan (AII antagonist) in a severe Hypertension model. *Proc. Int. Soc. Magn. Reson. Med.* **7,** 88.
48. Kayyem, J. F., Kumar, R. M., Fraser, S. E., and Meade, T. J. (1995) Receptor-targeted co-transport of DNA and magnetic resonance contrast agents. *Chem. Biol.* **2,** 615–620.
49. Louie, A. Y., Huber, M. M., Ahrens, E. T., et al. (2000) In vivo visualization of gene expression using magnetic resonance imaging. *Nat. Biotechnol.* **18,** 321–325.
50. Hogemann, D., Ntziachristos, V., Josephson, L., and Weissleder, R. (2002) High throughput magnetic resonance imaging for evaluating targeted nanoparticle probes. *Bioconjugate Chem.* **13,** 116–121.
51. Roussel, S. A., van Bruggen, N., King, M. D., Houseman, J., Williams, S. R., and Gadian, D. G. (1994) Monitoring the initial expansion of focal ischaemic changes by diffusion-weighted MRI using a remote controlled method of occlusion. *NMR Biomed.* **7,** 21–28.
52. Li, F., Han, S., Tatlisumak, T., et al. (1998) A new method to improve in-bore middle cerebral artery occlusion in rats: demonstration with diffusion- and perfusion-weighted imaging. *Stroke* **29,** 1715–1719.
53. Ishikawa, S., Yokoyama, K., Kuroiwa, T., and Makita, K. (2001) Evolution of cerebral ischaemia induced by thromboembolism in rats detected by early sequential MR imaging. *Br. J. Anaesth.* **87,** 469–476.
54. Gerriets, T., Li, F., Silva, M. D., et al. (2003) The macrosphere model: evaluation of a new stroke model for permanent middle cerebral artery occlusion in rats. *J. Neurosci. Methods* **122,** 201–211.
55. Kudo, M., Aoyama, A., Ichimori, S., and Fukunaga, N. (1982) An animal model of cerebral infarction. Homologous blood clot emboli in rats. *Stroke* **13,** 505–508.
56. Koizumi, J., Yoshida, Y., Nakazawa, T., and Ooneda, G. (1986) Experimental studies of ischemic brain edema, I: a new experimental model of cerebral embolism in rats in which recirculation can be introduced in the ischemic area. *Jpn. J. Stroke* **8,** 1–8.
57. Sauter, A. and Rudin, M. (1986) Calcium antagonists reduce the extent of infarction in rat middle cerebral artery occlusion model as determined by quantitative magnetic resonance imaging. *Stroke* **17,** 1228–1234.
58. Sauter, A., Rudin, M., and Wiederhold, K. H. (1988) Reduction of neural damage in irreversible cerebral ischemia by calcium antagonists. *Neurochem. Pathol.* **9,** 211–236.
59. Chandra, S., White, R. F., Everding, D., et al. (1999) Use of diffusion-weighted MRI and neurological deficit scores to demonstrate beneficial effects of isradipine in a rat model of focal ischemia. *Pharmacology* **58,** 292–299.
60. Reese, T., Porszasz, R., Baumann, D., et al. (2000) Cytoprotection does not preserve brain functionality in rats during the acute post-stroke phase despite evidence of non-infarction provided by MRI. *NMR Biomed.* **13,** 361–370.

61. Germano, I. M., Bartkowski, H. M., Berry, I., Moseley, M., Brant-Zawadzki, M., and Pitts, L. H. (1986) Magnetic resonance imaging in the evaluation of nimodipine-treated acute experimental focal cerebral ischemia. *Acta Radiol. Suppl.* **369,** 49–52.

62. Kucharczyk, J., Chew, W., Derugin, N., et al. (1989) Nicardipine reduces ischemic brain injury. Magnetic resonance imaging/spectroscopy study in cats. *Stroke* **20,** 268–274.

63. Chew, W., Kucharczyk, J., Moseley, M., Derugin, N., and Norman, D. (1991) Hyperglycemia augments ischemic brain injury: in vivo MR imaging/spectroscopic study with nicardipine in cats with occluded middle cerebral arteries. *AJNR Am. J. Neuroradiol.* **12,** 603–609.

64. Yenari, M. A., Palmer, J. T., Sun, G. H., de Crespigny, A., Mosely, M. E., and Steinberg, G. K. (1996) Time-course and treatment response with SNX-111, an N-type calcium channel blocker, in a rodent model of focal cerebral ischemia using diffusion-weighted MRI. *Brain Res.* **739,** 36–45.

65. Perez-Pinzon, M. A., Yenari, M. A., Sun, G. H., Kunis, D. M., and Steinberg, G. K. (1997) SNX-111, a novel, presynaptic N-type calcium channel antagonist, is neuroprotective against focal cerebral ischemia in rabbits. *J. Neurol. Sci.* **153,** 25–31.

66. Seega J. and Elger B. (1993) Diffusion- and T2-weighted imaging: evaluation of oedema reduction in focal cerebral ischaemia by the calcium and serotonin antagonist levemopamil. *Magn. Reson. Imaging* **11,** 401–409.

67. Reggiani, A., Pietra, C., Arban, R., et al. (2001) The neuroprotective activity of the glycine receptor antagonist GV150526: an in vivo study by magnetic resonance imaging. *Eur. J. Pharmacol.* **419,** 147–153.

68. Petty, M. A., Neumann-Haefelin, C., Kalisch, J., Sarhan, S., Wettstein, J. G., and Juretschke, H. P. (2003) In vivo neuroprotective effects of ACEA 1021 confirmed by magnetic resonance imaging in ischemic stroke. *Eur. J. Pharmacol.* **474,** 53–62.

69. Takano, K., Tatlisumak, T., Formato, J. E., et al. (1997) Glycine site antagonist attenuates infarct size in experimental focal ischemia. Postmortem and diffusion mapping studies. *Stroke* **28,** 1255–1262.

70. Qiu, H., Hedlund, L. W., Gewalt, S. L., Benveniste, H., Bare, T. M., and Johnson, G. A. (1997) Progression of a focal ischemic lesion in rat brain during treatment with a novel glycine/NMDA antagonist: an in vivo three-dimensional diffusion-weighted MR microscopy study. *J. Magn. Reson. Imaging* **7,** 739–744.

71. Lo, E. H., Pierce, A. R., Mandeville, J. B., and Rosen, B. R. (1997) Neuroprotection with NBQX in rat focal cerebral ischemia. Effects on ADC probability distribution functions and diffusion-perfusion relationships. *Stroke* **28,** 439–446.

72. Kucharczyk, J., Mintorovich, J., Sevick, R., Asgari, H., and Moseley, M. (1990) MR evaluation of calcium entry blockers with putative cerebroprotective effects in acute cerebral ischaemia. *Acta Neurochir. Suppl. (Wien).* **51,** 254–255.

73. Li, F., Carano, R. A., Irie, K., et al. (1999) Neuroprotective effects of a novel broad-spectrum cation channel blocker, LOE 908 MS, on experimental focal ischemia: a multispectral study. *J. Magn. Reson. Imaging* **10,** 138–145.

74. Allegrini, P. R. and Sauer, D. (1992) Application of magnetic resonance imaging to the measurement of neurodegeneration in rat brain: MRI data correlate strongly with histology and enzymatic analysis. *Magn. Reson. Imaging* **10,** 773–778.

75. Pschorn, U., Korperich, H., Heymans, L., Subramanian, S., and Kuhn, W. (1993) MRI and MRS studies on the time course of rat brain lesions and the effect of drug treatment: volume quantification and characterization of tissue heterogeneity by parameter selection. *Magn. Reson. Med.* **30,** 174–182.

76. Sauer, D., Martin, P., Allegrini, P. R., Bernasconi, R., Amacker, H., and Fagg, G. E. (1992) Differing effects of alpha-difluoromethylornithine and CGP 40116 on polyamine levels and infarct volume in a rat model of focal cerebral ischaemia. *Neurosci. Lett.* **141,** 131–135.

77. Sauer, D., Allegrini, P. R., Cosenti, A., Pataki, A., Amacker, H., and Fagg, G. E. (1993) Characterization of the cerebroprotective efficacy of the competitive NMDA receptor antagonist CGP40116 in a rat model of focal cerebral ischemia: an in vivo magnetic resonance imaging study. *J. Cereb. Blood Flow Metab.* **13,** 595–602.

78. Minematsu, K., Fisher, M., Li, L., et al. (1993) Effects of a novel NMDA antagonist on experimental stroke rapidly and quantitatively assessed by diffusion-weighted MRI. *Neurology* **43,** 397–403.

79. Minematsu, K., Fisher, M., Li, L., and Sotak, C. H. (1993) Diffusion and perfusion magnetic resonance imaging studies to evaluate a noncompetitive N-methyl-D-aspartate antagonist and reperfusion in experimental stroke in rats. *Stroke* **24,** 2074–2081.

80. Perez-Pinzon, M. A., Maier, C. M., Yoon, E. J., Sun, G. H., Giffard, R. G., and Steinberg, G. K. (1995) Correlation of CGS 19755 neuroprotection against in vitro excitotoxicity and focal cerebral ischemia. *J. Cereb. Blood Flow Metab.* **15,** 865–876.

81. Bochelen, D., Rudin, M., and Sauter, A. (1999) Calcineurin inhibitors FK506 and SDZ ASM 981 alleviate the outcome of focal cerebral ischemic/reperfusion injury. *J. Pharmacol. Exp. Ther.* **288,** 653–659.

82. Kozniewska, E., Roberts, T. P., Tsuura, M., Mintorovitch, J., Moseley, M. E., and Kucharczyk, J. (1995) NG-nitro-L-arginine delays the development of brain injury during focal ischemia in rats. *Stroke* **26,** 282–288.

83. Quast, M. J., Wei, J., and Huang, N. C. (1995) Nitric oxide synthase inhibitor NG-nitro-L-arginine methyl ester decreases ischemic damage in reversible focal cerebral ischemia in hyperglycemic rats. *Brain Res.* **677,** 204–212.

84. Haga, K. K., Gregory, L. J., Hicks, C. A., et al. (2003) The neuronal nitric oxide synthase inhibitor, TRIM, as a neuroprotective agent: effects in models of cerebral ischaemia using histological and magnetic resonance imaging techniques. *Brain Res.* **993,** 42–53.

85. Lee, J. H., Lee, Y. K., Ishikawa, M., et al. (2003) Cilostazol reduces brain lesion induced by focal cerebral ischemia in rats–an MRI study. *Brain Res.* **994,** 91–98.

86. Lesiuk, H., Sutherland, G., Peeling, J., Butler, K., and Saunders, J. (1991) Effect of U74006F on forebrain ischemia in rats. *Stroke* **22,** 896–901.

87. Muller, T. B., Haraldseth, O., Jones, R. A., et al. (1995) Perfusion and diffusion-weighted MR imaging for in vivo evaluation of treatment with U74389G in a rat stroke model. *Stroke* **26,** 1453–1458.

88. Imura, Y., Kiyota, Y., Nagai, Y., Nishikawa, K., and Terashita, Z. (1995) Beneficial effect of CV-4151 (Isbogrel), a thromboxane A2 synthase inhibitor, in a rat middle cerebral artery thrombosis model. *Thromb. Res.* **79,** 95–107.

89. Tatlisumak, T., Takano, K., Carano, R. A., and Fisher, M. (1996) Effect of basic fibroblast growth factor on experimental focal ischemia studied by diffusion-weighted and perfusion imaging. *Stroke* **27,** 2292–2297.

90. van Bruggen, N., Thibodeaux, H., Palmer, J. T., et al. (1999) VEGF antagonism reduces edema formation and tissue damage after ischemia/reperfusion injury in the mouse brain. *J. Clin. Invest.* **104,** 1613–1620.

91. Kent, T. A., Quast, M., Taglialatela, G., et al. (1999) Effect of NGF treatment on outcome measures in a rat model of middle cerebral artery occlusion. *J. Neurosci. Res.* **55,** 357–369.

92. Beech, J. S., Reckless, J., Mosedale, D. E., Grainger, D. J., Williams, S. C., and Menon, D. K. (2001) Neuroprotection in ischemia-reperfusion injury: an antiinflammatory approach using a novel broad-spectrum chemokine inhibitor. *J. Cereb. Blood Flow Metab.* **21,** 683–689.

93. Braunschweiger, P. G., Schiffer, L. M., and Furmanski, P. (1986) 1H-NMR relaxation times and water compartmentalization in experimental tumor models. *Magn. Reson. Imaging* **4,** 335–342.

94. Braunschweiger, P. G., Reynolds, K., Nelson, T. R., and Maring, E. (1987) The effect of dexamethasone on tissue water distribution and proton relaxation in Panc02 tumors. *Magn. Reson. Imaging* **5,** 483–492.

95. Furman, E., Margalit, R., Bendel, P., Horowitz, A., and Degani, H. (1991) In vivo studies by magnetic resonance imaging and spectroscopy of the response to tamoxifen of MCF7 human breast cancer implanted in nude mice. *Cancer Commun.* **3,** 287–297.

96. Wolf, W., Presant, C. A., Servis, K. L., et al. (1990) Tumor trapping of 5-fluorouracil: in vivo 19F NMR spectroscopic pharmacokinetics in tumor-bearing humans and rabbits. *Proc. Natl. Acad. Sci. USA* **87,** 492–496.

97. Shungu, D. C., Bhujwalla, Z. M., Wehrle, J. P., and Glickson, J. D. (1992) 1H NMR spectroscopy of subcutaneous tumors in mice: preliminary studies of effects of growth, chemotherapy and blood flow reduction. *NMR Biomed.* **5,** 296–302.

98. Rudin, M., Briner, U., and Doepfner, W. (1988) Quantitative magnetic resonance imaging of estradiol-induced pituitary hyperplasia in rats. *Magn. Reson. Med.* **7,** 285–291.

99. Siegel, R. A., Tolcsvai, L., and Rudin, M. (1988) Partial inhibition of the growth of transplanted dunning rat prostate tumors with the long-acting somatostatin analogue sandostatin (SMS 201-995). *Cancer Res.* **48,** 4651–4655.

100. Qin, Y., Van Cauteren, M., Osteaux, M., Schally, A. V., and Willems, G. (1992) Inhibitory effect of somatostatin analogue RC-160 on the growth of hepatic metastases of colon cancer in rats: a study with magnetic resonance imaging. *Cancer Res.* **52,** 6025–6030.

101. Checkley, D., Tessier, J. J., Kendrew, J., Waterton, J. C., and Wedge, S. R. (2003) Use of dynamic contrast-enhanced MRI to evaluate acute treatment with ZD6474, a VEGF signalling inhibitor, in PC-3 prostate tumours. *Br. J. Cancer* **89,** 1889–1895.

102. Checkley, D., Tessier, J. J., Wedge, S. R., et al. (2003) Dynamic contrast-enhanced MRI of vascular changes induced by the VEGF-signalling inhibitor ZD4190 in human tumour xenografts. *Magn. Reson. Imaging* **21,** 475–482.

103. Drevs, J., Muller-Driver, R., Wittig, C., et al. (2002) PTK787/ZK 222584, a specific vascular endothelial growth factor-receptor tyrosine kinase inhibitor, affects the anatomy of the tumor vascular bed and the functional vascular properties as detected by dynamic enhanced magnetic resonance imaging. *Cancer Res.* **62,** 4015–4022.

104. Cohen, S. M., Taber, K. H., Malatesta, P. F., et al. (1991) Magnetic resonance imaging of the efficacy of specific inhibition of 5 alpha-reductase in canine spontaneous benign prostatic hyperplasia. *Magn. Reson. Med.* **21,** 55–70.

105. Cohen, S. M., Werrmann, J. G., Rasmusson G. H., et al. (1995) Comparison of the effects of new specific azasteroid inhibitors of steroid 5 alpha-reductase on canine hyperplastic prostate: suppression of prostatic DHT correlated with prostate regression. *Prostate* **26,** 55–71.

106. Silva, M., Wen, S., Siebert, E., et al. (2004) Diffusion-weighted magnetic resonance imaging characterization of anti-tumor activity of MLN2704 in a bone metastatic cancer model. *Proc. Int. Soc. Magn. Reson. Med.* **12,** 2510.

107. Umemura, K., Zierhut, W., Rudin, M., et al. (1992) Effect of spirapril on left ventricular hypertrophy due to volume overload in rats. *J. Cardiovasc. Pharmacol.* **19,** 375–381.

108. McDonald, K. M., Rector, T., Carlyle, P. F., Francis, G. S., and Cohn, J. N. (1994) Angiotensin-converting enzyme inhibition and beta-adrenoceptor blockade regress established ventricular remodeling in a canine model of discrete myocardial damage. *J. Am. Coll. Cardiol.* **24,** 1762–1768.

109. Barone, F. C., Coatney, R. W., Chandra, S., et al. (2001) Eprosartan reduces cardiac hypertrophy, protects heart and kidney, and prevents early mortality in severely hypertensive stroke-prone rats. *Cardiovasc. Res.* **50,** 525–537.

110. Zierhut, W., Studer, R., Laurent, D., et al. (1996) Left ventricular wall stress and sarcoplasmic reticulum Ca(2+)-ATPase gene expression in renal hypertensive rats: dose-dependent effects of ACE inhibition and AT1-receptor blockade. *Cardiovasc. Res.* **31,** 758–768.

111. Ishikawa, M., Mori, T., Itoh, S., et al. (1995) Effects of OPC-18790, a new positive inotropic agent, on energetics in the ischaemic canine heart: a 31P-MRS study. *Cardiovasc. Res.* **30,** 299–306.

112. Lauerma, K., Saeed, M., Wendland, M. F., Derugin, N., Yu, K. K., and Higgins, C. B. (1996) Verapamil reduces the size of reperfused ischemically injured myocardium in hypertrophied rat hearts as assessed by magnetic resonance imaging. *Am. Heart J.* **131,** 14–23.

113. Watzinger, N., Lund, G. K., Higgins, C. B., Chujo, M., and Saeed, M. (2002) Noninvasive assessment of the effects of nicorandil on left ventricular volumes and function in reperfused myocardial infarction. *Cardiovasc. Res.* **54,** 77–84.

114. Thompson, K., Wisenberg, G., Sykes, J., and Thompson, R. T. (2003) MRI/MRS evaluation of cariporide in a canine long-term model of reperfused ischemic insults. Magnetic resonance imaging/magnetic resonance spectroscopy. *J. Magn. Reson. Imaging* **17,** 136–141.

115. Kupriyanov, V. V., Xiang, B., Sun, J., and Jilkina, O. (2002) The effects of drugs modulating K(+) transport on Rb(+) uptake and distribution in pig hearts following regional ischemia: (87)Rb MRI study. *NMR Biomed.* **15,** 348–355.

116. Faden, A. I., Knoblach, S. M., Cernak, I., et al. (2003) Novel diketopiperazine enhances motor and cognitive recovery after traumatic brain injury in rats and shows neuroprotection in vitro and in vivo. *J. Cereb. Blood Flow Metab.* **23,** 342–354.

117. Kroppenstedt, S. N., Stroop, R., Kern, M., Thomale, U. W., Schneider, G.H., and Unterberg, A. W. (1999) Lubeluzole following traumatic brain injury in the rat. *J. Neurotrauma* **16,** 629–637.

118. Petty, M. A., Poulet, P., Haas, A., Namer, I. J., and Wagner, J. (1996) Reduction of traumatic brain injury-induced cerebral oedema by a free radical scavenger. *Eur. J. Pharmacol.* **307,** 149–155.

119. Bradley, D. P., Smith, M. I., Netsiri, C., et al. (2001) Diffusion-weighted MRI used to detect in vivo modulation of cortical spreading depression: comparison of sumatriptan and tonabersat. *Exp. Neurol.* **172,** 342–353.

120. Lenhard, S. C., Nerurkar, S. S., Schaeffer, T. R., et al. (2003) p38 MAPK inhibitors ameliorate target organ damage in hypertension: Part 2. Improved renal function as assessed by dynamic contrast-enhanced magnetic resonance imaging. *J. Pharmacol. Exp. Ther.* **307,** 939–946.

121. de Souza, C. J., Eckhardt, M., Gagen, K., et al. (2001) Effects of pioglitazone on adipose tissue remodeling within the setting of obesity and insulin resistance. *Diabetes* **50,** 1863–1871.

122. Bradbeer, J. N., Kapadia, R. D., Sarkar, S. K., et al. (1996) Disease-modifying activity of SK&F 106615 in rat adjuvant-induced arthritis. Multiparameter analysis of disease magnetic resonance imaging and bone mineral density measurements. *Arthritis Rheum.* **39,** 504–514.

123. Badger, A. M., Griswold, D. E., Kapadia, R., et al. (2000) Disease-modifying activity of SB 242235, a selective inhibitor of p38 mitogen-activated protein kinase, in rat adjuvant-induced arthritis. *Arthritis Rheum.* **43,** 175–183.

124. Badger, A. M., Blake, S., Kapadia, R., et al. (2001) Disease-modifying activity of SB 273005, an orally active, nonpeptide alphavbeta3 (vitronectin receptor) antagonist, in rat adjuvant-induced arthritis. *Arthritis Rheum.* **44,** 128–137.

125. Borah, B., Francis, M. D., Hovancik, K., Boyce J. T., and Szeverenyi, N.M. (1995) A quantitative one-dimensional magnetic resonance imaging technique in adjuvant arthritis: the assessment of disease progression and indomethacin efficacy. *J. Rheumatol.* **22,** 855–862.

126. Beckmann, N., Bruttel, K., Schuurman, H., and Mir, A. (1998) Effects of Sandimmune neoral on collagen-induced arthritis in DA rats: characterization by high resolution three-dimensional magnetic resonance imaging and by histology. *J. Magn. Reson.* **131,** 8–16.

V

Novel Contrast Agents and Mechanisms

13

Hyperpolarized Gas and Oxygen-Enhanced Magnetic Resonance Imaging

Vu M. Mai

Summary

Unlike any other organ, imaging of lungs with magnetic resonance faces unique challenges owing to the complex microstructure and presence of gas–tissue interfaces. With the evolution of faster and stronger gradient systems leading to ultrafast imaging with ultrashort echo times, pulmonary magnetic resonance imaging (MRI) is no longer considered a technical challenge. In terms of functional evaluation, lungs are also associated with a unique function, *viz.* ventilation. Evaluation of ventilation is feasible with MRI either by using hyperpolarized noble gases or in an indirect fashion by performing oxygen-enhanced MRI. This chapter will provide an overview of these two methods.

Key Words: Lungs; ventilation; hyperpolarized gas; oxygen-enhanced MRI.

1. Introduction

Regional assessment of ventilation is crucial in the evaluation of pulmonary disorders because sufficient ventilation of the lung tissue is a major determinant of efficient gas exchange. Currently, lung ventilation imaging is performed using either radionuclide scintigraphy *(1,2)* or xenon computed tomography *(3)*. Both of these techniques have limitations; radionuclide scintigraphy needs administration of a radioactive tracer and suffers from poor spatial resolution, and xenon computed tomography involves exposure to ionizing radiation. Therefore, an alternate noninvasive ventilation imaging modality is clearly desirable. Magnetic resonance imaging (MRI) offers potential avenues for the assessment of ventilation in a noninvasive fashion. Conventional MRI is a powerful and versatile diagnostic imaging modality and has proven efficacious in diagnosing a host of pathologies in various organs. However, its application to the lung, until recently, has been limited because of the inherent properties of the lung, such as low proton density and large magnetic susceptibility difference arising from the air–tissue interfaces *(4,5)*. With the evolution of fast gra-

From: *Methods in Molecular Medicine, Vol. 124*
Magnetic Resonance Imaging: Methods and Biologic Applications
Edited by: P. V. Prasad © Humana Press Inc., Totowa, NJ

dient switching and ultrafast imaging, such as fast spin-echo techniques, pulmonary MRI is now feasible on most state-of-the-art commercial scanners. However, for both clinical and physiological studies, ability to perform additional functional studies, such as ventilation and perfusion are important.

There are two different approaches to performing ventilation MRI of the lungs. One is a direct method based on gas-phase imaging using hyperpolarized noble gases, such as ^{3}He and ^{129}Xe *(6–8)*. Alternatively, oxygen-enhanced MRI can serve as an indirect method of evaluating ventilation *(9,10)*. Oxygen-enhanced MRI does not image gas-filled spaces, but does allow for detecting ventilation defects. The key advantages of the latter technique are, of course, the fact that no specialized equipment is necessary and that oxygen is readily available in most MRI facilities.

In this chapter, we will present an overview of hyperpolarized gas and oxygen-enhanced MRI. We will describe the data acquisition methods, including technical and experimental procedures, as well as the postprocessing of the data, and provide a few examples to highlight potential applications. The goal is to provide interested readers with the sufficient technical and logistical background necessary to implement hyperpolarized gas and oxygen-enhanced ventilation imaging.

2. Hyperpolarized Gas MRI

The term hyperpolarized is used because the polarization of the nuclear spins is much greater, approx 5 orders of magnitude, than the polarization achieved using the magnetic field of a typical whole-body scanner. This leads to substantially high signal-to-noise ratio in the acquired images. Two noble gas isotopes, ^{3}He and ^{129}Xe, have been extensively used for hyperpolarized MRI studies because they possess a nuclear spin of 1/2. Although both gases have been used in the imaging of gas-filled spaces, ^{129}Xe can be of potential value for perfusion imaging because it is soluble in blood *(11,12)*. Because methodologies for ^{3}He and ^{129}Xe MRI are similar and more ^{3}He gas imaging studies have been conducted by various research groups, we will focus our discussion primarily on ^{3}He.

2.1. Hyperpolarization of ^{3}He

Hyperpolarized ^{3}He is produced by transferring the angular momentum from the circularly polarized light from a laser source to the nuclei of the gas. Currently, two techniques are being used: spin-exchange optical pumping (SEOP) and metastable-exchange optical pumping (MEOP). In both of these techniques, the polarization transfer occurs in two steps: from light (usually a laser tuned to the appropriate atomic transition frequency) to electron spins, and from electron spins to the nuclear spins of ^{3}He gas. Detailed descriptions of the

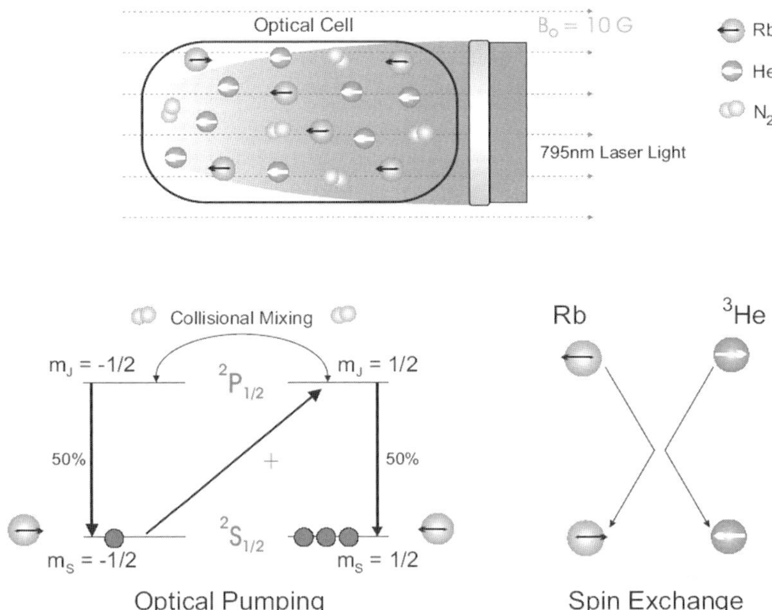

Fig. 1. Schematic representation of spin-exchange optical pumping (SEOP). Optical pumping with 795-nm laser light creates large electronic-spin polarization in the Rb atoms, which is transferred via spin-exchange collisions to the ^{3}He nuclei. A typical ^{3}He polarization-time constant is roughly 4 h for a 2 L batch.

two techniques are beyond the scope of this chapter. For interested readers, technical details of theoretical and practical considerations of SEOP and MEOP are described extensively elsewhere *(13–18)*. In SEOP, the laser light polarizes the valence electron of the vaporized alkali-metal atoms (Rb, K, or Cs) in a glass cell and excites the principal electric dipole transition of the valence electron from the $ns_{1/2}$ to the $np_{1/2}$ state. Because rubidium is the commonly used alkali metal, the wavelength of the laser light to facilitate this transition is tuned to 794.8 nm. The collisions between the excited valence electron of the alkali-metal atom and the noble gas atom facilitate the transfer of the electronic spin to the nuclear spin. The alkali-metal atom will then absorb another photon to embark on another spin-exchange cycle. A schematic diagram of the SEOP process is shown in **Fig. 1**. In MEOP, an intermediate alkali metal is not required. The laser light polarizes the valence electrons of the ^{3}He to a metastable $1s2s^3S_1$ state with a weak radio frequency discharge in which ^{3}He is maintained in a low-pressure environment (1–3 mbar). Optical pumping then occurs via the transition at 1083 nm light to the $1s2s^3P_0$ excited state, and decouples certain spin sublevels in the metastable state. Collisions between the

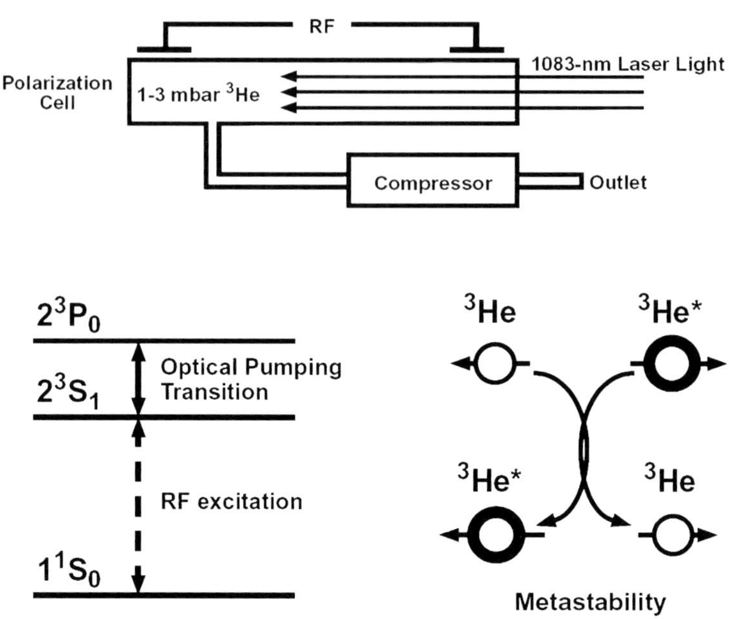

Fig. 2. Schematic representation of metastable-exchange optical pumping (MEOP). ^{3}He atoms at low pressure are excited into a metastable triplet state by a weak radio frequency discharge. Optical pumping of the metastable helium proceeds via absorption of 1083-nm light. Finally, a metastability-exchange collision results in a ground-state polarized ^{3}He atom.

polarized metastable and unpolarized atoms in the ground state will result in the nuclear polarization of the ^{3}He. The schematic diagram of the MEOP process is detailed in **Fig. 2**.

Once the polarizing process has stopped, MRI experiments can be performed on scanners equipped with broadband radio frequency transmitters and receivers. However, the longitudinal magnetization of hyperpolarized ^{3}He would continuously decay toward the equilibrium value. This decay rate, called the longitudinal relaxation time or T_1, has been measured to be several hours, but in the presence of oxygen it is dramatically reduced to several seconds *(19)*. Radio frequency pulses can also quickly destroy the longitudinal magnetization *(20)*. Therefore, efforts should be expended to optimize the use of radio frequency pulses. Automated frequency, transmitter, and receiver-gain adjustments that are routine on conventional MRI systems are not performed with hyperpolarized gas MRI. Instead, these calibrations are conducted using a glass cell containing a mixture of thermally polarized ^{3}He and 20% oxygen or a sufficiently small amount of hyperpolarized gas *(8)*. For the same reason, ac-

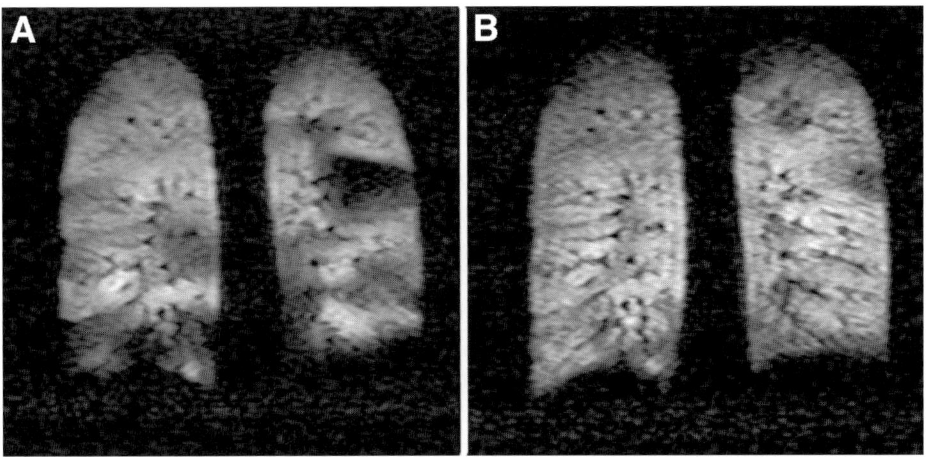

Fig. 3. Hyperpolarized [3]He magnetic resonance (MR) images from a confirmed asthmatic patient **(A)** before albuterol and **(B)** after albuterol administration. Note the ventilation defects in the before albuterol hyperpolarized [3]He images and the marked reduction in the number of defects in the after albuterol images. (Reproduced with permission from **ref. 27**.)

quisition of magnetic resonance (MR) hyperpolarized [3]He images are usually performed with flip angles of less than 10° when using gradient-echo or projection-reconstruction sequences *(6,11,21–23)*. However, a flip angle of 90° can be used when using single-shot techniques, such as echo planar imaging *(24)*.

2.2. Hyperpolarized Gas Imaging: Anatomic Evaluation

The first studies of hyperpolarized [3]He imaging were performed in animals *(6,21)*. Middleton et al. *(6)* and Black et al. *(21)* successfully imaged the lungs of the guinea pigs. These studies demonstrated that hyperpolarized [3]He retained significant polarization to allow for MR signal detection in the lung, and the acquired images exhibited detailed depiction of pulmonary air spaces, thus providing the impetus for in vivo human experimentation. Kauczor et al. *(25)* and MacFall et al. *(26)* were the first to conduct hyperpolarized [3]He imaging of the human lungs and found regional differences in signal intensity. Regional signal inhomogeneities with patchy or wedge-shaped defects were observed in patients with diseases such as chronic obstructive lung disease or bronchiectasis. Altes et al. *(27)* reported ventilation defects in asthmatic patients with [3]He imaging, even in cases in which the subjects showed normal pulmonary function testing because normal pulmonary function testing does not allow for regional assessment. They also demonstrated various degrees of reversal of ventilation defects after the administration of a bronchodilator (**Fig. 3**).

2.3. Hyperpolarized Gas Imaging: Functional Evaluation

Hyperpolarized gas imaging can potentially offer more than just elegant images of the gas space of the lung. Several investigators have explored the feasibility of deriving functional information using hyperpolarized gas imaging.

2.3.1. Dynamic Imaging

Johnson et al. *(28)* and Chen et al. *(29)* imaged the ^{3}He gas-flow dynamics in the lungs of guinea pigs using a radial pulse sequence. They demonstrated that high flip angles of the excitation radio frequency pulse enhanced the larger airways and that smaller flip angles progressively exhibited smaller airways. MacFall et al. *(26)* demonstrated real-time imaging of the gas-flow dynamics in the lungs of healthy subjects using a gradient-echo sequence and showed that inflow of gas was almost immediate at a temporal resolution of 1.8 s and a matrix size of 256 × 128. Ruppert et al. *(30)* applied a 2D fluoroscopic spiral sequence to image the slow inhalation of ^{3}He. Saam et al. *(24)*, detected ^{3}He signal in the distal lung within the first 200 ms at a temporal resolution of 122 ms and a reduced matrix size of 64 × 64. Real-time ^{3}He imaging studies of healthy and diseased lungs showed different patterns of signal enhancement. Wash-in and wash-out phases of the gas resulted in more uniform spatial distributions in healthy lungs, but appeared to be more heterogeneous and interspersed with ventilation defects in those diagnosed with smoking-related emphysema *(24,31,32)*.

2.3.2. Diffusion MRI

The high diffusion coefficient for gases and the fact that lungs have complex microarchitecture has led to an interest in performing diffusion imaging with hyperpolarized gases. The diffusion of ^{3}He is restricted by the sizes of the small airways and alveoli. Therefore, a diffusion-weighted MR study could characterize these pulmonary features and provide quantitative measures to identify early pathological changes in the microstructures of the lung. Apparent diffusion constants range from 0.17 to 0.28 cm^2/s in healthy subjects, as shown in **Fig. 4** *(20)*. However, in patients with emphysema, the values appear to be higher and the range of values broader (0.40–0.90 cm^2/s) *(33,34)*.

2.3.3. Oxygenation Maps

The interaction of ^{3}He with molecular oxygen in the lung accounts predominantly for the T_1 relaxation as mentioned in **Subheading 2.1.** Deninger et al. *(35,36)* have exploited this aspect to map the regional intrapulmonary oxygen concentration in subjects with apnea.

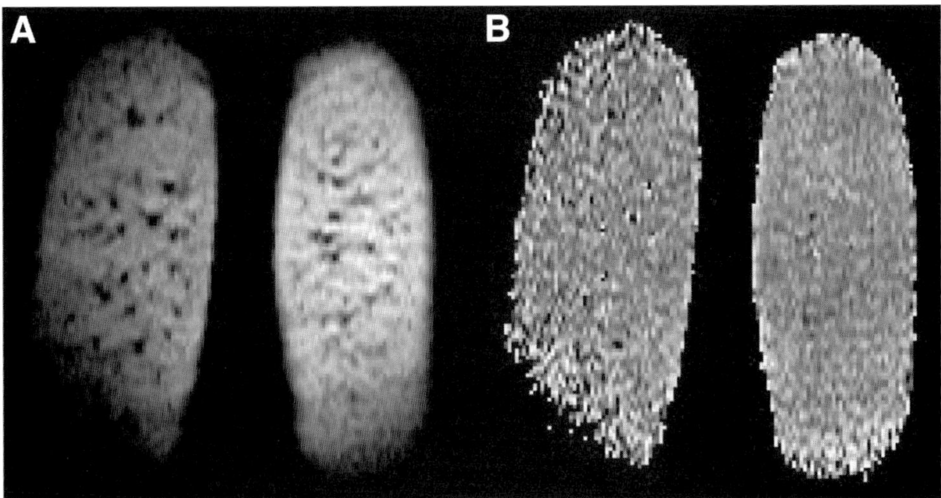

Fig. 4. **(A)** Representative 10-mm-thick ^{3}He base image and **(B)** the corresponding apparent diffusion coefficient map calculated from images acquired with four b values. The mean apparent diffusion coefficient in **(B)** was 0.25 cm^2/s. The base images were acquired using a 2D gradient-echo pulse sequence with an in-plane resolution of 2.0 × 3.8 mm.

3. Oxygen-Enhanced Ventilation MRI

Although the direct gas-phase imaging with hyperpolarized gases is desirable for ventilation imaging, there are several practical considerations that limit the more widespread application of the technology. These practical considerations include the need for a dedicated laser polarizing facility, and modifications to the scanner hardware (coils and associated electronics tuned to nonproton frequencies). Ability to obtain ventilation information based on proton MRI would be highly advantageous and would be readily available for widespread use. Oxygen-enhanced MRI has been shown to allow for an indirect method of evaluating lung ventilation. Before discussing the basics of oxygen-enhanced MRI, the challenges involved with proton MRI of the lung are briefly reviewed.

3.1. Proton MRI of the Lung

Until recently, detecting MR signal in the lung was particularly difficult because of the inherent architecture of the lung, because the lung is designed for efficient gas exchange and contains a significantly large number of alveoli. This produces large air-to-tissue interfaces, which, in turn, generate an inhospitable environment for MRI of the lung *(4,5)*. First, the numerous alveoli result in low proton density, which produces an inherently weak signal for detection relative to other organs in the body. Second, the air–tissue interfaces create large local magnetic field gradients that rapidly dephase the already weak MR signal and significantly reduce the apparent transverse relaxation time (T_2^*) to be approx 1.5 ms *(37)*. Lastly, the involuntary respiratory and cardiac motions potentially introduce artifacts to the image that may further degrade image quality. These make MRI of the lung highly challenging.

Early attempts to image the lung have focused on brute force approaches, such as shortening the echo times used with gradient-echo sequences in an effort to overcome the ultrashort T_2^* of the lung. Bergen et al. *(38)* proposed a back projection reconstruction imaging method, whereas Alsop et al. *(37)* designed a submillisecond echo time (TE) sequence using the advanced of gradient hardware technology. Although visualization of the lung has been demonstrated, the gradient-echo sequences are quite sensitive to magnetic susceptibility effects. The measured signal-to-noise ratio remains poor. Spin-echo sequences, on the other hand, are more immune to magnetic susceptibility differences and the signal is dictated by the transverse relaxation time (T_2), which is oftentimes significantly longer than that of T_2^*. However, the acquisition time of conventional spin-echo sequence is generally long, thus it is more prone to motion artifacts. Single-shot fast spin-echo sequences with an acquisition time on the order of hundreds of milliseconds are relatively immune to motion artifacts. Mayo et al. *(39)* were among the first to explore the use of spin-echo sequence for MRI of the lung, but visualization of the lung remained poor because of the bright signals from the surrounding tissues, such as fat and muscle. To enhance visualization of the lung tissue, the signal contributions from the thoracic muscle and fat should be suppressed. This was shown to be feasible using preparatory inversion recovery (IR) and multiple inversion recovery (MIR) pulses *(40–42)*. For the IR sequence, it was determined that a inversion time (TI) of 600 ms (at 1.5 T), which nulls the signal from thoracic muscle, is optimal for visualization of the lung *(40)*. To additionally suppress the MR signal from fat, a frequency-selective saturation pulse is used. On the other hand, two preparatory inversion radio frequency pulses are used in the MIR sequence to simultaneously suppress signals from fat and muscle by setting appropriate time delays. Assuming a T_1 of 250 ms for fat and of 1400 ms for the lung at 1.5 T, values of 800 and 150 ms have been used for the two inversion times in the MIR sequence *(41)*.

3.2. Paramagnetic Property of Oxygen

The weakly paramagnetic property of molecular oxygen caused by the presence of two unpaired electrons is the underling principle of oxygen-enhanced

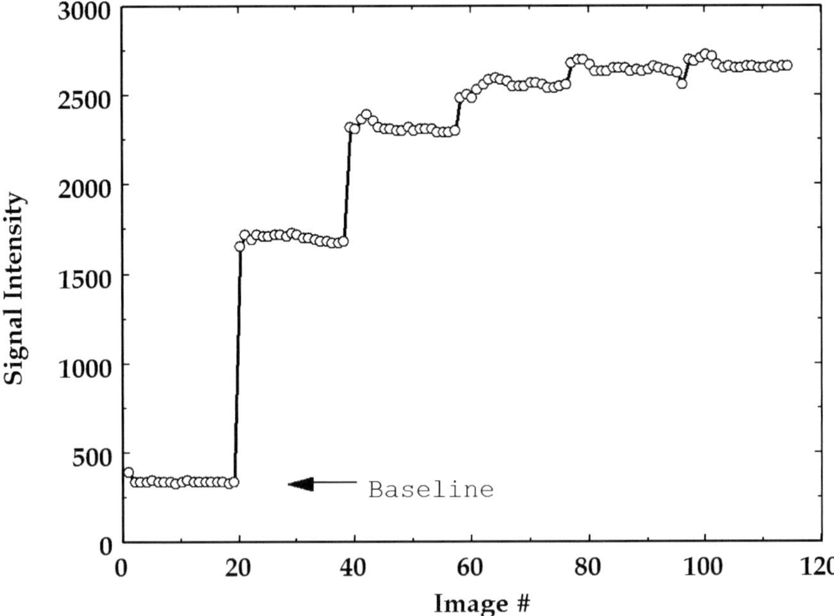

Fig. 5. Graded magnetic resonance (MR) signal changes corresponding to repeated oxygen bubbling periods of 30 s at a flow rate of 3 L/min. Signal intensity can be observed to plateau toward the end, indicating a saturation of concentration of oxygen in the solution.

ventilation imaging. Each electron has a magnetic moment that is 1000 times that of a nucleus, and the resulting fluctuating magnetic field can produce a greater dipole–dipole interaction than that of the neighboring nuclei, thus causing a faster rate of spin-lattice relaxation (R_1) $(=1/T_1)$. Chiarotti et al. *(43)* first reported that an increase in dissolved oxygen in water shortens its T_1. They also concluded that there exists a linear relationship between R_1 and the concentration of dissolved oxygen in water. A change in T_1 would, therefore, translate into a change in MR signal intensity on a T_1-weighted acquisition. **Fig. 5** shows the graded signal changes of the saline solution corresponding to different degrees of oxygen bubbling into the solution *(44)*. The signal plateau suggest of a saturation of dissolved oxygen in the saline solution.

Young et al. *(45)* extended Chiarotti's study to an in vivo application, and reported the shortening of T_1 and an increase in signal intensity of blood in the left ventricle of the heart after subjects inhaled 100% oxygen. Further expanding on these results, Edelman et al. *(9)* first proposed the use of oxygen for ventilation imaging in the lung. Although oxygen is only weakly paramagnetic, its overall effect on the lung is considerable given the large surface area of the lung and the large difference in partial pressures between room air and 100% oxygen. These two factors facilitate an environment that allows more oxygen to diffuse across the parenchyma and dissolve in blood. Generally, the oxygen-enhanced ventilation imaging technique involves the acquisition of series of images while the subjects alternately inhale room air (21% oxygen) and 100% oxygen *(9,10)*. The signal difference between the two reflects the change in the oxygen level dissolved in blood or lung tissues. The acquired images are then combined, and often subtracted, to produce the oxygen-enhanced ventilation image. Please note that this effect is different from the blood oxygenation level-dependent (BOLD) MRI that was discussed in Chapters 7 and 8.

3.3. Experimental Methods

Image acquisition of oxygen-enhanced studies involves two aspects: the MR sequence and the experimental protocol. To date, cardiac-triggered IR or MIR single-shot fast spin-echo sequences have often been used in oxygen-enhanced ventilation imaging because of their inherent advantages *(9,10,46)*. Cardiac triggering ensures that data acquisition would occur in late diastole *(46)* and in a reproducible fashion. The two TIs in the MIR sequence are usually set at 800 and 150 ms to concurrently suppress the signal from muscle and fat. This scheme improves the subtraction of the background tissues *(41,46)* compared with a single IR sequence. A single-shot fast spin-echo sequence with a short inter-echo spacing of 3.6 to 4.5 ms is commonly used with either centric reordering or half-Fourier acquisition. Subsequently, a time delay of 2 to 4 s is set to allow for the magnetization recovery.

The basic protocol of an oxygen-enhanced experiment uses alternating inhalation of room air and 100% oxygen by the subjects, who are asked to remain still and perform normal, quiet breathing during the MRI data acquisition *(9,10)*. The 100% oxygen flow is generally delivered at a rate of 15 L/min through a non-rebreathing ventilatory mask. Series of images (normally 20–30) are acquired during each period of inhalation of room air and 100% oxygen. Each of these periods typically lasts approx 3 min, and the whole procedure of image acquisition during alternated inhalation of room air and 100% oxygen can be repeated if necessary. Image acquisition during the oxygen-inhaling period can be obtained in either dynamic or steady-state schemes. In the steady-state scheme, at the end of the period of inhalation of room air, oxygen flow is initiated for approx 1 to 2 min before the start of image acquisition. This allows for the oxygen level in the lung to reach a steady state. Similarly, a delay of 1 to 2 min is applied at the end of 100% oxygen period before the next image acquisition during room air. On the other hand, image acquisition in the dynamic scheme would continue from the period of inhalation of room air into the period of inhalation of 100% oxygen as the oxygen

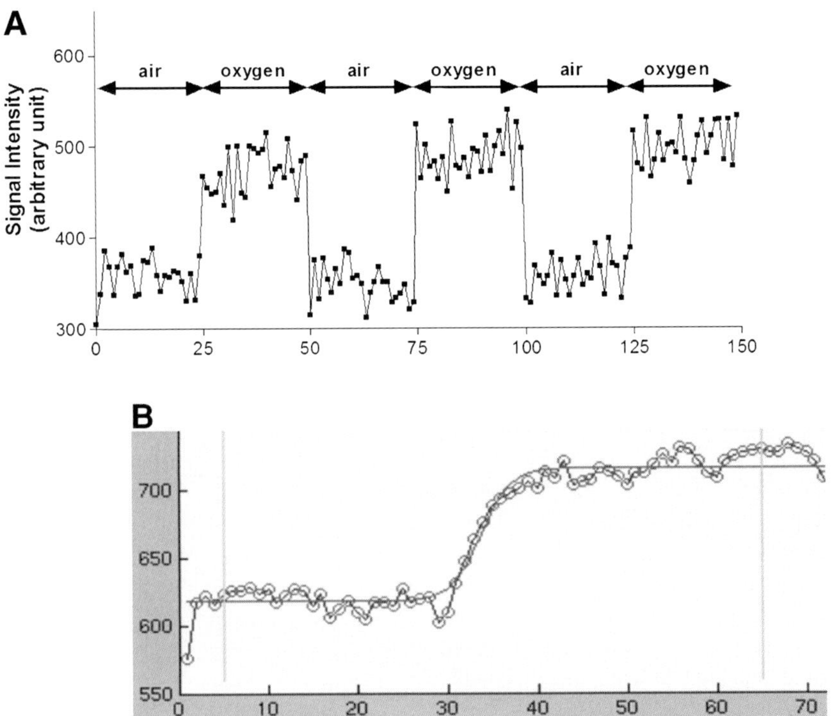

Fig. 6. **(A)** Time course of signal intensities of the lung during periods of inhalation of room air and 100% oxygen in a steady-state image acquisition. The average signal intensities were measured from a region of interest drawn in the upper right lung. Modulation of signal intensity between room air and 100% oxygen approximates the boxcar pattern. Note that for steady-state acquisitions, data is not obtained during the transition phase, hence, the apparent abrupt change in signal intensity. **(B)** The dynamic time course of oxygen-enhanced signal intensities of the up-slope ramp (room air to 100% oxygen). Signal intensity during the period of inhalation of room air progressively increases when 100% oxygen flow is initiated and subsequently reaches steady state. The solid line depicts the fit function, which was a hyperbolic tangent. From such fits, maps of slope, time-to-peak and time shift can be calculated on a pixel-by-pixel basis. These additional measures map allow for distinguishing partial from complete airway obstruction.

flow is initiated or ceased. This allows for acquiring the temporal response when switching between the breathing gases, as shown in **Fig 6B**. When similarly plotted, the steady-state scheme would result in an apparent immediate and abrupt transition in signal intensity between the periods of inhalation of room air and 100% oxygen (**Fig. 6A**), whereas the dynamic scheme would show a progressive rise in signal intensity from the room air to the 100% oxygen period until it reaches a steady state. Similar observations would also occur for the decrease in signal intensity in the transition period from 100% oxygen to room air when the flow ceases. The average signal intensities are usually measured using regions of interest drawn in the upper right or left lung, where effects of respiratory motion is minimal.

3.4. Data Analysis

Oxygen-enhanced ventilation images can be reconstructed by calculating the signal difference, percent difference, or statistical correlation on a pixel-by-pixel basis *(9,10,46–49)*. For calculating the difference and the percent difference images, the average of images acquired during breathing room air and 100% oxygen are first determined. To minimize mis-registration artifacts, a reference image (usually the one acquired at maximal expiration) is selected and only images from the steady-state segment of the series that match within a few pixels of the right lung–liver interface as reference are included. The difference image is then calculated by subtracting the average images obtained during the breathing room air period from the breathing 100% oxygen period. The percent difference image is obtained by dividing the difference image by the average image obtained during breathing of room air.

The qualitative correlation map is reconstructed by recognizing that the modulation of signal intensity between the images obtained during periods of breathing room air and breathing 100% oxygen approximates a boxcar pattern (**Fig. 6A**). This can be exploited to determine the correlation map using statistical analyses, which are being routinely applied in brain activation studies to localize regions of brain activation *(50,51)*. Pixel-by-pixel correlation maps of oxygen-enhanced ventilation can be generated by computing the cross-correlation between the time response function of each pixel and the ideal boxcar waveform that describes the expected time response. If the time response of each given pixel is denoted by the vector $\mathbf{A} = \{A_i\}$, where $i = 1$ to N, the number of images, and the expected time response is represented by the vector $\mathbf{B} = \{B_i\}$, the correlation coefficient, r, is computed using the following equation *(50,51)*:

$$r = \frac{\sum_{n=1}^{N}\left(A_i - \bar{A}\right)\left(B_i - \bar{B}\right)}{\sqrt{\sum_{n=1}^{N}\left(A_i - \bar{A}\right)^2}\sqrt{\sum_{n=1}^{N}\left(B_i - \bar{B}\right)^2}}, \qquad [1]$$

where $\bar{A}$ is the average value of vector $\mathbf{A}$, and $\bar{B}$ is the average value of the vector $\mathbf{B}$. The correlation coefficient reflects the degree to which the shapes of $\mathbf{A}$ and $\mathbf{B}$ are similar, but does not reflect their relative amplitudes.

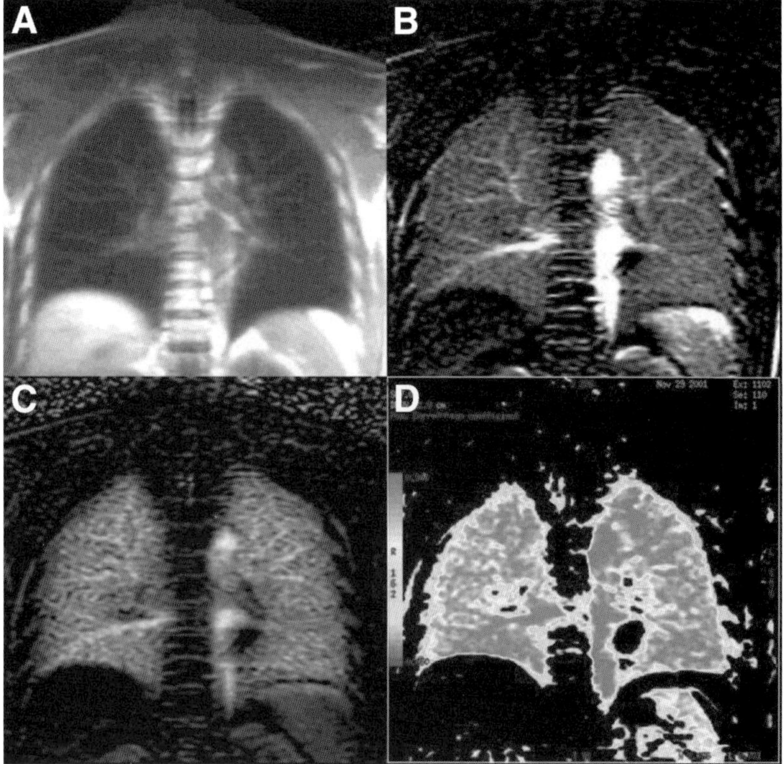

Fig. 7. Oxygen-enhanced ventilation images of a healthy volunteer obtained through different calculations. Shown are the **(A)** anatomical image, **(B)** difference image, **(C)** percent difference image, and **(D)** correlation map. Normal ventilation and similar pulmonary anatomy is observed among the images.

3.5. Applications

3.5.1. Steady-State Oxygen-Enhanced Imaging

The signal difference in oxygen-enhanced ventilation imaging has been reported in studies of healthy volunteers using IR or MIR sequences *(9,10,46–49)*. **Figure 7** shows IR oxygen-enhanced difference and percent difference images along with the correlation map, and **Fig. 8** shows MIR images along with their oxygen-enhanced difference images from three contiguous slices. Signal differences of pulmonary veins in **Figs. 7** and **8** are also observed and reflect the exchange of molecular oxygen from the airspace to pulmonary veins after inhalation of 100% oxygen. Similarly, the signal of the descending aorta, spleen, subclavian arteries, or the kidneys is indicative of the substantial increase in concentration of oxygen in the blood. The minimal change observed

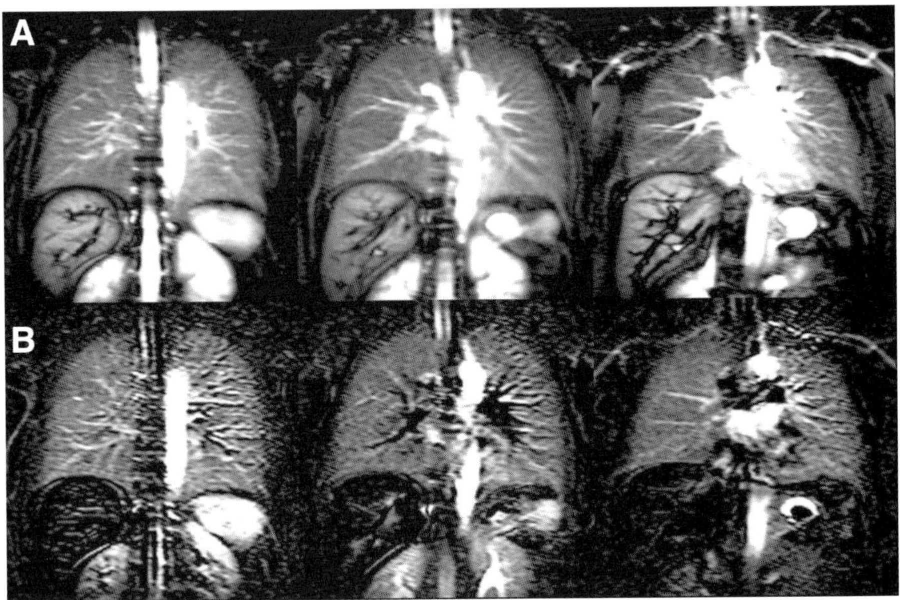

Fig. 8. Shown are three contiguous coronal multiple inversion recovery (MIR) anatomical images and their corresponding oxygen-enhanced difference images. Note that
the high signal difference occurs mainly in the lung parenchyma, pulmonary veins, the
descending aorta, the spleen, and the kidneys, but not in the pulmonary arteries. Excellent subtraction of the background tissues and a minimal presence of motion or spatial
mis-registration artifacts are observed.

in the pulmonary arteries is caused by the fact that it is the blood returning
from the rest of the body to the lungs and contains the least amount of oxygen.
Oxygen breathing leads to a difference in T_1 on the order of 100 to 200 ms
(10,47,52–54).

Despite the fact that oxygen-enhanced imaging is a recent development, it
has already been shown to successfully detect regional ventilation defects in
pulmonary diseases *(9,55,56)*. Edelman et al. *(9)* showed ventilation defects in
a patient with bullous emphysema. Nakagawa et al. *(55)* concluded that ventilation perfusion using oxygen-enhanced and bolus gadolinium contrast-enhanced techniques can be used to comprehensively assess pulmonary
ventilation–perfusion (V/Q) ratio abnormalities in patients with lung diseases.
Ohno et al. *(57)* studied patients with lung cancer who may or may not have
emphysema. Among the many findings reported, they found that the mean
slope of the signal enhancement was significantly lower in patients with lung
cancer than in healthy volunteers, and it was also significantly lower in lung
cancer patients with emphysema than in those without emphysema.

3.5.2. Dynamic Oxygen-Enhanced Imaging

The progressive increase in signal intensity in the dynamic data acquisition of oxygen-enhanced studies may provide potentially useful information regarding the ventilation, diffusion, and perfusion because the signal changes are the net result of these three factors. Ventilation determines the amount of oxygen being delivered to the lung; diffusion indicates the rate of oxygen crossing from the alveolar air space into blood; and perfusion, the rate of blood flow that carries the oxygenated blood away from the imaging slice. Muller et al. *(58)* showed that the mean slopes of the signal intensity are different between healthy volunteers and patients with pulmonary diseases, and that the slopes correlate with the diffusion capacity of the lung for carbon monoxide. Ohno et al. *(57,59)* also showed that mean relative enhancement ratios correlate with diffusion capacity of the lung for carbon monoxide and forced expiratory volume in 1 s.

Additional parameters, such as time shift and time to peak may be extracted from fitting the dynamic time course of the signal intensities to a mathematical function, such as hyperbolic tangent, as shown in **Fig. 6B**. Together, these may provide complementary and comprehensive regional information that may help in improving the specificity of the diagnosis of pulmonary diseases. Although the value of the maps of the difference and the slope has been established *(58,59)*, the maps of the time shift and time-to-peak may potentially differentiate between a complete and partial airway obstruction. However, there has not yet been any systematic study to evaluate the clinical use of this technique.

3.5.3. Ventilation–Perfusion Imaging

The matching of ventilation to pulmonary perfusion determines the efficiency of gas exchange in the lung. Ventilation and perfusion mismatching causes hypoxemia and impairs the gas exchange of both oxygen and carbon dioxide *(60–64)*. A thorough understanding of the distribution of V/Q ratio is, therefore, essential to elucidate the pathomechanisms leading to impaired gas exchange *(64)*. Pulmonary perfusion is an important physiological indicator in the evaluation of different lung diseases, such as pulmonary embolism (PE). However, an abnormal perfusion lung scan by itself is nonspecific because a variety of cardiorespiratory disorders, for example, chronic obstructive pulmonary diseases (COPD), can also result in pulmonary perfusion change. Consequently, a complementary ventilation scan is concurrently evaluated to ascertain patterns that reflect probabilities of PE and COPD. This is often referred as a V/Q scan. Generally, a mismatch in a V/Q scan (normal ventilation and abnormal perfusion) indicates a high probability of PE, and a matched V/Q (abnormal ventilation and perfusion) indicates a high probability of COPD.

Oxygen-enhanced ventilation imaging can be combined with either a gadolinium contrast-enhanced perfusion imaging or an arterial spin labeling (ASL) perfusion imaging technique to form an MR V/Q scan *(7,10,55,56,64–67)*. Contrast-enhanced perfusion imaging uses exogenous tracers, such as gadolinium chelates *(68–70)*, whereas ASL uses water in the blood as an endogenous and freely diffusible tracer *(71–74)*, which has been successfully demonstrated to image pulmonary perfusion *(75–77)*.

3.5.4. Mapping Partial Pressure of Oxygen in the Lung

Because the measured relaxation rate, R_1, is directly related to oxygen partial pressure *(43–45)*, in principle, measuring R_1 maps should allow one to create maps of oxygen pO_2.

However, additional information, such as the regional hematocrit, may be necessary before such maps can be derived. It has been previously shown that the T_1 changes are dependent on the hematocrit level *(78)*.

4. Conclusion

Hyperpolarized gas and oxygen-enhanced MRI of the lung are relatively new and exciting means to study gas exchange in the lung. They could also be potential clinical tools in the diagnosis of various pulmonary diseases. Although both techniques have been demonstrated to image ventilation, MR oxygen-enhanced ventilation imaging is different from hyperpolarized gas imaging in several aspects. The signal in hyperpolarized ^{3}He (or ^{129}Xe) gas imaging directly reflects the air spaces of the lung, whereas the signal of the oxygen ventilation imaging technique arises mainly from the pulmonary tissue or blood. As a result, oxygen-enhanced MRI is an indirect method of imaging ventilation. In addition, because oxygen plays a major role in the functional gas exchange within the lungs, the oxygen-enhanced ventilation imaging technique potentially provides a means to directly study oxygen transfer from the air space to the pulmonary vasculature. In more practical terms, oxygen is readily available as part of emergency equipment in most MR suites and is safe and inexpensive. The major drawbacks of hyperpolarized gas MRI include the high cost of the laser-polarizing unit, and the requirement for a non-proton imaging apparatus. The disadvantages of oxygen-enhanced imaging, however, are the relatively longer acquisition times and the need to perform subtraction or correlation analysis.

References

1. Amis, T. C., Crawford, A. B., Davison, A., and Engel, L. A. (1990) Distribution of inhaled ^{99m}Technetium labelled ultrafine carbon particle aerosol (Technegas) in human lungs. *Eur. Respir. J.* **3,** 679–685.

2. Hayes, M. and Taplin, G. V. (1980) Lung imaging with radioaerosols for the assessment of airway disease. *Semin. Nucl. Med.* **10,** 243–251.
3. Tajik, J. K., Chon, D., Won, C., Tran, B. Q., and Hoffman, E. A. (2002) Subsecond multisection CT of regional pulmonary ventilation. *Acad. Radiol.* **9,** 130–146.
4. Case, T. A., Durney, C. H., Ailion, D. C., Cutillo, A. G., and Morris, A. H. (1987) A mathematical model of diamagnetic line broadening in lung tissue and similar heterogeneous systems: calculations and measurements. *J. Magn. Reson.* **73,** 304–314.
5. Durney, C. H., Bertolina, J., Ailion, D. C., et al. (1989) Calculation and interpretation of inhomogeneous line broadening in models of lungs and other heterogeneous structures. *J. Magn. Reson.* **85,** 554–570.
6. Middleton, H., Black, R. D., Saam, B., et al. (1995) MR imaging with hyperpolarized 3He gas. *Magn. Reson. Med.* **33,** 271–275.
7. Bachert, P., Schad, L. R., Bock, M., et al. (1996) Nuclear magnetic resonance imaging of airways in humans with use of hyperpolarized 3He. *Magn. Reson. Med.* **36,** 192–196.
8. Mugler, J. P., 3rd, Driehuys, B., Brookeman, J. R., et al. (1997) MR imaging and spectroscopy using hyperpolarized 129Xe gas: preliminary human results. *Magn. Reson. Med.* **37,** 809–815.
9. Edelman, R. R., Hatabu, H., Tadamura, E., Li, W., and Prasad, P. V. (1996) Noninvasive assessment of regional ventilation in the human lung using oxygen-enhanced magnetic resonance imaging. *Nat. Med.* **2,** 1236–1239.
10. Chen, Q., Jakob, P. M., Griswold, M. A., Levin, D. L., Hatabu, H., and Edelman, R. R. (1998) Oxygen enhanced MR ventilation imaging of the lung. *MAGMA* **7,** 153–161.
11. Albert, M. S., Cates, G. D., Driehuys, B., et al. (1994) Biological magnetic resonance imaging using laser-polarized 129Xe. *Nature* **370,** 199–201.
12. Wagshul, M. E., Button, T. M., Li, H. F., et al. (1996) In vivo MR imaging and spectroscopy using hyperpolarized 129Xe. *Magn. Reson. Med.* **36,** 183–191.
13. Walker, T. G. and Happer, W. (1997) Spin exchange optical pumping of noble-gas nuclei. *Rev. Mod. Phys.* **69,** 629–642.
14. Happer, W. and van Wijngaarden, W. A. (1987) An optical pumping primer. *Hyperfine Interact.* **38,** 435–470.
15. Appelt, S., Ben-Amar Baranga, A., Erickson, C. J., Romalis, M. V., Young, A. R., and Happer, W. (1998) Theory of spin-exchange optical pumping of 3He and 129Xe. *Phys. Rev. A* **58,** 1412–1439.
16. Colegrove, F. D., Schearer, L. D., and Walters, G. K. (1963) Polarization of 3He gas by optical pumping. *Phys. Rev.* **132,** 2561–2572.
17. Gentile, T. R. and McKeown, R. D. (1993) Spin-polarizing 3He nuclei with an arclamp-pumped neodymium-doped lanthanum magnesium hexaluminate laser. *Phys. Rev. A* **47,** 456–467.
18. Stoltz, E., Meyerhoff, M., Bigelow, N., Leduc, M., Nacher, P. J., and Tastevin, G. (1996) High nuclear polarization in 3He and 3He-4He gas mixtures by optical pumping with a laser diode. *Appl. Phys. B* **63,** 629–633.
19. Saam, B., Happer, W., and Middleton, H. (1995) Nuclear relaxation of 3He in the presence of O2. *Phys. Rev. A* **52,** 862–865.

20. Moller, H. E., Chen, X. J., Saam, B., et al. (2002) MRI of the lungs using hyperpo-larized noble gases. *Magn. Reson. Med.* **47,** 1029–1051.
21. Black, R. D., Middleton, H. L., Cates, G. D., et al. (1996) In vivo He-3 MR im-ages of guinea pig lungs. *Radiology* **199,** 867–870.
22. Moller, H. E., Chen, X. J., Chawla, M. S., et al. (1999) Sensitivity and resolution in 3D NMR microscopy of the lung with hyperpolarized noble gases. *Magn. Reson. Med.* **41,** 800–808.
23. Mugler, J. P., 3rd. (1998) Optimization of gradient-echo sequences for hyperpo-larized noble gases MRI. *International Society of Magnetic Resonance in Medi-cine Annual Scientific Meeting, Sydney, Australia.*
24. Saam, B., Yablonskiy, D. A., Gierada, D. S., and Conradi, M. S. (1999) Rapid imaging of hyperpolarized gas using EPI. *Magn. Reson. Med.* **42,** 507–514.
25. Kauczor, H. U., Hofmann, D., Kreitner, K. F., et al. (1996) Normal and abnormal pulmonary ventilation: visualization at hyperpolarized He-3 MR imaging. *Radi-ology* **201,** 564–568.
26. MacFall, J. R., Charles, H. C., Black, R. D., et al. (1996) Human lung air spaces: potential for MR imaging with hyperpolarized He-3. *Radiology* **200,** 553–558.
27. Altes, T. A., Powers, P. L., Knight-Scott, J., et al. (2001) Hyperpolarized 3He MR lung ventilation imaging in asthmatics: preliminary findings. *J. Magn. Reson. Imaging* **13,** 378–384.
28. Johnson, G. A., Cates, G., Chen, X. J., et al. (1997) Dynamics of magnetization in hyperpolarized gas MRI of the lung. *Magn. Reson. Med.* **38,** 66–71.
29. Chen, X. J., Chawla, M. S., Hedlund, L. W., Moller, H. E., MacFall, J. R., and Johnson, G. A. (1998) MR microscopy of lung airways with hyperpolarized 3He. *Magn. Reson. Med.* **39,** 79–84.
30. Rupert, K., Brookeman, J. R., and Mugler, J. P., 3rd. (1998) Real-time MR imag-ing of pulmonary gas flow dynamics with hyperpolarized 3He. *International So-ciety of Magnetic Resonance in Medicine Annual Scientific Meeting, Sydney, Australia.*
31. Gierada, D. S., Saam, B., Yablonskiy, D., Cooper, J. D., Lefrak, S. S., and Conradi, M. S. (2000) Dynamic echo planar MR imaging of lung ventilation with hyperpo-larized (3)He in normal subjects and patients with severe emphysema. *NMR Biomed.* **13,** 176–181.
32. Salerno, M., Altes, T. A., Brookeman, J. R., de Lange, E. E., and Mugler, J. P., 3rd. (2001) Dynamic spiral MRI of pulmonary gas flow using hyperpolarized (3)He: preliminary studies in healthy and diseased lungs. *Magn. Reson. Med.* **46,** 667–677.
33. Saam, B. T., Yablonskiy, D. A., Kodibagkar, V. D., et al. (2000) MR imaging of diffusion of (3)He gas in healthy and diseased lungs. *Magn. Reson. Med.* **44,** 174–179.
34. Salerno, M., Brookeman, J. R., de Lange, E. E., Knight-Scott, J., and Mugler, J. P., 3rd. (2000) Detection of regional microstructural changes in lung in emphy-sema using hyperpolarized 3He diffusion MRI. *International Society of Magnetic Resonance in Medicine Annual Scientific Meeting, Denver, CO.*

35. Deninger, A. J., Eberle, B., Ebert, M., et al. (2000) (3)he-MRI-based measurements of intrapulmonary p(O2) and its time course during apnea in healthy volunteers: first results, reproducibility, and technical limitations. *NMR Biomed.* **13**, 194–201.

36. Deninger, A. J., Eberle, B., Ebert, M., et al. (1999) Quantification of regional intrapulmonary oxygen partial pressure evolution during apnea by (3)He MRI. *J. Magn. Reson.* **141**, 207–216.

37. Alsop, D. C., Hatabu, H., Bonnet, M., Listerud, J., and Gefter, W. (1995) Multislice, breathhold imaging of the lung with submillisecond echo times. *Magn. Reson. Med.* **33**, 678–682.

38. Bergin, C. J., Pauly, J. M., and Macovski, A. (1991) Lung parenchyma: projection reconstruction MR imaging. *Radiology* **179**, 777–781.

39. Mayo, J. R., MacKay, A., and Muller, N. L. (1992) MR imaging of the lungs: value of short TE spin-echo pulse sequences. *Am. J. Roentgenol.* **159**, 951–956.

40. Mai, V. M., Knight-Scott, J., Edelman, R. R., Chen, Q., Keilholz-George, S., and Berr, S. S. (2000) 1H magnetic resonance imaging of human lung using inversion recovery turbo spin echo. *J. Magn. Reson. Imaging* **11**, 616–621.

41. Mai, V. M., Knight-Scott, J., and Berr, S. S. (1999) Improved visualization of the human lung in 1H MRI using multiple inversion recovery for simultaneous suppression of signal contributions from fat and muscle. *Magn. Reson. Med.* **41**, 866–870.

42. Mai, V. M., Chen, Q., Li, W., Hatabu, H., and Edelman, R. R. (2000) Effect of respiratory phases on MR lung signal intensity and lung conspicuity using segmented multiple inversion recovery turbo spin echo (MIR-TSE). *Magn. Reson. Med.* **43**, 760–763.

43. Chiarotti, G., Cristiani, G., and Bliulotto, L. (1955) Proton relaxation in pure liquids and in liquids containing paramagnetic gases in solution. *Nuovo Cimento* **1**, 863–873.

44. Chen, Q., Levin, D. L., Mai, V. M., Edelman, R. R., and Hatabu, H. (1999) Magnetic resonance imaging using oxygen as a T1 contrast agent. *International Society of Magnetic Resonance in Medicine Annual Scientific Meeting, Philadelphia, PA.*

45. Young, I. R., Clarke, G. J., Bailes, D. R., Pennock, J. M., Doyle, F. H., and Bydder, G. M. (1981) Enhancement of relaxation rate with paramagnetic contrast agents in NMR imaging. *J. Comput. Tomogr.* **5**, 543–547.

46. Mai, V. M., Chen, Q., Bankier, A. A., and Edelman, R. R. (2000) Multiple inversion recovery MR subtraction imaging of human ventilation from inhalation of room air and pure oxygen. *Magn. Reson. Med.* **43**, 913–916.

47. Loffler, R., Muller, C. J., Peller, M., et al. (2000) Optimization and evaluation of the signal intensity change in multisection oxygen-enhanced MR lung imaging. *Magn. Reson. Med.* **43**, 860–866.

48. Muller, C. J., Loffler, R., Deimling, M., Peller, M., and Reiser, M. (2001) MR lung imaging at 0.2 T with T1-weighted true FISP: native and oxygen-enhanced. *J. Magn. Reson. Imaging* **14**, 164–168.

49. Mai, V. M., Tutton, S., Prasad, P. V., et al. (2003) Computing oxygen-enhanced ventilation maps using correlation analysis. *Magn. Reson. Med.* **49,** 591–594.
50. Bandettini, P. A., Wong, E. C., Hinks, R. S., Tikofsky, R. S., and Hyde, J. S. (1992) Time course EPI of human brain function during task activation. *Magn. Reson. Med.* **25,** 390–397.
51. Bandettini, P. A., Jesmanowicz, A., Wong, E. C., and Hyde, J. S. (1993) Processing strategies for time-course data sets in functional MRI of the human brain. *Magn. Reson. Med.* **30,** 161–173.
52. Stock, K. W., Chen, Q., Morrin, M., Hatabu, H., and Edelman, R. R. (1999) Oxygen-enhanced magnetic resonance ventilation imaging of the human lung at 0.2 and 1.5 T. *J. Magn. Reson. Imaging* **9,** 838–841.
53. Mai, V. M., Chen, Q., Bankier, A. A., Hatabu, H., and Edelman, R. R. (2000) Mapping T1 changes in oxygen-enhanced ventilation imaging in the human lung using MRI. *International Society of Magnetic Resonance in Medicine Annual Scientific Meeting, Denver, CO.*
54. Jakob, P. M., Hillenbrand, C. M., Wang, T., Schultz, G., Hahn, D., and Haase, A. (2001) Rapid quantitative lung (1)H T(1) mapping. *J. Magn. Reson. Imaging* **14,** 795–799.
55. Nakagawa, T., Sakuma, H., Murashima, S., Ishida, N., Matsumura, K., and Takeda, K. (2001) Pulmonary ventilation-perfusion MR imaging in clinical patients. *J. Magn. Reson. Imaging* **14,** 419–424.
56. Mai, V. M., Chen, Q., Gladstone, S., Li, W., Hatabu, H., and Edelman, R. R. (1999) Noninvasive ventilation-perfusion MR imaging using oxygen and FAIRER in humans and in a porcine model of airway obstruction. *International Society of Magnetic Resonance in Medicine Annual Scientific Meeting, Philadelphia, PA.*
57. Ohno, Y., Hatabu, H., Takenaka, D., Adachi, S., Van Cauteren, M., and Sugimura, K. (2001) Oxygen-enhanced MR ventilation imaging of the lung: preliminary clinical experience in 25 subjects. *Am. J. Roentgenol.* **177,** 185–194.
58. Muller, C. J., Schwaiblmair, M., Scheidler, J., et al. (2002) Pulmonary diffusing capacity: assessment with oxygen-enhanced lung MR imaging preliminary findings. *Radiology* **222,** 499–506.
59. Ohno, Y., Hatabu, H., Takenaka, D., Van Cauteren, M., Fujii, M., and Sugimura, K. (2002) Dynamic oxygen-enhanced MRI reflects diffusing capacity of the lung. *Magn. Reson. Med.* **47,** 1139–1144.
60. Krogh, A. and Lindhard, J. (1917) The volume of the dead space in breathing and the mixing of gases in the lungs of man. *J. Physiol.* **51,** 59–90.
61. Haldane, J. S. (1922) *Respiration*, Yale University Press, New Haven, CT.
62. Fenn, W. O., Rahn, H., and Otis, A. B. (1946) A theoretical study of the composition of alveolar air at altitude. *Am J. Physiol.* **146,** 637–653.
63. Riley, R. L. and Cournand, A. (1949) "Ideal" alveolar air and the analysis of ventilation-perfusion relationships in the lungs. *J. Appl. Physiol.* 825–847.
64. West, J. B. and Wagner, P. D. (1991) Ventilation-perfusion relationships, in *The Lung: Scientific Foundations* (Crystal, R. G., West, J. B., Barnes, P. J., Cherniack, N. S., and Weibel, E. R., eds.), Raven, New York, NY, pp. 1289–1305.

65. Chen, Q., Levin, D. L., Kim, D., et al. (1999) Pulmonary disorders: ventilation-perfusion MR imaging with animal models. *Radiology* **213,** 871–879.
66. Mai, V. M., Bankier, A. A., Prasad, P. V., et al. (2001) MR ventilation-perfusion imaging of human lung using oxygen-enhanced and arterial spin labeling techniques. *J. Magn. Reson. Imaging* **14,** 574–579.
67. Mai, V. M., Liu, B., Polzin, J. A., et al. (2002) Ventilation-perfusion ratio of signal intensity in human lung using oxygen-enhanced and arterial spin labeling techniques. *Magn. Reson. Med.* **48,** 341–350.
68. Hatabu, H., Gaa, J., Kim, D., Li, W., Prasad, P. V., and Edelman, R. R. (1996) Pulmonary perfusion: qualitative assessment with dynamic contrast-enhanced MRI using ultra-short TE and inversion recovery turbo FLASH. *Magn. Reson. Med.* **36,** 503–508.
69. Meaney, J. F., Weg, J. G., Chenevert, T. L., Stafford-Johnson, D., Hamilton, B. H., and Prince, M. R. (1997) Diagnosis of pulmonary embolism with magnetic resonance angiography. *N. Engl. J. Med.* **336,** 1422–1427.
70. Amundsen, T., Kvaerness, J., Jones, R. A., et al. (1997) Pulmonary embolism: detection with MR perfusion imaging of lung—a feasibility study. *Radiology* **203,** 181–185.
71. Detre, J. A., Leigh, J. S., Williams, D. S., and Koretsky, A. P. (1992) Perfusion imaging. *Magn. Reson. Med.* **23,** 37–45.
72. Edelman, R. R., Siewert, B., Darby, D. G., et al. (1994) Qualitative mapping of cerebral blood flow and functional localization with echo-planar MR imaging and signal targeting with alternating radio frequency. *Radiology* **192,** 513–520.
73. Kwong, K. K., Chesler, D. A., Weisskoff, R. M., et al. (1995) MR perfusion studies with T1-weighted echo planar imaging. *Magn. Reson. Med.* **34,** 878–887.
74. Kim, S. G. (1995) Quantification of relative cerebral blood flow change by flow-sensitive alternating inversion recovery (FAIR) technique: application to functional mapping. *Magn. Reson. Med.* **34,** 293–301.
75. Mai, V. M., Hagspiel, K. D., Christopher, J. M., et al. (1999) Perfusion imaging of the human lung using flow-sensitive alternating inversion recovery with an extra radiofrequency pulse (FAIRER). *Magn. Reson. Imaging* **17,** 355–361.
76. Mai, V. M., and Berr, S. S. (1999) MR perfusion imaging of pulmonary parenchyma using pulsed arterial spin labeling techniques: FAIRER and FAIR. *J. Magn. Reson. Imaging* **9,** 483–487.
77. Roberts, D. A., Gefter, W. B., Hirsch, J. A., et al. (1999) Pulmonary perfusion: respiratory-triggered three-dimensional MR imaging with arterial spin tagging—preliminary results in healthy volunteers. *Radiology* **212,** 890–895.
78. Silvennoinen, M. J., Kettunen, M. I., and Kauppinen, R. A. (2003) Effects of hematocrit and oxygen saturation level on blood spin-lattice relaxation. *Magn. Reson. Med.* **49,** 568–571.

14

Tissue pH Measurement by Magnetic Resonance Spectroscopy and Imaging

Natarajan Raghunand

Summary

Noninvasive techniques for measurement of tissue pH can be invaluable in assessing disease extent and response to therapy in a variety of pathological conditions, such as renal acidosis and alkalosis, and cancers. We present the details of three techniques for noninvasive measurement of tissue pH: magnetic resonance spectroscopy (MRS), magnetic resonance spectroscopic imaging (MRSI), and contrast-enhanced magnetic resonance imaging (MRI). These techniques exploit the pH-sensitivity of three different molecules, 3-aminopropylphosphonate (3-APP), (±) 2-imidazole-1-yl-3-ethoxycarbonyl propionic acid (IEPA), and 1,4,7,10-Tetraazacyclododecane-1,4,7,10-tetrakis(acetamidomethylenephosphonic acid) (Gd-DOTA-4AmP), to examine local extracellular pH in vivo. The level of detail presented will enable nonnovice users of MRS and MRI to reproduce these methodologies in their own laboratories.

Key Words: pH; magnetic resonance; spectroscopy; imaging; reporter; contrast agent; ^{1}H; ^{31}P; gadolinium; 3-aminopropylphosphonate; IEPA; Gd-DOTA-4AmP.

1. Introduction

The pH of bodily fluids affects the organism in many ways, especially through its effects on cellular and plasma proteins. Maintenance of acid–base homeostasis is critical, and occurs at several levels. The most immediate and local response to an acid or alkali load is through chemical processes, including intracellular, extracellular, and bone buffers. Buffering capacity is limited, and active and passive physiological responses are also required to maintain the acid–base balance. These physiological processes can be at the cellular level, such as through feedback changes in metabolism; and at the systemic level, involving adaptive changes to the excretion of volatile acids by the lungs and fixed acids by the kidneys *(1)*. In most tissues, the buffering capacity of intracellular and extracellular fluids are roughly equal, but the approx 1.5:1 greater volume of intracellular fluid compared with extracellular fluid results in a greater contribution of intracellular buffers to overall buffering in these tissues *(2)*.

From: *Methods in Molecular Medicine, Vol. 124*
Magnetic Resonance Imaging: Methods and Biologic Applications
Edited by: P. V. Prasad © Humana Press Inc., Totowa, NJ

Certain pathologies are associated with a perturbed pH homeostasis. For example, tumor interstitial fluid has a reduced buffering capacity compared with normal tissue and this, in combination with poor perfusion and increased lactic acid secretion by tumors *(3)*, is believed to result in an acidic extracellular pH (pHe) in tumors *(4)*. This situation is exacerbated by the lowered buffering capacity of bicarbonate at a more acid pH. This acidic pH of tumors has numerous consequences, including resistance to radiotherapy and chemotherapy *(5)*. Pathologically altered renal physiology can also manifest with perturbations in both systemic and renal pH. Hereditary defects and acquired deficiencies in renal tubular ion transport systems can result in systemic metabolic acidosis or alkalosis *(6,7)*. Therapies to correct these conditions include the use of alkalinizing or acidifying buffers. While novel gene therapies have also shown promise for the treatment of some of these diseases, there are still problems with heterogeneous gene delivery to the target tissue, and, over time, loss of corrective gene from the target tissue *(8,9)*. Methodologies to image the spatial distribution of tissue pH would have considerable biomedical and clinical relevance in such cases, by enabling the noninvasive assessment of disease extent, progression, and response to therapy.

Several methods have been proposed to measure tissue pH by magnetic resonance spectroscopy (MRS) and magnetic resonance imaging (MRI). Some exploit endogenous MRS peaks, whereas others require the administration of exogenous agents. Intracellular pH (pHi) in tissues can be estimated from the ^{31}P MRS peak of inorganic phosphate (P_i) *(3)*. The pH-sensitive ^{31}P MRS peak of 3-aminopropylphosphonate (3-APP) has been used by us and others to measure pHe of tumors and normal tissues in mice *(4,5,10)*. Molecules with pH-sensitive ^{19}F and ^{1}H resonances have also been reported. Ojugo et al. *(10)* report that pH measurements with excellent signal-to-noise per time period are possible with the extracellular ^{19}F-containing pH probe, ZK-150471. They list the lack of potentially interfering endogenous ^{19}F resonances and the higher nuclear magnetic resonance (NMR) and pH sensitivity of ZK-150471 as advantages of the ^{19}F probe compared with 3-APP. Both 3-APP and ZK-150471 are cell-impermeant and report only the pHe, although ^{31}P MRS of 3-APP offers the possibility of simultaneous measurement of pHi from the P_i resonance. Mason and coworkers have reported that a fluorinated derivative of vitamin B6, 6-fluoropyridoxol, readily enters cells and they have used this single molecule to measure both the pHi and pHe in rodent tumors by ^{19}F MRS *(11)*.

The ^{1}H nucleus offers the highest inherent sensitivity, and it is possible to image the spatial distribution of tissue pH in vivo by the use of probes with pH-sensitive ^{1}H resonances. We and others have used an exogenously administered imidazole, (±) 2-imidazole-1-yl-3-ethoxycarbonyl propionic acid (IEPA), for imaging breast *(12)* and brain *(13)* tumor pH in rodents by magnetic resonance spectroscopic imaging (MRSI) of the pH-sensitive resonance of the protons on the C-2 carbon in the imidazole ring. This resonance is in the 8 to 9 ppm region, with few interfering resonances. Endogenous imidazoles, such as histidine also have pH-sensitive ^{1}H resonances in this region, but their concentrations are too low to exploit. However, Vermathen et al. *(14)* have successfully measured brain pH in humans by localized ^{1}H MRS after oral administration of histidine. MRS and MRSI techniques for measuring pH suffer a disadvantage in sensitivity, and therefore spatial resolution, but have the advantage that the measurement is independent of the concentration of the pH probe.

A different approach to exploiting endogenous resonances to measure tissue pH has been proposed by Van Zijl and colleagues *(15)*. They point out that the region of the ^{1}H MR spectrum >5 ppm contains several very low and undetectable resonances from NH protons that are typically in fast exchange with solvent water. This exchange process renders these resonances nearly impossible to detect with pulse sequences that include a water presaturation pulse. However, using a pulse sequence that permits visualization of these resonances, Van Zijl et al. have demonstrated that it is possible to measure pH from the pH-sensitive rate of exchange with water protons of one or more of these protons. Ward and Balaban *(16)* demonstrated that a compound, such as 5,6-dihydrouracil, with multiple proton exchange sites, each with different pH dependencies, may be used to measure pH using a "ratiometric" method.

pH-sensitive gadolinium complexes *(17,18)* and gadolinium-containing pH-sensitive polyion complexes *(19)* offer the possibility of imaging pH with a spatial resolution comparable to standard MRI. However, the enhancement observed in an image will be dependent not only on the pH, but also on the local concentration of the agent. One approach to determine pH is to sequentially administer two contrast agents having identical tissue pharmacokinetics, one being insensitive to tissue pH and the other being pH-sensitive *(20)*. The distribution of the pH-insensitive agent can be used to predict the concentration of the pH-sensitive agent. In this chapter, we present details of pH measurement by ^{31}P MRS of 3-APP, ^{1}H MRSI using IEPA, and ^{1}H MRI using 1,4,7,10-Tetraazacyclododecane-1,4,7,10-tetrakis(acetamidomethylene-phosphonic acid) (Gd-DOTA-4AmP).

2. Materials

2.1. In Vivo pH Measurement by ^{31}P MRS

1. 245 m*M* Solution of 3-APP in ultrapure water, adjusted to pH 7.4.
2. 28-gage 1-mL Insulin syringe.
3. 26-gage, $^3/_4''$, Over-the-needle catheter.
4. Male Luer lock × $^1/_{16}''$ hose-barb tubing connector.
5. Female Luer lock × $^1/_{16}''$ hose-barb tubing connector.

6. PE-200 tubing.
7. 3-mL Syringe.
8. Mouse model of appropriate disease.
9. Ophthalmic eye ointment.
10. Transmitter/receiver radio frequency (RF) coil suitable for ^{31}P MRS.
11. Warm water or air system for maintaining mouse body temperature.
12. Temperature-monitoring system compatible with the MR magnet (optional, but highly recommended). For example, the Luxtron 790 Fluoroptic Thermometer (Luxtron Corporation, Santa Clara, CA).
13. Respiration rate monitoring system (optional).
14. Anesthesia of choice, for example one of the following:

    a. 1 to 4% Isoflurane plus oxygen delivery system, with face mask for mouse. Isoflurane vaporizer and oxygen mixing systems with scavenging pump and filters are available from a variety of vendors, such as Surgivet Inc., Waukesha, WI.
    b. 840 µL Ketamine (from 100 mg/mL stock) + 350 µL xylazine (from 20 mg/mL stock) + 700 µL acepromazine (from 10 mg/mL stock) + sterile saline to final volume of 10 mL.
    c. 233.3 µL Ketamine (from 100 mg/mL stock) + 233.3 µL midazolam (from 5 mg/mL stock) + sterile saline to final volume of 2 mL.

2.2. In Vivo pHe Imaging by ^{1}H MRSI

1. 284 m*M* Solution of IEPA in ultrapure water, adjusted to pH 7.4 (*see* **Note 1**). It can be ordered from Laboratorios Farmacéuticos ROVI, S.A, Madrid, Spain; www.rovi.es).
2. 28-gage Hypodermic needle with female Luer lock.
3. Male Luer lock × $^1/_{16}''$ hose-barb tubing connector.
4. Female Luer lock × $^1/_{16}''$ hose-barb tubing connector.
5. PE-200 tubing.
6. 1-mL Syringe.
7. Syringe pump capable of pumping at 0.15 mL/h.
8. Transmitter/receiver RF coil suitable for ^{1}H MRS of mouse.
9. Warm water or air system for maintaining normal mouse body temperature.
10. Surgical tape.
11. Mouse model of appropriate disease.
12. Ophthalmic eye ointment.
13. Fluoroptic temperature probe and meter (optional).
14. Respiration monitor (optional).
15. Anesthesia of choice.

2.3. In Vivo pHe Imaging by Gd-DOTA-4AMP-Enhanced ^{1}H MRI

1. 50 m*M* Solution of Gd-DOTP in injectable saline, adjusted to pH 7.4 (*see* **Note 2**). It can be obtained from Macrocyclics, Inc., Dallas, TX; www.macrocyclics.com.

2. 50 m*M* Solution of Gd-DOTA-4AmP in injectable saline, adjusted to pH 7.4 (*see* **Note 3**). Available from Macrocyclics, Inc.
3. Saline suitable for intravenous injection, containing 3000 U/mL of heparin.
4. 27-gage Hypodermic needle separated from Luer lock.
5. PE-20 tubing.
6. 30-gage Luer lock stub adapter.
7. Heparin plug.
8. Two 28-gage 1-mL insulin syringes.
9. Surgical tape.
10. Ophthalmic eye ointment.
11. Anesthesia of choice.
12. Fluoroptic physiological temperature-monitoring system.
13. Physiological respiration-monitoring system.
14. Transmitter/receiver RF coil suitable for ^{1}H MRI of mouse.
15. Warm water/air system for maintaining normal mouse body temperature.
16. Mouse model of appropriate disease.

3. Methods

3.1. In Vivo pH Measurement by ^{31}P MRS

1. Animal preparation.
   a. Preparing the ip catheter line. For MRS experiments lasting less than 2 h, a single 0.6 to 0.8 mL ip injection of 3-APP administered to a 20 to 25 g mouse immediately before the MRS experiment is sufficient. However, 3-APP is continuously cleared by the animal, and for longer experiments, it may be necessary to inject additional 3-APP into the animal. To be able to do so without removing the animal from the magnet in the middle of the experiment, prepare an ip catheter line as follows:
      i. Connect the male Luer lock/hose-barb fitting to one end of the PE-200 tubing (*see* **Note 4**), and the female Luer lock/hose-barb to the other end.
      ii. Attach the 3-mL syringe to the female Luer lock and fill the entire line and syringe with the 3-APP solution.
      iii. Insert the over-the-needle catheter into the peritoneal cavity of the anesthetized mouse.
      iv. Remove the needle from the over-the-needle catheter and attach the tubing filled with 3-APP from **step 1.a.ii.** to the catheter at the Luer lock fitting.

   Figure 1 shows the fully assembled line and catheter.

   b. Preparing animal for MRS:
      i. Anesthetize the mouse. We prefer inhaled isoflurane for anesthetizing mice, as this provides superior control over depth and duration of anesthesia. However, injected anesthetics can also be used.
      ii. Protect the eyes of the animal from dehydration with a coat of eye ointment.

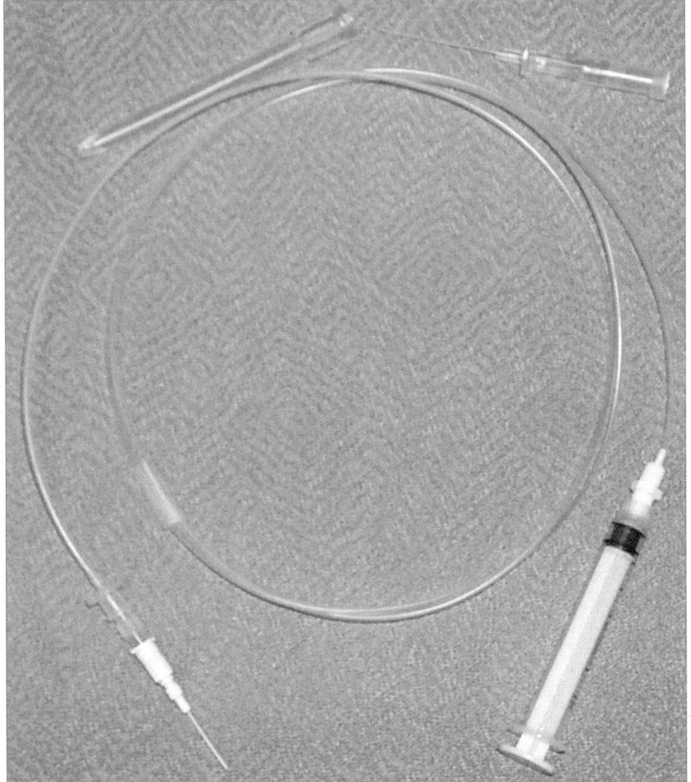

Fig. 1. The fully assembled ip catheter line for delivery of 3-aminopropyl-phosphonate (3-APP) to a mouse during a magnetic resonance spectroscopy experiment. The catheter (white) is shown already separated from the needle (top right). In practice, the catheter is to be inserted into the mouse, the needle removed, and then the tubing attached to the catheter via the Luer lock.

iii. We prefer to use a fluoroptic rectal thermometer to continuously monitor the body temperature of the mouse during the experiment. Temperature monitoring is optional but highly recommended.

iv. We prefer to use respiration monitoring to continuously track the status of the animal under anesthesia. Use of respiration monitoring is also optional but highly recommended.

v. Inject 0.7 mL of the 3-APP solution into the animal via the ip catheter line.

vi. Immobilize the animal in the transmitter/receiver RF coil with the tissue of interest appropriately positioned within the coil. Center the RF coil within the magnet.

vii. Adjust the circulating warm water or air system to maintain proper mouse body temperature.

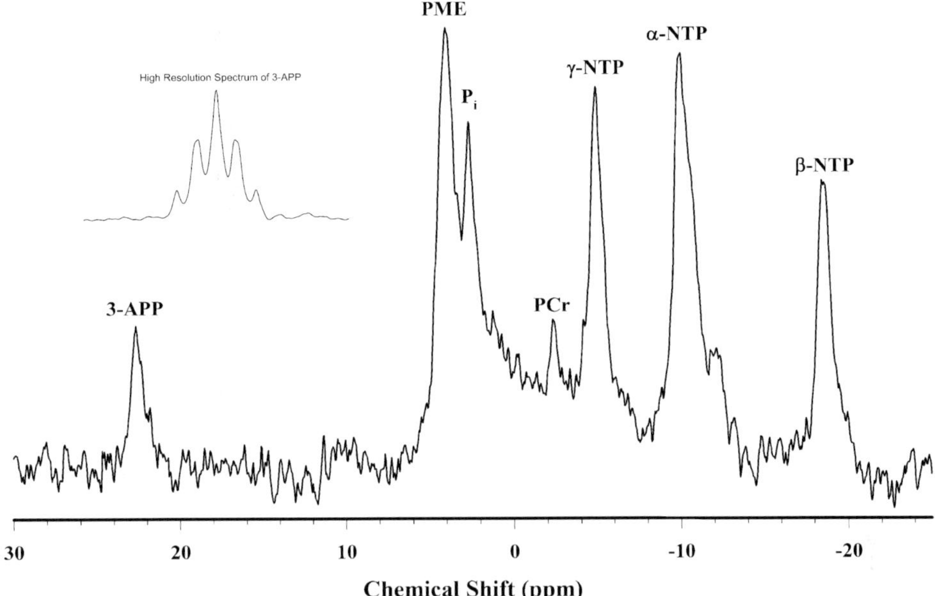

Fig. 2. In vivo ^{31}P magnetic resonance (MR) spectrum of a tumor xenograft in a SCID mouse. PME: phosphomonoesters; PCr: phosphocreatine; NTP: nucleoside triphosphates. The inset is a high-resolution in vitro spectrum of 3-aminopropyl-phosphonate (3-APP), depicting the multiplet nature of this resonance in proton-coupled ^{31}P MR spectra.

2. MR acquisition methods. The initial bolus of 3-APP provides sufficient signal during experiments shorter than 2 h in duration. Booster boluses of 3-APP may be administered via the ip catheter line, as needed, during longer experiments. Several pulse sequences for performing volume-localized MRS have been reported in the literature. Parameters to use at 4.7 T with two common sequences are as follows:

   a. Image-selected in vivo spectroscopy (ISIS) localization. Nucleus = [31]P; recycle time, TR = 10 s; spectral width = 80 ppm; and number of points = 8192. Adiabatic slice-selective and excitation pulses are highly recommended if a surface coil is used for RF transmission.
   b. Point-resolved spectroscopy (PRESS) localization. Nucleus = [31]P; recycle time, TR = 1.0 s; echo time, TE = as short as possible; spectral width = 80 ppm; and number of points = 8192.

Figure 2 shows an in vivo ^{31}P spectrum of a tumor xenograft in a SCID mouse, obtained at 4.7 T. The inset shows a high-resolution ^{31}P MR spectrum of 3-APP obtained in vitro at 11.7 T. The resonance of the single ^{31}P nucleus in 3-APP is revealed to be a multiplet, caused by couplings with protons in the molecule. This splitting of the 3-APP resonance is not observed in vivo at 4.7 T because of a combination of factors, including shorter T_2 relaxation times in vivo than in vitro, lower inherent spectral resolution at the lower field strength, and pH heterogeneity in vivo.

3. Data analysis. Fourier transform the time-domain data and apply appropriate apodization to the resulting spectrum. Carefully correct the phase of the spectrum. Calibrate chemical shifts by setting α-nucleoside triphosphate (NTP) to –10.05 ppm.

   a. Titratability of the Pi resonance. At physiological pH, Pi exists primarily in the forms $H_2PO_4^-$ and HPO_4^{2-}. The fast exchange of ^{31}P nuclei between these two forms results in a single resonance being observed between 0.58 ppm and 3.14 ppm, with the exact location of the resonance being determined by the relative amounts of the two forms. In turn, the relative amounts of these two forms is determined by pH. It has been shown that, in tumors, the Pi signal originates primarily from the intracellular space *(3)*. Thus, the pH sensitivity of the endogenous Pi resonance in ^{31}P MR spectra can be exploited to measure pHi in mouse tumors. The Henderson-Hasselbach equation relating pH and observed chemical shift of Pi (δ, relative to α-NTP at –10.05 ppm) is:

   $$pH = 6.85 + \log_{10}[(\delta - 0.58)/(3.14 - \delta)].\qquad [1]$$

   b. Titratability of the 3-APP resonance. Analogously, the chemical shift of the single ^{31}P nucleus in 3-APP (**Fig. 3**) is pH-dependent. It is cell-membrane impermeant, and, therefore, reports on the pHe in vivo. The Henderson-Hasselbach equation relating pH and observed chemical shift of 3-APP (δ relative to α-NTP at –10.05 ppm) is:

   $$pH = 6.91 - \log_{10}[(\delta - 21.10)/(24.32 - \delta)].\qquad [2]$$

   c. Correcting the intensity of the Pi peak. Copy the intensity vs chemical shift data from the portion of the ^{31}P MR spectrum between 0.58 and 3.14 ppm, and paste into a graphing or spreadsheet program. The relationship between pH and chemical shift of Pi is not linear (**Eq. [1]**). Consequently, the following transformation must be carried out to normalize the intensity of each point on the Pi resonance *(21)*. Here, I is the raw signal intensity of a given point on the Pi peak, I^{corr} is its corrected signal intensity, and δ is its chemical shift:

   $$I^{corr} = I \cdot (\delta - 0.58) \cdot (3.14 - \delta)/(3.14 - 0.58).\qquad [3]$$

   d. Correcting the intensity of the 3-APP peak. Copy the intensity vs chemical shift data from the portion of the ^{31}P MR spectrum between 21.10 and 24.32 ppm, and paste into a graphing or spreadsheet program. Analogous to the previous step, the following transformation must be carried out to normalize the intensity of each point on the 3-APP resonance. Here, I is the raw signal intensity of a given point on the 3-APP peak, I^{corr} is its corrected signal intensity, and δ is its chemical shift:

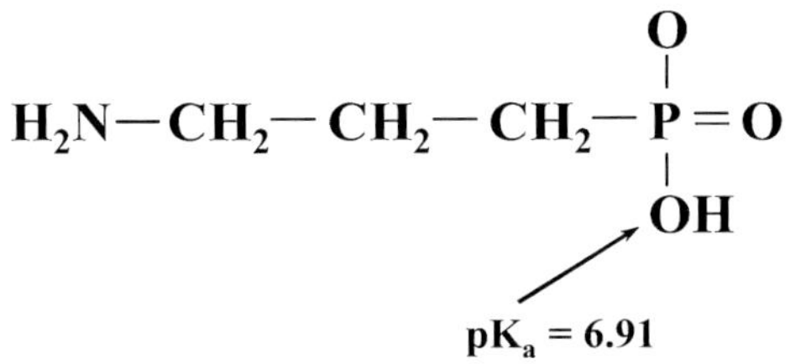

$$H_2N-CH_2-CH_2-CH_2-\overset{\displaystyle O}{\underset{\displaystyle OH}{P}}=O$$

$$pK_a = 6.91$$

Fig. 3. 3-aminopropylphosphonate (3-APP). The oxygen with a titratable proton is identified by the arrow.

$$I^{corr} = I \cdot (\delta - 21.1) \cdot (24.32 - \delta)/(24.32 - 21.1). \tag{4}$$

  e. Converting the chemical shift of Pi to pH. Take the I^{corr} vs δ data generated in **step 3.c.**, and apply **Eq. [1]** to convert the chemical shift numbers to pH. Because Pi is found in both the extracellular and intracellular fluids in most tissues, this pH is typically a weighted combination of pHi and pHe. For the specific case of tumors, Pi primarily reports the pHi *(3)*.

  f. Converting the chemical shift of 3-APP to pH. Take the I^{corr} vs δ data generated in **step 3.d.**, and apply **Eq. [2]** to convert the chemical shift numbers to pH. Because 3-APP is cell impermeant, this pH is the pHe.

Figures 4B and **D** depict the I^{corr} vs pH corresponding to the Pi and 3-APP peaks, respectively, from **Fig. 2**. **Fig. 4A** and **C** plot the corresponding raw intensity vs pH for these two resonances. The significant differences between the centers of gravity of the raw and normalized pH distributions demonstrates the importance of performing the intensity corrections described in **steps 3.c.** and **3.d.** It should be noted that the apparent spread of pH reported by Pi (**Fig. 4B**) incorporates both the true in vivo heterogeneity of pH, and the peak broadening caused by T_2 relaxation. In the case of 3-APP (**Fig. 4D**), additional peak broadening also results from the multiplet nature of this resonance (**Fig. 2**, inset).

3.2. In Vivo pHe Imaging by ^{1}H MRSI

1. Animal preparation.

  a. Preparing the iv catheter line. Connect the 28-gage needle and 1-mL syringe to the two ends of a length of PE-200 tubing using the Luer lock/barb fittings in a manner analogous to **Subheading 3.1.**, **step 1.a.** (also *see* **Notes 5** and **6**).

  b. Preparing mouse for iv infusion and MRSI:

    i. Inject 0.4 mL of the IEPA solution into the peritoneal cavity of the awake mouse 30 min before inducing anesthesia (*see* **Note 7**).

    ii. Connect the iv catheter line to the infusion pump and fill the line completely with the IEPA solution.

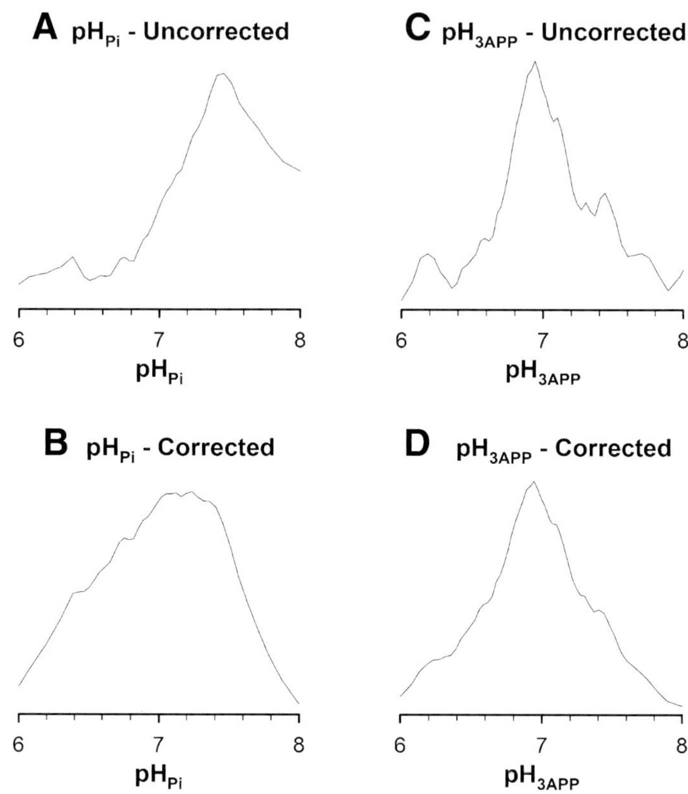

Fig. 4. Panels (**A**) and (**C**): conversion of the chemical shifts of inorganic phosphate and 3-aminopropylphosphonate (3-APP) to pH using **Eqs. [1]** and **[2]**, respectively. Panels (**B**) and (**D**) depict the same data as in (**A**) and (**C**), after normalization to the slopes of **Eqs. [1]** and **[2]**, respectively. The slopes of the titration **Eqs. [1]** and **[2]** are provided in **Eqs. [3]** and **[4]**, respectively.

   iii. Anesthetize the mouse and cannulate the tail vein with the iv line.

   iv. Protect the eyes of the animal from dehydration with a coat of eye ointment.

    v. Operate the infusion pump at 0.1 to 0.15 mL/kg/min (*see* **Note 8**).

   vi. Attach a fluoroptic rectal thermometer and respiration-monitoring pad, if desired.

  vii. Immobilize the animal in the transmitter/receiver RF coil with the tissue of interest appropriately positioned within the coil. Center the RF coil within the magnet.

 viii. Adjust the circulating warm water or air system to maintain proper mouse body temperature.

2. MR acquisition methods. It is possible to acquire MRSI data using more than one sequence. For the spin-echo BASSALE sequence *(22)*, suggested parameters to

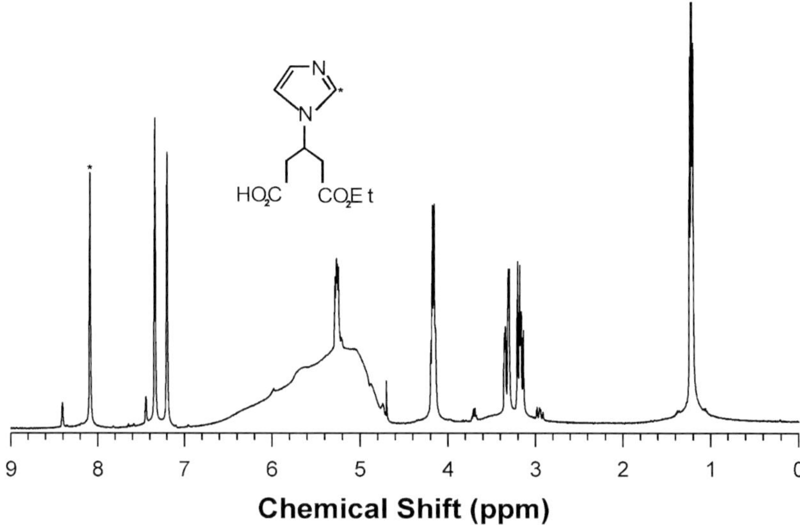

Fig. 5. A high-resolution ^{1}H magnetic resonance spectrum of (±) 2-imidazole-1-yl-3-ethoxycarbonyl propionic acid (IEPA) obtained in vitro at 37°C and 9.4 T. The inset shows the structure of IEPA. The asterisk indicates the pH-sensitive resonance on the spectrum and its location on the molecule.

use are: recycle time, TR = 2 s; echo time, TE = as short as possible; spectral width = 30 ppm; matrix resolution = 128 points; and averages = 8, with water-suppression. Fat suppression is highly desirable to improve baseline shape. Also acquire spectra of unsuppressed water with the same sequence and parameters for use in referencing chemical shift.

3. Data analysis. It may be necessary to write custom software to adequately process your MRSI data. A step-by-step description of data analysis is not possible, as that would depend on the exact sequence used to acquire the data. In general, some manner of filtering of the time-domain data as well as 3D Fourier transformation will be required. Calibrate chemical shifts relative to unsuppressed water at 4.7 ppm.

   a. Titratability of the C2 proton resonances. The chemical shift of the proton bonded to the C2 carbon of IEPA (**Fig. 5**, inset) is pH dependent. IEPA is cell-membrane impermeant, and, therefore, the chemical shift of this resonance reports the pHe in vivo. The Henderson-Hasselbach equation relating pH and observed chemical shift of this resonance (δ, relative to water protons at 4.7 ppm) is:

$$pH = 6.49 - \log_{10}[(\delta - 7.77)/(8.92 - \delta)]. \qquad [5]$$

Figure 5 also shows a high-resolution in vitro ^{1}H MR spectrum of IEPA. The pH-sensitive resonance and the C2 proton are indicated by the asterisk.

b. Normalizing the peak intensity to the slope of the titration curve. For each pixel, apply the following transformation to the portion of the ^{1}H MR spectrum between 7.77 and 8.92 ppm to normalize intensities to the slope of the titration curve, **Eq. [5]**, as follows. Here, I is the raw signal intensity of a given point on the peak, I^{corr} is its corrected signal intensity, and δ is its chemical shift:

$$I^{corr} = I \cdot (\delta - 7.77) \cdot (8.92 - \delta)/(8.92 - 7.77) \qquad [6]$$

c. Converting chemical shift to pH. For each pixel, take the I^{corr} vs δ data generated in **Subheading 3.2.**, **step 3.b.**, and apply **Eq. [5]** to convert the chemical shift numbers to pH. This will yield a pH distribution for each pixel, analogous to **Fig. 4B** and **D**. Identify the center of gravity of this pH distribution for each pixel. Because IEPA is cell impermeant, this pH is the weighted-average pHe in each pixel. Render the weighted-average pHe obtained from each pixel in image form, to create a pHe map corresponding to the tissue imaged.

3.3. In Vivo pHe Imaging by Gd-DOTA-4AMP-Enhanced ^{1}H MRI

1. Animal preparation.
   a. Preparing a low dead-volume iv catheter:
      i. Attach the blunt end of a 27-gage needle separated from the Luer lock to PE-20 tubing (*see* **Note 9**).
      ii. Attach the 30-gage stub adapter to the other end of the tubing. Attach the heparin plug to the Luer lock fitting on the stub adapter.

Figure 6 shows a fully assembled low dead-volume iv catheter line.

   b. Preparing the mouse for iv injection and MRI:
      i. Anesthetize the animal.
      ii. Protect the eyes of the animal from dehydration with a coat of eye ointment.
      iii. Flush the low dead-volume iv catheter line with heparinized saline. Cannulate the tail vein of the animal with this iv needle and secure the line to the tail with surgical tape or sutures.
      iv. Place the animal in a holder adapted to the dimensions of the RF transmitter/receiver coil.

Figure 7 shows a close-up of an RF coil, the fluoroptic end of the temperature probe, and a respiration-monitoring pressure pad. **Figure 8** shows a mouse in a holder with anesthesia face mask, tail-vein catheter, rectal temperature probe, and respiration monitoring in place. **Figure 9** shows the entire assembly in position in the RF coil. A jacket connected to circulating warm water is shown in place under the anesthesia mask and RF coil. Because RF coils can be purchased in a multitude of sizes and configurations, these pictures are meant only to be a general guide.

2. MRI methods.

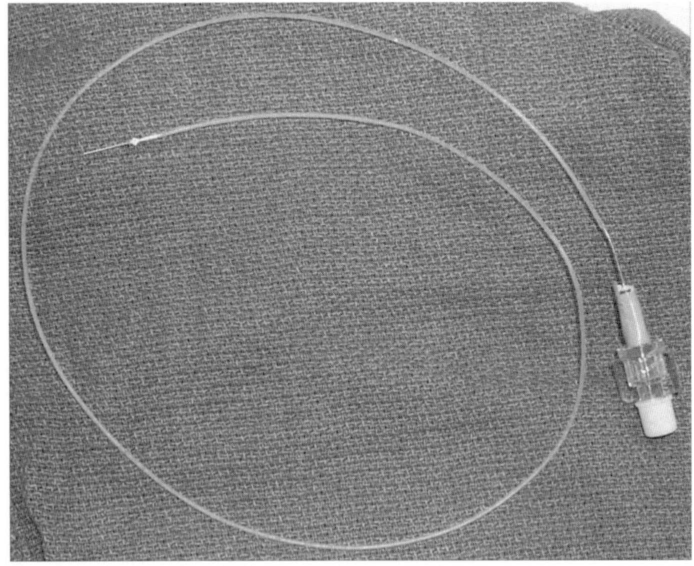

Fig. 6. A low dead-volume iv catheter line suitable for sequential injections of two different contrast agents into the animal.

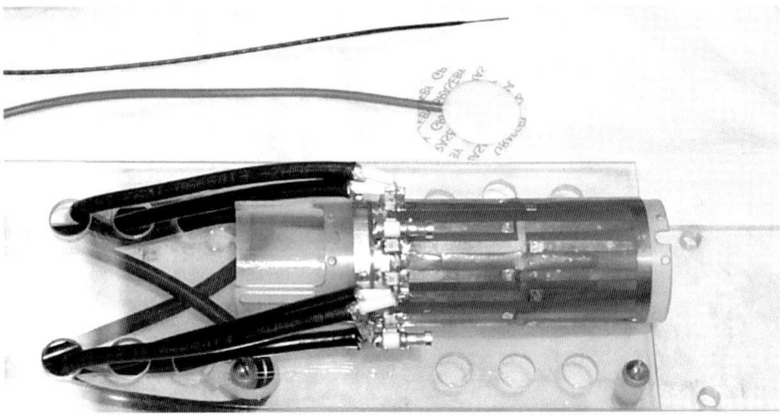

Fig. 7. Close-up of radio frequency coil, fluoroptic end of temperature probe, and pressure pad for monitoring respiration.

a. Plan slice position and geometry from scout scans. The final slice geometry should include not just the tissue of interest but also the cross-section of one or more major arteries (*see* **Note 10**).
b. Acquire a precontrast T_1 map with the final slice geometry.

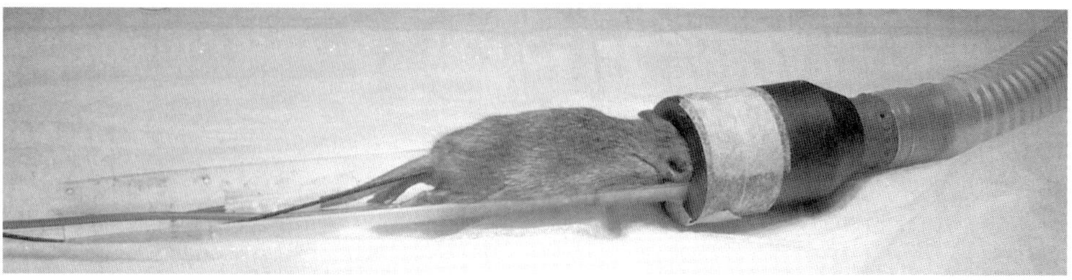

Fig. 8. Mouse in holder with anesthesia facemask, tail-vein catheter, rectal temperature probe, and respiration monitoring in place.

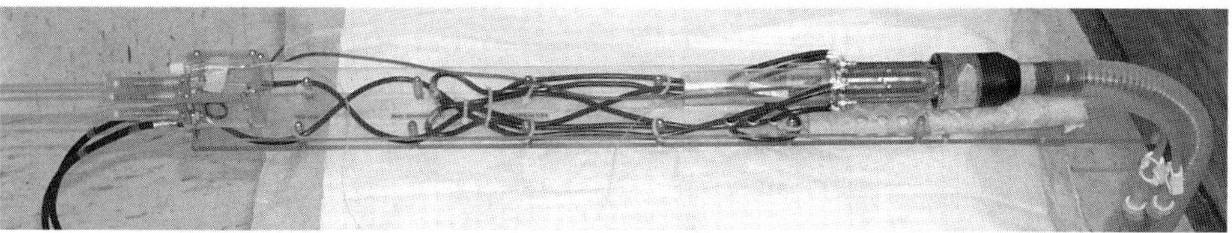

Fig. 9. The entire assembly in position in the radio frequency (RF) coil. A jacket connected to circulating warm water is shown in place under the anesthesia mask and the RF coil.

   c. Acquire a dynamic T_1-weighted series of spin-echo images with the following parameters: recycle time, TR = 80 ms; echo time, TE = as short as possible; and fat suppression = on. After four to eight images in the series have been collected, inject 0.03 to 0.1 mmol/kg of Gd-DOTP via the heparin plug and flush with enough saline to clear the iv catheter line of remaining gadolinium (*see* **Notes 11–13**).

   d. After significant wash-out of gadolinium has occurred, repeat **step 2.c.**, this time injecting Gd-DOTA-4AmP instead of Gd-DOTP (*see* **Note 14**).

3. Data analysis. It will be necessary to write custom software to perform the following manipulations on a pixel-by-pixel basis:

   a. pH dependence of the relaxivity of Gd-DOTA-4AmP. At 4.7 T and 37°C, pH in the range of 5.75 to 8.0 can be calculated from the in vivo relaxivity of Gd-DOTA-4AmP, r_1, by the following relationship:

$$pH = 1.62 + 4.5 \cdot (r_1) - 0.78 \cdot (r_1)^2. \tag{7}$$

   b. Measurement of the in vivo relaxivity of Gd-DOTA-4AmP. The in vivo pharmacokinetics of Gd-DOTP, the pH-insensitive tetraphosphonate analog of Gd-DOTA-4AmP, are used as a surrogate for the pharmacokinetics of Gd-DOTA-4AmP. **Figure 10** shows the structures of the two molecules.

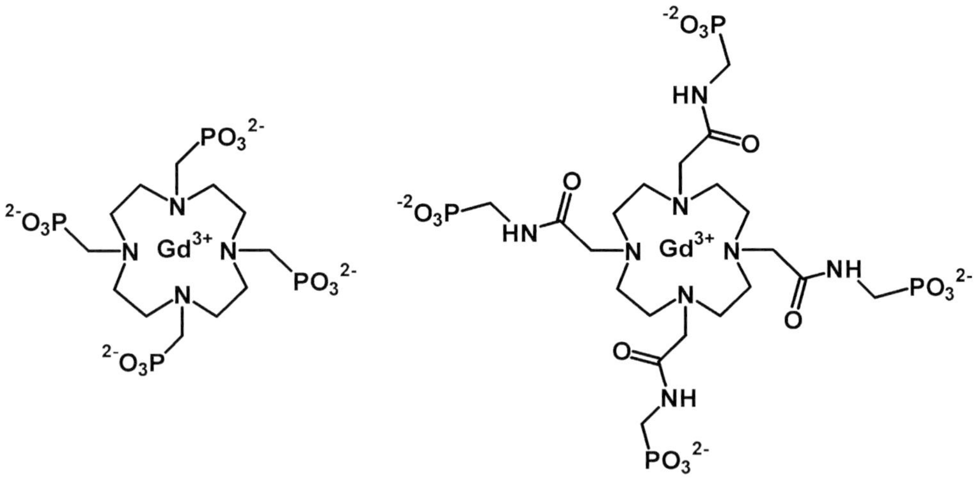

Fig. 10. Structures of Gd-DOTP *(left)* and Gd-DOTA-4AmP *(right)*.

c. Concentration from signal enhancement. Using the precontrast T_1 map acquired in **step 2.b.** and the four to eight precontrast images collected in **step 2.c.**, convert signal enhancement in this dynamic series to concentration of Gd-DOTP. Use a relaxivity of 3.0 mM^{-1}s^{-1} for Gd-DOTP at 37°C and 4.7 T, and assume a linear relationship between gadolinium concentration and relaxation rate.

d. Relaxation rate from signal enhancement. Using the precontrast T_1 map acquired in **step 2.b.** and the four to eight precontrast images collected in **step 2.d.**, convert signal enhancement in this dynamic series to relaxation rate.

e. Arterial input function (AIF) differences between injections. Identify pixels corresponding to arteries (*see* **Note 15**). Calculate an AIF for the Gd-DOTP bolus from the concentration maps computed in **step 3.c.** Assume an arterial pH for the animal, based on its metabolic status and physiology (pH 7.4 in normal mice), and use **Eq. 7** and this assumed pH to calculate an AIF for the Gd-DOTA-4AmP bolus from the relaxation rate maps computed in **step 3.d.** Correct for gadolinium dose and injection timing differences between the two boluses using these two AIFs. This will require pharmacokinetic modeling, the details of which are beyond the scope of this work.

f. We make the assumption that the pharmacokinetics of Gd-DOTP are a surrogate for the pharmacokinetics of Gd-DOTA-4AmP in a given animal. In other words, we assume that, at a given time after injection, in a given pixel, the concentration of Gd-DOTA-4AmP (from **step 2.d.**) is equal to the concentration of Gd-DOTP (from **step 2.c.**) at the same time after injection in the same pixel. This makes it possible to calculate a relaxivity of Gd-DOTA-4AmP for

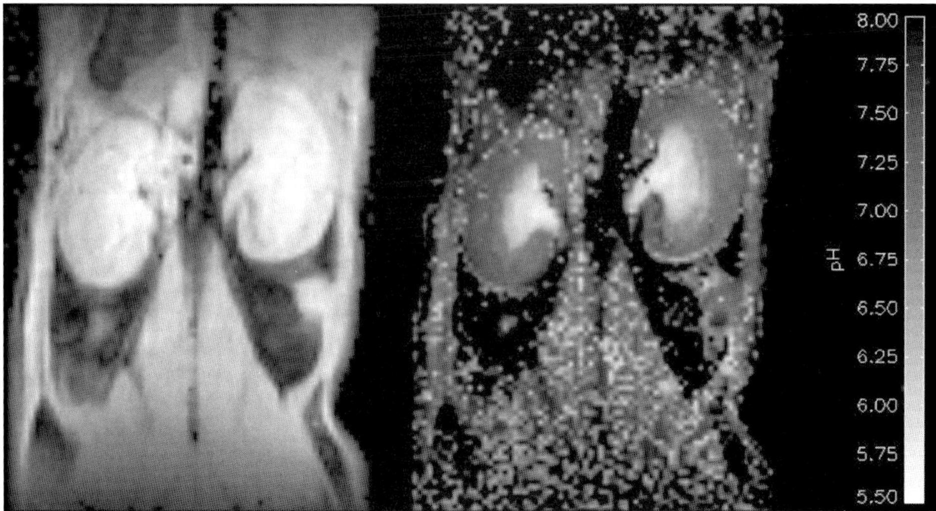

Fig. 11. The left panel is a proton density-weighted reference anatomic image obtained in the coronal plane from a female mouse. The kidneys and surrounding tissues are visible. The right panel depicts the corresponding calculated pH image. A low dose of contrast agents (0.03 mmol/kg) was used for optimal enhancement of the kidneys. The resulting low signal enhancement in nonrenal pixels greatly reduces sensitivity of pH measurement in those regions.

that pixel at that time after injection. Applying **Eq. [7]**, this relaxivity can be converted to a pH. By doing so on a pixel-by-pixel basis, it is possible to obtain a pH map corresponding to each imaged slice. **Figure 11** shows an anatomic reference image and pH map of kidneys and surrounding tissues in a female mouse.

4. Notes

1. Obtain formula weight from manufacturer for the actual batch of IEPA supplied.
2. Obtain formula weight from manufacturer for the actual batch of Gd-DOTP supplied.
3. Obtain formula weight from manufacturer for the actual batch of Gd-DOTA-4AmP supplied.
4. The length of the PE-200 tubing should be long enough that, with one end at the center of the magnet, the other end is accessible from either end of the magnet.
5. The length of the entire assembly must be sufficient to extend from the magnet mid-point to the syringe pump.
6. For safety, the syringe pump and other strongly ferromagnetic objects should be properly anchored several feet away from the magnet.
7. This concentration of IEPA is calculated to be normosmolal at pH 7.4, and amounts to a dose of 5.35 mmol/kg for a 21-g mouse. The purpose of this

preanesthesia bolus is to speed the attainment of steady-state plasma concentration of IEPA. Input of IEPA (via initial bolus plus maintenance infusion) and output (via renal clearance) produces a steady state concentration of IEPA in tissues in approx 15 min.

8. Higher infusion rates result in higher steady-state concentrations of IEPA, but carry the risk that IEPA (a buffer) may itself alter the pH that is sought to be measured.
9. The tubing should be long enough to extend from the magnet mid-point to the edge of the magnet bore.
10. Inclusion of the cross-section of at least one major artery permits the calculation of an AIF for each injection. AIFs can be used to correct for differences in dose and timing of the two gadolinium injections by use of an appropriate pharmacokinetic model.
11. The number of repetitions/images in the dynamic series can vary, but imaging should begin before injection of contrast and continue through significant washout of contrast from the tissue/organ of interest. The precontrast images in the series are used for calculation of the precontrast T_1 map.
12. The optimal dose of gadolinium used varies by tissue. We have found that 0.03 mmol/kg is optimal for pH imaging of mouse kidneys, whereas 0.1 mmol/kg is optimal for imaging muscle and tumors.
13. The flush volume of saline required to adequately clear the iv line of gadolinium is five times the dead volume of the line. Minimizing the dead volume of this line minimizes the fluid load to the animal from the two boluses required during the experiment.
14. The dose of gadolinium delivered should be identical to the dose of gadolinium administered in **Subheading 3.3.**, **step 2.c.** It is also very important to exactly match the timing of this second injection, relative to the start of the dynamic imaging series, with the timing of the injection in **Subheading 3.3.**, **step 2.c.**, relative to the start of that dynamic imaging series.
15. Pixels falling within arteries can be identified manually by reference to anatomical features, or automatically by thresholding the images on the basis of time to maximum enhancement.

References

1. Adrogue, H. E. and Adrogue, H. J. (2001) Acid–base physiology. *Respir. Care* **46,** 328–341.
2. Adrogue, H. J. and Wesson, D. E. (1994) *Acid–Base.* Blackwell Scientific, Boston, MA.
3. Stubbs, M., Bhujwalla, Z. M., Tozer, G. M., et al. (1992) An assessment of ^{31}P MRS as a method of measuring pH in rat tumours. *NMR Biomed.* **5,** 351–359.
4. Raghunand, N., Altbach, M. I., Van Sluis, R., et al. (1999) Plasmalemmal pH-gradients in drug-sensitive and drug-resistant MCF-7 human breast carcinoma xenografts measured by ^{31}P magnetic resonance spectroscopy. *Biochem. Pharmacol.* **57,** 309–312.

5. Raghunand, N., Mahoney, B., Van Sluis, R., Baggett, B., and Gillies, R.J. (2001) Acute metabolic alkalosis enhances response of C3H mouse mammary tumors to the weak base mitoxantrone. *Neoplasia* **3,** 227–235.

6. Paillard, M. (1997) Na+/H+ exchanger subtypes in the renal tubule: function and regulation in physiology and disease. *Exp. Nephrol.* **5,** 277–284.

7. Lai, L. W., Erickson, R. P., Venta,. P. J., Tashian, R. E., and Lien, Y. H. (1998) Promoter activity of carbonic anhydrase II regulatory regions in cultured renal proximal tubular cells. *Life Sciences* **63,** 121–126.

8. Shayakul, C., Breton, S., Brown, D., and Alper, S. L. (1999) Gene therapy of inherited renal tubular disease. *Amer. J. Kidney Diseases* **34,** 374–379.

9. Lien, Y.H. and Lai, L.W. (1997) Gene therapy for renal diseases. *Kidney Intl. Suppl.* **61,** S85–S88.

10. Ojugo, A. S., McSheehy, P. M., McIntyre, D. J., et al. (1999) Measurement of the extracellular pH of solid tumours in mice by magnetic resonance spectroscopy: a comparison of exogenous 19F and 31P probes. *NMR Biomed.* **12,** 495–504.

11. Mason, R. P. (1999) Transmembrane pH gradients in vivo: measurements using fluorinated vitamin B6 derivatives. *Curr. Med. Chem.* **6,** 481–499.

12. Van Sluis, R., Bhujwalla, Z. M., Raghunand, N., et al. (1999) Imaging of extracellular pH using 1H MRSI. *Magn. Reson. Med.* **41,** 743–750.

13. Garcia-Martin, M. L., Herigault, G., Remy, C., et al. (2001) Mapping extracellular pH in rat brain gliomas in vivo by 1H magnetic resonance spectroscopic imaging: comparison with maps of metabolites. *Cancer Res.* **61,** 6524–6531.

14. Vermathen, P., Capizzano, A. A., and Maudsley, A. A. (2000) Administration and 1H MRS detection of histidine in human brain: application to in vivo pH measurement. *Magn. Reson. Med.* **43,** 665–675.

15. Mori, S., Eleff, S. M., Pilatus, U., Mori, N., and Van Zijl, P. C. M. (1998) Sensitive detection of solvent-saturable resonances by proton NMR spectroscopy: a new approach to study pH effects. *Magn. Reson. Med.* **40,** 36–42.

16. Ward, K.M. and Balaban, R.S. (2000) Determination of pH using water protons and chemical exchange dependent saturation transfer (CEST). *Magn. Reson. Med.* **44,** 799–802.

17. Zhang, S., Wu, K., and Sherry, A. D. (1999) A novel pH-sensitive MRI contrast agent. *Angew. Chemie Intl. Ed.* **38,** 3192–3194.

18. Aime, S., Botta, M., Crich, S. G., Giovenzana, G., Palmisano, G., and Sisti, M. (1999) A macromolecular Gd(III) complex as pH-responsive relaxometric probe for MRI applications. *Chem. Commun.* **16,** 1577–1578.

19. Mikawa, M., Miwa, N., Brautigam, M., Akaike, T., and Maruyama, A. (2000) Gd(3+)-loaded polyion complex for pH depiction with magnetic resonance imaging. *J. Biomed. Mat. Res.* **49,** 390–395.

20. Raghunand, N., Howison, C., Sherry, A. D., Zhang, S., and Gillies, R.J. Renal and systemic pH imaging by contrast-enhanced MRI. *Magn. Reson. Med.* **49,** 249–257.

21. Graham, R. A., Taylor, A. H., and Brown, T. R. (1994) A method for calculating the distribution of pH in tissues and a new source of pH error from the 31P-NMR spectrum. *Am. J. Physiol.* **266,** R638–R645.

22. Shungu, D. C. and Glickson, J. D. (1994) Band-selective spin-echoes for in vivo localized 1H NMR spectroscopy. *Magn. Reson. Med.* **32,** 277–284.

15

Biological Applications of Manganese-Enhanced Magnetic Resonance Imaging

Robia G. Pautler

Summary

The manganese ion (Mn^{2+}) has long been used in biomedical research as an indicator of calcium (Ca^{2+}) influx in conjunction with fluorescent microscopy because it is well established that Mn^{2+} enters cells through voltage-gated Ca^{2+} channels. Mn^{2+} is also paramagnetic, resulting in a shortening of the spin-lattice relaxation time constant, T_1, which yields positive contrast enhancement in T_1-weighted magnetic resonance imaging (MRI), specific to tissues in which the ion has accumulated. Manganese-enhanced MRI (MEMRI) uses a combination of these properties of Mn^{2+} to elucidate anatomical information and to identify regions of cellular activity. The focus of this chapter will detail some of the current MEMRI methodologies and biological applications.

Key Words: Manganese ion; Mn^{2+}; magnetic resonance imaging; MRI; manganese-enhanced MRI; MEMRI; brain; mouse; rat; rodent; olfactory; neuronal tracts; tract tracing; cardiac; heart; calcium channels; Ca^{2+} influx; neuronal activation; neuronal connections.

1. Introduction

The manganese ion (Mn^{2+}) has long been used in biological research in conjunction with fluorescent dyes, such as fura-2, to monitor the influx of Ca^{2+} ions, because Mn^{2+} is a well-known Ca^{2+} analog *(1–6)*. Although useful information can be obtained using Mn^{2+} as a reporter of Ca^{2+} influx, it is important to note that, at high concentrations, Mn^{2+} is also a neurotoxin *(7,8)*. For example, it has been shown that welders can be exposed to high levels of inhaled Mn^{2+}, because the ion is a by-product in welding fumes, and excessive exposure to Mn^{2+} can result in manganism (manganese poisoning) *(9–11)*. The mechanism of Mn^{2+} toxicity includes the oxidation of dopamine, resulting in the depletion of the neurotransmitter and the generation of superoxide radicals that damages tissues. Individuals with manganism exhibit an enhanced accumulation of Mn^{2+} within the striatum and eventually exhibit symptoms, some

From: *Methods in Molecular Medicine, Vol. 124*
Magnetic Resonance Imaging: Methods and Biologic Applications
Edited by: P. V. Prasad © Humana Press Inc., Totowa, NJ

of which are similar to those observed in Parkinson's disease *(9–11)*. These symptoms include hallucinations, tremors, an awkward gait, abnormal balance, memory loss, impairment of motor skills, slurred speech, lack of facial expression, and sleep disorders *(9–11)*.

From a toxicology point of view, it was previously thought that Mn^{2+} accessed the brain systemically through the inhaled route of exposure—that is, welders would inhale Mn^{2+} and it would be taken up into the lungs and enter the bloodstream and subsequently enter the brain *(12,13)*. Using radioactive Mn^{2+} in the pike (fish) and later the rat, Tjälve et al. were the first to demonstrate that the ion actually has additional direct access to the brain via uptake and transport along olfactory receptor neurons *(14,15)*. In these studies, the Mn^{2+} traversed a synapse traveling from the olfactory receptor neurons to the olfactory bulb to the olfactory cortex *(14,15)*. This axonal transport feature has been verified by Sloot et al. using radioactive Mn^{2+} injected into the rat striatum *(16)*.

Another very important feature about the Mn^{2+} ion is that it is paramagnetic *(17–21)*. The paramagnetic properties of Mn^{2+} effectively shorten the spin-lattice relaxation time constant, T_1, in tissues where Mn^{2+} has accumulated *(17–21)*. This results in positive contrast enhancement in T_1-weighted MRI images where the ion has accumulated *(17–21)*.

These three features of Mn^{2+} prompted the initiation of a small MRI pilot study in the olfactory system of the mouse to determine whether the Mn^{2+} ion could be used to trace neuronal tracts in an activity-dependent manner:

1. Mn^{2+} can be used to measure Ca^{2+} influx.
2. Mn^{2+} can be transported along axons and traverse synapses.
3. Mn^{2+} is paramagnetic and, therefore, MRI detectable.

The initial study involved exposing mice to a nasal lavage of a concentrated Mn^{2+} solution and imaging at time points after exposure *(22)*. Similar to what Tjälve et al. observed with radioactive Mn^{2+} in the pike and later the rat, the olfactory pathway in the mouse exhibited contrast enhancement in T_1-weighted MRI images (**Fig. 1**) *(14,15,22)*. The peak signal intensity in the olfactory bulbs occured at 29 h after Mn^{2+} exposure, and after 72 to 96 h, the signal intensity returned to baseline *(22)*. The return to baseline signal intensity, indicating the wash-out of the ion from the tissue, allows for longitudinal studies to be performed in the same animal *(22)*. Additionally, it is important to note that the levels of Mn^{2+} used in these studies, and in all studies mentioned in this chapter, were all well below the neurotoxic levels and, indeed, no symptoms of manganism were ever observed in any of the test subjects.

An examination into the mechanism of the Mn^{2+} uptake and transport features is described in a current model that results from an integration of information from several research laboratories and is summarized in **Fig. 2**. Briefly,

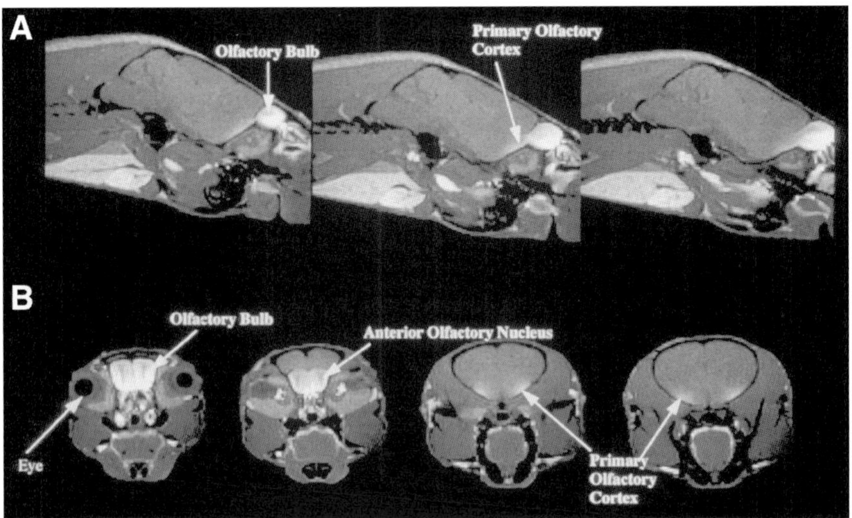

Fig. 1. MEMRI tract tracing in the mouse olfactory system. (**A**) Serial sagittal sections from a 3D T_1-weighted MRI data set. (**B**) Serial axial sections from the same 3D T_1-weighted MRI data set. Note the enhanced olfactory bulb as well as the primary olfactory cortex. (From **ref. 22**. © 1998, with permission from Wiley.)

Mn^{2+} enters cells through voltage-gated Ca^{2+} channels and accumulates in the endoplasmic reticulum (*6,23–25*). In the endoplasmic reticulum, Mn^{2+} is most likely packaged for transport and transported along microtubules to the synaptic cleft, where it is released and taken up by the next neuron in the circuit (*23,24*).

Because of this basic, initial olfactory experiment, MEMRI has been employed in a variety of settings, including tract tracing in the visual system (**Fig. 3**), activity-dependent tract tracing (**Fig. 4**), and tracing from deep brain nuclei, and MEMRI has evolved to include other species, including rats, songbirds, and nonhuman primates (*26–29*). Furthermore, MEMRI has been applied to other organ systems, such as the heart (*30*). This chapter provides details on how to perform basic MEMRI experiments in the brain and the heart, primarily in the rodent. Additionally, potential biological applications are discussed.

2. Materials

2.1. Tract Tracing the Olfactory System in Rodents—Anatomy and Activation

1. $MnCl_2$ (0.77 g in 1 mL of H_2O, *see* **Note 1**).
2. Sterile water.
3. 1-mL Tubes.
4. Vortexer.

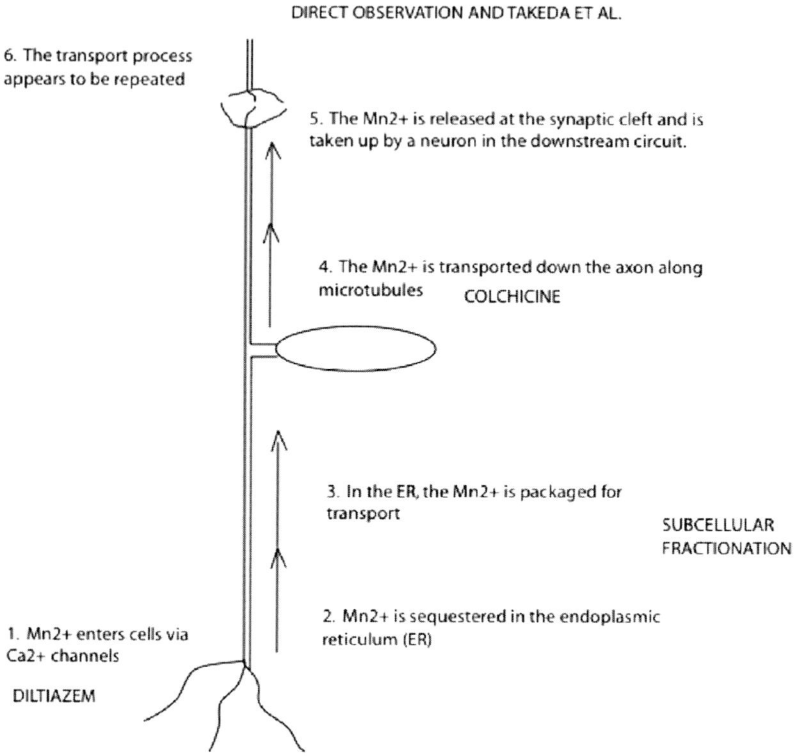

Fig. 2. The current model of Mn^{2+} uptake and transport is as follows: *1*, Mn^{2+} first enters cells through Ca^{2+} channels. Utilizing the Ca^{2+} channel blocking drug, diltiazem, prevents the uptake of Mn^{2+} into cells. This has been verified in brain as well as the heart *(2,5–6,24,30)*. *2,3*, After entry into the cell, the Mn^{2+} is sequestered into the endoplasmic reticulum where it is most likely packaged for transport. This has been verified utilizing subcellular fractionation obtained through sucrose gradient centrifugation and photometric sensitive Mn^{2+} assays on the collected subcellular fractions *(24)*. *4*, The Mn^{2+} is then transported along microtubules. This has been demonstrated with the use of colchicine. Upon disruption of the microtubules, the transport of the Mn^{2+} was halted *(16,24)*. *5,6*, After transport along the microtubules to the synaptic cleft, the Mn^{2+} is then released at the synaptic cleft and taken up by the next neuron in the circuit *(22–25)*. Quite interestingly, it has been shown that neurons that have been pre-loaded with Mn^{2+} co-release the ion with glutamate upon stimulation, indicating the possibility that Mn^{2+} is transported within synaptic vesicles *(23)*.

5. Mouse or rat.
6. 10-µL Pipetter.
7. Pipet tips.
8. Anesthesia (e.g., ketamine/xylazine, *see* **Note 2**).
9. Warming pad.

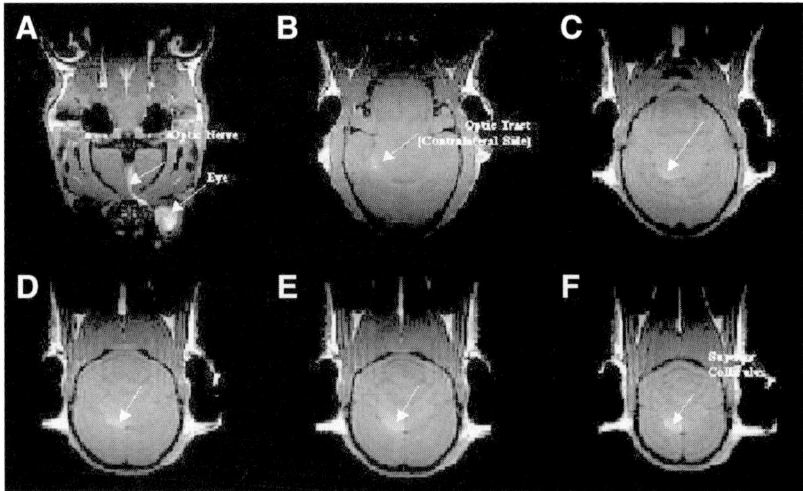

Fig. 3. MEMRI tract tracing in the visual system. **(A–F)** Serial horizontal sections starting at the base of the brain moving dorsally. Note the enhanced eye and optic nerve as well as the connections on the contralateral side of the brain ending in the superior colliculus. (From **ref. 22**. © 1998, with permission from Wiley.)

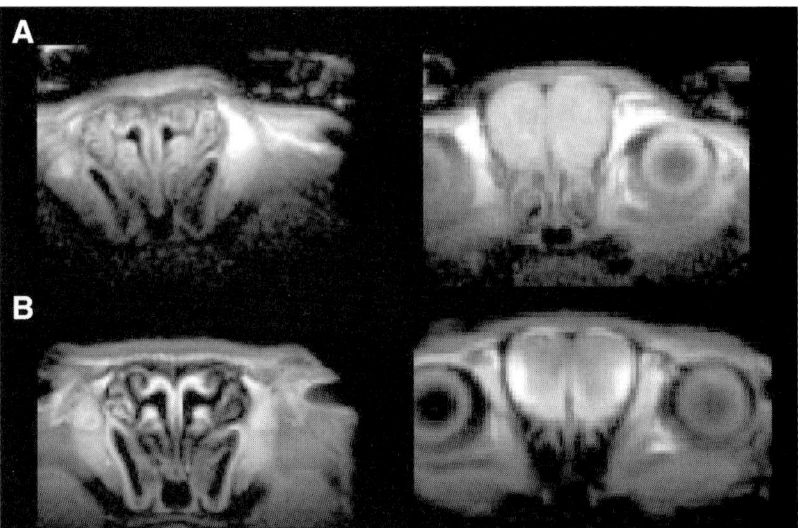

Fig. 4. Activity dependent MEMRI tract tracing in response to olfactory activation. All imaging took place 1.5 h post exposure. **(A)** Control mice exposed to aerosolized Mn^{2+} only. *Left,* turbinates; *right,* olfactory bulb. **(B)** Mice exposed to aerosolized Mn^{2+} and amyl acetate. *Left,* turbinates; *right,* olfactory bulb. Note the specific pattern of accumulation of Mn^{2+} in the nasal turbinates and olfactory bulbs of the mouse exposed to the aerosolized Mn^{2+} and amyl acetate. (From **ref. 24**. © 2002, with permission from Elsevier.)

10. Exposure chamber[*].
11. Aromatherapy device[*] or equivalent for aerosolizing the Mn^{2+}.
12. Proper safety precautions[*] to avoid exposure to aerosolized Mn^{2+} (mask, gloves, lab coat, and eye protection).

[*]For experiments specific to olfactory activation.

2.2. Tract Tracing the Visual System in Rodents

1. 0.8 mM $MnCl_2$ in 1 mL of H_2O (*see* **Note 1**).
2. Sterile water.
3. 1-mL Tubes.
4. Vortexer.
5. Mouse or rat.
6. 30-gage Needle and insulin syringe.
7. Dissecting scope.
8. Anesthesia (e.g., ketamine/xylazine, *see* **Note 2**).
9. Warming pad.

2.3. Stereotactic Brain Injections—Tracing from Brain Nuclei

1. 5 mM $MnCl_2$ made up in H_2O (*see* **Note 1**).
2. Sterile water.
3. Vortexer.
4. 1-mL Tube.
5. Stereotactic brain apparatus.
6. Glass-bead sterilizer.
7. Sterile surgical skin scrub/wash (e.g., chlorhexidine and sterile water).
8. Sterile cotton swabs.
9. Anesthesia (e.g., ketamine/xylazine, *see* **Note 2**).
10. Analgesic (e.g., bupivicaine).
11. Surgical tools—scalpel blade, scalpel handle, small scissors, small needle holder, curved forceps, and straight forceps.
12. Pura-lube or an equivalent eye ointment.
13. Warming pad.
14. Pulled quartz pipette needle (preferably with filament).
15. Picospritzer (e.g., Parker-Hannifin Picospritzer III).
16. Dissecting microscope mounted 90° from original position on a boom (*see* **Figs. 5** and **6**).
17. Small high-speed drill with associated bits.
18. Magnifying visor.
19. Calibrated gage for nanoliter injection volumes (*see* **Note 13** for specific details on the construction of a calibrated gage).

2.4. MEMRI in the Heart

1. 0.05 mM $MnCl_2$ made up in H_2O (*see* **Note 1**).
2. Beaker and warm water for warming the tail.
3. 27- or 30-gage Needle attached to a 1-mL syringe.

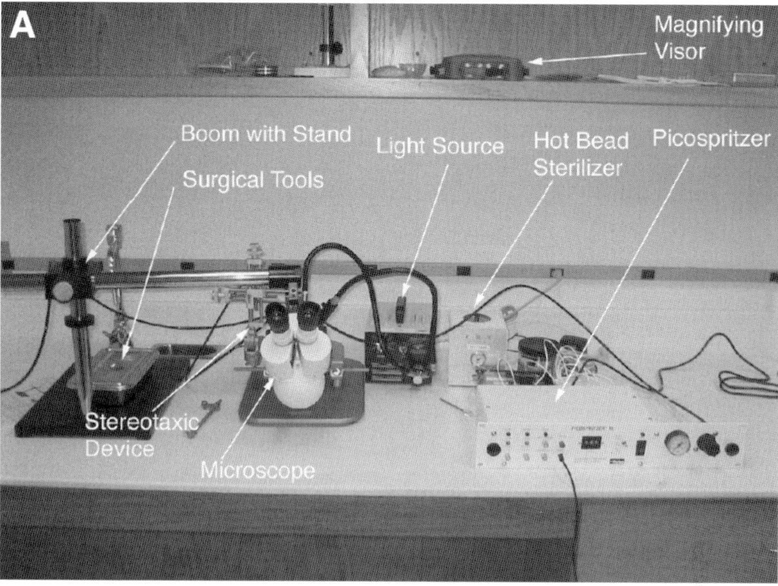

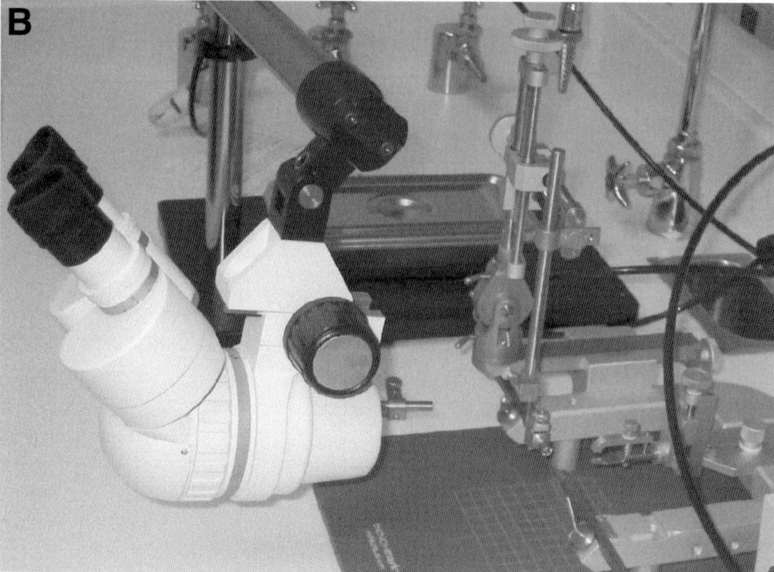

Fig. 5. (**A**) Example of a typical stereotaxic set up for rodent brain injections. Note that the dissecting microscope is mounted on a boom such that it can be swung out of the way. Photograph by R.G. Pautler. (**B**) Example of the orientation of the dissecting scope such that it can be utilized to view the meniscus of the solution in the pipette. Note that the scope is oriented 90° from the standard orientation. Photograph by R.G. Pautler.

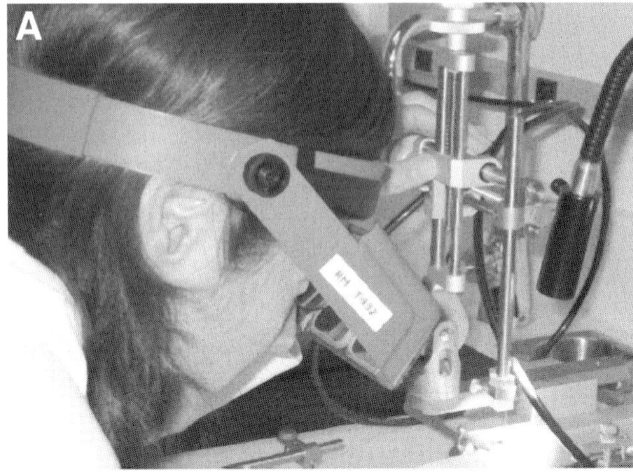

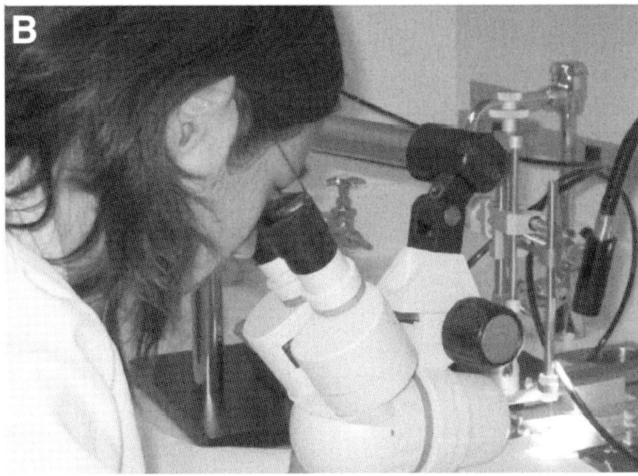

Fig. 6. (**A**) Example of how to utilize the magnifying visor to ascertain the injection site in addition for use during drilling into the skull. The use of a small dental mirror makes this process much easier. (**B**) Once the site has been identified and the hole bored into the skull, remove the magnifying visor, swing the dissecting scope back into place, and utilize it to watch the meniscus during injection. Photographs by R.G. Pautler.

4. Anesthesia (e.g., ketamine/xylazine, *see* **Note 2**).
5. Sterile saline solution.
6. Connector that can attach to the syringe head. Make sure that a tube prefilled with the contrast agent of choice is attached to this connector and that a 1-mL syringe is at the opposite end of this tubing.
7. Scissors.
8. Small hemostat.

9. 4.0-gage Silk suture.
10. Sports tape.
11. 1-mL Syringe.
12. Syringe pump capable of delivering 0.2 mL/h.

3. Methods

3.1. Tracing the Olfactory System

3.1.1. Anatomy vs Activity—Different Exposure Modalities

Two current exposure modalities exist for tracing the olfactory system that allow for either the anatomy or the activation of specific neurons to be traced. Anatomical olfactory tracings involve the mere pipetting of concentrated $MnCl_2$ into the naris (**Fig. 1**). Activity-dependent tracings involve the exposure of aerosolized Mn^{2+} (**Fig. 4**). The paradigm is as follows:

3.1.1.1. ANATOMICAL OLFACTORY TRACINGS

1. Dissolve 0.77 g of $MnCl_2$ into 1 mL of sterile H_2O. Vortex. The solution will be a faint pink.
2. Anesthetize a mouse and, on lack of a toe pinch reflex, pipet 1 µL of the $MnCl_2$ solution into the naris using a 10-µL pipetter (*see* **Note 2**). Pipet 1 µL into the contralateral naris (*see* **Notes 3** and **4**). Repeat as desired until up to 2 µL per naris have been applied.
3. Recover the mouse on a warming pad until the mouse awakens (*see* **Note 5**).

3.1.1.2. ACTIVITY-DEPENDENT OLFACTORY TRACINGS

1. Dissolve 15 g of $MnCl_2$ into 50 mL of H_2O.
2. For experiments involving the application of an odor, mix a 1:100 dilution of amyl acetate, for example, directly into the $MnCl_2$.
3. Place the humidifier into a plastic box (e.g., 3 in. × 1 in.) that has a closeable lid (*see* **Note 6**). This whole setup should be kept in a hood with a barrier that can be closed to prevent investigators from inhaling the aerosolized Mn^{2+}. It is also important to be able to turn the humidifier on/off from outside of the hood. Additionally, it is advised to observe proper safety precautions during experiments when the Mn^{2+} is aerosolized (mask, eye protection, gloves, lab coat, and so on).
4. Place the $MnCl_2$ solution into the heating chamber of a humidifier.
5. Anesthetized vs awake:
   a. For studies involving anesthetized mice, anesthetize the mouse with 0.1 mL/10 g of body weight of 75 mg/mL of urethane. Secure the mouse in a restraining device and place above the humidifier to allow exposure of the aerosolized Mn^{2+}.
   b. For studies in the awake animal, place the mouse into the plastic box that also housed the humidifier.
6. Close the box lid, close the hood, and turn on the humidifier.
7. Exposure: anesthetized vs awake:

    a. For the anesthetized mice, the exposure paradigm is 5-min on followed by 5-min off. This 5-min on followed by 5-min off procedure is repeated twice and then kept off for 1.5 h with the mouse still in the exposure chamber. It is important not to access the box at this time because aerosolized Mn^{2+} could still be present.

    b. For the awake paradigm, the device is turned on for 30 min and then turned off for 1.5 h with the mouse still in the exposure chamber. Again, it is important not to access the box at this time because aerosolized Mn^{2+} could still be present.

3.1.2. Imaging Parameters at Different Field Strengths

Two different field strengths have been investigated using tracing the olfactory pathway in mice, 7.0 T and 11.7 T. The optimal imaging parameters for these two field strengths using a T_1-weighted, spin-echo imaging sequence are:

3.1.2.1. 7.0 T

Repetition time (TR) = 300 ms; echo time (TE) = 8.7 ms; number of signal averages (NEX) = 2; and matrix = 128^2 with a 1-mm slice thickness, or matrix = 128^3 with a field of view (FOV) ranging from 1.5 to 2.5 cm^2 or 1.5 to 2.5 cm^3. As the hardware permits, feel free to push the resolution.

3.1.2.2. 11.7 T

TR = 504.1 ms; TE = 8.2 ms; NEX = 2; and matrix = 128^2 with a 1-mm slice thickness, or matrix = 128^3 with a FOV = 1.5 cm^3 or 1.0 cm^3.

- As with any type of mouse MRI, it is important to maintain the animal's physiology during scanning. The use of a heated water bath with an associated warming blanket is highly recommended.

3.1.3. Optimal Imaging Times

3.1.3.1. ANATOMICAL OLFACTORY TRACINGS

To view anatomical tracings to the pyriform and also entorhinal cortex, the optimal imaging time is 24 to 29 h after application of Mn^{2+}. Spin-echo, 3D, T_1-weighted imaging works best to obtain useable tracings.

3.1.3.2. ACTIVITY-DEPENDENT OLFACTORY TRACINGS

To view activity-dependent tracings to the olfactory bulbs, the optimal imaging time is 1.5 to 3 h after Mn^{2+} exposure. Either 2D or 3D images can be acquired, depending on the size of the activated area. For example, in studies using amyl acetate activation, 2D images were sufficient to obtain useable data. To get comparable results between mice, acquire a 1-mm sagittal slice that encompasses the middle of the olfactory bulbs. From this reference sagittal slice, line up four axial slices, with the first slice aligned with the posterior edge of the olfactory bulb.

However, because the size of the accessory olfactory bulb was smaller than the 1-mm slice thickness used in the amyl acetate studies, it was oftentimes masked in the 2D images. Therefore, it is necessary to obtain 3D data sets.

3.1.4. Expected Results

3.1.4.1. ANATOMICAL PROTOCOL

The expected results for the anatomical tract tracing are positive contrast enhancements starting from the olfactory epithelium, proceeding to the olfactory bulbs, to the primary olfactory cortex, and extending as far as the entorhinal cortex (**Fig. 1**). The peak signal intensity for the olfactory bulbs is at approx 29 h. For downstream structures, the signal intensity decreases with distance from the site of the nasal lavage.

3.1.4.2. ACTIVATION PROTOCOL

The expected results from the activity-dependent tract tracings are localized positive contrast enhancement starting from the olfactory epithelium and proceeding to the olfactory bulbs (**Fig. 4**). These results can be observed between 1.5 and 3 h. Extending the imaging time beyond this period could potentially elucidate the specificity within the olfactory cortex as well.

3.1.5. Applications in Neurobiology

3.1.5.1. OLFACTORY CONNECTIVITY

The gross anatomical tracings of the olfactory system can be used in several different ways. For example, they are useful to use as reference points in MRI images; and in determining volumes and surface areas of the olfactory cortex during development from infancy to adulthood, and during aging. Furthermore, olfactory tracings can be used to characterize changes in stereotaxic coordinates as well as for the verification of the stereotaxic coordinates. For example, olfactory tracings in the reeler mouse as compared with the control background strain (C57/bl6) exhibited a significant shift in the location of the primary olfactory cortex relative to baseline *(31)*. Another example includes the Pax-6 small-eyes mutant that exhibited a smaller area of activation in the olfactory bulbs when exposed to amyl acetate as compared with the associated controls *(31)*.

3.1.5.2. OLFACTORY ACTIVATION

The olfactory activation experiments can be used to elucidate the activation in the olfactory epithelium and the corresponding projections to the olfactory bulb. Such an analysis could potentially prove to be useful in the correlating receptors with trajectory patterns to the olfactory bulb as well as to downstream structures.

3.2. Tracing the Visual System

3.2.1. Intravitreal Injections

1. To inject Mn^{2+} into the vitreous of the rodent eye, first anesthetize the animal with 7.5 mg/mL of ketamine and 0.5 mg/mL of xylazine at a dose of 0.17 mL/10 g of body weight. Alternatively, 5 mg/mL of sodium pentobarbital can be used as an anesthesia at a dose of 0.1 mL / 10 g of body weight. During all injections, be sure to maintain the animal's body temperature on a heating pad.
2. Using an insulin syringe with a 30-gage needle, fill the syringe with the $MnCl_2$ solution. Be sure to clear the syringe of air bubbles by flicking the side of the syringe.
3. Carefully insert the needle into the mesolateral portion of the orbit of the eye.
4. After insertion, point the needle toward the back of the eye, where the retinal ganglion cells are located, and inject 1 to 2 μL of the Mn^{2+} solution. Be sure to do this injection very slowly to minimally perturb the interocular pressure.
5. To gage the success of an injection, the vitreal humor should appear bright on T_1-weighted MRI images. Evaluation of the integrity of the eye several hours after injection is advised.

3.2.2. Imaging Parameters at Different Field Strengths

Two different field strengths have been investigated using tracing the olfactory pathway in mice, 7.0 T and 11.7 T. The optimal imaging parameters for these two field strengths using a spin-echo imaging sequence are:

3.2.2.1. 7.0 T

TR = 300 ms; TE = 8.7 ms; NEX = 2; and matrix = 128^2 with a 1-mm slice thickness, or matrix = 128^3 with a FOV = 1.5 cm^3 or 1.0 cm^3. As the hardware permits, feel free to push the resolution.

3.2.2.2. 11.7 T

TR = 504.1 ms; TE = 8.3 ms; NEX = 2; and matrix = 128^2 with a 1-mm slice thickness, or matrix = 128^3 with a FOV = 1.5 cm^3 or 1.0 cm^3.

3.2.3. Optimal Imaging Times

The optimal imaging time for the visual system is approx 24 to 36 h after injection.

3.2.4. Expected Results

Expected results include contrast enhancement in the eye, optic nerve and tract, and superior colliculus (**Fig. 3**).

3.2.5. Applications in Neurobiology

Current applications have included using MEMRI tract tracing in the eye to evaluate radiation-induced damage to the optic nerve and validation of diffusion tensor imaging *(32,33)*. Additional uses could potentially include monitoring anatomical changes in neurodegenerative diseases, such as observed in experimental allergic encephalitis mice *(34)*. Experimental allergic encephalitis mice are a good model for multiple sclerosis *(34)*, and MEMRI could potentially be used to evaluate changes as disease progression ensues.

3.3. Stereotactic Brain Injections

3.3.1. Brain Injection Protocol

The brain injection protocol is as follows:

1. Anesthetize the mouse with 7.5 mg/mL of ketamine and 0.5 mg/mL of xylazine at a dose of 0.17 mL/10 g of body weight. Alternatively, 5 mg/mL of sodium pentobarbital can be used as an anesthesia at a dose of 0.1 mL/10 g of body weight.
2. On lack of a toe pinch reflex, put the mouse on a paper towel to trim the fur from the top of the head.

   - It is not trivial to remove the fur from the mouse's head before surgery. Mice are different from rats in that the use of an electric shaver to remove the hair does not work well (even electric moustache clippers have been tried with dismal results!). Two alternatives are available—either use scissors to trim away the excess fur or some researchers use a scalpel blade to scrape away the fur. Because the scalpel blade can oftentimes lead to the simultaneous removal of skin, it is strongly recommended to use scissors to trim the hair. Use the scissors to lift up the hair at the base of the roots such that the scissors are perpendicular to the plane of the head and trim as closely as possible to the scalp. Continue removing the hair on the entire top of the head, from the base of the skull to just behind the eyes, extending laterally to the ears.

3. Swing the microscope secured on the boom out of the way (*see* **Figs. 5** and **6** for the basic setup).
4. Place the mouse into the stereotaxic device, and secure the nose, tooth, and ear bars. At this point, put an eye ointment solution, such as Pura-lube onto the eyes, otherwise, they can dry out during the surgical procedure. To ensure the sterility of the surgical procedure, it is advisable to put sterile surgical drapes over the body of the mouse, leaving only the shaved head exposed. At this point, use surgical scrub and sterile cotton swabs to clean the head. After cleaning the scalp area, use a surgical rinse or sterile H_2O to remove the soap. To ensure sterility, this cleaning must be performed a total of three times.
5. Make sure that the head is level (*see* **Note 7**). Once the initial incision has been made and the skull has been dried of blood and fluids, the longitudinal and the lateral levelness of the head can be validated. Use the magnifying visor rather than the microscope during this procedure (**Fig. 6A**).
6. Secure a pulled pipet to the stereotaxic apparatus and use it to map out the stereotaxic coordinates relative to bregma (*see* **Notes 8–10**). Again, use the magnifying visor during this procedure (**Fig. 6A**).

- While wearing the magnifying visor, it is also helpful to use a small, hand-held dental mirror that can easily be placed at different locations to view the pipet from different angles. Once the site has been identified, use a fine, high-speed drill to drill a hole just through the skull, taking care not to touch the brain tissue with the drill bit (*see* **Note 11**).

7. Lower the filled needle into the correct coordinates in the brain. Set the injection pressure to approx 20 psi and set the injection time to about 5 ms.
8. Swing the microscope back toward the stereotaxic apparatus to watch the meniscus during the injection (*see* **Note 12**). Adjust the location and focus of the scope until the gage can be observed through the microscope (**Fig. 6B**). Zoom in as much as possible to the meniscus and use a gage attached to the back of the needle to monitor the injection volume (**Fig. 7**). With an initial injection time of 5 ms, adjust the injection timing (usually increase it) such that the meniscus only moves at the most 1/10 of a line width, as observed on the calibrated gage (*see* **Note 13**). Inject until the desired volume is expulsed. The optimal injection volume for tract tracings in the mouse brain appears to be 10 to 20 nL. Leave the needle in place for approx 5 min.
9. Before closing the wound, place a few drops of an analgesic (such as bupivicaine) underneath the scalp (typically on the side of the skull contralateral to where the hole was drilled). Be sure not to get this drug on the exposed brain tissue.
10. Use sterile wound clips or suture to close the wound. If wound clips are used, be sure to remove them before imaging.

3.3.2. Animal Recovery

Place the mouse on a warming pad as it recovers from the anesthesia and surgery. Once the mouse has awakened, it can be returned to its cage until it is to be imaged.

3.3.3. Imaging Parameters

It is advised to use the 3D MRI sequences as described in the olfactory and visual sections for the Mn^{2+} brain injections.

3.3.4. Expected Results

The expected results are multisynaptic tract tracings to multiple structures from the site of injection (*see* **Fig. 8**; **Note 14**). The contrast enhancement will diminish and is completely absent 10 d after injection (**Fig. 9**). Mice have been kept for up to 30 d after injection and observed for behavioral deficits. During this 30-d time period, mice remained consistently healthy and void of symptoms of manganism.

3.3.5. Applications in Neurobiology

Applications of the stereotaxic injection protocol include monitoring the changes in the projections before and after a specific paradigm and monitoring

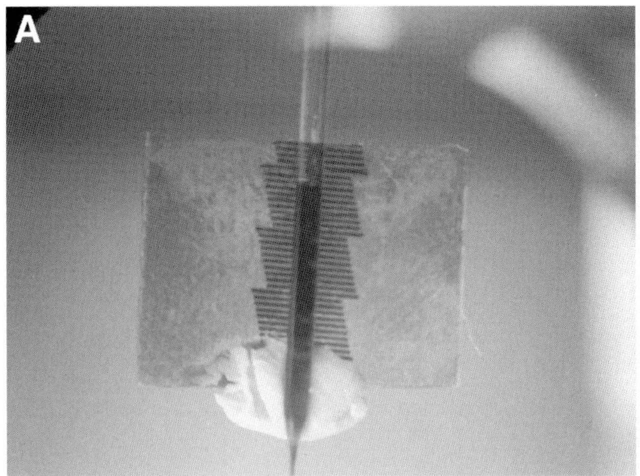

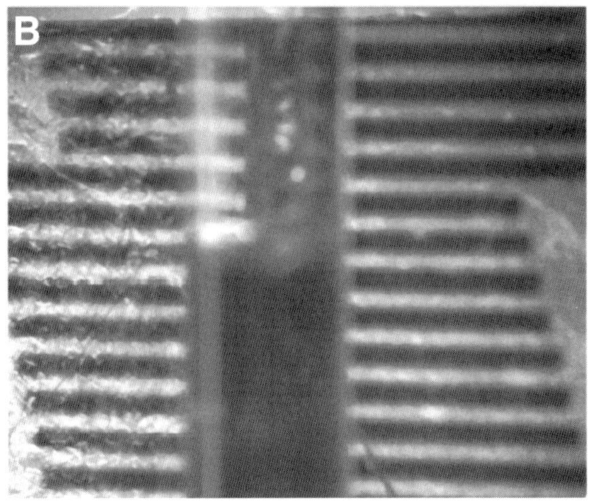

Fig. 7. (**A**) Gross view of the quartz pipet with the gage attached to the back. For this example, the pipet was filled with dye. (**B**) Meniscus and calibrated gage as viewed through the dissecting microscope. During injection, a starting pulse of 5 ms is recommended. Keep increasing the pulse length until the meniscus barely moves. Continue pulsing until the desired injection volume is obtained. Photographs by R.G. Pautler.

sexually dimorphic anatomical and functional differences in projections. For example, Van der Linden's group has used MEMRI to trace the anatomical connections in voice control nuclei in songbirds *(29)*. They were also able to observe functional differences in the rates of accumulation of the ion that were sexually dimorphic *(29)*.

Furthermore, the injection protocol has evolved to include nonhuman primates. For example, Logothetis was able to demonstrate MEMRI tract tracing

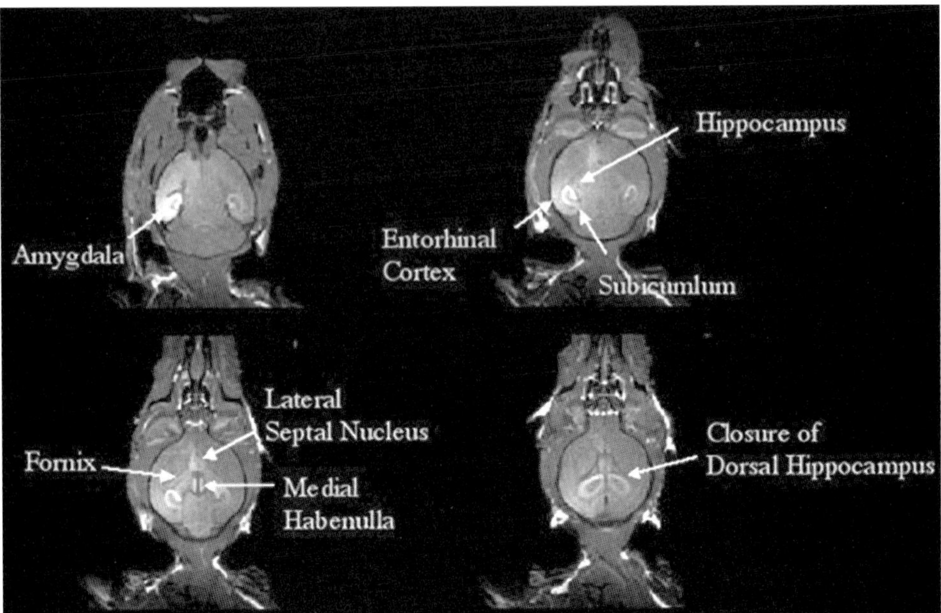

Fig. 8. MEMRI tract tracing from the amygdala. Serial horizontal sections starting at the level of the amygdala and moving dorsally. Note the enhancement starting at the level of the amygdala, extending into the entorhinal cortex, hippocampus, subiculum, fornix, lateral septal nucleus, and medial habenula. (From **ref. 25**. © 2003, with permission from Wiley.)

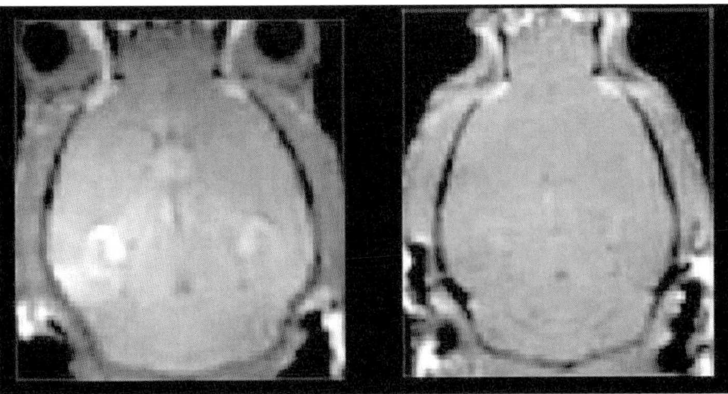

Fig. 9. MEMRI tract tracing from the amygdala. The same mouse is observed 2 d (left) and 10 d (right) post injection. Note that the contrast enhancement disapates with time thereby allowing for longitudinal studies involving repeated tracings to be pursued in the same animal. (From **ref. 25**. © 2003, with permission from Wiley.)

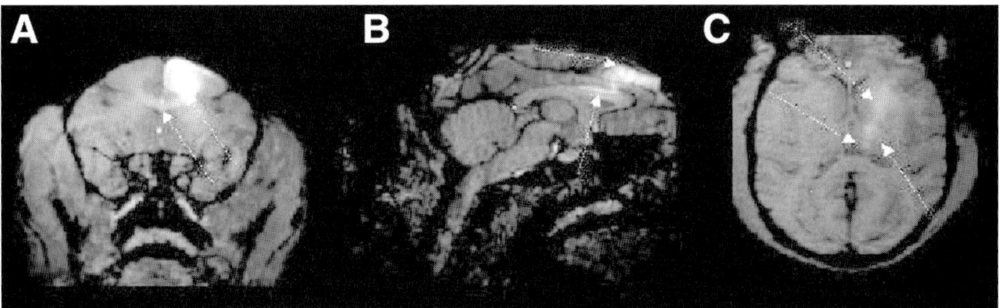

Fig. 10. Three-dimensional, T_1-weighted MRI, spin echo in vivo MEMRI images of the rhesus macaque. One milliliter of $MnCl_2$ was injected into the frontal cortex over the course of 8 min. The animal was allowed to recover for 36 h prior to imaging. **(A)** Axial image of the rhesus macaque brain. Note the site of injection as well as the tracing of the Mn^{2+} (as evidenced by the contrast enhancement) across the corpus callosum to the contralateral side of the brain. **(B)** Sagittal view of the same rhesus macaque. Note the striated, banded appearance of the frontal cortex and the tract leading to the corpus callosum. **(C)** Horizontal section of the same rhesus macaque. Note the tracings from the frontal cortex along the internal capsule to the thalamus. This macaque was imaged 1 wk post injection and all evidence of Mn^{2+} tracings had washed out. The macaque recovered from the imaging without any apparent detriment as evidenced by behavior and additional MRI scans. This work was performed in collaboration with Carl Olsen, Donald S. Williams, Chien Ho, and Alan Koretsky at Carnegie Mellon University.

in the visual system of rhesus macaques *(28)*. Additionally, Pautler et al. demonstrated tract tracing in the frontal cortical projections of the rhesus macaque **(Fig. 10)** *(31)*.

3.4. MEMRI in the Heart

3.4.1. Setting Up a Tail-Vein Line

1. Anesthetize the mouse with ketamine/xylazine or pentobarbital and keep it warm on the heating pad.

   • There are several ways of introducing a tail-vein line into the mouse for the infusion of contrast agents. These include:

   a. Insertion of a catheter attached to tubing, prefilled with contrast agent. This is not a highly recommended methodology because it is very easy to accidentally introduce agent into the mouse during the insertion of the needle before imaging.
   b. Insertion of a 27- or 30-gage needle into the tail vein attached to a 1-mL syringe filled with saline. After successful insertion into the tail vein, the syringe is removed and a connector attached to tubing filled with the contrast

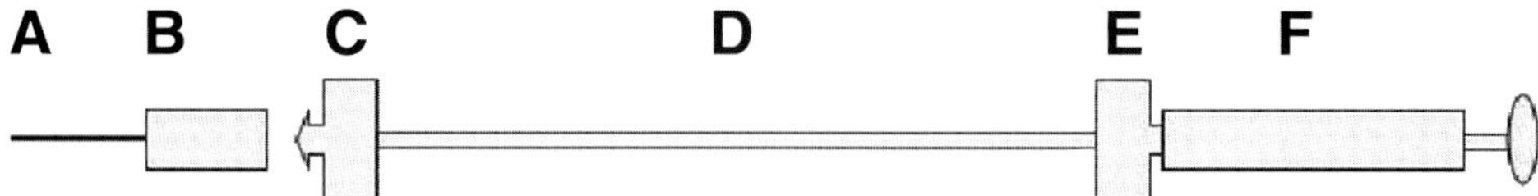

Fig. 11. Basic setup for intravenous infusion into the rodent via tail vein. (**A**) Metal part of the needle where the suture is tied. (**B**) Plastic part of the needle where the sports tape is placed. (**C**) Connector that attaches to the needle after the removal of the syringe. (**D**) Tubing that is prefilled with contrast agent. (**E**) Back connector that will allow for a 1-mL syringe to be conjoined to the tubing. (**F**) One-milliliter syringe also filled with contrast agent. See **ref. *30*** for the original description.

> agent is carefully fitted to the needle in the vein. This methodology will be detailed because it is the preferred mode.

2. Dip the mouse's tail into a beaker of warm water to dilate the tail vein.

    - Prefill the syringe (needle attached) with the saline solution. Do not attach the needle too tightly to the syringe because it will be very difficult to remove in later steps.

3. Place the mouse back onto the counter and insert the needle into the tail vein. Successful insertion into the tail vein is affirmed by the back-wash of blood into the saline-filled syringe.
4. Once the needle is in place, use a small square of sports tape (approx 1 cm wide and 2 cm long) to wrap around the plastic part of the needle and tail to hold the needle in place.
5. Place the suture underneath the tail and tie two knots around the tail and needle using the forceps and hemostats. At the end of this procedure, the plastic part of the needle will be held in place via the sports tape and the suture will be tied around the tail and hold the metal part of the needle in place. Note: the suture does not go through the skin.
6. Carefully remove the syringe and attach the connector/tubing to the needle head. Be sure not to introduce any air bubbles because the infusion of air bubbles intravenously can result in an embolism. *See* **Fig. 11** for a diagram of the final setup.
7. Place the syringe connected at the end of the tubing into the syringe pump and load the animal into the magnet.
8. During imaging, infuse a total volume of 0.1 mL of the $MnCl_2$ solution over a period of 30 min.

3.4.2. Imaging Parameters

The optimal imaging parameters at 7 T are to use a cardiac-gated fast, low angle shot imaging sequence with 16 segments, with each segment containing 4 phase encodes. TR = 300 ms; TE = 1.3 ms; matrix = 128 × 64; slice thickness = 1.0 mm; FOV = 2.5 cm; and number of averages (NA) = 8. It is always good to verify the enhanced results by varying the TR over a range to ensure that the signal enhancement is caused by accumulation of Mn^{2+} rather than variations in the TR that may have resulted from variations in the cardiac cycle, thereby altering the cardiac-gated image acquisition *(30)*. Additionally, other groups have had success with inversion recovery spin-echo sequences *(30)*.

3.4.3. Optimal Imaging Times

The optimal imaging times are before, during, and after the infusion of the $MnCl_2$ solution, until the signal intensity has reached a maximum. The typical acquisition experiment can last 70 min *(30)*.

3.4.4. Expected Results

The expected results are an incremental positive contrast enhancement in the cardiac muscle over time *(30,35)*.

3.4.5. Applications

Applications include using cardiac MEMRI to monitor inotropy and stunned myocardium *(30,35)*. Furthermore, the potential for MEMRI to be useful as a general research tool for the cardiac sciences lies in the realm of identification of areas of heart that work harder during specific stresses, monitoring the recovery of tissues after infarct, and studies centered on cardiac development.

4. Notes

1. Do not mix $MnCl_2$ with phosphate-based buffers. A precipitate will form, and injecting such solutions is quite toxic to the animals.
2. Ketamine/xylazine is a preferred anesthesia over pentobarbital because mice appear to recover more easily from the former.
3. Be careful not to damage the nasal epithelium when pipetting the $MnCl_2$ solution into the naris. If handled too roughly, the nose can bleed.
4. There is a structure called the nasal window that connects the two naris. Hence, at times, when a single naris is lavaged with the $MnCl_2$, both olfactory bulbs will exhibit enhancement.
5. Electronic heating pads from conventional drug stores can be used as warming-pads for the recovery of the mice.
6. The humidifier that was used in the olfactory activation experiments was actually a small aromatherapy device purchased from K-Mart for $20.00.
7. To insure that the head is level, it is highly recommended to use a two-pronged device that is spaced evenly from bregma to lambda on the skull. Your local machinist can easily make one.
8. Use quartz pipettes with filaments (e.g., Sutter Instruments). Outer diameter = 1.0 mm; inner diameter = 0.70 mm; and length = 10 cm.
9. When pulling quartz pipettes, a Sutter Instruments p2000 laser pipet puller works very well. The settings that work quite well in pulling these pipettes are: Heat = 700; Fil = 4; vel = 60; Del = 145; and Pul = 175.

10. When filling the pulled quartz pipette, it is very useful and advised to have the vacuum-loading feature on the Picospritzer. Set the pressure gage to 40 to 60 psi when vacuum loading.
11. During drilling, it is helpful to stabilize your arm by holding the drill with the opposite arm. This accounts for a much more stable drilling approach.
12. If the solution falls out of the quartz needle when it touches the brain, your needle tip is too large. Try a smaller needle tip.
13. Constructing a calibrated gage: create an Adobe Photoshop or equivalent file and use the appropriate tools to draw a single vertical line. To this vertical line, add a series of horizontal lines that are one pixel apart. Zoom in as much as possible to create the horizontal lines that are one pixel apart. Make sure that the document has the same output resolution as the printer that will be used. A printer with a resolution of 600 dpi works quite well. After obtaining or constructing such a file, print the file on negative film or onto a clear overhead. Trim away the excess media. Each space corresponds to 10 nL of fluid when using a 1.0-mm-diameter quartz pipet. *See* **Fig. 7**. Contact R. G. Pautler (rpautler@bcm.tmc.edu) to obtain a copy of a file if you are having trouble making your own.
14. If you see a black spot in your injection site, you injected too much Mn^{2+}. Although Mn^{2+} is traditionally a T1 contrast agent, at high concentrations, it can have T_2 effects.

Acknowledgments

Acknowledgments are given to Rita Schack, T. Pautler, E. L. Pautler, and Y. W. Pautler for help and support during the preparation of this manuscript. Additionally, acknowledgments are given to Raymond Mongeau for his help and guidance in constructing the gage for injections.

References

1. Merrit, J. E., Jacob, R., and Hallam T. J. (1989) Use of manganese to discriminate between calcium influx and mobilization from internal stores in stimulated human neutrophils. *J. Biol. Chem.* **264,** 1522–1527.
2. Simpson, P. B., Challiss, R. A., and Nahorski, S. R. (1995) Divalent cation entry in cultured rat cerebellar granule cells measured using Mn^{2+} quench of fura 2 fluorescence. *Eur. J. Neurosci.* **7,** 831–840.
3. Tisch-Idelson, D., Sharabani, M., Kloog, Y., and Aviram, I. (1999) Stimulation of neutrophils by prenylcysteine analogs: Ca^{2+} release and influx. *Biochim. Biophys. Acta.* **1451,** 187–195.
4. Wiemann, M., Busselberg, D., Schirrmacher, K., and Bingmann, D. (1998) A calcium release activated calcium influx in primary cultures of rat osteoblast-like cells. *Calcif. Tissue Int.* **63,** 154–159.
5. Du, C., MacGowan, G. A., Farkas, D. L., and Koretsky, A. P. (2001) Calibration of the calcium dissociation constant of Rhod(2) in the perfused mouse heart using manganese quenching. *Cell Calcium* **29,** 217–227.

6. Narita, K., Kawasaki, F., and Kita, H. (1990) Mn and Mg influxes through Ca channels of motor nerve terminals are prevented by verapamil in frogs. *Brain Res.* **510,** 289–295.

7. Aschner, M. and Aschner, J. (1991) Manganese neurotoxicity: cellular effects and blood brain barrier transport. *Neurosci. Biobehav. Rev.* **15,** 333–340.

8. Brurok, H., Schjitt, J., Berg, K., Karlsson, J. O., and Jynge, P. (1997) Manganese and the heart: acute cardiodepression and myocardial accumulation of manganese. *Acta Physiol. Scand.* **159,** 33–40.

9. Chandra, S. V., Shukla, G. S., Srivastava, R. S., Singh, H., and Gupta, V. P. (1981) An exploratory study of manganese exposure to welders. *Clin. Toxicol.* **18,** 407–416.

10. Pal, P. K., Samii, A., and Calne, D. B. (1999) Manganese neurotoxicity: a review of clinical features, imaging and pathology. *Neurotoxicology* **20,** 227–238.

11. McMillan, D. E. (1999) A brief history of the neurobehavioral toxicity of manganese: some unanswered questions. *Neurotoxicology* **20,** 499–507.

12. Bird, E. D., Anton, A. H., and Bullock, B. (1984) The effect of manganese inhalation on basal ganglia dopamine concentrations in rhesus monkey. *Neurotoxicology* **5,** 59–65.

13. Morganti, J. B., Lown, B. A., Stineman, C. H., D'Agostino, R. B., and Massaro, E. J. (1985) Uptake, distribution and behavioral effects of inhalation exposure to manganese (MnO2) in the adult mouse. *Neurotoxicology* **6,** 1–15.

14. Tjälve, H., Mejare, C., and Borg-Neczak, K. (1995) Uptake of manganese and cadmium from the nasal mucosa into the central nervous system via olfactory pathways in rats. *Pharm. Toxicol.* **77,** 23–31.

15. Tjälve, H., Henriksson, J., Tallkvist, J., Larsson, B., and Lindquist, N. (1996) Uptake of manganese and cadmium from the nasal mucosa into the central nervous system via olfactory pathways in rats. *Pharm. Toxicol.* **79,** 347–356.

16. Sloot, W. N. and Gramsbergen, J. P. (1994) Axonal transport of manganese and its relevance to selective neurotoxicity in the rat basal ganglia. *Brain Res.* **657,** 124–132.

17. Merritt, J. E., Jacob, R., and Hallam, T. J. (1989) Use of manganese to discriminate between calcium influx and mobilization from internal stores in stimulated human neutrophils. *J. Biol. Chem.* **25,** 1522–1527.

18. Cory, D. A., Schwartzentruber, D. J., and Mock, B. H. (1987) Ingested manganese chloride as a contrast agent for magnetic resonance imaging. *Magn. Reson. Imaging* **5,** 65–70.

19. Geraldes, C. F., Sherry, A. D., Brown, R. D. 3rd, and Koenig, S. H. (1986) Magnetic field dependence of solvent proton relaxation rates induced by Gd3+ and Mn2+ complexes of various polyaza macrocyclic ligands: implications for NMR imaging. *Magn. Reson. Med.* **3,** 242–250.

20. Mendonca-Dias, M. H., Gaggelli, E., and Lauterbur, P. C. (1983) Paramagnetic contrast agents in nuclear magnetic resonance medical imaging. *Semin. Nucl. Med.* **13,** 364–376.

21. Fornasiero, D., Bellen, J. C., Baker, R. J., and Chatterton, B. E. (1987) Paramagnetic complexes of manganese(II), iron(III), and gadolinium(III) as contrast agents for magnetic resonance imaging. The influence of stability constants on the biodistribution of radioactive aminopolycarboxylate complexes. *Invest. Radiol.* **22,** 322–327.

22. Pautler, R. G., Silva, A. C., and Koretsky, A. P. (1998) In vivo neuronal tract tracing using manganese-enhanced magnetic resonance imaging. *Magn. Reson. Med.* **40,** 740–748.

23. Takeda, A., Ishiwatari, A., and Okada, S. (1998) In vivo stimulation-induced release of manganese in rat amygdala. *Brain Res.* **811,** 147–151.

24. Pautler, R. G. and Koretsky, A. P. (2001) Tracing odor induced activation in the olfactory bulbs of mice using manganese enhanced magnetic resonance imaging (MEMRI). *Neuroimage* **16,** 441–448.

25. Pautler, R. G., Mongeau R., and Jacobs R. E. (2003) In vivo trans-synaptic tract tracing from the murine striatum and amygdala utilizing manganese enhanced MRI (MEMRI). *Magn. Reson. Med.* **50,** 33–39.

26. Watanabe, T., Michaelis, T., and Frahm, J. (2001) Mapping of retinal projections in the living rat using high-resolution 3D gradient-echo MRI with Mn2+-induced contrast. *Magnet. Reson. Med.* **46,** 424–429.

27. Saleem, K. S., Pauls, J. M., Augath, M., et al. (2002) Magnetic resonance imaging of neuronal connections in the macaque monkey. *Neuron* **34,** 685–700.

28. Van der Linden, A., Verhoye, M., Van Meir, V., et al. (2002) In vivo manganese-enhanced magnetic resonance imaging reveals connections and functional properties of the songbird vocal control system. *Neuroscience* **112,** 467–474.

29. Tindemans, I., Verhoye, M., Balthazart, J., and Van Der Linden, A. (2003) In vivo dynamic ME-MRI reveals differential functional responses of RA- and area X-projecting neurons in the HVC of canaries exposed to conspecific song. *Eur. J. Neurosci.* **18,** 3352–3360.

30. Hu, T. C. C., Pautler, R. G., MacGowan, G. A., and Koretsky, A. P. (2001) Manganese MRI enhancement of the mouse heart during changes in ionotropy. *Magn. Reson. Med.* **46,** 884–890.

31. Pautler, R. G., Olson, C., Williams, D. S., Ho, C., and Koretsky, A. P. (1990) Mn2+ enhanced MRI (MEMRI) in vivo tract tracing in mouse mutants and non-human primates. *Proc. Intl. Soc. Mag. Reson. Med.* **7,** 448.

32. Ryu, S., Brown, S. L., Kolozsvary, A., Ewing, J. R., and Kim, J. H. (2002) Noninvasive detection of radiation-induced optic neuropathy by manganese-enhanced MRI. *Radiat. Res.* **157,** 500–505.

33. Watanabe, T., Michaelis, T., and Frahm, J. (2001), Mapping of retinal projections in the living rat using high-resolution 3D gradient-echo MRI with Mn2+-induced contrast. *Magn. Reson. Med.* **46,** 424–429.

34. Lublin, F. D., Maurer, P. H., Berry, R. G., and Tippett, D. (1981) Delayed, relapsing experimental allergic encephalomyelitis in mice. *J. Immunol.* **126,** 819–822.

35. Krombach, G. A., Saeed, M., Higgins, C. B., Novikov, V., and Wendland, M. F. (2004) Contrast-enhanced MR delineation of stunned myocardium with administration of MnCl(2) in rats. *Radiology* **230,** 183–190.

16

Targeted Magnetic Resonance Imaging Contrast Agents

Shelton D. Caruthers, Patrick M. Winter, Samuel A. Wickline,
and Gregory M. Lanza

Summary

The era of personalized medicine is emerging as physicians attempt to diagnose disease in asymptomatic individuals and treat pathology early in its natural history. A novel tool in an emerging armamentarium, molecular imaging will allow noninvasive characterization and segmentation of patients for delivering custom-tailored therapy. Nanoparticulate agents, such as superparamagnetic agents, liposomes, perfluorocarbon nanoparticle emulsions, and dendrimers, are being intensively researched as formulation platforms for various targeted clinical applications. As exemplified by perfluorocarbon nanoparticles, these new agents, in combination with the rapid innovations in imaging hardware and software, will allow the emergence of new medical diagnostic and therapeutic paradigms.

Key Words: Personalized medicine; molecular imaging; gadolinium; iron oxides; nanoparticles; dendrimers; liposomes; targeted therapeutics; nanomedicine.

1. Introduction

This chapter addresses some of the current and imminent applications of magnetic resonance imaging (MRI) contrast agents that have unique applications for diagnosis, therapy, and monitoring through specific targeting. In general, the strategy is to recognize and characterize early disease, which otherwise would be difficult or impossible to detect using routine magnetic resonance (MR) techniques. In essence, the intent of biochemical imaging agents is to provide noninvasive assessments of pathology analogous to the use of immunohistochemistry. The strengths and weaknesses of various molecular imaging approaches are presented along with selected examples of cardiovascular and oncological applications.

2. MR Detectability

Although the binding affinity and specificity of the homing ligands are critical for targeting, robust MR detectability of the agent is required for usefulness

From: *Methods in Molecular Medicine, Vol. 124*
Magnetic Resonance Imaging: Methods and Biologic Applications
Edited by: P. V. Prasad © Humana Press Inc., Totowa, NJ

at clinical field strengths. Superparamagnetic agents can be sensitively assessed with MRI, but these particles may induce field inhomogeneity artifacts that compromise resolution and obscure proximal anatomic features. Conversely, contrast from paramagnetic formulations can be highly dependent on water flux within the targeted environment as well as the concentration of metal accumulated within each voxel *(1)*.

The concentration of metal within an MR voxel has been, until recently, the fundamental barrier to success of targeted paramagnetic agents. Inadequate numbers of available binding sites within an MRI voxel results in low concentrations of paramagnetic metals, which are unable to overcome partial-volume dilution effects. From the equipment side of the MR molecular-imaging equation, the ever-present trade-offs between voxel size, partial volume effects, signal-to-noise ratio, and imaging time must be optimally balanced. Because molecular targets are heterogeneously distributed at the microscopic level, reducing an imaging voxel to less than 100 µm on a side might seem highly desirable. However, the reduction in voxel volume to minimize partial-volume contrast dilution concurrently increases the imaging sensitivity to minute motion-related errors (including diffusion) and drastically reduces the signal-to-noise ratio. Increasing scan time to offset diminished signal-to-noise ratio may further prolong the opportunity for motion-related artifacts. Small fields of view and thin slices are highly desirable for most molecular-imaging applications, but focused scanning strategies require an optimized balance of major hardware features, including high-performance gradients and radio frequency (RF) systems, customized coils, and high magnetic field strength, which are usually the providence of small bore, high-field animal magnets (e.g., $\geq$ 4.7 T). However, the rapid evolution of the current state-of-the-art systems at 1.5 T and the increasing placement of high-field (i.e., 3.0 T) systems in clinical settings now allow noninvasive high-resolution imaging in humans. In many situations, *a priori* knowledge of the disease permits focused, small field-of-view imaging of important regions of interest. However, in some applications, large coverage imaging (e.g., whole-body screening) may be required to locate pathological tissues, and the contrast effects imparted by the targeted agent must be able to withstand larger partial-volume dilution effects. Clearly, a complex interplay of many factors must be weighed and balanced for successful molecular imaging.

Contrast agent selection must complement the anticipated application, which involves consideration of biosignature density, accessibility, and voxel resolution. For biochemical targets that exist in great abundance (e.g., fibrin in thrombus), an inherently weaker contrast agent may provide adequate detection, but for imaging of sparse epitopes (e.g., adhesion molecules), a strong signal influence from each bound particle is required. In certain situations, a differential imaging approach may be preferable, wherein a "switchable" or "on-off" system, such as a magnetization transfer agent, may be essential *(2)*.

3. Targeting Approaches

3.1. Passive Targeting Strategies

In vivo molecular imaging generally uses active or passive targeting approaches to provide contrast to tissues or biochemical markers expressed in or on cells. Passive targeting, as its name implies, uses differential permeability and natural clearance pathways to partition the contrast agents into the desired anatomic locations. For example, malignant brain lesions often disrupt the normally impermeable blood–brain barrier, which permits gadolinium-diethylenetriamine pentaacetic acid (Gd-DTPA) to penetrate the compromised barrier at pathological sites while excluding extravasation of the contrast agent elsewhere *(3)*. Conversely, prolonged retention of Gd-DTPA within myocardial scars relative to normal muscle regions allows infarcted territories to be readily differentiated from viable tissue *(4)*. Still other contrast agents are readily phagocytized by, and accumulate within, macrophages, which are prevalent around tumors *(5)*, in lymph nodes *(6–11)*, and within atherosclerotic plaques *(12,13)*. The reader is referred to companion chapters within this volume in which these and other passive contrast strategies are further discussed. This chapter focuses on active, ligand-directed targeting, which implies that contrast specificity results from the explicit interaction between homing molecules and pathognomonic biomarkers.

3.2. Active Targeting Strategies

Over the years, a common coupling method for active targeting has used the natural high affinity of avidin and biotin *(14,15)*. Contrast agents using avidin–biotin interactions may be linked *a priori* to homing ligands and given as a single-step injection or administered as two or three sequential components and assembled in vivo. Self-assembly in vivo uses a pretargeting strategy, in which a biotinylated antibody, for instance, is systemically administered and time is allowed for the antibody to localize and saturate a biochemical target. After adequate clearance of the nonbound, circulating ligand, avidin (from egg) or streptavidin (from bacteria) is injected, and it binds to the pretargeted, biotinylated antibody. Next, a biotinylated contrast agent is administered, which binds to the antibody–avidin complex, forming the complete targeted contrast construct. In some instances, avidin may be coupled to either the contrast agent or the homing ligand, reducing the number of required steps from three to two. Unfortunately, in vivo multistep methods are time-consuming and complicated to perform in a clinical setting. Moreover, endogenous biotin can interfere with in vivo self-assembly, and avidins, regardless of source, are immunogenic foreign proteins.

Direct covalent linkage between the homing molecule and the contrast agent is the most desirable strategy for clinical use in terms of convenience, efficacy, and safety. For particulate contrast agents, the number of targeting moieties can be varied from one to hundreds, depending on the diameter of the particle and the molecular weight of the homing ligand. Increasing the number of targeting ligands per contrast agent particle generally improves binding affinity and decreases the rate of dissociation. This "stick-and-stay" effect is commonly referred to as avidity.

4. Targeting Ligands

The revolution of genomic and proteomic science continues to unmask a myriad of possible targets to which new ligands, predominantly antibodies, are quickly being developed *(16–18)*. Any high affinity and high-specificity ligand directed toward a unique biochemical epitope or intracellular constituent may be used to target contrast agents. Immunoglobin-γ-class monoclonal antibodies, primarily of murine origin, are a common example from the vast possibilities. These relatively large (160 kDa) proteins may be attached to particles in low numbers, typically less than 25 to 50 per nanoparticle, for molecular imaging. For clinical utility, antibodies often require humanization by chimerizing the bioactive binding sites with a human antibody backbone or by conservative amino acid substitution of T-cell recognition sites. Humanization procedures can be effective from an immunological standpoint, but reductions in biological activity are possible. Moreover, repetitive display of large proteins on the surface of a particle can also be immunostimulatory and, in some instances, further accelerate biological clearance of the conjugated complex. A common alternative to intact monoclonal antibodies are $F_{(ab)}$ and $F_{(ab)2}$ fragments, which eliminate the Fc region interference and retain similar binding affinities per binding site. Other small molecule ligands may be identified using various combinatorial technologies, including phage display peptides *(19–26)* and aptamers (i.e., nucleic acid constructs) *(27)*. For physico–chemically defined receptors, computer-assisted molecular modeling may be employed to facilitate the organic synthesis of small peptidomimetics. In other situations, natural products, such as asialoglycoproteins and polysaccharides, may be used to achieve highly selective targeting. Regardless of the homing mechanism employed, the success of assessing the molecular information through noninvasive in vivo imaging relies on a robust signal amplification strategy *(1)*.

5. Contrast Platforms for Molecular Imaging and Personalized Medicine

5.1. Superparamagnetic Agents

Just as there are a variety of targeting techniques, so there are a variety of methods to use the techniques in creating targeted contrast agents. Some contrast agents employ both active and passive targeting techniques *(28–34)*, such as ultrasmall superparamagnetic iron oxides (USPIO) or dextran-crosslinked monocrystalline iron oxides (CLIO), which may be functionally modified with targeting monoclonal antibodies, fragments, peptides, and so on. Ultrasmall superparamagnetic iron oxides have been coupled with RGD peptides to target GP IIbIIIa receptors of platelets for thrombus-targeted contrast *(35)*. Dextran-crosslinked monocrystalline iron oxides have been used with a variety of ligands, including Twin-arginine translocation (Tat) peptides *(36,37)*, e-selectin *(38)*, and annexin V *(39)*, to target and image cells in culture. Additional examples include commercially available streptavidin-conjugated superparamagnetic nanoparticles used to target Her-2/neu-expressing breast cancer cells in a two-step administration sequence *(40)*, and iron oxide poly-acrylamide pebbles passively targeted to brain tumors *(41)*. The latter have also been adapted to identify angiogenic vasculature using arginine-glycine-aspartic acid (RGD) peptides.

A common theme for all paramagnetic agents is high surface payload when important but sparse biochemical epitopes are to be imaged. Although dendrimers can bear high numbers of metal atoms to a target site *(42,43)*, their usefulness as targeted agents in vivo has not been demonstrated. The advent of nanoparticles, by virtue of their inherently high surface area, has been demonstrated to be the most effective platform, with two classes predominating the literature: liposomes *(44–46)* and emulsions *(41,47)* (*see* **Fig. 1**).

5.2. Paramagnetic Liposomes

Initially pursued as a means to overcome the partial-volume dilution problem discussed in **Subheading 2.**, paramagnetic liposomes are vesicles that enclose high payloads of gadolinium in an aqueous volume entirely entrapped by lipid bilayer membrane(s). Unfortunately, the limited diffusivity of water across the stabilized liposomal membranes greatly minimizes the efficacy of the encapsulated paramagnetic chelates *(48,49)*. The synthesis of amphipathic paramagnetic chelates has more recently supported the direct incorporation of gadolinium into lipid membranes *(50,51)*, which greatly improves communication between the relaxation agent and surrounding water, while simultaneously augmenting r_1 relaxivity resulting from the slower particle tumbling rate.

Sipkins et al. *(52)* first reported a paramagnetic polymerized liposome targeted to $\alpha_v\beta_3$ for the detection of angiogenesis in the Vx-2 tumor model, 24 h after injection. This biotinylated liposome system, complexed through avidin, exploited a biotinylated LM-609 antibody and provided early in vivo demonstration that sparse pathological biomarkers, such as integrins, were accessible to MR molecular imaging with ultraparamagnetic particles. Later, Hood et al. *(53,54)* reported that a cationic polymerized version of this construct coupled to an $\alpha_v\beta_3$-integrin-targeting peptide could selectively deliver a mutant Raf gene, ATPmu-Raf, to angiogenic blood vessels of M21-L melanoma implanted subcutaneously in athymic mice and thereby induce tumor regression.

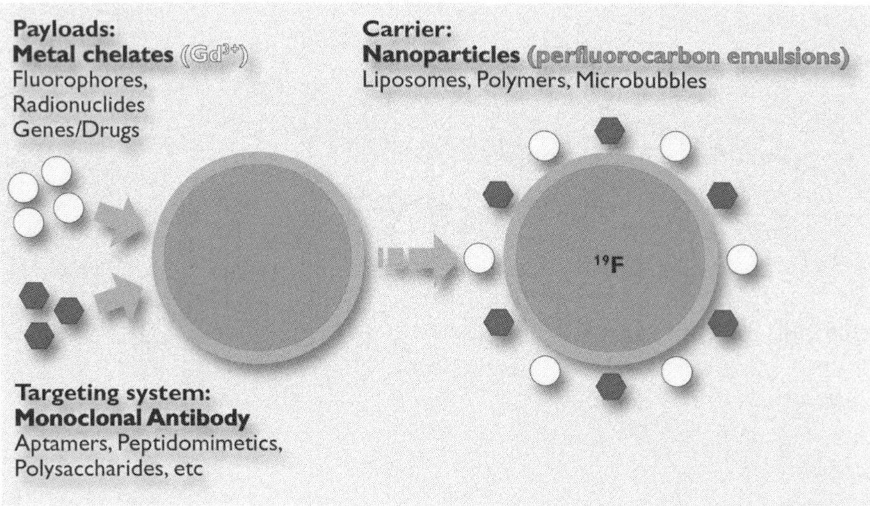

Fig. 1. Generalized paradigm for targeted contrast agents based on the nanoparticle technique. The core—which can be liposomes, fluid-filled nanoparticles, and so on—provides a skeleton on which multiple copies of the targeting system, imaging payload, and even therapeutic agents can be placed. Amplification strategies such as this permit magnetic resonance molecular imaging to be feasible when targeting sparse epitopes. (Reproduced courtesy of *Medicamundi*, **ref. *73*.**)

5.3. Paramagnetic Nanoparticle Emulsions

The second major class of paramagnetic nanoparticles are emulsions, the most notable being a liquid perfluorocarbon-based emulsion that has been targeted to multiple cardiovascular and oncological markers. The first in vivo demonstration of such a system specifically used the inherent acoustic contrast of bound perfluorocarbon nanoparticles to detect intravascular thrombus in canines *(47)*. Later, this acoustic agent was further modified for MR molecular imaging by inclusion of high payloads of gadolinium chelates within the lipid shell (*see* **Fig. 2**) *(55)*. Although the fibrin targets offer an abundance of binding sites that may be relatively easily detected on T_1-weighted MR images, these ultraparamagnetic nanoparticles had sufficient payloads (50,000–100,000 gadolinium-chelate molecules per nanoparticle) *(56)*, which permitted picomolar concentrations of the targeted agent *(57)* to be conspicuously visualized.

The usefulness of paramagnetic perfluorocarbon nanoparticle to image the expression of $\alpha_v\beta_3$ integrin on angiogenic vessels associated with nascent tumors and early atherosclerosis *(58–65)* has been demonstrated in vivo *(66–70)*. In New Zealand White rabbits, Vx-2 tumors were implanted into the hindlimb and the induced neovasculature was imaged 12 d later with $\alpha_v\beta_3$-targeted

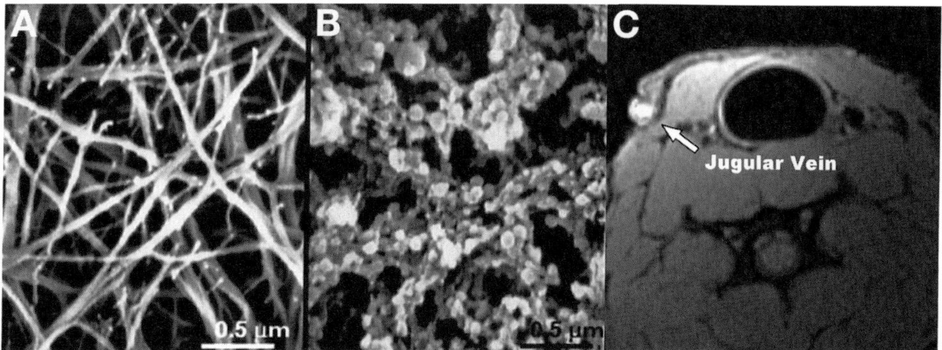

Fig. 2. A scanning electron microscope image shows the fibrin tendrils (**A**) of a clot. When targeted to the fibrin, paramagnetic nanoparticles densely decorate the fibrin (**B**), bringing more than 50,000 gadolinium chelates per binding site. The effect, in this canine model (**C**) is a very visible enhancement (arrow) on this T_1-weighted image, as compared with the control clot in the contralateral vein. (Reprinted with permission from *Circulation* **ref. 55**.)

paramagnetic nanoparticles injected intravenously *(68)*. Using a clinical 1.5 T MRI (Intera CV, Philips Medical Systems) and dedicated surface receiver coils, high-resolution (250 μm × 250 μm × 500 μm) 3D T_1-weighted images were acquired dynamically to track the accumulation of nanoparticles within the tumor vs the surrounding musculature. The signal intensity enhancement increased over time for the 2 h imaged, and the targeted contrast enhancement of the neovasculature increased 126% from baseline. This was twice the change in MR signal caused by extravascular leakage alone. Nearby skeletal muscle exhibited no signal enhancement with either the targeted or the nontargeted paramagnetic nanoparticles. The enhancement was observed in heterogeneous patterns, typically asymmetrically located around the tumor capsule, at interfaces between tumor and muscle, and in neighboring vasculature (*see* **Fig. 3**). Importantly, in vivo competitive-binding experiments, wherein the $\alpha_v\beta_3$-integrins were presaturated with targeted nonparamagnetic nanoparticles (i.e., invisible on MRI) then followed by $\alpha_v\beta_3$-targeted paramagnetic nanoparticles, further demonstrated receptor specificity of the targeted agent. Similar studies with equivalent results further substantiated these findings in a second independent tumor model of human melanoma (C-32) implanted into athymic mice *(69)*.

As briefly discussed in this chapter the capability to target and image specific molecular markers with particles provides the unique opportunity to

1. Segment patient populations for the presence and severity of disease based on the expression of specific biosignatures.

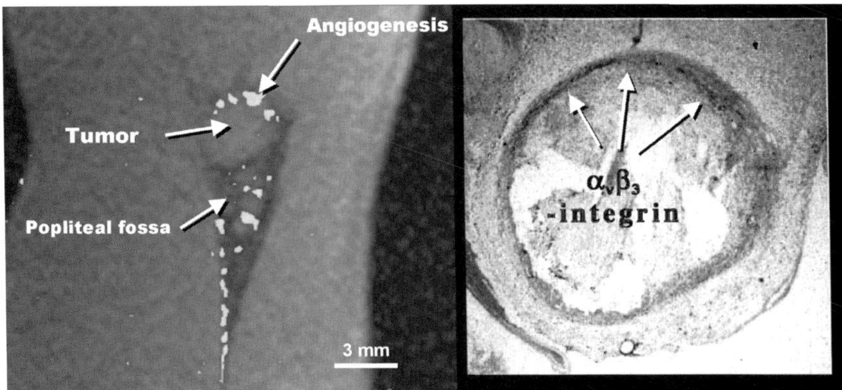

Fig. 3. In this Vx-2 tumor model, the T_1-weighted signal enhancement from the $\alpha_v\beta_3$-targeted paramagnetic nanoparticle is overlaid on the baseline image (**A**). The integrin is expressed heterogeneously around the 3-mm tumor capsule and other nearby areas of angiogenesis. The histology (**B**) corroborates the heterogeneous distribution of $\alpha_v\beta_3$-integrin (dark stain). (Reproduced by courtesy of *Medicamundi* **ref. 73.**)

2. Deliver potent individualized therapy directly to disease sites.
3. Monitor the treatment response through MRI *(70,71)*.

This emerging paradigm of personalized medicine has been demonstrated in several animal models using $\alpha_v\beta_3$-targeted therapeutic nanoparticles and MRI. As an example *(72)*, atherosclerotic rabbits fed high cholesterol diets for 80 d develop early expansion of the vasa vasorum in the adventia of the coronary and aortic arteries, which continues to fuel plaque progression as the diffusional limits from the arterial lumen are exceeded. $\alpha_v\beta_3$-targeted paramagnetic nanoparticles laden with fumagillin, an antiangiogenic drug, markedly pruned the nascent vessels from the vasa vasorum when measured 1 wk later (with drug-free, $\alpha_v\beta_3$-targeted paramagnetic nanoparticles) (*see* **Fig. 4**). Control rabbits given $\alpha_v\beta_3$-targeted paramagnetic nanoparticles without drug at baseline had no change in angiogenic vessel concentration 1 wk after treatment. Moreover, nontargeted fumagillin nanoparticles had no significant effect on the neovasculature density. By way of corroboration, histological assessments showed that the level of angiogenesis in animals receiving targeted drug-laden nanoparticles was significantly reduced in comparison with the vasa vasorum expansion noted in rabbits receiving nontargeted or targeted drug-free nanoparticles.

5.4. Safety and Use in Humans

Although the application of this technology has already proven useful in studying pathophysiology in animal models, the ultimate purpose is for per-

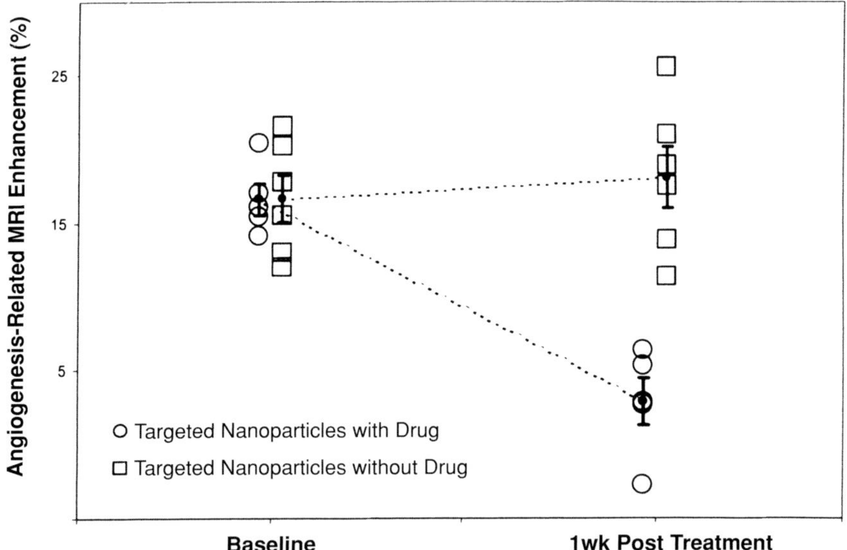

Fig. 4. Use of $\alpha_v\beta_3$-targeted paramagnetic nanoparticles allows both the detection of angiogenesis and the delivery of antiangiogenic therapy. At the time of treatment (baseline) the level of angiogenesis is the same in both groups of cholesterol-fed atherosclerotic rabbits, plotted as individuals (hollow markers) and mean ± SEM (bars). One week after the single treatment, the effect of the drug is clear, but animals receiving drug-free nanoparticles exhibit no therapeutic effects.

sonalized medicine in humans. Thus, targeted contrast agents must exhibit appropriate biocompatibility and pharmacokinetics, which are affected by many factors, including surface chemistry, in vivo stability, and size. For example, perfluorocarbon nanoparticles, which are approx 200 nm, are unique from other oil-based emulsions because of the properties of perfluorocarbons, resulting in robust stability against handling, pressure, heat, and shear. The carbon–fluorine bond is chemically and thermally stable and essentially biologically inert. Biocompatibility data abounds for liquid fluorocarbons, having been used for liquid ventilation, oxygen delivery, and imaging. Most, even at large doses, are innocuous and physiologically inactive. Regarding pure fluorocarbons within the range of molecular weight 460 to 520, no toxicity, carcinogenicity, mutagenicity, or teratogenic effects have been reported. For very large doses of perfluorocarbon emulsions (i.e., blood transfusion dosages), increased pulmonary residual volumes have been reported in rabbits, swine, and macaque; but not in mouse, dog, or human.

Perfluorocarbon nanoparticle distribution and clearance data fit well into a biexponential function with an estimated circulatory half-life in excess of 1 h. Fluorocarbons are not metabolized but are slowly reintroduced to the circulation in dissolved form by lipid carriers, and ultimately exhaled. They have long tissue half-life residencies, ranging from 4 d for perfluorooctylbromide to as much as 65 d for perfluorotripropylamine.

6. Summary

MR is emerging as an advantageous technique for molecular imaging, given its high spatial resolution and unique capability to extract both anatomical and physiological information simultaneously. Targeted superparamagnetic agents exploit the expansive effects of magnetic susceptibility artifacts produced by iron oxides, which appear on T_2-weighted imaging as dark contrast voids. Alternatively, development of ultraparamagnetic nanoparticles or liposomes, which multiply their effect by carrying high paramagnetic payloads to each targeted site, exert a bright contrast influence on T_1-weighted images, even when the biomarkers are present at nanomole concentrations. Importantly, targeted nanoparticles, particularly paramagnetic nanoparticles, can serve as a unique platform to diagnose, treat, and monitor therapy in early disease. With its initial feasibility demonstrated, molecular imaging, using targeted MR contrast agents, may soon be included in our clinical armamentarium, thereby helping to usher in the era of personalized medicine.

References

1. Weissleder R. (1999) Molecular imaging: exploring the next frontier. *Radiology* **212,** 609–614.
2. Zhang, S., Winter, P., Wu, K., and Sherry, A. D. (2001) A novel europium(III)-based MRI contrast agent. *J Am. Chem. Soc.* **123,** 1517–1518.
3. Runge, V. M., Schoerner, W., Niendorf, H. P., et al. (1985) Initial clinical evaluation of gadolinium DTPA for contrast-enhanced magnetic resonance imaging. *Magn. Reson. Imaging* **3,** 27–35.
4. Kim, R. J., Fieno, D. S., Parrish, T. B., et al. (1999) Relationship of MRI delayed contrast enhancement to irreversible injury, infarct age, and contractile function. *Circulation* **100,** 1992–2002.
5. Enochs, W. S., Harsh, G., Hochberg, F., and Weissleder, R. (1999) Improved delineation of human brain tumors on MR images using a long-circulationg, superparamagnetic iron oxide agent. *J. Magn. Reson. Imaging* **9,** 228–232.
6. Weissleder, R., Elizondo, G., Wittenberg, J., Lee, A. S., Josephson, L., and Brady, T. J. (1990) Ultrasmall superparamagnetic iron oxide: an intravenous contrast agent for assessing lymph nodes with MR imaging. *Radiology* **175,** 494–498.
7. Harisinghani, M. G., Saini, S., Weissleder, R., et al. (1999) MR lymphangiography using ultrasmall superparamagnetic iron oxide in patients with primary abdominal and pelvic malignancies: radiographic-pathologic correlation. *Am. J. Roentgenol.* **172,** 1347–1351.
8. Torchia, M. G., Nason, R., Danzinger, R., Lewis, J. M., and Thliveris, J. A. (2001) Interstitial MR lymphangiography for the detection of sentinel lymph nodes. *J. Surg. Oncol.* **78,** 151–156.

9. Lind, K., Kresse, M., Debus, N. P., and Muller, R. H. (2002) A novel formulation for superparamagnetic iron oxide (SPIO) particles enhancing MR lymphography: comparison of physicochemical properties and the in vivo behaviour. *J. Drug Target.* **10,** 221–230.

10. Michel, S. C., Keller, T. M., Frohlich, J. M., et al. (2002) Preoperative breast cancer staging: MR imaging of the axilla with ultrasmall superparamagnetic iron oxide enhancement. *Radiology.* **225,** 527–536.

11. Bellin, M. F., Lebleu, L., Meric, J. B. (2003) Evaluation of retroperitoneal and pelvic lymph node metastases with MRI and MR lymphangiography. *Abdom. Imaging* **28,** 155–163.

12. Schmitz, S. A., Coupland, S. E., Gust, R., et al. (2000) Superparamagnetic iron oxide-enhanced MRI of atherosclerotic plaques in Watanabe hereditable hyperlipidemic rabbits. *Invest. Radiol.* **35,** 460–471.

13. Ruehm, S. G., Corot, C., Vogt, P., Kolb, S., and Debatin, J. F. (2001) Magnetic resonance imaging of atherosclerotic plaque with ultrasmall superparamagnetic particles of iron oxide in hyperlipidemic rabbits. *Circulation* **103,** 415–422.

14. Paganelli, G., Magnani, P., Zito, F., et al. (1991) Three-step monoclonal antibody tumor targeting in carcinoembryonic antigen-positive patients. *Cancer Res.* **51,** 5960–5966.

15. Paganelli, G., Magnani, P., and Fazio, F. (1993) Pretargeting of carcinomas with the avidin-biotin system. *Int. J. Biol. Markers.* **8,** 155–159.

16. Britz-Cunningham, S. H. and Adelstein, S. J. (2003) Molecular targeting with radionuclides: state of the science. *J. Nucl. Med.* **44,** 1945–1961.

17. Rosebrough, S. F. (1996) Two-step immunological approaches for imaging and therapy. *Q. J. Nucl. Med.* **40,** 234–251.

18. Colcher, D., Pavlinkova, G., Beresford, G., Booth, B. J., Choudhury, A., and Batra, S. K. (1998) Pharmacokinetics and biodistribution of genetically-engineered antibodies. *Q. J. Nucl. Med.* **42,** 225–241.

19. de Bruin, R., Spelt, K., Mol, J., Koes, R., and Quattrocchio, F. (1999) Selection of high-affinity phage antibodies from phage display libraries. *Nat. Biotechnol.* **17,** 397–399.

20. Stadler, B. (1999) Antibody production without animals. *Dev. Biol. Stand.* **101,** 45–48.

21. Wittrup, K. (1999) Phage on display. *Trends Biotechnol.* **17,** 423–424.

22. Pasqualini, R., Koivunen, E., Kain, R., et al. (2000) Aminopeptidase N is a receptor for tumor-homing peptides and a target for inhibiting angiogenesis. *Cancer Res.* **60,** 722–727.

23. Ruoslahti E. (2000) Targeting tumor vasculature with homing peptides from phage display. *Semin. Cancer. Biol.* **10,** 435–442.

24. Ruoslahti, E. and Rajotte, D. (2000) An address system in the vasculature of normal tissues and tumors. *Annu. Rev. Immunol.* **18,** 813–827.

25. Arap, W., Haedicke, W., Bernasconi, M., et al. (2002) Targeting the prostate for destruction through a vascular address. *Proc. Natl. Acad. Sci. USA* **99,** 1527–1531.

26. Essler, M. and Ruoslahti, E. (2002) Molecular specialization of breast vasculature: a breast-homing phage-displayed peptide binds to aminopeptidate P in breast vasculature. *Proc. Natl. Acad. Sci. USA* **99,** 2252–2257.

27. Conrad, R. C., Giver, L., Tian, Y., and Ellington, A. D. (1996) In vitro selection of nucleic acid aptambers that bind proteins. *Meth. Enzymol.* **267,** 336–367.

28. Anzai, Y., McLachlan, S., Morris, M., Saxton, R., and Lufkin, R. B. (1994) Dextran-coated superparamagnetic iron oxide: an MR contrast agent for assessing lymph nodes in the head and neck. *Am. J. Neuroradiol.* **15,** 87–94.

29. Anzai, Y. and Prince, M. R. (1997) Iron oxide-enhanced MR lymphography: the evaluation of cervical lymph node metastases in head and neck cancer. *J. Magn. Reson. Imaging* **7,** 75–81.

30. Jung, C. W. and Jacobs, P. (1995) Physical and chemical properties of superparamagnetic iron oxide MR constrast agents: ferumoxides, ferumoxtran, ferumoxsil. *Magn. Reson. Imaging* **13,** 661–674.

31. Schmitz, S. A., Taupitz, M., Wagner, S., Wolf, K. J., Beyersdorff, D., and Hamm, B. (2001) Magnetic resonance imaging of atherosclerotic plaques using superparamagnetic iron oxide particles. *J. Magn. Reson. Imaging* **14,** 355–361.

32. Sigal, R., Vogl, T., Casselman, J., et al. (2002) Lymph node metastases from head and neck squamous cell carcinoma: MR imaging with ultrasmall superparamagnetic iron oxide particles (Sinerem MR)—results of a phase-III multicenter clinical trial. *Eur. Radiol.* **12,** 957–958.

33. Dardzinski, B. J., Schmithorst, V. J., Holland, S. K., et al. (2001) MR imaging of murine arthritis using ultrasmall superparamagnetic iron oxide particles. *Magn. Reson. Imaging* **19,** 1209–1216.

34. Kanno, S., Wu, Y. J., Lee, P. C., et al. (2001) Macrophage accumulation associated with rat cardiac allograft rejection detected by magnetic resonance imaging with ultrasmall superparamagnetic iron oxide particles. *Circulation* **104,** 934–938.

35. Johansson, L. O., Bjornerud, A., Ahlstrom, H. K., Ladd, D. L., and Fujii, D. K. (2001) A targeted contrast agent for magnetic resonance imaging of thrombus implications of spatial resolution. *J. Magn. Reson. Imaging* **13,** 615–618.

36. Josephson L., Tung C. H., Moore A., and Weissleder R. (1999) High efficiency intracellular magnetic labeling with novel superparamagnetic-Tat peptide conjugates. *Bioconjug. Chem.* **10,** 186–191.

37. Dodd, C. H., Hsu, H. C., Chu, W. J., et al. (2001) Normal T-cell response and in vivo magnetic resonance imaging of T cells loaded with HIV transactivator-peptide-derived superparamagnetic nanoparticles. *J. Immunol. Methods* **256,** 89–105.

38. Kang, H. W., Josephson, L., Petrovsky, A., Weissleder, R., and Bogdanov, A., Jr. (2002) Magnetic resonance imaging of inducible E-selectin expression in human endothelial cell culture. *Bioconjug. Chem.* **13,** 122–127.

39. Schellenberger, E. A., Bogdanov, A., Jr., Hogemann, D., Tait, J., Weissleder, R., and Josephson, L. (2002) Annexin V-CLIO: a nanoparticle for detecting apoptosis by MRI. *Mol. Imaging* **1,** 102–107.

40. Artemov, D., Mori, N., Okollie, B., and Bhujwalla, Z. M. (2003) MR molecular imaging of the Her-2/neu receptor in breast cancer cells using targeted iron oxide nanoparticles. *Magn. Reson. Med.* **49,** 403–408.

41. Moffat, B. A., Reddy, G. R., McConville, P., et al. (2003) A novel polyacrylamide magnetic nanoparticle contrast agent for molecular imaging using MRI. *Mol. Imaging* **2,** 324–332.

42. Quintana, A., Raczka, E., Piehler, L., et al. (2002) Design and function of a dendrimer-based therapeutic nanodevice targeted to tumor cells through the folate receptor. *Pharm. Res.* **19,** 1310–1316.
43. Kobayashi, H. and Brechbiel, M. W. (2003) Dendrimer-based macromolecular MRI contrast agents: characteristics and application. *Mol. Imaging* **2,** 1–10.
44. Navon, G., Panigel, R., and Valensin, G. (1986) Liposomes containing paramagnetic macromolecules as MRI contrast agents. *Magn. Reson. Med.* **3,** 876–880.
45. Unger, E. C., Porter, T., Culp, W., Labell, R., Matsunaga, T., and Zutshi, R. (2004) Therapeutic applications of lipid-coated microbubbles. *Adv. Drug Deliv. Rev.* **56,** 1291–1314.
46. Li, K. C. and Bednarski, M. D. (2002) Vascular-targeted molecular imaging using functionalized polymerized vesicles. *J. Magn. Reson. Imaging* **16,** 388–393.
47. Lanza, G. M., Wallace, K. D., Scott, M. J., et al. (1996) A novel site-targeted ultrasonic contrast agent with borad biomedical application. *Circulation* **94,** 3334–3340.
48. Fossheim, S., Fahlvik, A., Klaveness, J., and Muller, R. (1999) Paramagnetic liposomes as MRI contrast agents: influence of liposomal physiochemical properties on the in vitro relaxivity. *Magn. Reson. Imaging* **17,** 83–89.
49. Koenig, S. H., Ahkong, Q. F., Brown, R. D., et al. (1992) Permeability of liposomal membranes to water: results from the magnetic field dependence of T1 of solvent protons in suspensions of vesicles with entrapped paramagnetic ions. *Magn. Reson. Med.* **23,** 275–286.
50. Grant, C. W., Karlik, S., and Florio, E. (1989) A liposomal MRI contrast agent: phosphatidylethanolamine-DTPA. *Magn. Reson. Med.* **11,** 236–243.
51. Kabalka, G., Davis, M., Holmberg, E., Maruyama, K., and Huang, L. (1991) Gadolinium-labeled liposomes containing amphiphilic Gd-DTPA derivatives of varying chain length: targeted MRI contrast enhancement agents for the liver. *Magn. Reson. Imaging* **9,** 373–377.
52. Sipkins, D. A., Cheresh, D. A., Kazemi, M. R., Nevin, L. M., Bednarski, M. D., and Li, K. C. (1998) Detection of tumor angiogenesis in vivo by alphaVbeta3-targeted magnetic resonance imaging. *Nat. Med.* **4,** 623–626.
53. Hood, J. D. and Cheresh, D. A. (2002) Targeted delivery of mutant Raf kinase to neovessels causes tumor regression. *Cold Spring Harb. Sym.* **67,** 285–291.
54. Hood, J. D., Bednarski, M., Frausto, R., et al. (2002) Tumor regression by targeted gene delivery to the neovasculature. *Science* **296,** 2404–2407.
55. Flacke, S., Fischer, S., Scott, M. J., et al. (2001) Novel MRI contrast agent for molecular imaging of fibrin: implications for detecting vulnerable plaques. *Circulation* **104,** 1280–1285.
56. Winter, P. M., Caruthers, S. D., Yu, X., et al. (2003) Improved molecular imaging contrast agent for detection of human thrombus. *Magn. Reson. Med.* **50,** 411–416.
57. Morawski, A. M., Winter, P. M., Crowder, K. C., et al. (2004) Targeted nanoparticles for quantitative imaging of sparse molecular epitopes with MRI. *Magn. Reson. Med.* **51,** 480–486.
58. Tenaglia, A. N., Peters, K. H., Sketch, M. H., Jr., and Annex, B. H. (1998) Neovascularization in atherectomy specimens from patients with unstable angina: implications for pathogenesis of unstable angina. *Am. Heart J.* **143,** 164–172.

59. Falcioni, R., Cimino, L., Gentileschi, M., et al. (1994) Expression of β1, β3, β4 and β5 integrins by human lung carcinoma cells of different histotypes. *Exp. Cell Res.* **210,** 113–122.
60. Brooks, P. C., Stromblad, S., Klemke, R., Visscher, D., Sarkar, F. H., and Cheresh, D. A. (1995) Antiintegrin $\alpha_v\beta_3$ blocks human breast cancer growth and angiogenesis in human skin. *J. Clin. Invest.* **96,** 1815–1822.
61. Felding-Habermann, B., Mueller, B. M., Romerdahl, C. A., and Cheresh, D. A. (1992) Involvement of integrin α_v gene expression in human melanoma tumorigenicity. *J. Clin. Invest.* **89,** 2018–2022.
62. Natali, P. G., Hamby, C. V., Felding-Habermann, B., et al. (1997) Clinical significance of $\alpha_v\beta_3$ integrin and intercellular adhesion molecule-1 expression in cutaneous malignant melanoma lesions. *Cancer Res.* **57,** 1554–1560.
63. Gladson, C. L. and Cheresh, D. A. (1991) Glioblastoma expression of vitronectin and $\alpha_v\beta_3$ integrin. Adhesion mechanism for transformed glial cells. *J. Clin. Invest.* **88,** 1924–1932.
64. Eliceiri, B. P. and Cheresh, D.A. (2000) Role of alpha v integrins during angiogenesis. *Cancer J.* **6,** S245–249.
65. Bishop, G. G., McPherson, J. A., Sanders, J. M., et al. (2001) Selective $\alpha_v\beta_3$-receptor blockade reduces macrophage infiltration and restenosis after balloon angioplasty in the atherosclerotic rabbit. *Circulation* **103,** 1906–1911.
66. Anderson, S. A., Rader, R. K., Westlin, W. F., et al. (2000) Magnetic resonance contrast enhancement of neovasculature with $\alpha_v\beta_3$-targeted nanoparticles. *Magn. Reson. Med.* **44,** 433–439.
67. Winter, P. M., Morawski, A. M., Caruthers, S. D., et al. (2003) Molecular imaging of angiogenesis in early-stage atherosclerosis with $\alpha_v\beta_3$-integrin-targeted nanoparticles. *Circulation* **108,** 2270–2274.
68. Winter, P. M., Caruthers, S. D., Kassner, A., et al. (2003) Molecular imaging of angiogenesis in nascent Vx-2 rabbit tumors using a novel $\alpha_v\beta_3$-targeted nanoparticle and 1.5 tesla magnetic resonance imaging. *Cancer Res.* **63,** 5838–5843.
69. Schmieder, A. H., Winter, P. M., Caruthers, S. D., et al. (2005) MR molecular imaging of melanoma angiogenesis with $\alpha_v\beta_3$-targeted paramagnetic nanoparticles. *Magn. Reson. Med* **53,** 621–627.
70. Chenevert, T. L., Meyer, C. R., Moffat, B. A., et al. (2002) Diffusion MRI: a new strategy for assessment of cancer therapeutic efficacy. *Mol. Imaging* **1,** 336–243.
71. Lanza, G. M., Yu, X., Winter, P. M., et al. (2002) Targeted antiproliferative drug delivery to vascular smooth muscle cells with a magnetic resonance imaging nanoparticle contrast agent: implications for rational therapy of restenosis. *Circulation* **106,** 2842–2847.
72. Winter, P. M., Morawski, A. M., Caruthers, S. D., et al. (in press) A combined therapeutic and molecular imaging agent for treatment and monitoring of plaque angiogenesis in atherosclerosis. *J. Am. Coll. Cardiol.*
73. Lanza, G. M., Lamerichs, R., Caruthers, S., and Wickline, S. A. (2003) Molecular Imaging in MR with targeted paramagnetic nanoparticles. *Medicamundi* **47,** 34–39.

17

Design and Characterization of Magnetic Resonance Imaging Gene Reporters

Angelique Louie

Summary

We review the current status for magnetic resonance contrast agents that are designed to act as gene reporters. The basic concepts behind magnetic resonance and contrast enhancement are discussed, and factors that influence design of activatable contrast agents are presented. Several designs for magnetic resonance imaging (MRI) gene reporters are described, including contrast agents that are activated by β-galactosidase, and marker genes that code for proteins that sequester iron. Methods to characterize the uptake and delivery of contrast agents are outlined.

Key Words: Contrast agent; activatable contrast agent; molecular imaging; MRI gene marker; gene expression.

1. Gene Reporters and In Vivo Imaging

A reporter gene must be used to study expression of a gene of interest, unless the gene of interest produces a protein product with an identifiable handle. The reporter gene produces a protein product with a uniquely identifiable and/ or quantifiable phenotype; historically, these largely have been genes encoding for enzymes. The activity of the enzymes, for example, alkaline phosphatase or β-galactosidase (β-gal), is then measured by processing of a substrate that yields a measurable change on cleavage. The disadvantage of these types of reporters has been that the introduction of substrate typically requires permeabilization of the tissue of interest through fixation, or that the observable change in the substrate involves production of an opaque, insoluble (toxic) precipitate; therefore these reporters have not been useful for examining dynamic changes in living systems *(1,2)*. Observing changes in gene expression in vivo was revolutionized in the 1990s with the cloning of green fluorescent protein (GFP).

GFP was first identified in the bioluminescent *Aequorea* jellyfish. In the jellyfish, GFP is a fluorescence energy transfer partner with the protein,

From: *Methods in Molecular Medicine, Vol. 124*
Magnetic Resonance Imaging: Methods and Biologic Applications
Edited by: P. V. Prasad © Humana Press Inc., Totowa, NJ

aequorin. Aequorin fluoresces blue, however, the jellyfish bioluminesces green through transfer of energy from aequorin to GFP. GFP was first reported in 1962, but its application as a gene reporter was not explored until the gene was cloned in 1992 *(3)* and, shortly thereafter, shown to retain fluorescence activity when expressed in other organisms *(4,5)*. No cofactors are required to produce the fluorescence, fortuitously the GFP gene contains all of the information needed to produce fluorescence *(6)*. GFP has shown no toxicity effects in most of the systems in which it has been expressed, and GFP has made the use of optical imaging methods for interrogating gene expression in living systems almost a routine procedure. However, as with all optical techniques, the usefulness of GFP for monitoring gene expression ends where light propagation ends, so other techniques must be devised to examine gene expression in deeper tissues and opaque systems.

Recently, advances in imaging probe development have led to the use of clinical imaging modalities, such as positron emission tomography (PET) or magnetic resonance imaging (MRI) to monitor gene expression in living systems. These two modalities have unlimited depth of interrogation, are noninvasive, and are capable of high-resolution (MRI) and high-sensitivity (PET) imaging. In this review, we focus on recent developments in contrast agents for MRI that allow visualization of gene expression in vivo.

2. MRI Contrast Agents

Contrast agents are exogenous molecules that can be introduced to a system to increase image contrast. This increase in contrast can be achieved by increasing or decreasing signal intensity for tissues containing the contrast agent compared with neighboring tissues. Relaxation agents work by modifying the rate of relaxation and tend to affect both T_1 and T_2, but certain types or concentrations of agents may be more effective at influencing one type of relaxation time and thus are used more often in images weighted for that type of relaxation. Effects on relaxation times are concentration dependent—the more agent present, the greater the effect. To compare between agents it is useful to define a term, relaxivity (R), which is a concentration-independent description of the efficiency of the contrast agents at enhancing the relaxation times of water protons.

2.1. Relaxation Agents

2.1.1. T_1 Agents

In the presence of T_1 relaxation agents, the T_1 relaxation time is shortened. In other words, a perturbed net magnetic moment of the observed nuclei relaxes back to equilibrium faster in the presence of a T_1 agent. This shortened T_1 results in increased signal intensity in regions containing contrast agent. ProHance (Bracco Diagnostics, Princeton, NJ) and Magnevist (Berlex, Wayne,

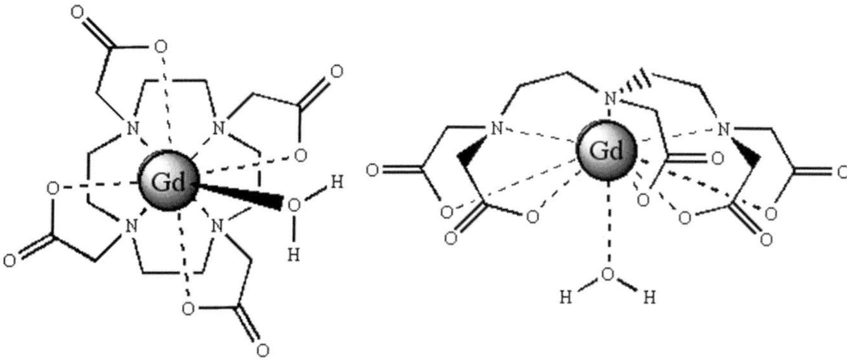

Fig. 1. Clinical contrast agents. ProHance (left) and Magnevist (right) are commercially available contrast agents used in the clinic. Both consist of paramagnetic gadolinium ions chelated by organic molecules. Both are considered extracellular agents—i.e., they leave the lumen of blood vessels and distribute in the interstitial space. They do not enter intact cells.

NJ) are examples of T_1 contrast agents currently used in the clinic. Typically, these agents consist of gadolinium ions bound by a chelating group *(7,8)*. Chelation of the gadolinium groups is vital because free gadolinium can substitute for calcium in the body and be quite toxic. For ProHance, the chelator is a ring-like structure known as a macrocycle; whereas, for Magnevist, the chelator is an open configuration. Both chelators contain carboxylic acid arms. Gadolinium has an affinity for nitrogen and oxygen groups and binds to the chelators through the nitrogens and the carboxyl groups (**Fig. 1**).

Gadolinium(III) is the most widely used paramagnetic ion in T_1 agents and is selected based on its high magnetic moment and large number of unpaired electrons (seven—the most of any stable ion). The effect of gadolinium on signal intensity requires direct interaction between unpaired electrons in the ion and water protons. Thus, contrast agents are designed with open sites for coordination of water to gadolinium. Gadolinium has nine coordination sites, meaning that it can bind to nine other atoms. In ProHance, eight of the coordination sites are occupied by the chelator, with one site open for interaction with water. This degree of chelation makes for a very stable complex with little chance of release of gadolinium from the complex in vivo. Similarly, in Magnevist, three coordination sites are occupied by nitrogens and five by carboxyl groups, leaving one site available to bind to water. Other paramagnetic ions, such as manganese (with five unpaired electrons), may be used as T_1 agents but these can be less effective. Manganese is the topic of Chapter 15 in this volume.

2.1.2. T_2 Agents

A large class of T_2 agents are composed of superparamagnetic species, such as iron *(9,10)*. Typical agents consist of an iron-oxide core, coated by a water-soluble shell, such as dextran. These agents affect contrast by introducing a large, regional magnetic field gradient in the vicinity of the superparamagnetic cores. Thus, their effect is more long range than that for gadolinium, which requires direct interaction with water protons. In high concentrations, ions such as manganese also act as T_2 agents. Both Mn(II) and Fe(III) have five unpaired electrons compared with gadolinium's seven. The shortening of T_2 relaxation time caused by the agents results in a decrease of signal intensity in tissues containing the agents, resulting in contrast enhancement compared with neighboring tissues. However, because the contrast enhancement comes from a signal decrease rather than a signal increase, T_1 agents are considered to provide images with larger dynamic range.

Superparamagnetic iron oxide particles are prepared in a variety of size ranges that are generally classed as small (>50 nm) or ultrasmall (<50 nm). As particles increase further in size, they tend to lose their superparamagnetic properties. Ultrasmall superparamagnetic iron oxide particles have a longer residence time in the blood, being less subject to removal by the reticuloendothelial system and lymphatic system. When accumulation in the liver is desirable, to image hepatocytes, for example, the larger, superparamagnetic iron oxide particles may be used. The larger particles also may experience greater uptake efficiency in phagocytic cell types *(11–14)*.

2.2. Modifying Agents for Functional Response

2.2.1. What Influences Effectiveness of T_1 Contrast Agents?

Signal intensity in MRI depends on many factors and can be described by a complex expression with numerous terms (Solomon-Bloembergen-Morgan), some of which are dependent on the environment around the agent. Therefore, unlike PET or CT agents, which have fixed physical properties providing signal for imaging, there is a possibility for designing MRI contrast agents that have varying signal enhancement in response to the environment. Some of the factors that influence signal intensity in a magnetic resonance (MR) image include *(8,15)*:

1. Magnetic field strength. As field strength increases, the energy difference between the high and low energy states of magnetic moments increases. This results in increased signal intensity from relaxation of the water protons at higher fields (note that the signal-to-noise ratio has a more complicated relation to field strength). However, the effectiveness of paramagnetic contrast agents (relaxivity) on images has a complex relationship with field strength that tends to decrease

with increasing field strength in a sigmoidal fashion *(16,17)*. Therefore, there is a tradeoff between the increased resolution capability offered at higher field strengths caused by properties of the water protons at higher fields vs the decreased efficiency of contrast agents, which must be taken into consideration when imaging with contrast agents.

2. Hydration state. As described in **Subheading 2.1.1.**, enhancement of signal intensity for T_1 agents requires direct interaction between the unpaired electrons in paramagnetic ions and water protons. Therefore, the hydration state of the contrast agent, the number of water molecules coordinated, has a direct effect on signal intensity. Agents can be designed that block access of water to the paramagnetic ion to modulate contrast. This will be seen in greater detail as we discuss agents sensitive to gene expression. Changing the hydrophilicity of an agent can cause it to partition to lipid rich regions that are low in water content, thus reducing signal enhancement.

3. Water exchange rate. Similarly, it is not only the number of water protons in contact with the paramagnetic ion at a given moment in time, but the number of water protons that can be interacted with over time that affects signal intensity *(18)*. The more water molecules that can be relaxed by the contrast agent per unit time, the greater the change in signal intensity.

4. Rotation. Larger molecules generally have a slower rotational correlation time, which translates to increased relaxivity. However, this is not necessarily true for large flexible molecules; therefore, the rigidity of a contrast agent also affects relaxivity *(18)*. Agents can be designed that aggregate under specific conditions to act as indicators. This has been used for developing MRI contrast agents sensitive to iron concentrations.

2.2.2. Designing "Smart" Contrast Agents as Gene Expression Indicators

The factors described in **Subheading 2.2.1.** can be exploited to develop activatable MRI contrast agents that respond to gene expression with a change in relaxivity. This is a key benefit for MRI T_1 agents compared with probes for other clinical imaging modalities, such as computed tomography (CT) and PET. For the latter imaging agents, the detectable signals, X-ray opacity and radioactive decay, respectively, cannot be turned off. If a CT or PET agent is present, signal is always produced and cannot be attenuated by chemical means.

2.3. Current Examples of MRI Gene Reporters

How does gene expression activate a contrast agent? Alternatively, how can MRI signal be enhanced by gene expression? We will explore some examples of MRI indicators of gene expression in this section.

2.3.1. "Smart" Contrast Agents: β-Gal Indicator

The first example of an MRI contrast agent that is activated by gene expression was an enzyme-sensitive agent developed in the laboratory of Thomas

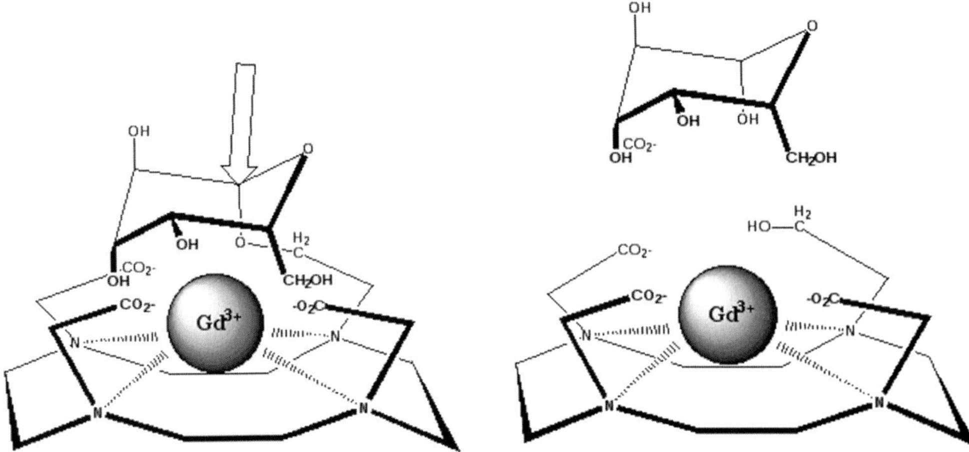

Fig. 2. Enzyme-activatable contrast agent: *Egad*. This agent is also based on a macrocycle-chelated gadolinium group, but with the addition of a galactose moiety that is connected to the macrocycle through one of the arms. The galactose moiety is attached through a bond that is cleavable by β-galactosidase (left image, vertical bond at point of arrow). In the presence of β-galactosidase, the galactose residue is removed, opening a site of access for water to the gadolinium ion (right).

Meade, then at the California Institute of Technology. This agent, **Fig. 2**, consisted of gadolinium bound by a macrocylic ligand that had been modified with an appended galactose group *(19)*. Attachment of the galactose group to the macrocycle was through a β-gal-cleavable linker. The galactose group interacted with gadolinium to block water access. In the presence of β-gal, the galactose group was enzymatically removed, which opened access for water to gadolinium. This change in hydration state resulted in a 20% change in relaxivity for the molecule after cleavage. This change was insufficient to produce significant contrast in in vivo models, however. Further development of the contrast agent led to a modified structure that introduced a methyl group on the linker attaching the galactose to the macrocycle (**Fig. 3**). It is hypothesized that this methyl group acts to restrict the motion of the galactose group and to stabilize its position to block water more effectively. The introduction of this relatively small structural modification resulted in an increase in the change of relaxivity after cleavage to 55%. In in vivo studies, this agent was able to detect expression of β-gal both from introduced RNA and DNA forms of the lacZ gene *(20)* (**Figs. 4** and **5**).

Additional studies on this contrast agent indicated that it is taken up by cells via asialoglycoprotein receptors, presumably through recognition of the galactose residue on the molecule *(21)*. The idea that the galactose moiety was re-

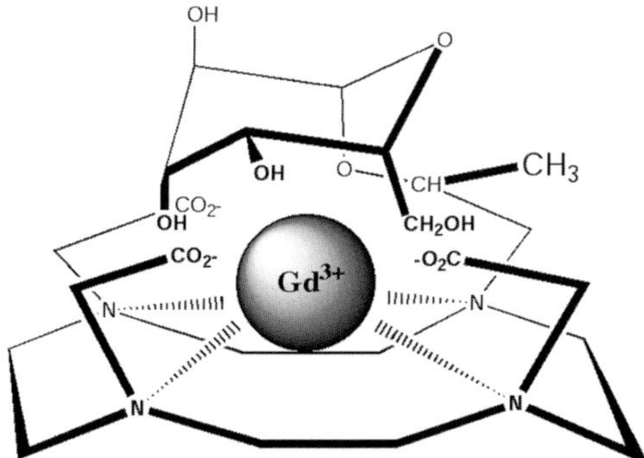

Fig. 3. Improved enzyme-activatable contrast agent: *EgadMe*. The addition of a methyl group to the linker arm of the agent described in **Fig. 2** significantly improved contrast enhancement between uncleaved and cleaved states. It is hypothesized that the methyl group stabilizes the galactose moiety's position, so that water blocking is more efficient in the uncleaved state.

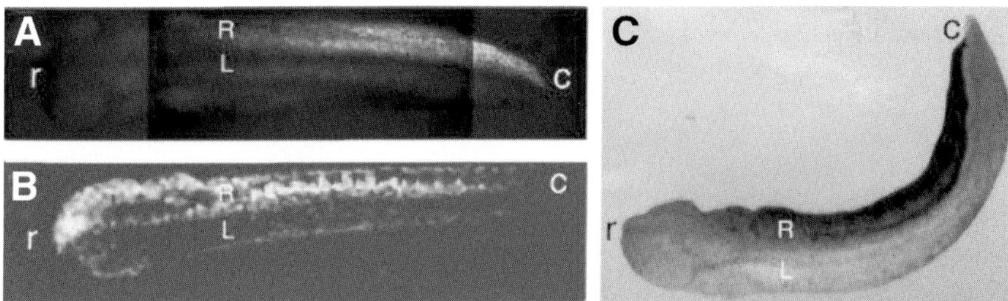

Fig. 4. Detection of mRNA expression in *Xenopus* system. One cell of a *Xenopus* embryo at the two-cell stage was injected with mRNA for β-galactosidase (β-gal) and coinjected with mRNA for nGFP (green fluorescent protein) as a marker of injection efficiency. Both cells were injected with EgadMe (*see* **Fig. 3**). Embryos were kept at 16°C until after gastrulation and then moved to room temperature for 24 h before imaging. The first cleavage approximates the future midline for the animal. Thus, half of the animal contains β-gal, whereas the contrast agent is distributed throughout. (**C**) Shows that histological staining for β-gal is restricted to the right side of the animal. This correlates with the expression of nGFP on the right side shown in a fluorescence image (**A**). The region of high signal intensity by magnetic resonance imaging is also localized to the right side (**B**). Thus, in the half of the animal containing β-gal, the agent is activated, whereas in the half lacking β-gal, the agent is silent. R, right; L, left; r, rostral; c, caudal. (From **ref. 20**, with permission.)

sponsible not only for enzyme recognition but for receptor-mediated uptake by cells suggests the possibility for attachment of other types of moieties to 1,4,7,10-Tetraazacyclododecane-1,4,7,10-tetraacetic acid (DOTA)-like mol-

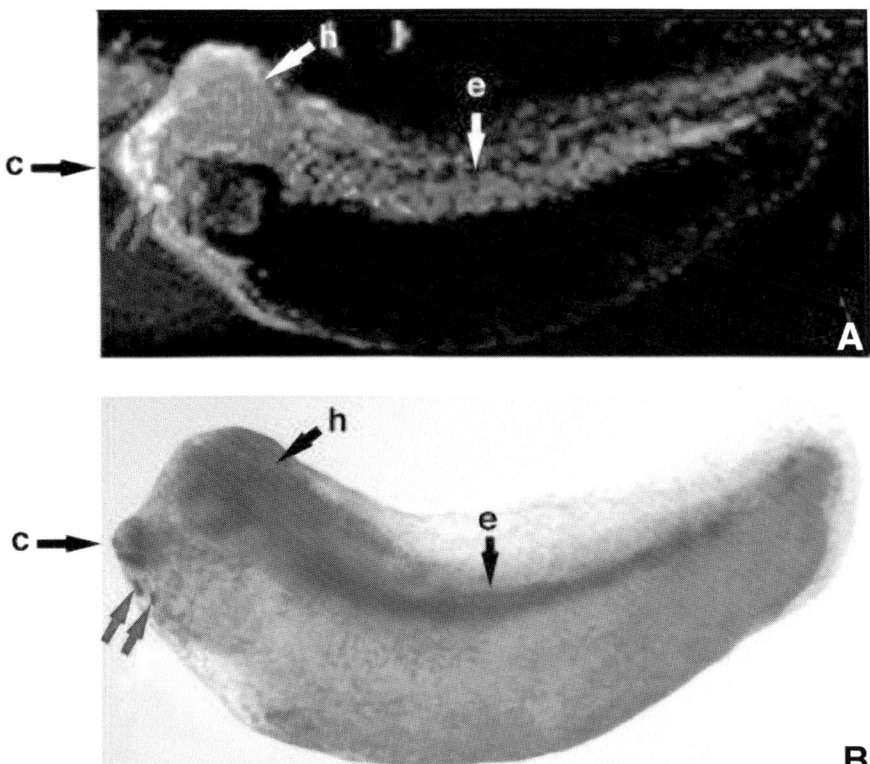

Fig. 5. Detection of gene expression in *Xenopus* embryos. Experiments identical to those described in **Fig. 4** were performed, but with the injection of linearized plasmid carrying lacZ rather than mRNA. **(B)** Histological staining for β-galactosidase (β-gal) is found in a broad strip of endoderm and in two distinct spots ventral to the cement gland (arrows). This matches the pattern of signal intensity in the magnetic resonance image **(A)**. Activation of the contrast agent localizes with presence of β-gal. e, endoderm, h, head, c, cement gland. (From **ref. *20***, with permission.)

ecules to direct uptake or enzymatic processing. Methods for delivering the contrast agents to cells that do not express asialoglycoprotein receptors must be developed before this system can be used as a general indicator of gene expression.

2.3.2. Tyrosinase Gene

A different approach to imaging gene expression by MRI is to use a marker gene that codes for a protein that will sequester paramagnetic ions. Weissleder and colleagues *(22)* applied this concept to introduce melanins as a gene marker. In this system, the gene for tyrosinase is used as a marker gene.

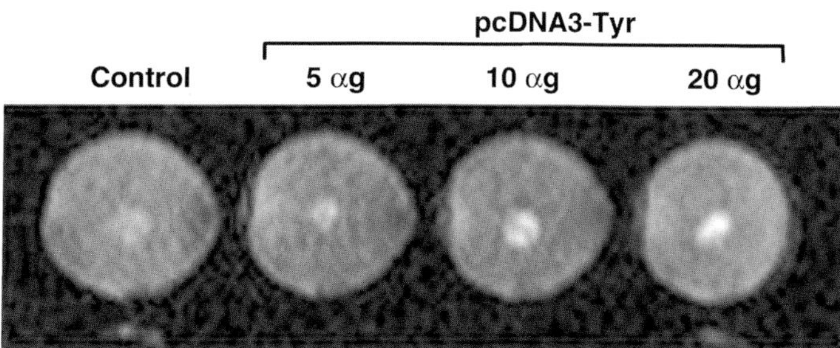

Fig. 6. Increased magnetic resonance imaging signal intensity in cells expressing tyrosinase. L929 mouse fibroblasts were transfected with varying amounts of human tyrosinase (mammalian expression vector pcDNA3-Tyr). Cells transfected with the greatest amount of tyrosinase showed the highest signal intensity. It is hypothesized that the increase in tyrosinase activity results in an increased production of iron-binding melanin, and that the scavenging of paramagnetic iron results in the enhanced magnetic resonance contrast in transfected cells. (From **ref. *22***, with permission.)

Melanins are a heterogeneous group of pigment proteins of high molecular mass, the biosynthesis of which occurs in melanocytes. These pigment proteins are capable of binding relatively large amounts of iron *(23)*, and cultured melanotic cells have show increased MRI contrast compared with amelanotic controls *(24)*. Melanogenesis, the biochemical pathway for melanin synthesis, involves a number of metalloenzymes, the most critical of which is tyrosinase. Tyrosinase is a copper-dependent enzyme of molecular weight 60 to 75 kDa that catalyzes the first two rate-limiting steps in the conversion of L-tyrosine to eumelanin or pheomelanin *(25)*. Melanin polymers were investigated earlier for use as contrast agents *(26)*.

In the melanin induction system, the idea is to use the gene for tyrosinase as a marker gene fused to the gene of interest. As the gene of interest is synthesized, tyrosinase is also synthesized, leading to an increase in tyrosinase activity and upregulated production of iron-binding melanin. Initial experiments in a cell culture system show significantly higher MRI signal from cells transfected with tyrosinase compared with nontransfected cells (**Fig. 6**). However, this system has limited use as a general marker for gene expression because toxic metabolites are produced during melanogenesis, and melanin itself can be toxic *(15,27)*. It could be useful for tracking gene therapy intended to kill the targeted cells, such as in cancer therapy.

2.3.3. Transferrin Indicator

In an interesting variation of the use of iron-sequestering proteins as markers for gene expression, Weissleder and colleagues also investigated the use of the transferrin uptake system to load cells with contrast-enhancing iron. Transferrin is an approx 80-kDa glycoprotein that binds two Fe^{3+} ions and is responsible for iron transport in the blood. Transferrin is taken up by cells through transferrin receptors expressed on the cell surface in a classic feedback system—the presence of iron inside the cell downregulates the expression of the receptor. The nucleotide sequence of transferrin receptor mRNA has several iron regulatory elements (IRE) in the 3' untranslated region. Under low iron conditions, an IRE-binding protein binds to these IREs. In the presence of iron, the IRE-binding protein binds to iron instead of RNA, and the mRNA is rapidly degraded.

To harness the transferrin system for imaging, a gene encoding transferrin receptors that lacks the iron-regulatory region is used as a marker gene. Lacking the regulatory elements, these receptors are constitutively overexpressed. Iron oxide nanoparticles conjugated to transferrin are introduced to load cells expressing the receptors with iron. Contrast enhancement using this system has been demonstrated in cells in culture *(28)*. In a mouse tumor model, tumors derived from cells transfected with the engineered transferrin receptors showed detectable contrast enhancement compared with tumors derived from control-transfected cells (**Fig. 7**) *(29)*. However, the use of this endogenous gene as a marker could have ramifications for cellular iron homeostasis and toxicity that remain to be determined. As with the tyrosinase system described in **Subheading 2.3.2.**, the transferrin receptor system may be limited to cytotoxic gene therapy.

2.3.4. Tyramide (Mramp) System

Recently, another route to imaging gene expression has been investigated that takes advantage of the dependence of relaxivity on rotational correlation time *(30)*. In this system, a primary antibody–digoxygenin and secondary anti-digoxygenin–peroxidase conjugate is used to label the gene product (**Fig. 8**). The attached peroxidase catalyzes the reduction of peroxide using a chelated gadolinium complex coupled to hydroxytyramine, D-DOTA(Gd), as the electron donor. The authors demonstrated that, in solution, the oxidized D-DOTA(Gd) self-polymerizes to form large, paramagnetic polymers, with increased relaxivity compared with the monomer complexes (**Figs. 9** and **10**). This is a modified version of the fluorescent tyramide signal-amplification system that is used for histology *(31)* and is named Mramp for "magnetic resonance imaging signal amplification."

Experiments with the contrast agent and enzyme in vitro demonstrate increased MR contrast that is dependent on concentration of primary antibody and concentration of peroxidase. In experiments on HUVEC cells overexpressing E-selectin, signal intensity is higher than controls (experiments

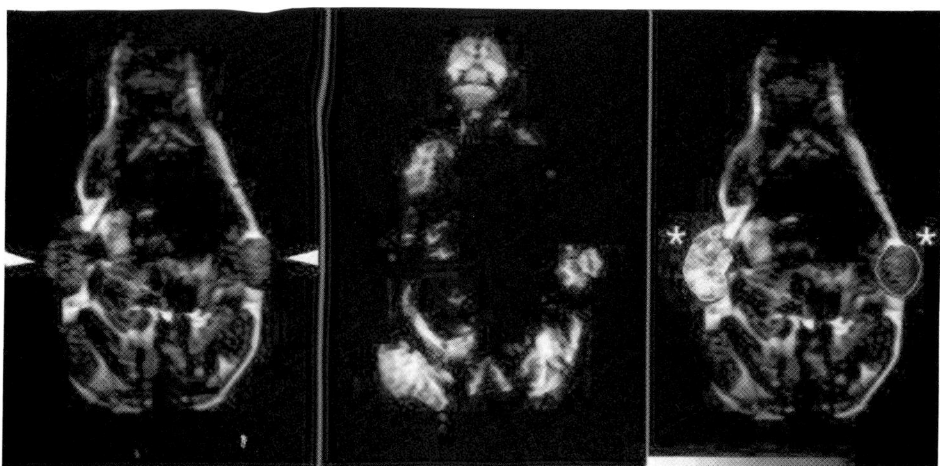

Fig. 7. Magnetic resonance image (MRI) of tumors overexpressing transferrin receptor in mouse model. Tumors derived from cells engineered to overexpess transferrin receptor (ETR$^+$) or control transfected (ETR$^-$) cells were grown in the flanks of nude mice. No difference was seen between the tumors by MRI, indicating that endogenous iron scavenging was insufficient to produce measurable contrast. Transferrin-conjugated, superparamagnetic iron oxide particles were then introduced by tail-vein injection. No difference between the tumor types is seen in the T_1-weighted image (left panel; ETR$^+$, left arrowhead; ETR$^-$, right arrowhead), but T_2-weighted images show enhanced contrast (middle panel) in the ETR$^+$ tumor, in which the accumulation of nanoparticles decreases the signal intensity. The right panel shows a T_1-weighted image for anatomical detail overlaid with a T_2 relaxivity difference map. The greatest changes in R_2 are seen in the ETR$^+$ tumor. (From **ref. 29**, with permission.)

with unstimulated cells or stimulated cells lacking primary antibody), but the difference between cells labeled with the Mramp system and cells incubated with a standard solution of 50 μM GdCl$_3$ is not dramatic. Although the monomers polymerize in solution, it remains to be confirmed whether hydroxytyraminyl-glycylmethyl Gd-DOTA (D-DOTA[Gd]) polymers form in environments that are rich with other proteins. In fluorescence applications, the highly reactive, short-lived tyramide radicals are believed to bind to phenol moieties of tyrosine residues and do not appear to self-aggregate—which would cause self-quenching in the fluorescent system. The balance between tyrosine interactions and self-polymerization will likely be a function of substrate concentration and needs to be demonstrated with greater rigor for the MRI agents. Although the self-polymerization of Gd-1,4,7,10-tetraazacyclododecane-1,4,7,10-tetraaceticacid (Gd-DOTA)-tyramine proposed in this system is a novel concept, binding to tyrosines may preclude the use of this system for in

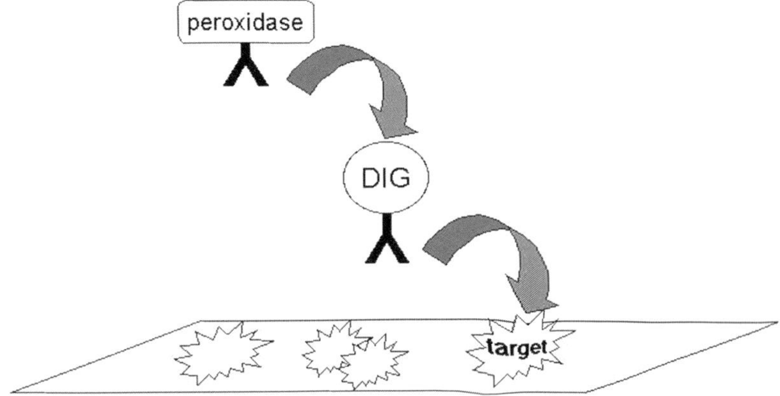

Fig. 8. Magnetic resonance imaging signal amplification (Mramp) gene product labeling. Primary antibody to the target gene product is labeled with digoxygenin (DIG). A secondary antibody against DIG carrying peroxidase is used to amplify the signal, and additional amplification occurs as the bound peroxidase oxidizes the Mramp agent.

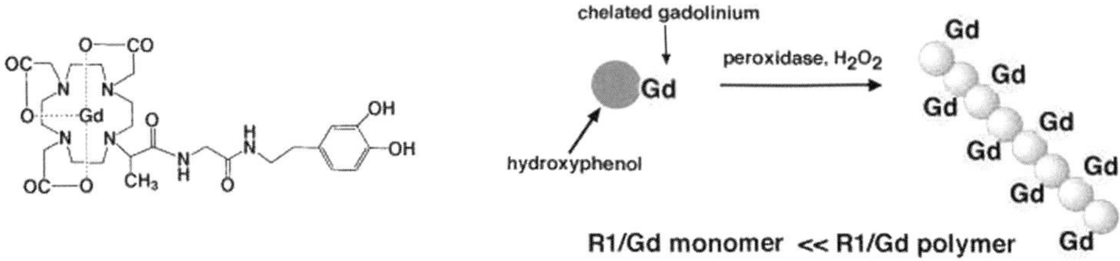

Fig. 9. Hydroxytyraminyl-glycylmethyl Gd-DOTA [D-DOTA(Gd)]. D-DOTA(Gd) (left) is oxidized by peroxidase, leading to a highly reactive molecule that can self-polymerize (right). (From **ref. 30**, with permission.)

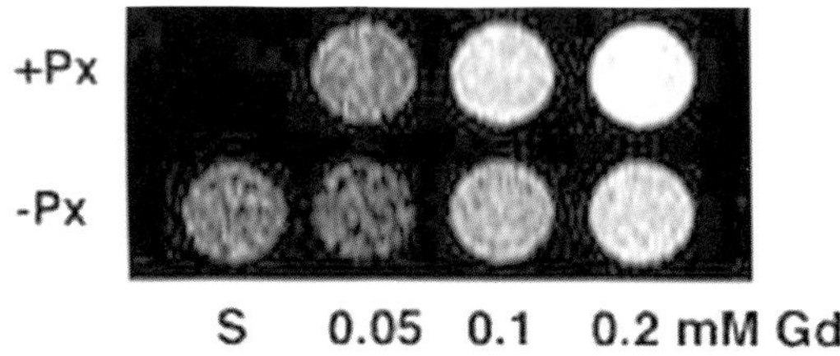

Fig. 10. Concentration dependence of Mramp signal enhancement. Varying concentrations of D-DOTA(Gd) were incubated with or without peroxidase (Px) and imaged by magnetic resonance imaging. There is background signal from the D-DOTA(Gd) that increases with increasing concentration, however, the presence of peroxidase increases the signal significantly above this background. (From **ref. 30**, with permission.)

vivo imaging, because modifications of tyrosines can alter protein function. The usefulness of MRI for histological applications is not clear. Fluorescence microscopy can provide much higher resolution and sensitivity in the types of systems amenable to tyramide signal amplification.

3. Uptake and Delivery of Contrast Agents

3.1. Evaluating Cell Uptake

One of the stepping stones to evaluating the efficiency of contrast agents for future in vivo applications is characterizing their behavior in cells in culture. The amount of contrast agent taken up by cells is used to determine dosimetry—how much contrast agent must be given to obtain a sufficient concentration for detection in an image. Because MRI lacks the resolution to interrogate subcellular events and is nonquantitative (it is difficult to calculate contrast agent concentration based on signal intensity), one must rely on other methods to investigate uptake.

3.1.1. Confocal and Multiphoton Microscopy

If the contrast agents can be labeled with fluorophores they can be tracked by fluorescence microscopy techniques. Alternatively, one can use europium as a substitute for gadolinium in the contrast agent *(32)*. Chelated europium has fluorescence excitation in the ultraviolet range and emits at multiple wavelengths in the green–red range. The exact excitation and emission wavelengths depend on the structure of the contrast agent. Ultraviolet laser, blue light-emitting diode, or multiphoton microscopy can be used to provide the appropriate excitation for imaging. Two-photon excitation at approx 750 to 800 nm will excite Eu-DOTA type complexes, for example.

3.1.2. Nuclear Magnetic Resonance

Relative uptake of the contrast agent can be assessed in cell lysates using nuclear magnetic resonance (NMR) relaxometry. Cells are incubated with varying concentrations of contrast agent, precise numbers of cells are lysed, and relaxation times T_1 or T_2 determined by NMR. These can be compared with standards of known concentrations mixed into control cell lysates for a more quantitative estimate of contrast agent concentration.

3.2. Evaluating In Vivo Applications: Biodistribution Studies

Distribution of contrast agent can be more quantitatively assessed using radioactive techniques. For such studies, a radioactive ion, such as ^{111}In is substituted for gadolinium and introduced by intravenous injection to the animal model of choice. After varying times after injection, the animal is euthanized and tissues of interest are harvested and analyzed by γ-counting. The radioactive derivative of the contrast agent may also be used to assess clearance through the kidney by collecting periodic urine samples, and serum half-life can be determined by collecting periodic blood samples *(21)*.

3.3. The Question of Delivery

A question that always plagues the use of MRI for imaging gene expression is whether enough contrast agent can be accumulated for detection. Uptake of contrast agents needs to be more efficient and more uniformly distributed through tissues for general use in vivo. It is beyond the scope of this chapter, but many methods are in development to enhance the uptake and accumulation of small molecule-based and nanoparticle-based contrast agents, including attachment of membrane translocating peptide sequences *(33–35)*.

4. Discussion

The ability of MRI to acquire 3D images noninvasively and without the use of ionizing radiation make it an attractive technology for in vivo imaging of gene expression—but it does suffer from limitations. Compared with radioactive imaging techniques, MRI is far less sensitive and, therefore, requires higher concentrations of contrast agent for visualization, but the higher resolution of MRI makes it an attractive modality for molecular imaging applications. In recent years, it has become increasingly clear that combinations of imaging modalities may need to be used to obtain information of interest. In fact, emerging technologies are in development to combine modalities, such as PET and MR imaging capabilities, in the same instrument to combine the strengths of each *(36)*.

The specific gene expression-imaging systems described in this chapter have all been tested using genes that are highly expressed. However, what about genes that are not highly expressed? The activatable contrast agent holds the promise of signal amplification, but its use in detecting low-level expression needs to be demonstrated. The iron-sequestering methodologies could accumulate iron over longer times, but that also needs to be determined, and delays between expression of the gene and accumulation of detectable quantities of iron could make data interpretation more difficult. All of the methods lack the ability to dynamically sense gene expression—they turn "on" when the gene of interest is expressed, but when gene expression turns "off," the contrast agent (or sequestered iron) must be cleared by normal cellular pathways to restore the signal to baseline. This is also a drawback of traditional optical markers for gene expression. Future research in development of probes that can also be switched off would greatly improve the usefulness for MR markers of gene expression. Finally, as for optically based gene reporters, the in vivo markers respond at the level of translation as opposed to transcription. Biological activity arising from gene expression involves a complex interplay between the number of transcripts made, the number of proteins produced from each tran-script, and the stability of both the transcripts and the protein products. Ideally, it would be desirable to monitor all of these components to come to a more complete understanding of gene expression and regulation as it relates to biochemical effects. One important application for in vivo monitoring of gene expression is in gene therapy. Understanding where, when, and the level at which introduced genes are expressed could shed light on the mechanisms behind failure or success of gene therapy.

In the quest for in vivo markers for gene expression, new probes should be designed that:

1. Amplify possibly low signal levels.
2. Respond dynamically.
3. Are able to monitor expression at different points in the pathway from gene to protein.

Only the future can tell whether this is possible. The novel systems described in this chapter demonstrate the proof of principle and show the promise of contrast agents for general use in MRI of gene expression.

References

1. New, D., Miller-Martini, D., and Wong, Y. (2003) Reporter gene assays and their application to bioassays of natural products. *Phytother. Res.* **17,** 439–448.
2. Naylor, L. (1999) Reporter gene technology: the future looks bright. *Biochem. Pharmacol.* **58,** 749–757.
3. Prasher, D., Eckenrode, V., Ward, W., Prendergast, F., and Cormier, M. (1992) Primary structure of the aquorea-victoria green fluorescent protein *Gene* **111,** 229–233.
4. Inouye, S. and Tsuji, F. (1994) Evidence for redox forms of the aequorea green fluorescent protein. *FEBS Lett.* **341,** 277–280.
5. Chalfie, M., Tu, Y., Euskirchen, G., Ward, W., and Prasher, D. (1994) Green fluorescent protein as a marker for gene-expression *Science* **263,** 802–805.
6. Tsien, R. (1998) The green fluorescent protein. *Ann. Rev. Biochem.* **67,** 509–544.
7. Tweedle, M. F. (1992) Physicochemical properties of gadoteridol and other magnetic resonance contrast agents. *Invest. Radiol.* **27,** S2–S6.
8. Lauffer, R. (1987) Paramagnetic metal complexes as water proton relaxation agents for NMR imaging: theory and design. *Chem. Rev.* **87,** 901–927.
9. Kawaguchi, T. and Hasegawa, M. (2000) Structure of dextran-magnetite complex: relation between conformation of dextran chains covering core and its molecular weight. *J. Matl. Sci. Matl. Med.* **11,** 31–35.
10. Landfester, K. and Ramirez, L. (2003) Encapsulation of magnetite particles for biomedical application. *J. Phys. Condens. Matter* **15,** S1345–S1361.
11. Paul, K., Frigo, T., Groman, J., and Groman, E. (2004) Synthesis of ultrasmall superparamagnetic iron oxides using reduced polysaccharides. *Bioconjug. Chem.* **15,** 394–401.
12. Kehagias, D., Gouliamos, A., Smyrniotis, V., and Vlahos, L. (2001) Diagnostic efficacy and safety of MRI of the liver with superparamagnetic iron oxide particles (SH U 555 A). *J. Mag. Res. Med.* **14,** 595–601.

13. Hauger, O., Delalande, C., Deminiere, C., et al. (2000) Nephrotoxic nephritis and obstructive nephropathy: evaluation with MR imaging enhanced with ultrasmall superparamagnetic iron oxide—preliminary findings in a rat model. *Radiology* **217,** 819–826.

14. Bowen, C., Zhang, X., Saab, G., Gareau, P., and Rutt, B. (2002) Application of the static dephasing regime theory to superparamagnetic iron-oxide loaded cells. *Mag. Res. Med.* **48,** 52–61.

15. Jacques, V. and Desreux, J. (2002) New classes of MRI contrast agents. *Top. Curr. Chem.* **221,** 123–164.

16. Aime, S. and Nano, R. (1988) Factors determining the proton T1 relaxivity in solutions containing Gd-DTPA. *Invest. Radiol.* **23(Suppl. 1),** S264–S266.

17. Roche, A., Gillis, P., Ouakssim, A., and Muller, R. (1999) Proton magnetic relaxation in superparamagnetic aqueous colloids: a new tool for the investigation of ferrite crystal anisotropy. *J. Magn. Mag. Matl.* **201,** 77–79.

18. Nicolle, G., Toth, E., Schmitt-Willich, H., Raduchel, B., and Merbach, A. (2002) The impact of rigidity and water exchange on the relaxivity of a dendritic MRI contrast agent. *Chem. Eur. J.* **8,** 1040–1048.

19. Moats, R., Fraser, S., and Meade, T. (1997) A "smart" magnetic resonance imaging agent that reports on specific enzyme activity. *Angew Chem. Int. Ed.* 726–728.

20. Louie, A. Y., Huber, M. M., Ahrens, E. T., Rothbacher, U., Moats, R., Jacobs, R. E., Fraser, S. E., and Meade, T. J. (2000) In vivo visualization of gene expression using magnetic resonance imaging. *Nat. Biotechnol.* **18,** 321–325.

21. Alauddin, M., Louie, A., Shahinian, A., Meade, T., and Conti, P. (2003) Receptor mediated uptake of a radiolabeled contrast agent sensitive to β-galactoside activity. *Nucl. Med. Biol.* **30,** 261–265.

22. Weissleder, R., Simonova, M., Bogdanova, A., Bredow, S., Enochs, W., and Bogdanov, A. (1997) MR imaging and scintigraphy of gene expression through melanin induction. *Radiology* **204,** 425–429.

23. Wunderbaldinger, P., Bogdanov, A., and Weissleder, R. (2000) New approaches for imaging in gene therapy. *Eur. J. Radiology* **34,** 156–165.

24. Enochs, W., Petherick, P., Bogdanova, A., Mohr, U., and Weissleder, R. (1997) Paramagnetic metal scavenging by melanin: MR imaging. *Radiology* **204,** 417–423.

25. Sulaimon, S. and Kitchell, B. (2003) The biology of melanocytes. *Vet. Dermatol.* **14,** 57–65.

26. Williams, R., Siegle, R., Salman, M., et al. (1996) Substrate modification of melanin polymers to increase effectiveness of contrast agents for magnetic resonance imaging. *Acad. Radiol.* **3,** S365–S369.

27. Graham, D., Tiffany, S., and Vogel, F. (1978) The toxicity of melanin precursors. *Invest. Derm.* **70,** 113–116.

28. Hogemann, D., Josephson, L., Weissleder, R., and Basilion, J. P. (2000) Improvement of MRI probes to allow efficient detection of gene expression. *Bioconjug. Chem.* **11,** 941–946.

29. Weissleder, R., Moore, A., Mahmood, U., et al. (2000) In vivo magnetic resonance imaging of transgene expression. *Nat. Med.* **6,** 351–354.

30. Bogdanov, A., Matuszewski, L., Bremer, C., Petrovsky, A., and Weissleder, R. (2002) Oligomerization of paramagnetic substrates result in signal amplification and can be used for MR imaging of molecular targets. *Mol. Imaging* **1,** 16–25.
31. vanGijlswijk, R., Zijlmans, H., Wiegant, J., et al. (1997) Fluorochrome-labeled tyramides: use in immunocytochemistry and fluorescence in situ hybridization. *J. Histo. Cyto.* **45,** 375–382.
32. Toth, E., Burai, L., and Merbach, A. (2001) Similarities and differences between the isoelectric Gd(III) and Eu(II) complexes with regard to MRI contrast agent applications. *Coord. Chem. Rev.* **216,** 363–382.
33. Aime, S., Dastru, W., Crich, S., Gianolio, E., and Mainero, V. (2003) Innovative magnetic resonance imaging diagnostic agents based on paramagnetic Gd(III) complexes. *Biopolymers* **66,** 419–428.
34. Allen, M. and Meade, T. (2003) Synthesis and visualization of a membrane-permeable MRI contrast agent. *J. Biol. Inorg. Chem.* **8,** 746–750.
35. Josephson, L., Tung, C., Moore, A., and Weissleder, R. (1999) High-efficiency intracellular magnetic labeling with novel superparamagnetic-Tat peptide conjugates. *Bioconjug. Chem.* **10,** 186–191.
36. Jacobs, R. and Cherry, S. (2001) Complementary emerging techniques: high resolution PET and MRI. *Curr. Opin. Neurobiol.* **11,** 621–629.

18

Intracellular Endosomal Magnetic Labeling of Cells

Jeff W. M. Bulte

Summary

Cellular imaging encompasses the noninvasive and repetitive imaging of targeted cells and cellular processes in living organisms. Magnetic resonance imaging (MRI), with its excellent spatial resolution, is ideally suited to provide unique information on the location and migration of cells after transplantation or transfusion. This approach requires magnetic prelabeling of the cells of choice. In this chapter, several methods and techniques will be described that can be applied for an efficient intracellular magnetic labeling of cells. In addition, a few basic protocols for the analysis and evaluation of cell labeling will be provided. The chapter will focus on the use of superparamagnetic iron oxides, because they are biocompatible and have strong effects on T_2^* relaxation. With the currently available magnetic labeling methods, it is anticipated that cellular MRI will find broad applications in biology and medicine.

Key Words: MR contrast agent; superparamagnetic iron oxide; macrophage; stem cell; transplantation; dendrimer; transfection agent; poly-L-lysine; monoclonal antibody.

1. Introduction

The transplantation or transfusion of (therapeutic) cells has been pursued as a very active research area over the last decade, and, for progenitor and stem cell therapy, a remarkable progress has been obtained in animal disease models. To further develop cell-based therapies into the clinic, noninvasive cellular imaging techniques are warranted. These imaging techniques are needed to provide detailed information on the biokinetics of administered cells (either transplanted or transfused); cell–tissue interactions, including preferred pathways of migration; and cell survival. In addition, within the hematological and immunological community, there is now also increasing interest in the spatiotemporal dynamics of cell "homing" after intravenous injection of hematopoietic and white blood cells.

Several image modalities now fulfill the requirement of being able to noninvasively and repetitively image targeted cells and cellular processes in

From: *Methods in Molecular Medicine, Vol. 124*
Magnetic Resonance Imaging: Methods and Biologic Applications
Edited by: P. V. Prasad © Humana Press Inc., Totowa, NJ

living organisms. Among these are single-photon emission computed tomography *(1)* and positron emission tomography *(2)*, which both use radioactive labels, and bioluminescence imaging *(3)* and magnetic resonance imaging (MRI) *(4)*. When these four modalities are compared, only MRI offers near-cellular resolution, with the ability of detecting only a few cells. Although initial studies were aimed at MRI cell tracking in disorders of the central nervous system, i.e., dysmyelination *(5,6)*, neuroinflammation *(7)*, and stroke *(8,9)*, studies have now also been performed in muscle disorders *(10)* and swine models of myocardial infarction, using X-ray fluoroscopy-guided injection *(11–14)*. An example of MRI cell tracking is illustrated in **Fig. 1**.

For cells to be visualized on magnetic resonance (MR) images, they need to be magnetically labeled to be discriminated from the surrounding native tissue. Because of their biocompatibility and strong effects on T_2^* relaxation, superparamagnetic iron oxides (SPIO) are currently the preferred magnetic label. SPIOs provide the targeted cell with a large magnetic moment, which creates substantial disturbances in the local magnetic field, leading to a rapid dephasing of protons, including those not directly in the vicinity of the targeted cell. MRI techniques, such as gradient-echo techniques, that do not compensate for dephasing are particularly sensitized to detect the presence of SPIOs. In general, iron oxide nanoparticles require stabilization to prevent aggregation. Most commonly, this is accomplished by a surface coating of dextran. Dextran-coated iron oxides include the products Feridex® and Endorem (Berlex Laboratories, Wayne, NJ; and Guerbet, Paris, France, respectively), the ultrasmall superparamagnetic iron oxides (USPIO) Combidex® and Sinerem (Berlex Laboratories and Guerbet, respectively), monocrystalline iron oxide nanoparticles, and crosslinked iron oxide. The presence of dextran on the outer surface represents a suitable platform for further biochemical manipulation. Dextran-coated SPIOs were first introduced for hepatic imaging *(15,16)*. After intravenous injection, the particles are rapidly taken up by liver Kupffer cells, which appear hypointense or black on the MR images. In areas in which the normal liver architecture is disturbed (i.e., lack of Kupffer cells), such as exists in the presence of a primary liver tumor or liver metastasis, the signal intensity remains unaltered and, thus, stands out from the normal surrounding tissue. Subsequently, USPIOs were developed that have a longer blood half-life and are normally taken up by macrophages, including those in lymph nodes *(17,18)*.

The challenge for magnetic labeling of cells has been to develop methods and protocols that achieve an efficient magnetic labeling of nonphagocytic cells in culture. It appears that this issue has now largely been resolved. In this chapter, several protocols will be provided for intracellular endosomal magnetic labeling of nonphagocytic cells. First, a generic protocol for the preparation of USPIOs will be provided. A further modification of these particles is then de-

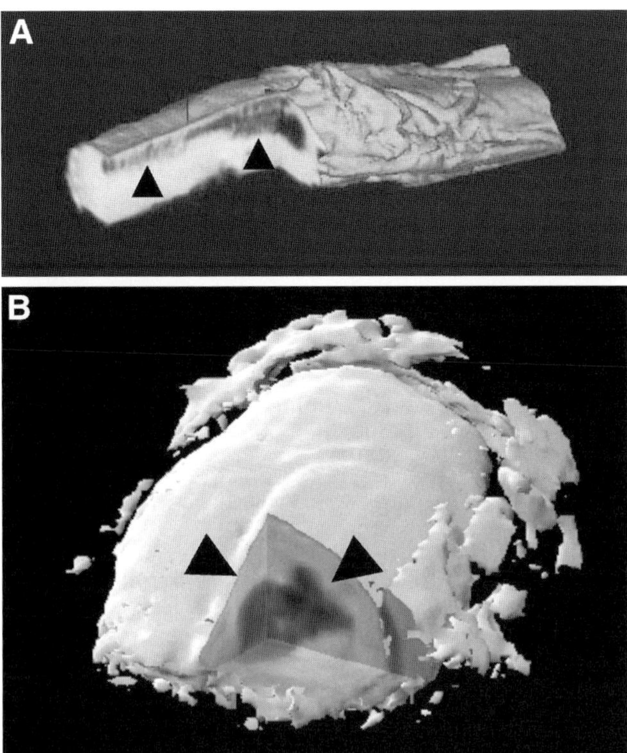

Fig. 1. **(A)** 3D reconstructed ex vivo magnetic resonance (MR) image (78-µm resolution) of dysmyelinated rat spinal cord showing distribution of magnetically labeled oligodendrocyte progenitors 10 d after transplantation. Note the migration along the dorsal column away from the injection site (arrowheads). **(B)** 3D reconstructed in vivo MR image (313-µm resolution) of dysmyelinated rat brain showing distribution of magnetically labeled oligodendroglial progenitors at 6 wk after transplantation. Note the migration of cells into the parenchyma away from the ventricle (arrowheads). For details, *see* **Ref. 4**.

scribed, which, after addition to cultured cells, leads to an efficient intracellular incorporation into endosomes. Methods for three different particle modifications are provided:

1. Covalent conjugation of dextran-coated SPIOs to internalizing monoclonal antibodies (moabs).
2. Synthesis and coating of SPIOs in the presence of carboxyl-terminated dendrimers, leading to the formation of magnetodendrimers.
3. The formation of SPIO–transfection agent (TA) complexes through electrostatic interactions.

Finally, several methods will be described that can serve as a starting point for the analysis and evaluation of magnetic labeling.

2. Materials

2.1. Preparation of USPIOs

1. Ferrous and ferric chloride.
2. Dextran T-10 (Pharmacia/Amersham).
3. Upright stirrer.
4. Ultrasonicator.
5. Ammonium hydroxide or sodium hydroxide.
6. Sodium citrate.
7. Ultracentrifuge.
8. Chromatography system (columns, peristaltic pump, ultraviolet [UV] monitor, and fraction collector).
9. Amicron microconcentrator.
10. Sodium azide.

2.2. Preparation of Monoclonal Antibody–USPIO Conjugates

1. USPIO and moab.
2. Sodium citrate.
3. Dialysis bags (10-kDa cutoff).
4. Sodium bicarbonate.
5. Sodium periodate.
6. Rotating shaker.
7. Chromatography system (columns, peristaltic pump, UV monitor, and fraction collector).
8. Amicon Centriprep-30 concentrator tubes.
9. Sodium cyanoborohydride.
10. Sodium azide.

2.3. Preparation of Magnetodendrimers

1. Carboxyl-terminated dendrimers (Sigma-Aldrich, Dendritech).
2. Methanol.
3. Nitrogen gas.
4. Ferrous ammonium sulfate.
5. Trimethylamine.
6. Syringe pump, syringes, and tubing.
7. pH-Stat instrument (i.e., Brinkmann) with software connected to a computer.
8. Autotitrator.
9. Sodium citrate.
10. Sodium azide.
11. Amicon Centriprep-30 concentrator tubes.

2.4. SPIO-Transfection Agent Complexes

1. Ferumoxide with negative ζ-potential (i.e., Feridex or Endorem, available from Berlex Laboratories or Guerbet, respectively).
2. Transfection agent (i.e., poly-L-lysine [PLL], heat-activated dendrimer, or cationic lipid-based transfection agent).
3. Rotating shaker.

2.5. Characterization of Magnetically Labeled Cells

1. Gelatin.
2. Sodium azide.
3. Hemocytometer.
4. Ultrapure perchloric and nitric acid.
5. Tube-heating device ("dry bath").
6. Relaxometer.
7. Ferrous chloride.
8. Carbon dioxide gas.
9. Ammonium iron (II) sulfate hexahydrate.
10. Hydrogen peroxide.
11. Eppendorf tube clamp, water bath.
12. Hydroxylamine.
13. 3-(2-Pyridyl)-5,6-diphenyl-1,2,4-triazine-4',4"-disulfonic acid (Ferrozine).
14. Pyridine ("Photrex®," Baker).
15. UV-VIS spectrophotometer.
16. Glutaraldehyde.
17. Neutral fast red (NFR).
18. Potassium ferrocyanide.
19. Hydrochloric acid.
20. 3',3"-Diaminobenzidine (DAB).
21. Aluminum sulfate.
22. Thymol.
23. 3-[4,5-dimethylthiazol-2-yl]-2,5-diphenyl tetrazolium bromid (MTT).
24. Propietary solubilization solution (Roche Diagnostics, together with MTT, available as a kit).
25. Microplate reader.
26. Trypan blue.

3. Methods

3.1. Generic Protocol for the Preparation of USPIOs

Many different protocols have been described for the preparation of dextran-coated USPIO particles. Variations in the protocol will lead to different physicochemical properties, including overall size (as determined by laser light scattering), core size (as determined by electron microscopy), magnetic susceptibility (measured by susceptometer), and T_1 and T_2 relaxivity (measured by relaxometer). An important aspect of the preparation is the production of a fairly uniform preparation, i.e., monodisperse rather than polydisperse, and the stability for a prolonged storage time without the formation of aggregates or precipitates. The procedure described below is optimized for the preparation of ultrasmall, monocrystalline USPIOs *(19)*.

1. Deionized, ultrapure water has to be used throughout these procedures.
2. Dissolve 1.51 g of $FeCl_3 \cdot 6H_2O$ and 0.64 g of $FeCl_2 \cdot 4H_2O$ in 100 mL of water (*see* **Note 1**).
3. Add 10 mg of dextran T-10 (molecular weight, MW, 10 kDa).
4. Heat the solution under continuous stirring using a metal or glass stirring rod (*see* **Note 2**).
5. Under continuous sonification (i.e., MSE ultrasonic power unit at 1.5–1.7 A) and stirring, raise the pH to 12.0 by the addition of approx 2.0 mL of 7.5% w/v NH_4OH (*see* **Note 3**).
6. Resuspend the sediment in 88.2 g of sodium citrate and 7.5 g of dextran T-10 in 300 mL of water (*see* **Note 4**).
7. Centrifuge the preparation for 10 min at 1000*g*.
8. Decant supernatant and resuspend solution in 88.2 g of sodium citrate and 7.5 g of dextran T-10 in 300 mL of water.
9. Adjust pH to 8.0.
10. Ultracentrifuge solution at 13,000*g* for 60 min.
11. Sonicate the supernatant for 30 min.
12. Separate USPIOs from SPIOs using a Sephadex column.
13. Elute in 10 m*M* phosphate buffer, pH 7.2 to 7.4 with 75 m*M* sodium citrate.
14. Concentrate USPIOs using an Amicon microconcentrator or Amicon Centriprep-30 tubes.
15. Add 0.02% sodium azide as a preservative and store the preparation at 4°C (do not freeze) (*see* **Note 5**).

3.2. Magnetic Labeling Using Moab–USPIO Conjugates

After binding to certain surface receptors, moabs can be internalized into cells. Substances that have been conjugated to internalizing moabs may enter the cell as well. An example of such an internalizing antibody is the anti-transferrin receptor, moab OX-26 *(20)*. When USPIOs are covalently linked to this moab and the preparation is added to cells in culture, the USPIO particles will be internalized into endosomes (**Fig. 2**) *(5)*. Moabs can be covalently linked to the dextran polysaccharide coat of a USPIO using a periodate–oxidation/borohydride–reduction method, which, through the formation of Schiff bases as intermediates, covalently links the amine (lysine) groups of the moab to the alcohol groups of the dextran *(21,22)*. This is schematically illustrated in **Fig. 3**. A protocol for making moab–SPIO constructs using 25 mg of protein starting material (*see* **Note 6**) follows:

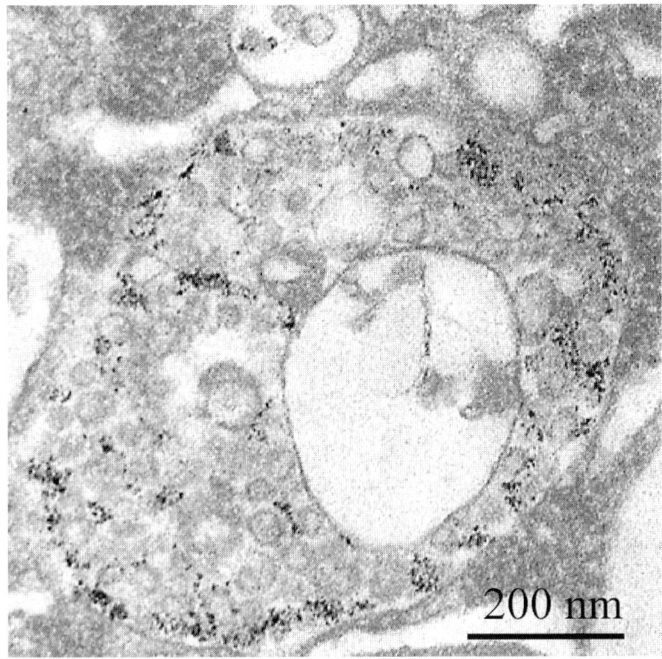

Fig. 2. Endosomal corporation of ultrasmall superparamagnetic iron oxides (MION-46L) particles into cells using an internalizing monoclonal antibody (moab). The particles are electrodense, similar to ferritin or gold particles used in immunoelectron microscopy. Individual iron oxide particles are visible, with a core diameter of approx 5 nm, mostly associated with the endosomal membrane. For details, *see* **Ref. 5**.

1. Using 10 mM sodium citrate and pH-8.4 buffer, prepare a 10-mL solution of USPIO containing 2.5 mg Fe/mL and dialyze this for 24 h against 1000 mL of 10 mM citrate, pH 8.4. Refresh the dialysis buffer twice.
2. Using a 200 mM sodium bicarbonate, pH 6.5 buffer, prepare a 25-mL solution of moab containing 1 mg protein/mL and dialyze this for 24 h against 1000 mL of 200 mM sodium bicarbonate buffer, pH 6.5. Refresh the dialysis buffer twice (*see* **Note 7**).
3. Collect the dialyzed USPIO and add 25 mg $NaIO_4$ (freshly prepared, 5 mg/mL water). Wrap the test tube in aluminum foil and incubate for 24 h at 4°C (cold room) using a rotating shaker.
4. Prepare a Sephadex G-100 (Pharmacia/Amersham) column, 45 cm in length and equilibrate with water.
5. Purify the oxidized USPIO on the Sephadex G-100 column. Elute with deionized water. Collect 4-mL fractions (approx 50), monitor the extinction and separate the USPIO from free dextran (*see* **Note 8**).
6. Reconcentrate the USPIO to 10 to 25 mL using Amicon Centriprep microcencentrator tubes (30-kDa MW cut-off) (*see* **Note 9**).

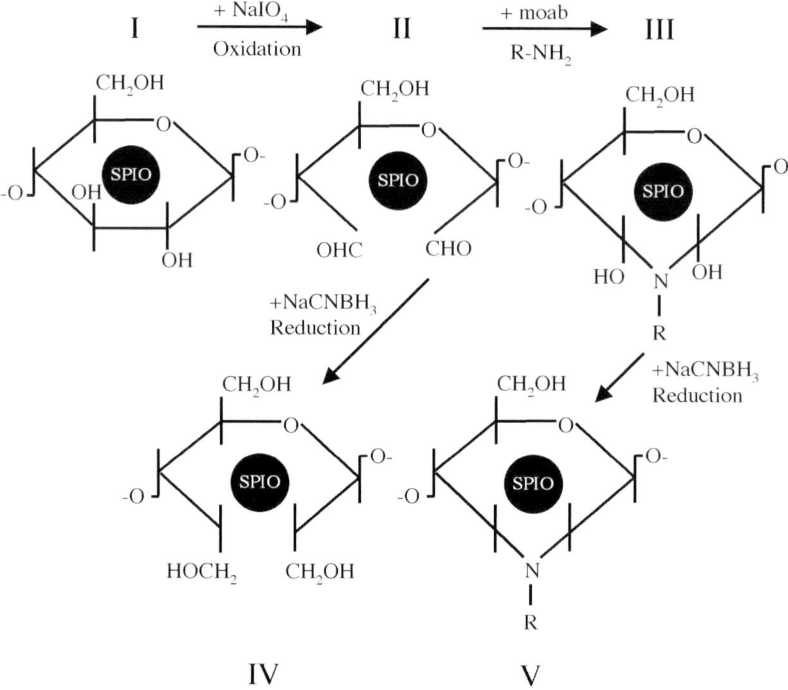

Fig. 3. Scheme for the conjugation of monoclonal antibodies (moab, R) to dextran-coated superparamagnetic iron oxides (SPIO) (I) using the periodate oxidation/borohydride reduction technique. The aldehyde groups of the oxidized dextran of the SPIO (II) react with the lysine residues of the moab to form intermediate Schiff bases (III). Borohydride reduction blocks unreacted dextran–SPIO and forms a covalent moab–SPIO construct (V).

7. Check the pH of the concentrated USPIO solution. The pH should be 6.5. If necessary, add a few milliliters of 200 m*M* sodium bicarbonate buffer, pH 6.5, to adjust the pH.
8. Mix the concentrated USPIO with the 25 mL of moab solution and incubate for 16 h at 4°C (cold room) on a rotating shaker with the test tube wrapped in aluminum foil.
9. Equilibrate the Sephadex G-100 column with 10 m*M* citrate in 0.9% NaCl, pH 7.5, plus 0.02% sodium azide.
10. Using facemask and gloves, weigh 25 mg of NaCNBH$_3$ and dissolve in 2.5 mL (*see* **Note 10**).
11. Add the cyanoborohydride solution to the USPIO–moab solution and incubate for 4 h at room temperature on a rotating shaker with the test tube wrapped in aluminum foil.

12. Purify the SPIO–moab conjugate on the Sephadex G-100 column. Elute fractions with 10 m*M* citrate in 0.9% saline, pH 7.5 to 8.0, plus 0.02% sodium azide. Collect USPIO–moab fractions and pool together.
13. Dialyze conjugates for 16 h against 10 m*M* citrate in 0.9% saline, pH 7.5 to 8.0, plus 0.02% sodium azide.
14. Concentrate the SPIO–moab solution to 5.0 to 7.5 mL using Amicron Centriprep-30 microconcentrator tubes.
15. Rinse or clean Sephadex G-100 column and store in H_2O plus 0.02% sodium azide. The column can be reused several times.

After the synthesis of the moab–SPIO construct, the final iron concentration is determined using a Ferrozine-based spectrophotometric assay *(6,23,24)*, described in **Subheading 3.5.1.** For intracellular magnetic labeling of cells, the moab–SPIO construct is dialyzed against 10 m*M* phosphate buffer. The preparation is then simply added to the culture medium at a final concentration of 10 to 25 μg Fe/mL *(5,7)*. Cells are then incubated for 24 to 48 h (shorter incubation times will induce less uptake).

3.3. Magnetic Labeling Using Magnetodendrimers

Magnetodendrimers do not have the specificity of moabs and can nonspecifically label a variety of cells, thus offering advantages as a versatile label for cells from different animal species. At the other hand, they cannot be used for specific labeling of cellular subsets in mixed cell populations. As in the case of internalizing moab–SPIO conjugates, magnetodendrimers pass across cell membranes and are incorporated into endosomes *(6)*. Below is a protocol for the preparation of magnetodendrimers that are loaded with an initial Fe to dendrimer ratio of 100:1 *(25)*, termed MD-100, but higher generation dendrimers and loading factors may be used.

1. Prepare a solution of 10 mg of a polyamidoamine dendrimer, generation = 4.5 (Sigma-Aldrich) in methanol (*see* **Note 11**).
2. Remove the methanol using a stream of N_2 for 20 min.
3. Dissolve the dendrimer in 30 mL of deaerated H_2O.
4. Add 0.1 *M* NaCl and adjust the solution to pH 8.5.
5. For further deaeration, bubble N_2 through the solution for 20 min and maintain anaerobism by continuing to use N_2 throughout the reactions.
6. Prepare a deaerated solution of $(NH_4)_2Fe(SO_4)$ (25 m*M*, 1.58 mL) and the two-electron oxidant, Me_3NO (25 m*M*, 1.58 mL).
7. Using a syringe pump, add the 3.16 mL of Fe^{2+}/Me_3NO to the dendrimer solution at a fixed rate of 0.5 mL/min.
8. Maintain the solution pH by titration of H^+ using a pH-Stat instrument and an autotitrator (*see* **Note 12**).

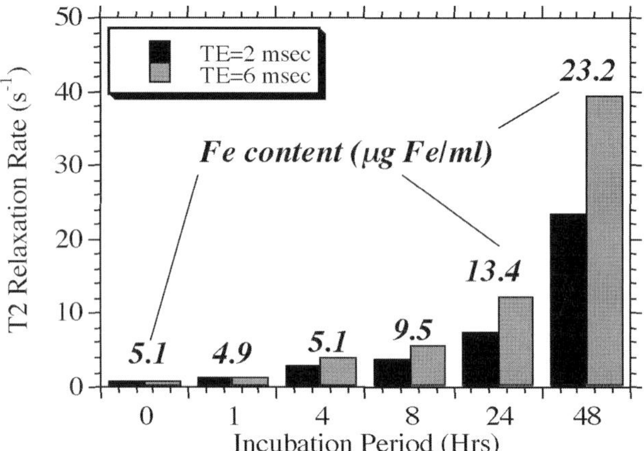

Fig. 4. Effect of incubation time on the amount of uptake of magnetic label and the effect on the increase of $1/T_2$ of cell suspensions in gelatin. HeLa (human cervix carcinoma) cells were seeded in culture flasks at similar cell densities and incubated with 25 μg Fe/mL MD-100 for 1 to 48 h (0 h represents unlabeled control). Cells were then collected and washed, gelatin samples were prepared, and the $1/T_2$ was measured at 1.0 T at room temperature for an echo time (TE) of 2 and 6 ms. The iron content in these samples was then determined using the quantitative iron assays, as described in **Subheading 3.5.1.** The increase of $1/T_2$ with increasing TE is a hallmark of clustering of particles in endosomes or cells, changing the size regimen of the magnetic inhomogeneities that cause the increase of $1/T_2$. The rapid increase from 24 to 48 h is partially caused by the growing number of cells (the cell doubling time = approx 24 to 36 h), increasing the total MD-100 uptake.

9. After the completion of the reaction, add 35 mM sodium citrate to remove any unmineralized Fe to prevent precipitation of nondendrimer-coated iron species (**Note 13**).
10. Dialyze the MD-100 preparation several times against deionized, distilled H_2O.
11. Concentrate the preparation 50-fold by ultrafiltration using a 100-kDa MW cutoff filter.
12. Add 0.02% sodium azide as a preservative and store the magnetodendrimer at 4°C.

After the synthesis of the MD-100, the final iron concentration is determined using a Ferrozine-based spectrophotometric assay *(6,24)* adapted from *(23)* and described further in **Subheading 3.5.1.**

For intracellular magnetic labeling of cells, the MD-100 construct is dialyzed against a 10 mM phosphate buffer. The preparation is then simply added to the culture medium at a final concentration of 10 to 25 μg Fe/mL *(6,7,10,26)*. Cells are incubated for 24 to 48 h (shorter incubation times will induce less uptake, *see* **Fig. 4**).

3.4. Magnetic Labeling Using SPIO–Transfection Agent Complexes

A disadvantage of the magnetodendrimers is that they have been synthesized in an academic setting (laboratory of Dr. T. Douglas) and are, in fact, a sort of "home-brew," without large scale production and continuous quality control. Because they have not yet been commercially developed, they are not widely available. Extrapolating from the concept of using dendrimers as transfection agents to chaperone SPIOs into cells, a simple and straightforward magnetic-labeling method has recently been developed that is based on the use of a commercially available USPIO formulation, i.e., Feridex or Sinerem, mixed with a TA *(8,27,28)*. Here, the iron oxide is not synthesized in the presence of the dendrimer, as in the case of magnetodendrimers, but the TA is added after particle synthesis. An added advantage is that the TAs are also commercially available, thus allowing anyone interested in using this method of intracellular magnetic labeling to proceed on their own. TAs are highly charged macromolecules, usually cationic in nature, and are used primarily to transfect DNA into cells. TAs, such as PLL, low- and high-MW heat-inactivated dendrimers, and lipofectamine, have positive ζ-potentials of up to 65 mV, whereas dextran-coated Ferumoxides and USPIOs with hydroxyl groups on the surface of the dextran coating of the nanoparticle have negative ζ-potentials *(29)*. After incubation of cells with TA–SPIO complexes, the particles accumulate in endosomes. A proposed mechanism of the complex formation and intracellular uptake is given in **Fig. 5**. In general, SPIOs exhibit a higher negative surface charge than USPIOs, allowing stronger complexing with cationic TAs, resulting in a higher uptake *(28)*. Because, in general, they also have a higher magnetic susceptibility and T_2 relaxivity, the use of SPIOs is preferred over USPIOs. A simple procedure for the labeling of cells using TA–SPIO complexes is given. Feridex and PLL are used as an example. The given amounts of PLL and Feridex used for labeling allow the detection of stem cells in vivo *(30)*.

1. Use sterile culture medium, specific for the cell type being used, and add 2.2 µL Feridex stock (11.2 mg Fe/mL, Berlex) to prepare a medium solution containing 25 µg Fe/mL. Mix well (**Notes 14–16**).
2. Prepare a stock solution of 1.5 mg/mL PLL in sterile water. This can be aliquoted in small portions and stored at –20°C for prolonged times.
3. Add transfection agent to the Feridex medium at the appropriate concentration, i.e., 375 ng/mL (250 nL/mL medium using the 1.5 mg/mL stock). Mix well (**Notes 15** and **16**).
4. Incubate the PLL–Feridex medium for 60 min at room temperature using a rotating shaker. This allows the formation of PLL–Feridex complexes through electrostatic interactions.

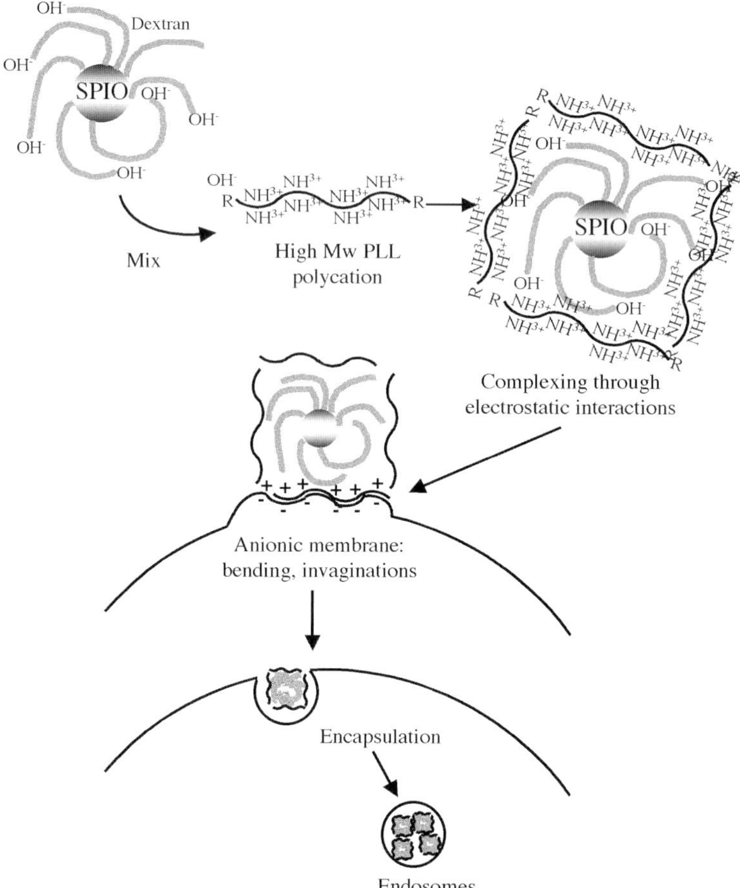

Fig. 5. Proposed mechanism for intracellular magnetic labeling using poly-L-lysine (PLL)–Feridex complexes. The dextran coating of the superparamagnetic iron oxides (SPIO) has a negative surface charge (ζ-potential of -41 mV) *(29)*, whereas the cationic transfection agent, PLL, has a positive charge. When SPIO and PLL are mixed before incubation with cells, the PLL will coat the SPIO through electrostatic interactions, and the SPIO will obtain a net positive charge. After adding the complexes to cells in culture, the SPIO–PLL complexes will bind to the anionic cell membrane at multiple places (because of the large size of the SPIO–PLL complexes, in the megadalton range), causing membrane bending and membrane disruption. The cell membrane then forms invaginations, encapsulating the complexes, after which, the outer ends of the cell membrane fuse, resulting in the formation of endosomes. The concept of the binding of PLL to cell membranes is similar to the use of PLL in allowing cells to adhere to glass slides, in which the positively charged PLL is an intermediate between the negatively charged glass slides and the anionic cell membrane through van der Waals forces.

5. For adherent cells, remove the old medium and add the PLL–Feridex-containing medium. For floating cells, spin the cells down at 400*g* and resuspend the pellet in the PLL–Feridex medium. For cells that are very sensitive to (autocrine) growth factors and supplements in the medium, spin the cells down at 400*g*, resuspend the cells in 50% old medium, and add 50% PLL–Feridex medium containing 50 µg Fe/mL Feridex and 750 ng/mL PLL.
6. Incubate cells for 24 to 48 h. Shorter incubation times will induce less uptake.

3.5. Characterization of SPIO Solutions and Magnetically Labeled Cells

3.5.1. Quantitative Determination of Iron Concentration in SPIO Solutions and Magnetically Labeled Cell Preparations

In this assay, the solution or cell preparation is first completely acid digested to produce free iron atoms *(6,24)*. The quantative iron assay is based on binding of ferric ion (any ferrous ion in the samples is converted to the three-spin state using the hydrogen peroxide oxidative step) to Ferrozine, that forms a purple complex after the addition of pyridine. By using appropriate standards in the range of 0.1 to 1.0 m*M* Fe, the iron concentration in the sample can be deducted from a standard (calibration) curve. Depending on the total initial amount of cells, the assay has a sensitivity of about 1 to 3 µg Fe/500 µL acid-digested cell suspension (*see* **steps 10–12**), or 30 µg/50 µL original sample. This is a much lower sensitivity than other (expensive) assays, such as atomic absorption spectrophotometry or inductively coupled plasma atomic absorption spectrophotometry, but the latter assays require very careful preparation of diluted samples and are prone to contamination, increasing the chance of errors. As an alternative, a relaxometric iron assay is described here that is as nearly as sensitive as the Ferrozine iron assay *(6)*. Examples of the results obtained using both quantitative assays are shown in **Fig. 6**. The first protocol for the acid digestion is given, followed by the relaxometric and spectrophotometric procedures.

1. Prepare a 4% w/v gelatin solution in 10 m*M* phosphate-buffered saline by bringing the solution slowly to a boil. Add 0.02% sodium azide as a preservative and store at 4°C.
2. Prewarm gelatin to 60 to 70°C before use.
3. Collect and wash cells three times after magnetic labeling. Include unlabeled cells as a reference standard for endogenous iron.
4. Count cells using a hemocytometer.
5. Resuspend cells in 500 µL of 4% w/w warm gelatin per test tube at a density greater than 1×10^7 cells/mL.
6. Cool samples on ice.
7. If desired, perform T_1 and T_2 relaxometry of the gelatin cell suspensions.
8. Dry the gelatin cell suspensions at 110°C for 16 h.
9. Perform the procedures below in a fume hood.

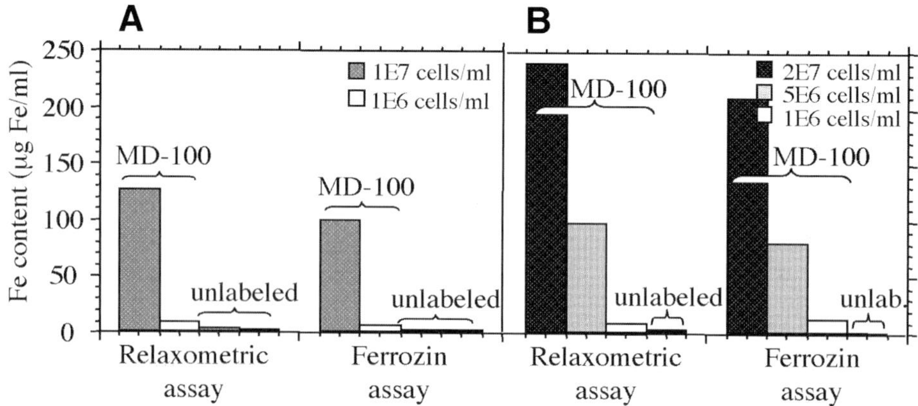

Fig. 6. Example of the quantitative assessment of intracellular magnetic labeling of cells by a T_2 relaxometric and Ferrozine-based assay, respectively. In this case, MD-100 was used as the magnetic label. Shown are the results for rat oligodendrocyte progenitor (CG-4) cells (**A**) and human cervix carcinoma (HeLa) cells (**B**). Shaded bars in (**A**) panels represent 1×10^7 cells/mL, white bars represent 1×10^6 cells/mL; in (**B**), dark bars represent 2×10^7 cells/mL, shaded bars 5×10^6 cells/mL, and white bars 1×10^6 cells/mL. By correcting for cell density, the amount of iron per cell can be obtained (in this case, between 10 and 20 pg of iron per cell). These examples are taken from **ref. 6**, in which the original assays are described.

10. Add 375 µL of 70% ultrapure perchloric acid (containing <2 ppb Fe) to each sample (*see* **Note 17**).
11. Add 125 µL of 100% ultrapure nitric acid (<0.6 ppb Fe) to each sample and mix.
12. Incubate samples for 3 h at 60°C, using a heating block.

The two methods of iron quantification can be applied to these 500-µL samples. For the relaxometric method:

1. Measure the $1/T_2$ at room temperature and a fixed magnetic field strength (i.e., 0.47 T).
2. Include samples of calibration standards, containing ferrous chloride solutions of 0.2 to 10.0 mM Fe, dissolved in the same 500-µL acid mixture as described above.
3. Plot the $1/T_2$ of the samples (diluted as necessary in the acid mixture) vs standards. The relationship between $1/T_2$ and Fe concentration is linear for the entire Fe range, with a slope of approx 12 to 13 s^{-1}/mM Fe.
4. Calculate the total amount of iron in the original sample and divide by the counted number of cells (using a hemocytometer) to determine the iron content per cell (*see* **Note 18**).
5. Discard contents of samples as chemically hazardous waste.

For the spectrophotometric method:

1. Perform the procedures below in a fume hood.
2. Throughout, use deionized water that has been boiled for 15 min to remove CO_2.
3. Pipette triplicate 50-μL samples (i.e., iron oxide preparations or magnetically labeled cells) from the 500-μL acid-digested solutions in 1.5-mL eppendorf tubes. Include water samples as blanks to zero the absorbance measurements.
4. For iron-containing test samples of unknown concentration without an estimate, include various dilutions, i.e., 1:10, 1:100, and 1:1000 to determine a workable range.
5. Include tubes with 50-μL iron calibration standards (ammonium iron (II) sulfate hexahydrate), adjusted to contain between 0.1 and 1.0 mM Fe.
6. Add 50 μL of 60% perchloric acid (*see* **Note 17**) and 50 μL of 30% hydrogen peroxide and mix.
7. Close eppendorf tubes, secure in a tube-clamping device, and boil for 30 min using a water bath.
8. Cool tubes down on ice and then centrifuge at 1000g for 2 min in a minicentrifuge.
9. Prepare a fresh solution of 10% w/v hydroxylamine and slowly add 100 μL to each tube, using safety glasses (the mixture is very reactive).
10. Incubate for 30 min at room temperature and then add 50 μL of hydroxylamine.
11. Incubate for 10 min at room temperature.
12. Add 500 μL of 0.5% w/v Ferrozine and 500 μL of pyridine ("Photrex" reagent), close tubes, and mix well using a vortexer.
13. Incubate for 50 min and switch on the UV-VIS spectrophotometer.
14. Transfer samples to disposable cuvettes.
15. Set spectrophotometer to a wavelength of 562 nm.
16. Starting with the water samples, auto-zero (blank) the absorbance.
17. Measure the absorbance of the samples at 562 nm and plot against standards. The absorption coefficient using a 1-cm light path is approx 1.15 mM^{-1}.
18. Calculate the total amount of iron in the original sample and divide by the counted number of cells (using the hemocytometer) to determine the iron content per cell.
19. Discard samples as chemically hazardous waste.

3.5.2. Histochemical Stain for Iron (Perls' Reaction)

An important qualitative method of analysis is Prussian Blue staining or Perls' staining. The method is based on binding of the cellular ferric iron to the ferrocyanide salt at low pH, forming a deep (Prussian) blue complex that can be further enhanced with DAB. Examples of labeled, stained cells are given in **Figs. 7** and **8**.

1. After magnetic labeling, wash cells three times and prepare cytospins or plate cells overnight on chamberslides.
2. Prepare an NFR solution: dissolve 100 mg NFR in 100 mL deionized water.
3. Add 5 g of aluminum sulfate and bring to a boil while stirring.
4. Cool and filter the NFR counterstain solution and add a grain of thymol as a preservative. The NFR solution is good for several weeks.
5. Fix slides with 4% glutaraldehyde for 10 min.

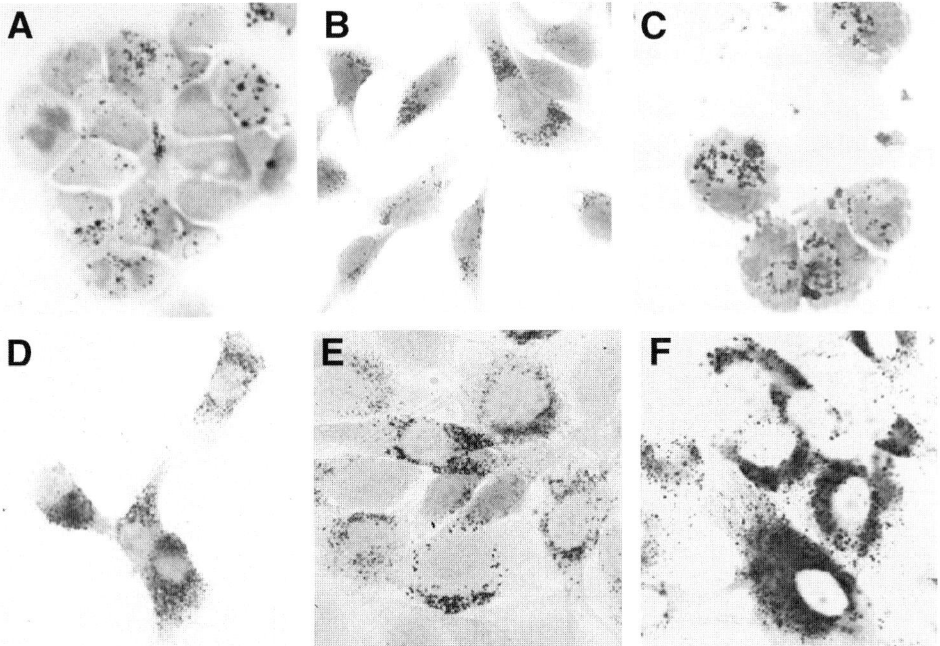

Fig. 7. Example of the qualitative assessment of intracellular MD-100 magnetic labeling of cells by nonenhanced Prussian blue staining **(A–E)** and diaminobenzidine (DAB)-enhanced Prussian blue staining **(F)**. **(A)** GLC-28 human small cell lung carcinoma cells **(B)**, HeLa human cervix carcinoma cells, **(C)** CG-4 rat oligodendrocyte progenitor cells, **(D)** 3T3 mouse fibroblasts, and **(E,F)** C2C12 mouse muscle progenitor cells. The iron is present in intracellular endosomes and absent in the nucleus. The binding and uptake of MD-100 labeling is nonspecific and allows cellular magnetic labeling of cells from different species. Note that the DAB-enhancement provides a higher sensitivity of detection, compare **(E)** with **(F)**. These examples are taken from **ref. 6**.

6. In the dark, incubate slides for 30 min with 2% potassium ferrocyanide in 6% HCl.
7. Wash cells and counterstain with NFR for about 5 min (depending on freshness of NFR).
8. Embed slides and apply coverslip.
9. For DAB-enhanced Prussian Blue staining, instead of NFR staining the slides are incubated with unactivated 14% w/v DAB solution (in deionized water) for 15 min in the dark.
10. In the dark, incubate slides with activated 14% w/v DAB, containing 0.03% H_2O_2, for 15 min.
11. Wash slides and counterstain with either NFR or hematoxylin. For optimal sensitivity of detection, noncounterstained slides are preferred.
12. Embed slides and apply coverslip.

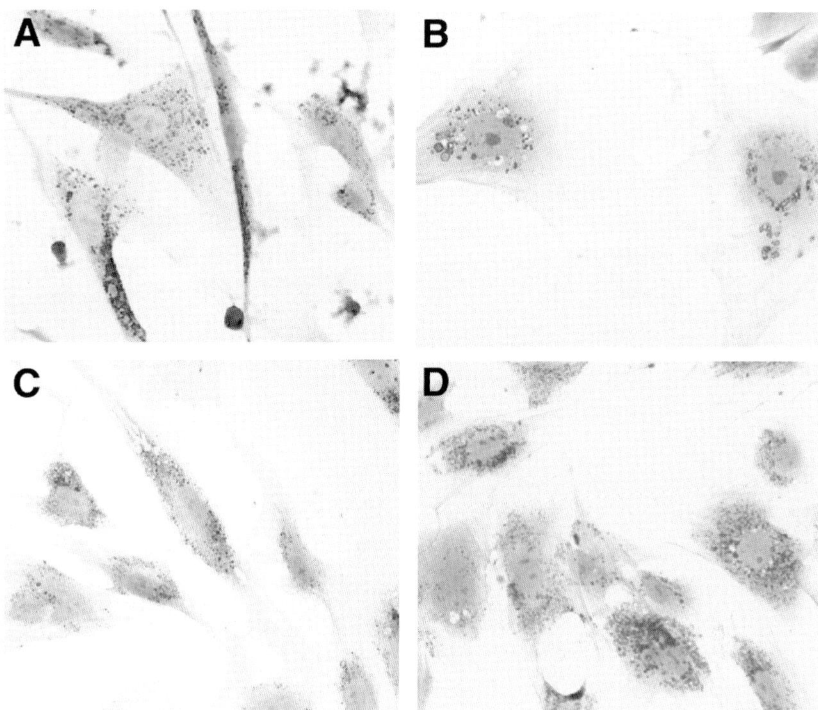

Fig. 8. Example of the qualitative assessment of intracellular poly-L-lysine (PLL)–Feridex magnetic labeling of cells by nonenhanced Prussian blue staining. (**A**) Human embryonic germ–embryoid body-derived SDEC stem cells *(33)*; (**B**) Mouse D3–embryonic stem cell-derived neural progenitors; (**C**) human mesenchymal stem cells; and (**D**) swine mesenchymal stem cells. Again, the iron is present in intracellular endosomes and absent in the nucleus. At equal Fe labeling concentrations, the binding and uptake of PLL–Feridex is comparable to MD-100, both qualitatively and quantitatively, and also allows cellular magnetic labeling of cells from different species.

3.5.3. Assessment of Cellular Viability and Proliferation

In addition to trypan blue staining, which simply reveals whether a cell is dead or alive based on dye exclusion, the actual assimilation and proliferation of cells after magnetic labeling should be assessed. One commonly used assay is based on the use of MTT (3-[4,5-dimethylthiazol-2-yl]-2,5-diphenyl tetrazolium bromide), which is converted by mitochondrial assimilation to a colored formazon product. The obtained MTT measures should be compared with unlabeled controls under similar culture conditions *(6)*. The number of cells should be very accurately determined and kept constant among the different samples:

1. In triplicate, seed cells in flat-bottom well plates at 1.5×10^4 cells per well in 90 µL of medium.
2. Include water blanks to auto-zero the absorbance measured using the plate spectrophotometric reader (*see* **step 8**).
3. Add the magnetic label at the appropriate concentration(s).
4. Incubate for 24 to 48 h in an incubator in a humidified atmosphere and 5% CO_2.
5. Add 10 µL of MTT at a final concentration of 0.5 mg/mL medium during the last 4 h of culture (*see* **Note 19**).
6. Initiate reaction by adding 100 µL of solubilization solution (Roche Molecular Biochemicals).
7. Incubate plates overnight at 37°C.
8. Measure blank wells, auto-zero the 96-well plate spectrophotometer, and measure the formazon product at a wavelength of 570 nm with 750 nm as a subtracted reference.
9. Plot the measured extinction as percent of controls (unlabeled cells).

4. Notes

1. The ratio of Fe^{2+}/Fe^{3+} may be varied, but this will lead to the formation of SPIOs with different sizes. In general, higher Fe^{3+} ratios will favor USPIOs with single cores, whereas lower Fe^{3+} ratios favor larger SPIOs containing multiple iron crystals. In addition, higher dextran to iron ratios favor smaller clusters of particles.
2. When a magnetic plate stirrer is used with magnetic stirring bars, a significant amount of iron oxides iron oxides may stick to the stirring bar. Instead, an upright metal or glass, nonmagnetic stirring rod should be used.
3. The original Molday and MacKenzie protocol uses ammonium hydroxide *(31)*, but sodium hydroxide can be used instead to avoid the strong odor of ammonia.
4. During storage, free Fe ions may be released. These can rapidly flocculate and form iron oxyhydroxides or other iron species that aggregate. The addition of citrate is essential to bind and sequester the released iron, preventing precipitation.
5. If plain, unmodified USPIOs are used for in vivo injections, the sodium azide and citrate have to be removed by dialysis.
6. For the moab–USPIO conjugation using the periodate-oxidation method other amounts of moab maybe used, but the ratio USPIO to protein should always be 1 mg Fe:1 mg protein.
7. The 200 m*M* sodium bicarbonate buffer used for dialysis for the moab needs to be readjusted to pH 6.5 several times as CO_2 degasses from the buffer over time.
8. Small aggregates will form after the borohydride reduction that will not pass through the Sephadex G-100 column. These can be removed later from the mesh filter on the top of the column.
9. Make sure filtrate is clear; occasionally the filter membranes are leaky.
10. Sodium cyanoborohydride is very toxic and care should be taken when working with this chemical.
11. Carboxyl-terminated dendrimers need to be used. The more commonly used amine-terminated dendrimers will not bind and sequester Fe atoms on their surface.

12. The use of the pH-Stat instrument eliminates the need to use contaminating buffers and allows monitoring of the progress of the reaction. The change in pH that occurs is, in part, caused by the acidic nature of the Fe(II) added and also caused by H^+ generated by the oxidative hydrolysis reaction to form the iron oxide mineral.

13. As mentioned in **Note 4** for the dextran-coated USPIO synthesis, during magnetodendrimer storage, free Fe ions may be released. These can rapidly flocculate and form iron oxyhydroxides or other iron species that aggregate. The addition of citrate is essential to bind and sequester the release iron, preventing precipitation.

14. Instead of using complete medium, PLL–Feridex complex formation may also be carried out in serum-free medium *(32)*.

15. The amount of TA should be carefully titrated and optimized for each cell type. The suggested concentration of 375 ng/mL is only a guideline; this amount has been found to provide sufficient SPIO endocytosis without affecting cell proliferation or differentiation for most cell types.

16. It is extremely important to first add the Feridex to the medium and mix very well before adding the PLL or other TA. If this is not done, formation of large TA–SPIO aggregates and precipitation will occur.

17. For rapid pipetting using many samples, use a repetitive pipetter rather than standard pipetter in the quantitative assays.

18. In general, the amount of endogenous iron is below 1 pg per cell (i.e., near or below the sensitivity of the assay). For the magnetic labeling procedures described here, i.e., incubation with 25 µg Fe/mL, the iron content is generally between 5 and 15 pg of Fe per cell. For the determination of iron content, increasing the number of cells per 500 µL of gelatin (before acid digestion) will increase the lower detection limit of the quantitative iron assays.

19. Alternatively, the proliferation and viability of labeled cells can be determined after (i.e., not during) labeling, mimicking the situation in vivo.

Acknowledgments

For **Fig. 8**, the human embryoid body-derived embryonic germ and mouse embryonic stem cell-derived neural progenitors were provided by Dawn Agnew, John Gearhart, and Mike Shamblott. The human and swine mesenchymal stem cells were obtained from Osiris Therapeutics, Inc., Baltimore, MD. The author is supported, in part, by RO1 NS045062 and PP0922 (Multiple Sclerosis Society).

References

1. Chin, B. B., Nakamoto, Y., Bulte, J. W., Pittenger, M. F., Wahl, R., and Kraitchman, D. L. (2003) [111]In oxine labeled mesenchymal stem cell SPECT after intravenous administration in myocardial infarction. *Nucl. Med. Commun.* **24,** 1149–1154.

2. Koehne, G., Doubrovin, M., Doubrovina, E., et al. (2003) Serial in vivo imaging of the targeted migration of human HSV-TK-transduced antigen-specific lymphocytes. *Nat. Biotechnol.* **21,** 405–413.

3. Hardy, J., Francis, K. P., DeBoer, M., Chu, P., Gibbs, K., and Contag, C. H. (2004) Extracellular replication of Listeria monocytogenes in the murine gall bladder. *Science* **303,** 851–853.

4. Bulte, J. W. M., Duncan, I. D., and Frank, J. A. (2002) In vivo magnetic resonance tracking of magnetically labeled cells after transplantation. *J. Cereb. Blood Flow Metab.* **22,** 899–907.

5. Bulte, J. W. M., Zhang, S., van Gelderen, P., et al. (1999) Neurotransplantation of magnetically labeled oligodendrocyte progenitors: magnetic resonance tracking of cell migration and myelination. *Proc. Natl. Acad. Sci. USA* **96,** 15,256–15,261.

6. Bulte, J. W. M., Douglas, T., Witwer, B., et al. (2001) Magnetodendrimers allow endosomal magnetic labeling and in vivo tracking of stem cells. *Nat. Biotechnol.* **19,** 1141–1147.

7. Bulte, J. W. M., Ben-Hur, T., Miller, B. R., et al. (2003) MR microscopy of magnetically labeled neurospheres transplanted into the Lewis EAE rat brain. *Magn. Reson. Med.* **50,** 201–205.

8. Hoehn, M., Kustermann, E., Blunk, J., et al. (2002) Monitoring of implanted stem cell migration in vivo: a highly resolved in vivo magnetic resonance imaging investigation of experimental stroke in rat. *Proc. Natl. Acad. Sci. USA* **99,** 16,267–16,272.

9. Zhang, Z. G., Jiang, Q., Zhang, R., et al. (2003) Magnetic resonance imaging and neurosphere therapy of stroke in rat. *Ann. Neurol.* **53,** 259–263.

10. Walter, G. A., Cahill, K. S., Huard, J., et al. (2004) Noninvasive monitoring of stem cell transfer for muscle disorders. *Magn. Reson. Med.* **51,** 273–277.

11. Dick, A. J., Guttman, M. A., Raman, V. K., et al. (2003) Magnetic resonance fluoroscopy allows targeted delivery of mesenchymal stem cells to infarct borders in swine. *Circulation* **108,** 2899–2904.

12. Garot, J., Unterseeh, T., Teiger, E., et al. (2003) Magnetic resonance imaging of targeted catheter-based implantation of myogenic precursor cells into infarcted left ventricular myocardium. *J. Am. Coll. Cardiol.* **41,** 1841–1846.

13. Kraitchman, D. L., Heldman, A. W., Atalar, E., et al. (2003) In vivo magnetic resonance imaging of mesenchymal stem cells in myocardial infarction. *Circulation* **107,** 2290–2293.

14. Hill, J. M., Dick, A. J., Raman, V. K., et al. (2003) Serial cardiac magnetic resonance imaging of injected mesenchymal stem cells. *Circulation* **108,** 1009–1014.

15. Stark, D. D., Weissleder, R., Elizondo, G., et al. (1988) Superparamagnetic iron oxide: clinical application as a contrast agent for MR imaging of the liver. *Radiology* **168,** 297–301.

16. Weissleder, R. (1994) Liver MR imaging with iron oxides: toward consensus and clinical practice. *Radiology* **193,** 593–595.

17. Weissleder, R., Elizondo, G., Wittenberg, J., Lee, A. S., Josephson, L., and Brady, T. J. (1990) Ultrasmall superparamagnetic iron oxide: an intravenous contrast agent for assessing lymph nodes with MR imaging. *Radiology* **175,** 494–498.

18. Harisinghani, M. G., Barentsz, J., Hahn, P. F., et al. (2003) Noninvasive detection of clinically occult lymph-node metastases in prostate cancer. *N. Engl. J. Med.* **348,** 2491–2499.

19. Weissleder, R. (1996) Monocrystalline iron oxide particles for studying biological processes. *US Patent*, Vol. 5,492,814.
20. Jefferies, W. A., Brandon, M. R., Hunt, S. V., Williams, A. F., Gatter, K. C., and Mason, D. Y. (1984) Transferrin receptor on endothelium of brain capillaries. *Nature* **312**, 162–163.
21. Dutton, A. H., Tokuyasu, K. T., and Singer, S. J. (1979) Iron-dextran antibody conjugates: general method for simultaneous staining of two components in high-resolution immunoelectron microscopy. *Proc. Natl. Acad. Sci. USA* **76**, 3392–3396.
22. Sanderson, C. J. and Wilson, D. V. (1971) A simple method for coupling proteins to insoluble polysaccharides. *Immunology* **20**, 1061–1065.
23. Stookey, L. L. (1970) Ferrozine—a new spectrophotometric reagent for iron. *Anal. Chem.* **42**, 779–781.
24. Bulte, J. W., Miller, G. F., Vymazal, J., Brooks, R. A., and Frank, J. A. (1997) Hepatic hemosiderosis in non-human primates: quantification of liver iron using different field strengths. *Magn. Reson. Med.* **37**, 530–536.
25. Strable, E., Bulte, J. W. M., Moskowitz, B. M., Vivekanandan, K., Allen, M., and Douglas, T. (2001) Synthesis and characterization of soluble iron oxide-dendrimer complexes. *Chem. Mater.* **13**, 2201–2209.
26. Lee, I. H., Bulte, J. W., Schweinhardt, P., Douglas, T., Trifunovski, A., Hofstetter, C., Olson, L., Spenger, C. (2004) In vivo magnetic resonance tracking of olfactory ensheathing glia grafted into the rat spinal cord. *Exp. Neurol.* **187**, 509–516.
27. Frank, J. A., Zywicke, H., Jordan, E. K., et al. (2002) Magnetic intracellular labeling of mammalian cells by combining (FDA-approved) superparamagnetic iron oxide MR contrast agents and commonly used transfection agents. *Acad. Radiol.* **9(Suppl. 2)**, S484–S487.
28. Frank, J. A., Miller, B. R., Arbab, A. S., et al. (2003) Clinically applicable labeling of mammalian and stem cells by combining superparamagnetic iron oxides and transfection agents. *Radiology* **228**, 480–487.
29. Kalish, H., Arbab, A. S., Miller, B. R., et al. (2003) Combination of transfection agents and magnetic resonance contrast agents for cellular imaging: relationship between relaxivities, electrostatic forces, and chemical composition. *Magn. Reson. Med.* **50**, 275–282.
30. Kraitchman, D. L., Heldman, A. W., Atalar, E., et al. (2003) In vivo magnetic resonance imaging of mesenchymal stem cells in myocardial infarction. *Circulation* **107**, 2290–2293.
31. Molday, R. S. and MacKenzie, D. (1982) Immunospecific ferromagnetic iron-dextran reagents for the labeling and magnetic separation of cells. *J. Immunol. Methods* **52**, 353–367.
32. Arbab, A. S., Bashaw, L. A., Miller, B. R., Jordan, E. K., Bulte, J. W., and Frank, J. A. (2003) Intracytoplasmic tagging of cells with ferumoxides and transfection agent for cellular magnetic resonance imaging after cell transplantation: methods and techniques. *Transplantation* **76**, 1123–1130.
33. Shamblott, M. J., Axelman, J., Wang, S., et al. (1998) Derivation of pluripotent stem cells from cultured human primordial germ cells. *Proc. Natl. Acad. Sci. USA* **95**, 13,726–13,731.

Index